Mosby's

Emergency Nursing Reference

Mosby's
Emergency Nursing Reference

Third Edition

Julia Fultz
RN, BSN, CEN, CFRN
Nurse Educator
Central Baptist Hospital
Flight Nurse
University of Kentucky Air Medical Service
Lexington, Kentucky

Patty A. Sturt
RN, MSN, CEN
Emergency Department Educator
St. Joseph Hospital
Lexington, Kentucky

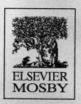

ELSEVIER
MOSBY

ELSEVIER MOSBY

11830 Westline Industrial Drive
St. Louis, Missouri 63146

MOSBY'S EMERGENCY NURSING REFERENCE ISBN 0-323-03150-1
Copyright © 2005, Mosby Inc.

NOTICE

Previous editions copyrighted 2000, 1996

International Standard Book Number 0-323-03150-1

Executive Editor: Susan R. Epstein
Senior Developmental Editor: Jean Sims Fornango
Publishing Services Manager: John Rogers
Senior Project Manager: Beth Hayes
Senior Designer: Kathi Gosche

Working together to grow
libraries in developing countries
www.elsevier.com | www.bookaid.org | www.sabre.org

ELSEVIER BOOK AID International Sabre Foundation

Printed in the United States of America

Last digit is the print number: 9 8 7 6 5 4 3 2 1

This book is dedicated to Pam Kidd. Pam is the primary reason this book is in existence, and her memory guided this revision. Pam was a wise and trusted mentor, friend, and role model. She empowered emergency nurses to aim higher and accomplish more than they thought possible. Pam had an uncanny ability to communicate and impart knowledge to nurses of all levels of education and experience. Pam made us think! She wanted emergency nurses to know they could do anything—even publish. Pam spoke quietly, and when people listened to Pam they learned. What they learned from Pam empowered and motivated them. When reading back over what we have written, Pam seems too good to be true—she was. She was all of the above and more. We respected and admired Pam. We greatly miss her! It is our hope that all of you will have a "Pam Kidd" in your life as a mentor, motivator, and friend.

In loving memory of Dr. Pamela S. Kidd, September 16th, 1957 to December 25, 2002.

contributor and editor

Billie Jean Walters, RN, MSN, CEN
Nurse Educator, Emergency Services
Central Baptist Hospital
Lexington, Kentucky

contributors

Deborah M. Anderson, RN, MSN, CIC
Infection Control Coordinator
Central Baptist Hospital
Lexington, Kentucky

Mary Rose Bauer, RN, BSN
University of Kentucky Medical Center
Emergency Department
Lexington, Kentucky

Cyndi Baxter, RN, BSN, CCRN, CEN
Director, Emergency and Dialysis Services
Central Baptist Hospital
Lexington, Kentucky

Kathy M. Blanton, RN
Registered Nurse
Central Baptist Hospital
Lexington, Kentucky

Maggie Borders, RN, BSN, CEN
Flight Nurse
University of Kentucky Emergency
Transport Service
Lexington, Kentucky

Erin Chiswell, RN, BSN, SANE
Clinical Coordinator, Emergency Department
Central Baptist Hospital
Lexington, Kentucky

Elizabeth Clark
Flight Nurse
Veterans Administration Hospital
Lexington, Kentucky

Lisa, Collins-Brown, RN
Staff Nurse
Veterans Administration Hospital
Lexington, Kentucky

Carlos Coyle, NREMT-P, AS
Flight Paramedic
University of Kentucky Air Medical Services
Lexington, Kentucky

Edward Crews, NREMTP
Firefighter Paramedic
Lexington, Kentucky
Flight Paramedic
University of Kentucky Air Medical Services
Lexington, Kentucky

Jill Dinsmore, RN, BSN
Flight Nurse
University of Kentucky Air Medical Services
Lexington, Kentucky

Lisa Fryman, RN
Staff Nurse
University of Kentucky Emergency and Trauma Services
Lexington, Kentucky

Brigette Holleran Ganahl, RN, BSN
Emergency Department Staff Nurse
Central Baptist Hospital
Lexington, Kentucky

Kelly Gandee, RN, BSN, CM
Clinical Manager, Emergency Department
St. Joseph Hospital
Lexington, Kentucky

Lee Garner, RN
Emergency/Trauma Services
University of Kentucky Hospital
Lexington, Kentucky

Theresa M. Glessner, RN, MSN, SRNP-BC, CCRN
Nurse Practitioner, Emergency Department
Highland Hospital
Rochester, New York

Ronald Stewart Gray, RN, CBE
Registered Nurse
Central Baptist Hospital
Lexington, Kentucky

Amy Herrington, RN, BSN, CEN, NR-EMT/B
Clinical Faculty
Lexington Community College
Lexington, Kentucky

Tammy R. Higgins, RN, BSN
Emergency Department,
University of Kentucky Hospital
Lexington, Kentucky

Joseph Hill, RN
Night Supervisor
Clark Regional Medical Center
Staff Nurse, University of Kentucky
Chairman, University of Kentucky
    Hazmat Committee
Mt. Sterling, Kentucky

Donna Arvin Isfort, RN, BSN
Eastern Kentucky University
Richmond, Kentucky
Marcum and Wallace Memorial Hospital
Irvine, Kentucky

John W. Isfort, BS, NREMT-P
University of Kentucky Hospital
Air Medical Service
Lexington, Kentucky
Marcum and Wallace Memorial Hospital
Irvine, Kentucky

Jo Ann Mathews, MSN, ARNP
University of Kentucky Hospital
Lexington, Kentucky

Jo Lynn McKee, RN
Flight Nurse
University of Kentucky Hospital
Lexington, Kentucky

Linda Murray, RN, ADNIII
Emergency Room and Neurosurgery Nurse
University of Kentucky Medical Center
Central Baptist Hospital

Terry Nalle, RN
Flight Nurse
University of Kentucky Hospital
Lexington, Kentucky

Naomi North, ADN
Staff Nurse/Emergency Department
University of Kentucky Hospital
Lexington, Kentucky

Mark B. Parshall, PhD, RN
Professor, University of New Mexico
College of Nursing
Albuquerque, New Mexico

Annette M. Rossman, RN, ADN
Nurse, Emergency Department
University of Kentucky Hospital
Lexington, Kentucky

Debbie Smothers, RN, MSN
Vascular Access Case Manager
University of Kentucky Medical Center
Lexington, Kentucky

Jeff Sotski, RN
Emergency Department
St. Joseph Hospital
Lexington, Kentucky

Pam Talbert, RN, NREMT
Chief Flight Nurse
Carolina Air Care
University of North Carolina Hospitals
Chapel Hill, North Carolina

Steve Talbert, PhD, RN
Assistant Professor
Director, Acute Care Program
Duke University School of Nursing
Durham, North Carolina

Bruce W. Walters, RRT, NR-EMT-P
Paramedic, Critical Care Transport
Central Baptist Hospital
Lexington, Kentucky

Ellen Williams, BSN, EMBA
Clinical Manager, Emergency Department
University of Kentucky Medical Center
Lexington, Kentucky

reviewers

Colleen Andreoni, APN, CNP, CEN, CCNS
QI Specialists, EMSC
Loyola University Medical Center
Maywood, Illinois

Susan Engman Lazear, RN, MN
Director
Specialists in Medical Education
Woodinville, Washington

Linda Scott, RN, MSN, PhD, C-FNP
Marshall University
College of Nursing and Health Professions

Russell Wilshaw, RN, MS, CEN
Trauma Coordinator, Emergency Department
Utah Valley Regional Medical Center
Provo, Utah

Lisa Beth Valente, RN, BSN
Emergency Department Staff Nurse
Massachusetts General Hospital
Boston, Massachusetts

preface

The world and environment in which we work is continually changing. This book has been revised to reflect these changes. The third edition was developed by people who practice in the emergency setting. Our ultimate purpose is to provide the nurse clinician in the emergency setting with a resource for accessing information related to the many and varied aspects of emergency nursing—after all, we are special! From newborn to 110 years of age, emergency nurses are there providing care, comforting, and teaching.

Reference material has been added or updated to reflect changes in practice.

- Cardiac resuscitation guidelines
- DKA and HHS treatment guidelines
- Expanded blood administration guidelines and transfusion reaction
- Safety in the emergency department
- Stroke algorithm

The essence and role of triage is essential to our practice of emergency nursing. Triage occurs at the time of initial contact, so we have pulled the triage information from each respective chapter and placed it together in one section. Subjective and objective triage assessment, triage acuity, and special considerations are covered in this new section. Long-time emergency nurses with years of triage experience collaborated to formulate a list of triage pearls. Pam loved to triage—she loved the challenge so we have chosen to call this section "Pam's Pearls for Triage." We hope to keep adding to this list.

Chapters in the third edition have the same features as in the second edition, such as the nursing alerts highlighting critical information; however, some of you requested we alter the format to make the information easier to locate. Your input was important, and we made the changes. The chapter format has been revised to facilitate accessing information quickly. For example, the specific conditions included in a chapter have been listed alphabetically. Distinct headings will assist in finding key information. We asked the authors to bullet key ideas for easy identification. The chapters are organized in the same way care evolves for a patient in the emergency department. The need for a quick reference source related to biologic, chemical, and radioactive agents was recognized. A chapter has been added that addresses care of the patient with potential or actual exposure to a hazardous substance.

New procedures have been added at your request.

- Advanced airway management
- Capillary blood sampling
- Decontamination of a patient
- EKG: 12-, 15-, and 18-lead monitoring
- External jugular intravenous access
- Nebulizer treatment
- Pediatric IM medication administration
- Preparation of a patient for interfacility transport
- Visual acuity

We know the challenges of caring for a greater volume of increasingly complex patients with limited hospital and community resources. We hope this book will help your efficiency and effectiveness in providing care to patients in the emergency setting.

acknowledgments

Deborah Bryant, RN, MSN, for her contribution to the Triage Section

Julie Max, RN, for her contribution to the Abuse chapter

Pam Cox, RN, and **Sonata Bohen, RN, MSN** for their contributions to the Behavioral chapter

Ralph Cooksey, RN, for his contribution to the Exposure: Chemical, Radiation, Biologic chapter

Dr. John Barton for his review of the Obstetric and Gynecologic Conditions chapter

Susan Summerville RN, for her review of the Intracranial Pressure Monitoring procedure

Lonnie Wright and **Lori Bailey,** librarians at Central Baptist Hospital, for their help in literature searches and locating those hard to find references that are needed when updating a book

Mendy Blair, the Director of Education at Central Baptist Hospital for her support and understanding during this project

contents

UNIT FOUR   PROCEDURES, 739

unit one

Reference Guides

REFERENCE GUIDE 1

Advanced Cardiac Resuscitation Guidelines: Adult

Advanced Cardiac Resuscitation Guidelines: Adult—Asystole

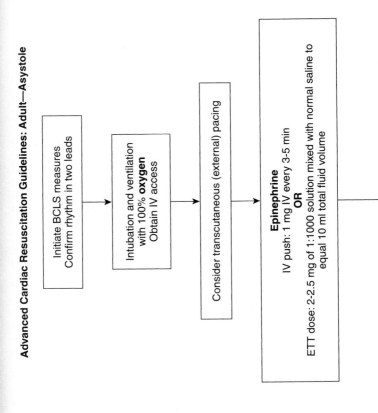

Initiate BCLS measures
Confirm rhythm in two leads

→

Intubation and ventilation
with 100% **oxygen**
Obtain IV access

→

Consider transcutaneous (external) pacing

→

Epinephrine
IV push: 1 mg IV every 3-5 min
OR
ETT dose: 2-2.5 mg of 1:1000 solution mixed with normal saline to
equal 10 ml total fluid volume

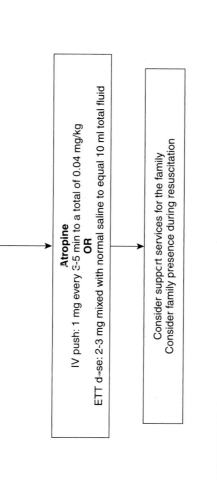

Atropine
IV push: 1 mg every 3-5 min to a total of 0.04 mg/kg
OR
ETT dose: 2-3 mg mixed with normal saline to equal 10 ml total fluid

Consider support services for the family
Consider family presence during resuscitation

Data from American Heart Association: *Advanced Cardiac Life Support: principles and practice*, Dallas, 2003, The Association.
ETT, Endotracheal tube.

Bradycardia: Symptomatic
(rate less than 60 or rate less than expected for patient condition)

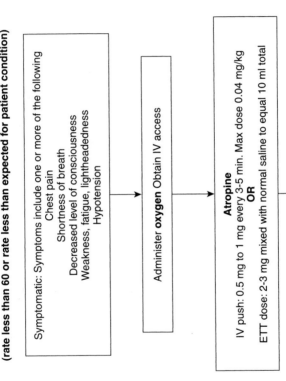

Symptomatic: Symptoms include one or more of the following
Chest pain
Shortness of breath
Decreased level of consciousness
Weakness, fatigue, lightheadedness
Hypotension

↓

Administer **oxygen** Obtain IV access

↓

Atropine
IV push: 0.5 mg to 1 mg every 3-5 min. Max dose 0.04 mg/kg
OR
ETT dose: 2-3 mg mixed with normal saline to equal 10 ml total

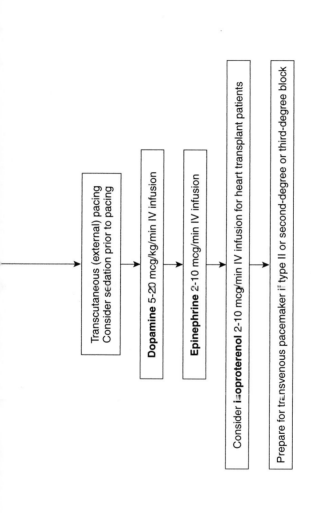

Transcutaneous (external) pacing
Consider sedation prior to pacing

Dopamine 5-20 mcg/kg/min IV infusion

Epinephrine 2-10 mcg/min IV infusion

Consider **isoproterenol** 2-10 mcg/min IV infusion for heart transplant patients

Prepare for transvenous pacemaker if type II or second-degree or third-degree block

Data from American Heart Association: *Advanced Cardiac Life Support: principles and practice*, Dallas, 2003, The Association.
ETT, Endotracheal tube.

Pulseless Electrical Activity (PEA)

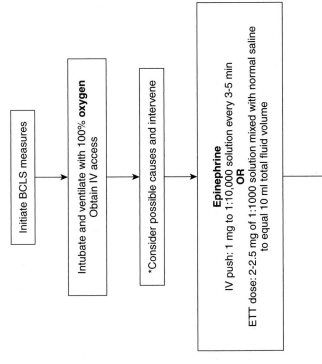

Initiate BCLS measures

↓

Intubate and ventilate with 100% **oxygen**
Obtain IV access

↓

*Consider possible causes and intervene

↓

Epinephrine
IV push: 1 mg to 1:10,000 solution every 3-5 min
OR
ETT dose: 2-2.5 mg of 1:1000 solution mixed with normal saline
to equal 10 ml total fluid volume

Atropine

IV push: 1 mg every 3-5 min to a maximum dose of
0.04 mg/kg if PEA rate less than 60

OR

ETT dose: 2-3 mg mixed with normal saline to equal 10 ml
total fluid volume

*Possible causes	Treatment
Hypovolemia	• IV fluids • Blood products
Hypoxia Acidosis	• Ventilation with 100% oxygen • Effective ventilation • Possible sodium bicarbonate
Hyperkalemia	• Sodium bicarbonate • Glucose and insulin • Calcium chloride IV • Kayexalate/sorbitol • Dialysis
Hypokalemia	• IV infusion of potassium
Hypothermia	• Warming measures
Overdose	• Appropriate antidotes
Tension pneumothorax	• Needle thoracostomy
Pericardial tamponade	• Pericardiocentesis

ETT, Endotracheal tube.

Stable Tachydysrhythmias

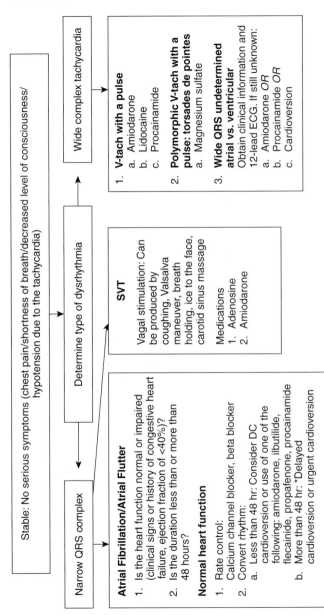

Stable: No serious symptoms (chest pain/shortness of breath/decreased level of consciousness/ hypotension due to the tachycardia)

Determine type of dysrhythmia

Narrow QRS complex

Atrial Fibrillation/Atrial Flutter

1. Is the heart function normal or impaired (clinical signs or history of congestive heart failure, ejection fraction of <40%)?
2. Is the duration less than or more than 48 hours?

Normal heart function

1. Rate control:
   Calcium channel blocker, beta blocker
2. Convert rhythm:
   a. Less than 48 hr: Consider DC cardioversion or use of one of the following: amiodarone, ibutilide, flecainide, propafenone, procainamide
   b. More than 48 hr: *Delayed cardioversion or urgent cardioversion

SVT

Vagal stimulation: Can be produced by coughing, Valsalva maneuver, breath holding, ice to the face, carotid sinus massage

Medications
1. Adenosine
2. Amiodarone

Wide complex tachycardia

1. **V-tach with a pulse**
   a. Amiodarone
   b. Lidocaine
   c. Procainamide

2. **Polymorphic V-tach with a pulse: torsades de pointes**
   a. Magnesium sulfate

3. **Wide QRS undetermined atrial vs. ventricular**
   Obtain clinical information and 12-lead ECG. If still unknown:
   a. Amiodarone *OR*
   b. Procainamide *OR*
   c. Cardioversion

Impaired heart function

1. Rate control:
   Diltiazem, amiodarone, or digoxin
2. Convert rhythm:
   a. Less than 48 hr: Amiodarone, consider cardioversion
   b. More than 48 hr: *Delayed cardioversion or early cardioversion

*Delayed cardioversion: Anticoagulation therapy for 3 wk before cardioversion, for 48 hr in conjunction with cardioversion, and for 4 wk after successful cardioversion
Urgent cardioversion: IV heparin immediately, transesophageal echo prior to cardioversion to rule out atrial thrombus, cardioversion within 24 hr, anticoagulation for 4 wk post cardioversion

Drug Dosages (Administration)

Adenosine: 6 mg IV push over 1-3 seconds, if no change in rhythm within 1-2 min, administer 12 mg IVP, may repeat × 1 in 1-2 min if needed.

Amiodarone: 150 mg IV over 10 min, repeat every 10 min as needed. After conversion, maintenance infusion: 1 mg/min × 6 hr, then 0.5 mg/min × 18 hr.

Procainamide: 20 mg/min IV infusion to a max dose of 17 mg/kg, hypotension occurs, QRS widens 50% of original width, dysrhythmia resolves. Maintenance infusion: 1-4 mg/min

Cardizem: 15-20 mg IV over ≥ min. May repeat in 15 min at 20-25 mg over 2 min. Maintenance infusion: 5-15 mg/hr

Lidocaine: 0.5-1.5 mg/kg IVP repeat at 0.5-0.75 mg/kg every 5-10 min to a maximum dose of 3 mg/kg. Then maintenance infusion of 1-4 mg/min.

Magnesium: 1-2 g in 50-100 ml D_5W over 5-60 min IV

Data from American Heart Association: Advanced Cardiac Life Support: principles and practice, Dallas, 2003, The Association.

Unstable Tachycardia
Synchronized Cardioversion
(serious symptoms: Chest pain, shortness of breath, decreased level of consciousness, hypotension due to the tachycardia)

Oxygen, IV, monitor
Suction available
Consider patient/family teaching if time available

Prepare for cardioversion
May give trial of medications such as adenosine, amiodarone, or lidocaine based on the rhythm, especially if rate is less than 150 beats/min.
Administer sedation (diazepam, midazolam, etomidate, or ketamine) and an analgesic (fentanyl, morphine, or meperidine) if at all possible.

Press the synchronization button before each cardioversion attempt. The flagged R wave will indicate synchronization mode is activated.

Type of rhythm determines the number of joules used; use the following monophasic energy sequence for each rhythm **(or equivalent biphasic energy level)**.

SVT: 50 joules (J), 100 J, 200 J, 300 J, 360 J
Atrial flutter: 50 J, 100 J, 200 J, 300 J, 360 J
Atrial fibrillation: 100 J, 200 J, 300 J, 360 J
Ventricular tachycardia with a pulse: 100 J, 200 J, 300 J, 360 J

If patient goes into ventricular fibrillation or pulseless ventricular tachycardia, turn off the synchronization and prepare to defibrillate.

Post cardioversion care
Verify rhythm and pulse
Continue to monitor oxygenation, ventilation, and perfusion
Administer antidysrhythmics and/or anticoagulants as ordered
12-Lead ECG

Data from American Heart Association: *Advanced Cardiac Life Support: principles and practice*, Dallas, 2003, The Association.

Ventricular Fibrillation (VF)/Pulseless Ventricular Tachycardia (VT)

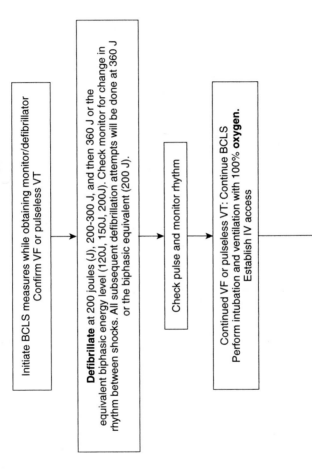

Initiate BCLS measures while obtaining monitor/defibrillator
Confirm VF or pulseless VT

↓

Defibrillate at 200 joules (J), 200-300 J, and then 360 J or the equivalent biphasic energy level (120J, 150J, 200J). Check monitor for change in rhythm between shocks. All subsequent defibrillation attempts will be done at 360 J or the biphasic equivalent (200 J).

↓

Check pulse and monitor rhythm

↓

Continued VF or pulseless VT: Continue BCLS
Perform intubation and ventilation with 100% **oxygen.**
Establish IV access

Continued VF or pulseless VT: Continue BCLS
Epinephrine 1 mg IV push every 3-5 min
(ETT dose: 2-2.5 mg of 1:1000 solution mixed with normal saline to equal 10 ml total fluid volume)

OR

Vasopressin (one time only) 40 units IV push followed in 30-60 sec by defibrillation
If vasopressin is administered, epinephrine 1 mg IV push may be given in 10-20 min and repeated every 3-5 min as needed

Administer antidysrhythmic and follow each dose with defibrillation

Amiodarone 300 mg in 20-30 ml D$_5$W IV push. May repeat dose of 150 mg IV push in 3-5 min for persistent VF or pulseless VT. Max dose 2.2 g/24 hr

Lidocaine 1.0-1.5 mg/kg IV push. May repeat 0.5-0.75 mg/kg IV push every 5-10 min. Max dose 3 mg/kg. (ETT dose: 2-4 mg/kg mixed with normal saline to equal 10 ml total fluid volume)

Magnesium sulfate 1-2 g diluted in 10 ml D$_5$W IV push over 1-2 min for torsades de pointes and/or hypomagnesemia

Data from American Heart Association: *Advanced Cardiac Life Support: principles and practice*, Dallas, 2003, The Association.
ETT, Endotracheal tube

REFERENCE GUIDE 2

Arterial Blood Gas Interpretation

Normal Arterial and Venous Blood Gas Values

Parameter	Arterial	Venous
PH	7.35-7.45	7.35-7.45
P_{CO_2}	35-45 mm Hg	40-45 mm Hg
P_{O_2}*	80-100 mm Hg	40-50 mm Hg
Oxygen saturation	96%-100%	60%-85%
Bicarbonate (HCO_3^-)	22-26 mEq/L	22-30 mEq/L
Base excess	−2 to +2 mEq/L	−2 to +2 mEq/L

*Decreases above sea level and with increasing age.

Interpretation of Arterial Blood Gas Values

Condition	pH	P_{CO_2}	HCO_3^-
Uncompensated respiratory acidosis	↓	↑	Normal
Respiratory acidosis with partial metabolic compensation	↓	↑	↑
Uncompensated metabolic acidosis	↓	Normal	↓
Metabolic acidosis with partial respiratory compensation	↓	↓	↓
Metabolic and respiratory acidosis	↓	↑	↓
Uncompensated respiratory alkalosis	↑	↓	Normal
Uncompensated metabolic alkalosis	↑	Normal	↑
Metabolic alkalosis with partial respiratory compensation	↑	↑	↑
Metabolic and respiratory alkalosis	↑	↓	↑

Data from: Horne M and Bond E: Fluid, electrolyte, and acid-base balance. In Lewis S, Heitkemper M, and Dirksen S, eds: *Medical surgical nursing*, ed 5, St Louis, 2000, Mosby.

REFERENCE GUIDE 3

Blood Component Administration Guidelines: Adult and Pediatric

Blood Component	Uses	Infusion Rate	Filter*	Volume	Pediatric Doses and Considerations	Comments
Albumin	Replace/increase intravascular volume, hypoalbuminemia	–2 ml/min for normovolemic patients	Vented administration set supplied with product	Varies	Albumin 5%: Usual dose is 1 g/kg or 20 ml/kg administered at 1-2 ml/min. Albumin 25%: Usual dose 1 g/kg or 4 ml/kg administered at 0.2-0.4 ml/min.	Prepared from plasma, comes in 5% and 25% solutions, can increase intravascular volume quickly; infuse cautiously and monitor for fluid overload. Does not have to be ABO-compatible.
Cryoprecipitate	Bleeding due to fibrinogen and factor XIII deficiencies. As a second-line therapy for	Use within 6 hr of thawing if closed single unit, use within 4 hr if system is open or	Standard blood infusion set*	Approximately 15 ml/unit. Pooled units will have volume	Rarely used in children. Four bags/10 kg.	Source of factor VIII, fibrinogen, vWF, and factor XIII. Compatibility testing not

Continued

15

Blood Component	Uses	Infusion Rate	Filter*	Volume	Pediatric Doses and Considerations	Comments
	von Willebrand disease and hemophilia A (factor VIII deficiency).	units have been pooled.		indicated on label and the volume of 9% NS added.		necessary, ABO-compatible material is preferred. Rh type need not be considered. Each unit contains approximately 80 international units of factor VIII and 150 mg of fibrinogen. When units are pooled, 0.9% sodium chloride is added to ensure complete removal of all material from container.
Fresh frozen plasma	Replace plasma proteins,	Less than 4 hr	Standard blood	Varies, will be listed	Usual dose to treat hemorrhage is	Must be ABO compatible with

	including all coagulation factors		infusion set*	on the label	15-30 ml/kg; for clotting deficiencies 10-15 ml/kg	recipient's red blood cells. Takes 20 min to thaw. Infuse immediately.
Granulocytes	Used in neutropenic patients	1 unit over 2-4 hr	Standard blood infusion set*	200-300 ml	Rarely used in children. Usual dose depends on WBC counts and clinical condition, 10-15 ml/kg/day initially over 2-4 hr because of fever and chills, common side effects associated with infusion.	Used in neutropenic patients in whom eventual marrow recovery is expected, who have documented infections and who have not responded to antibiotic therapy. Must be ABO-compatible with recipient's antibodies.
Leukocyte reduced red blood cells	Increase oxygen-carrying capacity in patients with history of recurrent febrile nonhemolytic	Infuse initial portion slowly to detect reactions. Then increase rate to infuse within	Standard blood infusion set*	Varies, will be listed on the label.	Same as packed red blood cells	Used to reduce the occurrence of febrile transfusion reactions due to leukocyte antibodies. Monitor for hypotension if

Continued

Blood Component	Uses	Infusion Rate	Filter*	Volume	Pediatric Doses and Considerations	Comments
	transfusion reactions.	4 hr. Can infuse rapidly if emergency situation exists.				leukocyte reduction is being done at the bedside.
Packed red blood cells, most of plasma removed	Increase oxygen-carrying capacity. Increases intravascular volume.	Infuse initial portion slowly to detect reactions. Then increase rate to infuse within 4 hr. Can infuse rapidly if emergency situation exists.	Standard blood infusion set*	225-350 ml	Usual dose is 10 ml/kg, not to exceed 15 ml/kg. Administer 5 ml/kg/hr or 2 ml/kg/hr if congestive heart failure develops. 1 ml/kg will increase Hct approximately 1%.	Prepared from whole blood, allowing remaining components in the plasma to be used for other purposes. Processing and/or storage of unit depletes the therapeutic effect of white cells and platelets. Raises HGB by approximately 1 g/dl; raises the HCT by approximately 3%.
Platelets	Platelet replacement	Less than 4 hr	Standard blood infusion set*	40-70 ml per unit, usual adult	Usual dose 1 unit for every 7-10 kg. Or 6 units/m². Administer	Prepared from fresh whole blood. Used to provide adequate

Transfusion Reaction	Symptoms	Treatment
Allergic Reaction: Sensitivity to soluble substance in donor plasma.	• Hives • Itching • Local erythema	• Stop transfusion. • Medicate with an antihistamine. • If symptoms are mild, may restart transfusion after localized urticarial reactions clear.
Delayed Hemolytic Reaction: Occurs 2-14 days post transfusion.	• Unexplained fever • Positive DAT (direct antiglobulin test) • Unexplained decrease in HGB/HCT • Elevation of LDH or bilirubin may be seen.	• No treatment required; course usually benign.
Circulatory overload: Occurs with any blood component administered at a rate more rapid than the recipient's cardiac output can accommodate.	• Dyspnea • Cough • Cyanosis • Severe headache • Peripheral edema • Systolic hypertension • Congestive heart failure	• Oxygen • Diuretics • Phlebotomy • Concentrate products • Monitor patient's tolerance of infusion.
Transfusion Related Acute Lung Injury (TRALI): Rare, massive leakage of fluids and protein into alveolar spaces and interstitium due to increased permeability of microcirculation.	• Cyanosis • Pulmonary white-out • Fever	• Aggressive respiratory support • Usually resolves in 72 hours

Information from: Circular of Information for the Use of Human Blood and Blood Components, American Association of Blood Banks, America's Blood Centers, and the American Red Cross, July, 2002.

number of platelets to prevent or stop bleeding. Each unit contains no fewer than 5.5×10^{10} platelets. One unit of platelets increases platelet count of a 70-kg adult by 5000-10,000/mcl and an 18-kg child by 20,000/mcl. Platelet units may contain trace amounts of RBCs and will appear pink tinged. Compatibility testing not necessary in routine transfusion. Should be ABO-compatible for infants or for large volumes.

dose is 4-8 units

10 ml/kg/hr, or over 1 hr, or as fast as patient can tolerate. Each unit will increase platelet count by 50,000/mm³.

Rarely used in children. 20 ml/kg initially.

450-500 ml

Standard blood infusion set*

Infuse initial portion slowly

Increase oxygen-carrying capacity, red

Whole blood, contains red

Processing and/or storage of unit

Continued

Blood Component	Uses	Infusion Rate	Filter*	Volume	Pediatric Doses and Considerations	Comments
cells and plasma constituents	increase intravascular volume.	for 15-30 min to detect reactions. Increase rate to complete infusion within 4 hr of initiation. Can infuse rapidly if emergency situation exists.			Usually reserved for massive hemorrhage.	depletes the therapeutic effect of white cells and platelets. Raises HGB by approximately 1 g/dl; raises the HCT by approximately 3%.

*All blood components must be transfused through a 170-mcm to 260-mcm filter (standard blood filter), designed to remove clots and aggregates. Use strict sterile technique.

Do not routinely administer medications or solutions with blood (except 0.9% sodium chloride injection) unless documentation is available attesting to the safety of the drug/blood combination.

Initiate infusion within 30 min of blood product leaving the blood bank.

Blood components expire 4 hr after opening.

Warm blood during massive transfusion with an FDA-cleared warming device to avoid causing hemolysis.

Monitor all patients for fluid overload.

Data from Circular of Information for the Use of Human Blood and Blood Components, American Association of Blood Banks, America's Blood Center, and The American Red Cross, July, 2002; and Hockenberry MJ: *Wong's nursing care of infants and children*, ed 7, St Louis, 2003, Mosby, p 1543.

REFERENCE GUIDE 4

Blood Transfusion Reactions

Transfusion Reaction	Symptoms	Treatment
Acute hemolytic reaction: Caused by ABO incompatibility. Immunologic destruction of transfused red cells. Will usually occur within 15 minutes.	• Fever/chills (most common presenting symptom) • Flushing • Tachycardia • Dyspnea • Headache • Nausea • Chest, back, or infusion site pain • Diffuse pain • Abnormal bleeding • Hypotension/shock • Hemoglobinemia • Hemoglobinuria • Oliguria/anuria/renal failure • Cardiac arrest	• Stop infusion! • Treat hypotension with normal saline. • Correct coagulopathy monitor for DIC. • Promote and maint... renal perfusion (Mannitol). • Urinary catheter t... monitor urine ou...
Anaphylactic reaction: Caused by sensitivity to plasma proteins; Develops after very small amounts of IgA-containing plasma in any blood component.	• Hypotension/shock • Respiratory distress • Abdominal cramps • Coughing/bronchospasm • Pulmonary/laryngeal edema • Nausea/vomiting • Diarrhea • Cardiac arrest	• Stop the tra... • Epinephrine subcutaneo... intramuscu... patient is i... then give i... • Treat hyp... with nor... • Protect t... • Adminis... and ant...
Febrile nonhemolytic reaction: Most often caused by leukocyte incompatibility or action of cytokinins.	• Temperature elevation of $\geq 1° C$ or $2° F$ with no other explanation • Chills/flushing • Headache	• Stop th... • Rule o... reactio... • Antip... • Repe... may... leuk... blo...

Steps in investigating transfusion reactions:

- Stop the transfusion! Keep a line open with saline.
- Check paperwork and blood bag for clerical errors.
- Send prereaction recipient blood or get type and crossmatch results from prereaction recipient blood.
- Send a postreaction recipient blood specimen for comparison to pretransfusion specimen. Check for hemoglobinemia.
- Send donor blood being administered at time of reaction.
- Send a posttransfusion urine sample; check for hemoglobinuria.
- Diagnosis is confirmed by direct antiglobulin testing (DAT) (a positive result on the Coombs' test) and separation of the offending antibody from red blood cells.

REFERENCE GUIDE 5

Calculations and Conversions
Conversions Volume
5 ml = 1 teaspoon (tsp)
15 ml = 1 tablespoon (T or T bsp)
30 ml (exact is 29.57 ml) = 1 ounce (oz) = 2 T
500 ml (exact is 473.16 ml) = 1 pint (pt)
1000 ml = 1 quart (qt)
1000 ml = 1 liter (L)
Milliter (ml) = 0.001 L

Weight
1 kilogram (kg) = 1000 grams (g)
1 kg = 2.2 pounds (lb)
1 g = 1000 milligrams (mg)
1 milligram (mg) = 0.001 gram (g)
1 mg = 1000 micrograms (mcg)
1 grain (gr) = 64.8 mg
5 grains = 324 mg
1/100 gr = 0.6 mg
1/150 gr = 0.4 mg

Weight Conversion Chart

lb	kg	lb	kg	lb	kg	lb	kg
1	0.5	35	15.9	110	49.9	250	113.5
2	0.9	40	18.2	120	54.5	260	118
3	1.4	45	20.4	130	59	270	122.6
4	1.8	50	22.7	140	63.6	280	127.1
5	2.3	55	25	150	68.1	290	131.7
6	2.7	60	27.2	160	72.6	300	136.2
7	3.2	65	29.5	170	77.2	310	140.7
8	3.6	70	31.8	180	81.7	320	145.3
9	4.0	75	34	190	86.3	330	149.9
10	4.5	80	36.3	200	90.8	340	154.3
15	6.8	85	38.6	210	95.3	350	158.9
20	9.1	90	40.9	220	99.9	360	163.4
25	11.3	95	43.1	230	104.4	370	168
30	13.6	100	45.4	240	109	380	172.5

1 lb = 0.454 kg.
1 kg = 2.2 lb.

Temperature Conversion Table

Centigrade (Celsius)	Fahrenheit	Centigrade (Celsius)	Fahrenheit	Centigrade (Celsius)	Fahrenheit
30	86	34.4	93.9	38.8	101.8
30.2	86.4	34.6	94.2	39	102.2
30.4	86.7	34.8	94.6	39.2	102.6
30.6	87.1	35	95	39.4	102.9
30.8	87.4	35.2	95.4	39.6	103.2
31	87.6	35.4	95.7	39.8	103.6
31.2	88.1	35.6	96.1	40	104
31.4	88.5	35.8	96.4	40.2	104.4
31.6	88.8	36	96.8	40.4	104.7
31.8	89.2	36.2	97.2	40.6	105
32	89.6	36.4	97.5	40.8	105.4
32.2	90	36.6	97.9	41	105.8
32.4	90.3	36.8	98.2	41.2	106.1

Continued

Temperature Conversion Table—cont'd

Centigrade (Celsius)	Fahrenheit	Centigrade (Celsius)	Fahrenheit	Centigrade (Celsius)	Fahrenheit
32.6	90.7	37	98.6	41.4	106.5
32.8	91.0	37.2	99	41.6	106.9
33	91.4	37.4	99.3	41.8	107.2
33.2	91.8	37.6	99.6	42	107.6
33.4	92.1	37.8	100	42.2	108
33.6	92.5	38	100.4	42.4	108.3
33.8	92.8	38.2	100.8	42.6	108.7
34	93.2	38.4	101.1	42.8	109
34.2	93.6	38.6	101.5	43	109.4

Length
2.5 centimeters (cm) = 1 inch
1 meter (m) = 3.28 feet
1 cm = 10 millimeters (mm)
1 m = 100 cm

Pressure
1 mm Hg = 1.36 cm H_2O

Temperature
C = (F − 32) × 5/9 or C = (F − 32) × 0.5555
F = (C × 9/5) + 32 or F = (C × 1.8) + 32

Critical Care Calculations
1 mg = 1000 mcg
1 g = 1000 mg

Drug concentrations in mg/ml or mcg/ml:
To determine the amount of drug in one milliliter: Divide the amount of drug in solution by the amount of solution.

Formula: mg/ml = $\dfrac{\text{amount of drug in the solution (mg)}}{\text{volume of solution (ml)}}$

Ex· 200 mg of drug in 500 ml.
To determine mg/ml:
$\dfrac{200 \text{ mg}}{500 \text{ ml}}$ = 0.4 mg/ml
To determine mcg/ml, first change mg to mcg.
200 mg × 1000 mcg/mg = 200,000 mcg
Then divide mcg by ml of solution:
$\dfrac{200,000 \text{ mcg}}{500 \text{ ml}}$ = 400 mcg/ml

Calculating mcg/kg/min
You must know:
the patient wt in kg (1 kg = 2.2 lb; see weight chart on p. 24)
the infusion rate (ml/hr)
drug concentration
Multiply the drug concentration by the infusion rate and divide by the patient wt × 60 min/hr

Formula: mcg/kg/min = $\dfrac{\text{mcg/ml} \times \text{ml/hr}}{\text{kg} \times 60 \text{ min/hr}}$

Ex: A 75-kg patient is receiving dopamine at 20 ml/hr. There is 250 mg of dopamine in 250 ml of D5W.
To determine dosage being given in mcg/kg/min,
First change mg to mcg:
250 mg = 250,000 mcg

Then divide the dose by the amount of solution:

$$\frac{250,000 \text{ mcg}}{250 \text{ ml}} = 1000 \text{ mcg/ml}$$

Now all three parameters are known.

$$\begin{aligned}
\text{mcg/kg/min} &= \frac{\text{mcg/ml} \times \text{ml/hr}}{\text{kg} \times 60 \text{ min/hr}} \\
&= \frac{1000 \times 20}{75 \times 60} \\
&= \frac{20,000}{4500} \\
&= 4.44 \text{ mcg/kg/min}
\end{aligned}$$

Calculating the Amount of Fluid to Infuse

You must know:

the patient weight in kg (1 kg = 2.2 lb; see above chart)

The dose ordered by the MD in mcg/kg/min

The drug concentration in mcg/min

Multiply the dose ordered by the patient weight × 60 minutes and divide by the drug concentration.

Formula: $\text{ml/hr} = \dfrac{\text{mcg/kg/min ordered} \times \text{kg} \times 60 \text{ min}}{\text{mcg/ml}}$

Ex: A 70-kg patient is to receive dopamine at 6 mcg/kg/min. There is 400 mg of dopamine in 250 ml of D5W.

To determine the infusion rate in ml:

First change the mg to mcg/mg.

400 mg = 400,000 mcg

Then divide the dose by the amount of solution:

$$\frac{400,000 \text{ mcg}}{250 \text{ ml}} = 1600 \text{ mcg/ml}$$

Now all three parameters are known.

$$\begin{aligned}
\text{ml/hr} &= \frac{\text{mcg/kg/min ordered} \times \text{kg} \times 60 \text{ min}}{\text{mcg/ml}} \\
&= \frac{6 \times 70 \times 60}{1600} \\
&= \frac{25,200}{1600} \\
&= 16 \text{ ml/hr}
\end{aligned}$$

Adapted from Stillwell SB: *Critical care nursing reference,* ed 3, St Louis, 2002, Mosby.

Diabetic Ketoacidosis (DKA): Adult

CLINICAL PRESENTATION

Symptoms: Polyuria, polydipsia, polyphagia, weight loss, vomiting, abdominal pain

Signs: Dehydration, weakness, altered mental status, hypothermia, tachycardia, hypotension, Kussmaul respirations (DKA), coma (more common in hyperosmolar hyperglycemia state [HHS]).

Diagnostic Criteria for DKA and HHS

	DKA			HHS
	Mild	Moderate	Severe	
Plasma glucose (mg/dl)	>250	>250	>250	>600
Arterial pH	7.25-7.30	7.00-7.24	<7.00	>7.30
Serum bicarbonate (mEq/L)	15-18	10-<15	<10	>15
Urine ketones*	Positive	Positive	Positive	Small
Serum ketones*	Positive	Positive	Positive	Small
Effective serum osmolality (mOsm/kg)†	Variable	Variable	Variable	>320
Anion gap‡	>10	>12	>12	Variable
Alteration in sensorium or mental obtundation	Alert	Alert/drowsy	Stupor/coma	Stupor/coma

*Nitroprusside reaction method.
†Calculation: 2(measured Na [mEq/L]) + glucose (mg/dl)/18.
‡Calculation: $(Na^+) - (Cl^- + HCO_3^-)$ (mEq/l).
From ADA: Hyperglycemic crises in patients with diabetes mellitus, *Diabetes Care* 26 (suppl 1), January, 2003.

Management of the adult patient with DKA and HHS

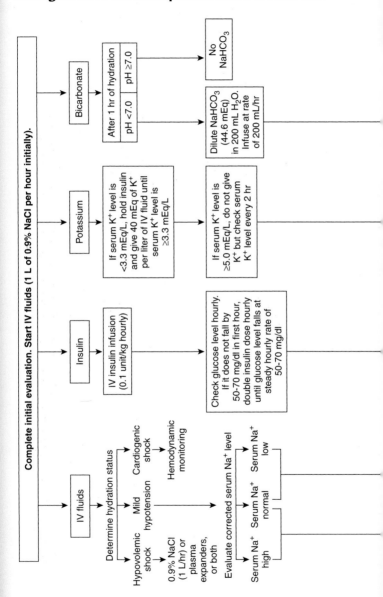

Complete initial evaluation. Start IV fluids (1 L of 0.9% NaCl per hour initially).

IV fluids

Determine hydration status

- Hypovolemic shock → 0.9% NaCl (1 L/hr) or plasma expanders, or both
- Mild hypotension
- Cardiogenic shock → Hemodynamic monitoring

Evaluate corrected serum Na+ level

- Serum Na+ high
- Serum Na+ normal
- Serum Na+ low

Insulin

IV insulin infusion (0.1 unit/kg hourly)

Check glucose level hourly. If it does not fall by 50-70 mg/dl in first hour, double insulin dose hourly until glucose level falls at steady hourly rate of 50-70 mg/dl

Potassium

If serum K+ level is <3.3 mEq/L, hold insulin and give 40 mEq of K+ per liter of IV fluid until serum K+ level is ≥3.3 mEq/L

If serum K+ level is ≥5.0 mEq/L, do not give K+ but check serum K+ level every 2 hr

Bicarbonate

After 1 hr of hydration

pH <7.0	pH ≥7.0

- pH ≥7.0 → No NaHCO$_3$
- pH <7.0 → Dilute NaHCO$_3$ (44.6 mEq) in 200 mL H$_2$O. Infuse at rate of 200 mL/hr

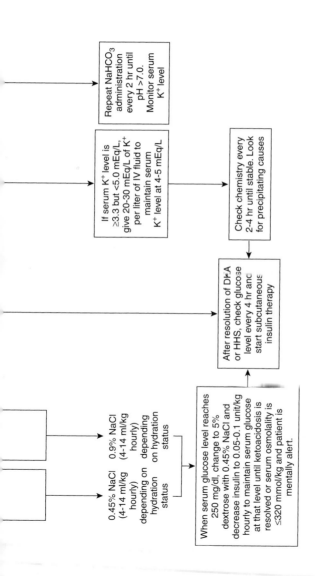

Repeat NaHCO₃ administration every 2 hr until pH >7.0. Monitor serum K⁺ level

If serum K⁺ level is ≥3.3 but <5.0 mEq/L, give 20-30 mEq/L of K⁺ per liter of IV fluid to maintain serum K⁺ level at 4-5 mEq/L

Check chemistry every 2-4 hr until stable. Look for precipitating causes

After resolution of DKA or HHS, check glucose level every 4 hr and start subcutaneous insulin therapy

0.45% NaCl (4-14 ml/kg hourly) depending on hydration status

0.9% NaCl (4-14 ml/kg hourly) depending on hydration status

When serum glucose level reaches 250 mg/dl, change to 5% dextrose with 0.45% NaCl and decrease insulin to 0.05-0.1 unit/kg hourly to maintain serum glucose at that level until ketoacidosis is resolved or serum osmolality is ≤320 mmol/kg and patient is mentally alert.

From Chiasson, J, et al: *Canadian Med Assoc J,* 168(7) •••, 2003 Copyright © 2003 American Diabetes Association. From *Diabetes Care* 26(1 Suppl):S10€–S117, 2003. Reprinted and adapted with permission from The American Diabetes Association.
DKA, Diabetic ketoacidosis; *HHS,* hyperosmolar hyperglycemia state.

REFERENCE GUIDE 7

Electrocardiogram (ECG) and Cardiac Marker Changes Associated With Myocardial Infarction (MI)

ECG Lead Correlation With MI Location

Location of Infarction	Lead Changes
Anterior	V_3, V_4
Anterolateral	I, aVL, V_3, V_4, V_5, V_6
Anteroseptal	V_1, V_2, V_3, V_4
Inferior	II, III, aVF
Lateral	High lateral: I, aVL
	Low lateral: V_5, V_6
Septal	V_1, V_2

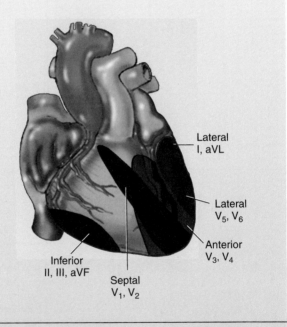

Lateral
I, aVL

Lateral
V_5, V_6

Anterior
V_3, V_4

Inferior
II, III, aVF

Septal
V_1, V_2

Data from: American Heart Association: *Advanced cardiac life support manual,* Dallas, 2001, the association. Stillwell SB: *Critical care nursing reference,* ed 3, St Louis, 2002, Mosby.

Cardiac Marker Elevations Associated With MI

Cardiac Marker	Onset	Peak	Return to Normal
Myoglobin	1-2 hr	6-9 hr	18-24 hr
Troponin I	4-6 hr	12-18 hr	~6 days
Troponin T	~4 hr	~12 hr	4-8 days
CK	3-8 hrs	12-24 hr	3-4 days
CK-MB	4-6 hr	12-24 hr	2-3 days

Data from: Karras DJ, and Kane DL: Serum markers in the emergency department diagnosis of acute myocardial infarction, *Emerg Med Clin North Am* 19(2):321-327, 2001.

REFERENCE GUIDE 8

Fluid Resuscitation Summary

Fluid Type	Description/Indication	Actions
Crystalloid		
Crystalloids: Ringer's lactate or normal saline is the fluid of choice for initial resuscitation of hemorrhagic and nonhemorrhagic shock.		
0.9% Normal saline (NS)	Isotonic	• May produce fluid overload† • 25% of volume administered will remain in vascular space • May produce hyperchloremic acidosis • May cause hypernatremia
Ringer's lactate solution	Isotonic, similar in composition to plasma, contains multiple electrolytes and lactate	• May produce fluid overload† • May promote lactic acidosis in prolonged hypoperfusion with decreased liver function • Lactate metabolizes to acetate; may produce metabolic alkalosis when large volumes are transfused
0.45% Normal saline	Hypotonic, moves fluid from vascular space to interstitial and intracellular spaces	• Decreases blood viscosity • May promote hypovolemia • May promote cerebral edema
5% Dextrose	Hypotonic	• 7.5 ml/100 ml infused will remain in vascular space • Inadequate for fluid resuscitation
Hypertonic saline (7.5%)	Hypertonic, pulls fluid from interstitial and intracellular spaces into vascular space	• Can be used to treat refractory hypovolemic shock—use controversial • Requires smaller amount to restore blood volume

34

- Increases cerebral oxygen while reducing ICP
- May promote hypernatremia
- May promote intracellular dehydration
- May promote osmotic diuresis

Synthetic Colloids

Dextran

Comes in 40, 70, and 75 molecular weight; similar to human albumin; expands plasma volume by drawing fluid from the interstitial to the intravascular space

- Expands plasma volume in hypovolemic shock or impending shock
- Associated with anaphylaxis
- Reduces factor VIII, platelets, and fibrinogen function so increases bleeding time
- May interfere with blood crossmatching and typing, glucose and erythrocyte sedimentation levels
- Risk of fluid overload‡
- Contraindicated in renal failure
- Used if blood products are not available

Hetastarch

Similar to human albumin; expands plasma volume

- Expands plasma volume
- May increase serum amylase levels
- May decrease hematocrit
- Associated with coagulopathy
- Risk of fluid overload‡
- Contraindicated in renal failure
- Maximum dose is approximately 20 ml/kg/day

Continued

Fluid type	Description/Indication	Actions
Natural Colloids		
Fresh frozen plasma	Contains all clotting factors	• Potential to transmit blood-borne pathogens • Can cause hypersensitivity reaction • Not used for volume expansion, only to increase clotting factors. Will increase clotting factors by 2% to 3% per unit infused
Plasmanate (plasma protein fraction)	Does not contain clotting factors, expands blood volume	• May cause hypersensitivity reaction • If given too rapidly (>10 ml/min), may cause hypotension • Blood volume expander
Albumin	5% Isooncotic; 25% hyperoncotic; "salt poor"	• Preferred as volume expander when risk from producing interstitial edema is great (e.g., pulmonary and heart disease) • Can give rapidly • May cause hypocalcemia

Whole blood	Can be administered without normal saline	• Compatible with LR, NaCl, Ringer's • 5% may be given undiluted, 25% may be given diluted or undiluted • Hyperkalemia, hypothermia, and hypocalcemia • May require greater amount than packed RBCs to increase oxygen-carrying capacity of blood • Rarely used, not cost-effective
Packed RBCs	Administer with normal saline	• Deficient in 2,3-diphosphoglycerate so may increase oxygen affinity to hemoglobin and may reduce oxygen delivery to tissue • Hypothermia, hyperkalemia, and hypocalcemia

*Dosages are not listed because of variability in patient response and reed.

†Fluid overload may occur when these agents are used because of large amounts of fluid required to replace lost volume (3:1 ratio).

‡Fluid overload may occur when these agents are used in cases of preexisting pulmonary or heart disease.

REFERENCE GUIDE 9

Formulas Used in Fluid Administration*

Basal fluid maintenance
1500 ml/m² BSA/24 hr = ml/24 hr (calculate as ml/hr)

General guidelines: Up to 10 kg = 100 ml/kg/24 hr
11-20 kg = 50 ml/kg/24 hr plus
100 ml/kg for first 10 kg
>20 kg = 20-25 ml/kg/24 hr plus
50 ml/kg for each kg
11 through 20 plus
100 ml/kg for first 10 kg

Volume replacement with crystalloids
Administer 3 ml for every ml lost. For fluid challenges
administer:
IV bolus 20 ml/kg NS RL in children
IV bolus of 200-300 ml RL in adult surgical patients
IV bolus of 200-300 ml NS in adult medical patients

Volume replacement with colloids
Administer 1 ml for every cc lost

Volume replacement for measured losses
Gastric losses: Replace 1 ml for every ml lost q 4 hr.
D5½ NS 30 mEq K/L
Intestinal losses: Replace 1 ml for every ml lost q 4 hr.
Use D5% LR.

Basal urine output
Up to 30 kg = 40 ml/kg/24 hr (2 ml/kg/hr)
>30 kg = 1-2 ml/kg/hr

---

*See Chapter 4, pp. 164-165 for burn resuscitation formulas.
NS, Normal saline; RL, Ringer's lactate.

REFERENCE GUIDE 10

Glasgow Coma Score: Adults

(For more detailed description of responses, see below.)

Glasgow Coma Scale

Category	Response	Score
Best eye-opening response	Opens eyes spontaneously	4
	Opens eyes to verbal stimuli	3
	Opens eyes to painful stimulus	2
	No eye opening	1
Best motor response	Follows commands	6
	Localizes to pain/purposeful movement	5
	Withdrawal in response to pain	4
	Abnormal flexion in response to pain	3
	Abnormal extension in response to pain	2
	No response to pain	1
Best verbal response	Oriented and converses	5
	Confused and converses	4
	Inappropriate words	3
	Incomprehensible sounds	2
	No verbal response	1
Possible point total is 3 to 15.	Total	

Category	Response	Description and Technique	Score
Eye response	Opens eyes spontaneously	Opens eyes without verbal or tactile stimuli	4
	Opens eyes to verbal stimuli	Opens eyes on command or when called by name. Start with a normal tone of voice and increase the loudness as necessary.	3
	Opens eyes to painful stimuli	Squeeze the trapezius muscle, the inner aspect of the arm or the thigh; do not rub the sternum with your knuckle, skin in this area is thin and fragile and bruises easily (especially in a geriatric patient); avoid twisting or pinching the nipples; do not apply pressure to the supraorbital area in head-injured patients. NOTE: These techniques to elicit pain also apply to the motor and verbal categories.	2
	No eye opening	Does not open eyes to painful stimuli	1
Motor response	Follows commands	Raises arms or holds up specific number of fingers on request. Do not ask patients to grasp hand; hand grasp may be a reflexive response.	6
	Localizes pain	Cannot follow commands but locates the painful stimulus and attempts to remove it with hand.	5
	Withdraws from pain	Does not actually locate source of pain with a hand but does withdraw from the pain; for example, may flex arm to withdraw from painful stimulus of a pinch.	4
	Abnormal flexion (to noxious or painful stimuli)	Adducts shoulders, flexes and pronates arms, flexes wrist, and makes a fist (decorticate posturing)	3

Category	Response	Description and Technique	Score
	Abnormal extension (to noxious or painful stimuli)	Adducts and internally rotates shoulders, extends forearm, and flexes wrist (decerebrate posturing)	2
	No response	Flaccid, no response to maximally applied painful stimuli	1
Verbal response	Oriented	Able to converse and oriented to person, place, and time	5
	Confused	Able to converse but is not fully oriented or demonstrates confusion	4
	Inappropriate words	Words are recognizable but make little or no sense; words verbalized in a disorganized manner	3
	Incomprehensible words	Words are not recognizable— moans, groans	2
	None	Does not make any sound in response to pain	1

REFERENCE GUIDE 11

Hemodynamic Formulas and Values

Parameter	Formula	Normal Range
Cardiac output (CO)	HR × SV	4-8 L/min
Cardiac index (CI)	$\dfrac{CO}{BSA}$	2.2-4.0 L/min/m²
Stroke volume (SV)	$\dfrac{CO \times 1000}{HR}$	60-150 ml/beat
Stroke volume index (SVI)	$\dfrac{CI \times 1000}{HR}$	30-65 ml/beat/m²
Mean arterial pressure	$\dfrac{2(DBP) + SBP}{3}$	70-105 mm Hg
Central venous pressure (CVP)	Measured	2-6 mm Hg
Systemic vascular resistance (SVR)	$\dfrac{(MAP - CVP) \times 80}{CO}$	800-1200 dynes/sec/cm⁵
Pulmonary artery systolic pressure (PAS)	Measured	20-30 mm Hg
Pulmonary artery diastolic pressure (PAD)	Measured	8-15 mm Hg
Mean pulmonary artery pressure (mean PAP)	$\dfrac{PAS + 2(PAD)}{3}$	10-20 mm Hg
Pulmonary artery wedge pressure (PAWP) or pulmonary artery occlusive pressure (PAOP)	Measured mean	6-12 mm Hg
Pulmonary vascular resistance (PVR)	$\dfrac{\left(\text{mean PAP} - \text{mean PAWP}\right) \times 80}{CO}$	< 250 dynes/sec/cm⁵
Right atrial pressure (RAP)	Measured	4-6 mm Hg
Left atrial pressure (LAP)	Measured	8-12 mm Hg
Right ventricular pressure (RVP)	Measured	$\dfrac{25}{0\text{-}5}$ mm Hg
Coronary artery perfusion pressure (CAPP)	DBP − PAWP	60-80 mm Hg
Cerebral perfusion pressure (CPP)	MAP − ICP	70-100 mm Hg

BSA, Body surface area, *DBP*, diastoic blood pressure, *HR*, heart rate, *ICP*, intracranial pressure, *SBP*, systolic blood pressure.
Data from Lewis SM, Heitkemper MM, and Dirkson SR: *Medical surgical nursing*, ed 5, St Louis, 2000, Mosby; and Swearingen PL and Keen JH: *Manual of critical care nursing*, ed 4, St Louis, 2001, Mosby.

REFERENCE GUIDE 12

Ischemic Chest Pain Algorithm

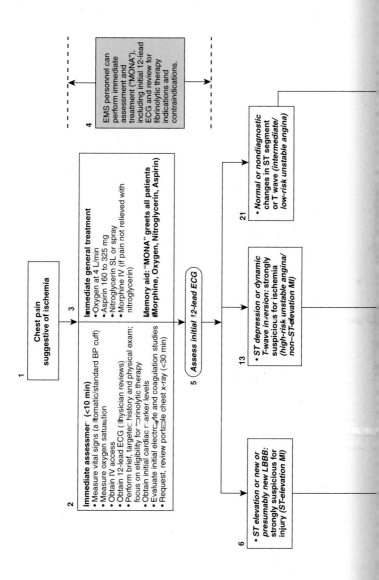

1
Chest pain suggestive of ischemia

2
Immediate assessment (<10 min)
• Measure vital signs (automatic/standard BP cuff)
• Measure oxygen saturation
• Obtain IV access
• Obtain 12-lead ECG (physician reviews)
• Perform brief, targeted history and physical exam; focus on eligibility for fibrinolytic therapy
• Obtain initial cardiac marker levels
• Evaluate initial electrolyte and coagulation studies
• Request, review portable chest x-ray (<30 min)

3
Immediate general treatment
• Oxygen at 4 L/min
• Aspirin 160 to 325 mg
• Nitroglycerin SL or spray
• Morphine IV (if pain not relieved with nitroglycerin)

Memory aid: "MONA" greets all patients
(Morphine, Oxygen, Nitroglycerin, Aspirin)

4
EMS personnel can perform immediate assessment and treatment ("MONA"), including initial 12-lead ECG and review for fibrinolytic therapy indications and contraindications.

5 Assess initial 12-lead ECG

6
• ST elevation or new or presumably new LBBB: strongly suspicious for injury (ST-elevation MI)

13
• ST depression or dynamic T-wave inversion: strongly suspicious for ischemia (high-risk unstable angina/non–ST-elevation MI)

21
• Normal or nondiagnostic changes in ST segment or T wave (intermediate/low-risk unstable angina)

43

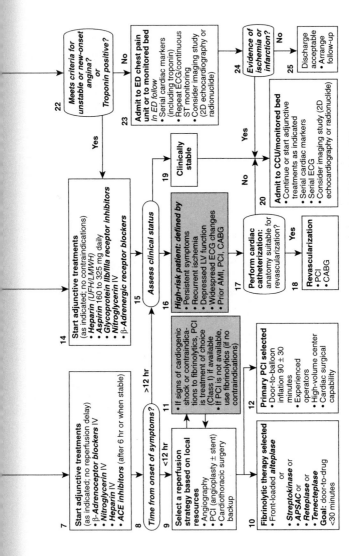

7
Start adjunctive treatments
(as indicated; no reperfusion delay)
- β-Adrenoceptor blockers IV
- Nitroglycerin IV
- Heparin IV
- ACE inhibitors (after 6 hr or when stable)

8
Time from onset of symptoms?

9 <12 hr

11 >12 hr

- If signs of cardiogenic shock or contraindications to fibrinolytics, PCI is treatment of choice (Class I) if available
- If PCI is not available, use fibrinolytics (if no contraindications)

10
Select a reperfusion strategy based on local resources
- Angiography
- PCI (angioplasty ± stent)
- Cardiothoracic surgery backup

Fibrinolytic therapy selected
- Front-loaded **alteplase**
  or
- **Streptokinase** or
- **APSAC** or
- **Reteplase** or
- **Tenecteplase**
- Goal: door-to-drug <30 minutes

12
Primary PCI selected
- Door-to-balloon inflation 90 ± 30 minutes
- Experienced operators
- High-volume center
- Cardiac surgical capability

14
Start adjunctive treatments
(as indicated; no contraindications)
- Heparin (UFH/LMWH)
- Aspirin 160 to 325 mg daily
- Glycoprotein IIb/IIIa receptor inhibitors
- Nitroglycerin IV
- β-Adrenergic receptor blockers

15
Assess clinical status

16
High-risk patient: defined by
- Persistent symptoms
- Recurrent ischemia
- Depressed LV function
- Widespread ECG changes
- Prior AMI, PCI, CABG

17
Perform cardiac catheterization: anatomy suitable for revascularization?

18 Yes
Revascularization
- PCI
- CABG

19
Clinically stable

20
Admit to CCU/monitored bed
- Continue or start adjunctive treatments as indicated
- Serial cardiac markers
- Serial ECG
- Consider imaging study (2D echocardiography or radionuclide)

22
Meets criteria for unstable or new-onset angina?
or
Troponin positive?

Yes
No

23
Admit to ED chest pain unit or to monitored bed
In ED follow
- Serial cardiac markers (including troponin)
- Repeat ECG/continuous ST monitoring
- Consider imaging study (2D echocardiography or radionuclide)

24
Evidence of ischemia or infarction?

Yes
No

25
- Discharge acceptable
- Arrange follow-up

Data from American Heart Association: *Advanced cardiac life support: Principles and practice.* Dallas, 2003, AHA.

REFERENCE GUIDE 13

Organ and Tissue Donation: Care of the Patient

Organ and tissue donation can be accepted from patients who:
- are diagnosed with brain death.
- have been pronounced dead because of a non-beating heart (i.e., cardiopulmonary arrest or having been removed from life support).

This reference guide is concerned with the patient who is a potential donor and will likely meet brain death criteria. These patients will require care until the organ and tissue recovery can occur.

The Medicare Conditions of Participation of August 21, 1998, require that all deaths and imminent deaths of potential donors be referred to the Organ Procurement Organization (OPO) in a timely manner. For imminent deaths (potential brain deaths), the OPO should be notified when the Glasgow Coma Scale score is ≤4 and before brain death determination. The role of the OPO is to:
1. Assess potential donors' medical suitability
2. Discuss donation with families
3. Obtain consent
4. Arrange for placement and recovery of tissue and organs

Potential Organ and Tissue Donations

Organs	Tissues
Heart	Cornea
Kidneys	Skin
Pancreas	Bone
Lungs	Bone marrow
Liver	Connective tissue
Intestines	Heart valves

NOTE: Tissue donation is possible up to 24 hours after the heart stops beating.

Typical Causes of Brain Death
- Head trauma (e.g., closed head injuries, gunshot wounds to the head, shaken child syndrome)
- Massive bleeding in the brain (e.g., cerebrovascular accident [CVA], subarachnoid hemorrhage [SAH], intracranial bleed [ICB], or subdural hemorrhage [SDH])
- Anoxia (e.g., after CPR, near drowning, or prolonged seizures)
- Brain tumors (primary central nervous system [CNS] tumors or brain metastasis)

- Infection (e.g., meningitis, brain abscess)
- Encephalopathies (metabolic disorders)

Criteria for Organ and Tissue Donation Referral to OPO

- Severe brain injury with the potential for brain death to occur
- Any age
- Need for ventilator to maintain oxygenation and ventilation

Preliminary Requirements to Make a Determination of Brain Death

- Knowledge of the cause of brain death
- Absence of toxic CNS depression (sedatives, alcohol, neuromuscular blockades)
- Absence of metabolic CNS depression (hypothermia: less than 90° F or 32.2° C; hypotension, acidosis)
- Negative screen for diabetic ketoacidosis (DKA), hyperosmolar hyperglycemic syndrome (HHS) and seizure activity

One of the following three types of testing must be met to determine brain death:

1. *Clinical examination:* Discloses the absence of cerebral and brainstem function. Cannot be used if toxic or metabolic CNS depression exists.
   - Unresponsive to any verbal or painful stimuli (comatose)
   - No pupil reflex (nonreactive pupils)
   - No doll's eyes (oculocephalic reflex)
   - No response to ice water caloric (oculovestibular reflex)
   - No corneal reflex
   - No gag reflex
   - No cough reflex

   NOTE: Spinal reflexes may be present, but all of the above reflexes must be absent.

   - Apnea ($Pco_2 \geq 60$ mm Hg) after observation of no respiratory activity with no respiratory assistance given. (The patient is ventilated for 10-20 minutes with 100% oxygen. Mechanical ventilations are withdrawn, and passive 100% oxygen is administered. Lack of spontaneous respirations in the face of hypercarbia [$Pco_2 \geq 60$ mm Hg] results in a positive apnea test supporting the clinical determination of brain death.)

   OR

2. EEG: Confirms lack of electrical activity during 30 minutes of recording

   (Cannot use if toxic or metabolic CNS depression exists.)

   Clinical examination must confirm brainstem death because EEG assesses only cerebral activity.

   OR

3. **Cerebral blood flow tests:** No blood flow to the brain, determined by one of the following (cannot use if systolic blood pressure ≤80 mm Hg):
   - Cerebral angiogram
   - Cerebral nuclear flow study (technetium 99 m brain scan)
   - Transcranial Doppler ultrasonography

   NOTE: These tests are often called confirmatory tests. Absence of blood flow to the brain is indicative of brain death, regardless of the cause.

   After brain death has been determined and the patient is deemed suitable for donation, the hospital in collaboration with the OPO must ensure that the family of the potential donor is informed of its options to donate. The individual designated by the hospital to make the request must be an organ procurement representative or a trained designated requester (an individual trained by the OPO on how to request a donation). If the patient is suitable for donation, the hospital must maintain the patient hemodynamically until necessary testing and recovery of organs occurs.

Patient Care Management for the Patient Determined Suitable for Organ and Tissue Transplantation

1. Provide hemodynamic support.
   - Monitor for dysrhythmias
   - Inotrope support (dopamine) if needed to maintain systolic blood pressure > 90 mm Hg
   - If possible, avoid potent vasoconstrictors (e.g., epinephrine); however, long-term hypotension is more damaging than the use of potent vasoconstrictors
   - Replace blood loss to maintain hematocrit ≥30%
   - Sodium nitroprusside for hypertension
   - Initiate IV crystalloid or colloids to maintain adequate intake
   - Monitor urine output: maintain 0.5 ml/kg/hr or greater
   - Low-dose dopamine (2-5 mcg/kg/min) can be used to increase renal perfusion
   - Monitor the patient for diabetes insipidus (DI). (Urine output greater than 200 ml/hr, rising serum sodium level, specific gravity less than or equal to 1.005)
   - If the patient develops DI, treat with vasopressin or desmopressin acetate (DDAVP, a synthetic analog of vasopressin) to keep urine output greater than 100 ml/hr and less than 200 ml/hr
   - Monitor for fluid overload
   - Monitor for disseminated intravascular coagulation (DIC) (see Chapter 14)

2. Provide temperature support.

   Maintain temperature of 35.6° to 37.8° C (96° F to 100° F)
   - Heating and cooling blankets
   - Adequate room temperature
   - Warm gastric lavage
   - Head coverings
   - Warmed oxygen temperatures
   - Antipyretics as ordered

3. Provide ventilatory support.
   - Use FiO_2 as appropriate to maintain $PaO_2 \geq 100$ mm Hg.
   - Tidal volume 12-15 ml/kg of ideal body weight.
   - Set ventilatory rate to maintain PCO_2 35-45 mm Hg.
   - Place all patients on PEEP of 5 cm H_2O.
   - Turn and suction patient q 1-2 hr to maintain optimal lung clearance and function.

4. Provide supportive care to family.
   - Involve supportive staff (e.g., chaplain, patient advocate staff, family liaisons) to assist families during the patient's hospital stay.
   - Donation should *not* be discussed or mentioned to the family until they have an *understanding and acknowledgment* that death is imminent and there is no hope for the patient's survival (decoupling).
   - The Medicare Conditions of Participation require that only OPO staff or individuals trained by the OPO should discuss donation with the family.[1] Research indicates that consent for donation is improved if families feel they have been provided supportive care.

   NOTE: Be aware of the state or country OPO policies and the hospital policies where you are working. In the United States, hospitals are required to make policies consistent with the practice of their organ procurement organization. The Medicare Conditions of Participation should lead the policies and practice. Federal regulations are mandates and take precedence over any state law. Each countrys policies may differ.

---

[1]Federal Register. Medicare and Medicaid programs: hospital condition of participation; identification of potential organ, tissue and eye donors, Health Care Financing Administration, June 22, 1998.

Oxygen Delivery Devices

Supplemental Adjunct	Flow Rate	O$_2$ Concentration	Indications	Comments	Pediatric Considerations*
Nasal cannula	1-6 L/min	24%-44%	Patients with minimal or no respiratory or oxygenation problem	A low-flow system in which the tidal volume is mixed with room air; for each L/min of flow increase, O$_2$ concentration increases by approximately 4%	Determination of actual inspired O$_2$ concentration from flow rate is unreliable because of influence of nasal and oropharyngeal resistance and volume, tidal volume, inspiratory flow rate; to avoid frightening child, start flow on O$_2$ after cannula is in place.
Face mask	6-10 L/min	35%-60%	Patients who require a concentration of O$_2$ greater than a nasal cannula can provide	Tidal volume is mixed with room air; requires an O$_2$ flow of at least 6 L/min to prevent an accumulation of exhaled air in mask.	Allow child to hold mask before putting it in place; mask should extend from bridge of the nose to the cleft of chin for proper sizing. Minimum of at least

Continued

Supplemental Adjunct	Flow Rate	O_2 Concentration	Indications	Comments	Pediatric Considerations*
Face mask with O_2 reservoir (also known as a nonrebreather mask or partial nonrebreather mask)	6-15 L/min	60% to almost 100%	Patients who need the highest possible O_2 concentration but are not candidates for endotracheal intubation	Mask should fit face snugly; monitor patient closely if level of consciousness is diminished; vomiting into the mask may result in aspiration; exhaled air escapes through a flapper valve on each side of the mask; O_2 flow rate should be such that the reservoir bag does not empty completely during inhalation.	6 L/min of flow must be used to prevent rebreathing exhaled carbon dioxide. Not available for a neonate; mask should extend from the bridge of the nose to the cleft of chin for proper sizing; if child is not tolerating a mask, blow-by oxygen through corrugated tubing held close to child's face may work*; O_2 flow rate should be such that the reservoir bag does not empty completely during inhalation.
Venturi mask	3-15 L/min	24%-50%	Moderate to severe hypoxemia; useful in patients who retain CO_2	More controlled O_2 concentration delivery; O_2 diluter and O_2 flow used dictate O_2	Not used on children

Device	Oxygen concentration	Indications	Notes
		such as with COPD	concentration being delivered.
			Must have a mask that fits child's face and obtain a good seal; tidal volume delivered should be sufficient to see chest rise visibly; gastric inflation common; applying cricoid pressure may help reduce the possibility of regurgitation and subsequent aspiration.
Pocket mask	Expired room air 17%; room air 10 L/min 50%; 15 L/min 80%	To support ventilation in the patient with inadequate or absent respiratory effort	Must obtain a good seal with mask; pocket mask has been shown to provide better tidal volumes than bag-valve mask; gastric inflation common; applying cricoid pressure may help reduce the possibility of regurgitation and subsequent aspiration.
Bag-valve mask	Room air 21%; 15 L/min 100%	Need for ventilatory assistance secondary to shallow ineffective respiratory effort; apnea	Adult bag-valve device volume is approximately 1600 ml; can be difficult to obtain effective seal to deliver appropriate tidal volume; place an oral airway in patients without a gag reflex and nasal airway in patients with a gag reflex to improve O$_2$ delivery; gastric inflation delivery; gastric inflation. Pediatric bag valve device volume is approximately 650 ml; term infant to child bag volume: 450 ml; neonate bag: 250 ml; tidal volume delivered should be sufficient to see chest rise visibly; popoff valves should be easily bypassed; mask should fit correctly to reduce under-mask volume and thus dead space; coordinate

Continued

Supplemental Adjunct	Flow Rate	O$_2$ Concentration	Indications	Comments	Pediatric Considerations*
				is common; applying cricoid pressure may help reduce the possibility of regurgitation and subsequent aspiration; administering slow ventilations will avoid high pressures that increase gastric inflation; coordinate assisted breaths with patient's effort; bag must be compressed to gain increased levels of oxygen, otherwise, patient will receive oxygen concentrations of only 21%.	assisted breaths with patient's effort.

*If a pediatric patient resists oxygen therapy, you must balance the need for oxygen against the increased oxygen demand caused by the resistance or agitation. Multiple types of adjuncts and delivery styles may need to be tried to find the balance.
Data from: American Heart Association: *ACLS: Principles and practice*, Dallas, 2003, American Heart Association; *Advanced pediatric life support textbook*, Dallas, 2002, American Heart Association.

Pain Scales

Pain Scale/Description	Instructions	Recommended Age
Faces scale: Consists of six cartoon faces ranging from very happy, smiling face for "no pain," to tearful face for "worst pain"	***Original instructions:*** Explain to child that each face is for a person who feels happy because there is no pain (hurt) or sad because there is some or a lot of pain. FACE 0 is very happy because there is no hurt. FACE 1 hurts just a little bit. FACE 2 hurts a little more. FACE 3 hurts even more. FACE 4 hurts a whole lot, but FACE 5 hurts as much as you can imagine, although you don't have to be crying to feel this bad. Ask the child to choose the face that best describes his or her own pain. Record the number under chosen face on pain assessment record.	Children as young as 3 yr Using same instructions without affect words, such as *happy* or *sad*, results in same pain rating, probably reflecting child's rating of pain intensity.

0	1	2	3	4	5
No hurt	Hurts little bit	Hurts little more	Hurts even more	Hurts whole lot	Hurts worst

Continued

Pain Scale/Description	Instructions	Recommended Age
Simple descriptive scale: Uses descriptive words (may vary according to scale) to denote varying intensities of pain	Explain to child, "This is a line with words to describe how much pain you may have." This side of the line means no pain and over here the line means worst possible pain." (Point with your finger where "no pain" is and run your finger along the line to "worst possible pain" as you say it.) "If you have pain, you would mark somewhere along the line, depending on how much pain you have" (show example). "The more pain you have, the closer to worst pain you should mark. The worst	Children age 4 to 17 yr

pain possible is marked like this" (show example). "Show me how much pain you have right now by marking with a straight, up-and-down line anywhere along the line to show how much pain you have right now." With a millimeter rule, measure from the "no pain" end to the mark and record this measurment as the pain score.

No pain

Little pain

Medium pain

Large pain

Worst possible pain

From Hockenberry MJ: *Wong's nursing care of infants and children*, ec 7, St. Louis, 2003, Mosby.

Pain Scale/Description	Instructions	Recommended Age
Numeric scale: Uses straight line with end points identified as "no pain" and "worst pain", divisions along line are marked in units from "0" to "10" (high number may vary)	Explain to child that at one end of line is "0", which means that person feels no pain (hurt); at the other is 10, which means person feels worst pain imaginable, numbers 1 to 9 are for very little pain to whole lot of pain; ask child to choose number that best describes own pain	Children as young as 5 yr, provided they can count and have some concepts of numbers and their values in relation to other numbers.

No pain

|—|—|—|—|—|—|—|—|—|—|
0   1   2   3   4   5   6   7   8   9   10

Worst pain

From Hockenberry MJ: *Wong's nursing care of infants and children*, ed 7, St. Louis, 2003, Mosby.

REFERENCE GUIDE 16

Pediatric and Infant Coma Scale

Activity	Infants (< 1 year)	Points	Children
Eye opening	Spontaneous	4	Spontaneous
	To voice	3	To voice
	To pain	2	To pain
	No response	1	No response
Motor	Normal spontaneous movement	6	Obeys commands
	Localizes to pain/purposeful movement	5	Localizes to pain/purposeful movement
	Withdraws to pain	4	Withdraws to pain
	Abnormal flexion to pain	3	Abnormal flexion to pain
	Abnormal extension to pain	2	Abnormal extension to pain
	No response	1	No response
Verbal	Coos, babbles, cries appropriately	5	Appropriate words and phrases
	Irritable, appropriate crying	4	Inappropriate words
	Inappropriate crying, screaming	3	Persistent crying or screaming
	Grunts or moans to pain	2	Grunts or moans to pain, incomprehensible words
	No verbal response	1	No verbal response
Point total:			

Possible point range is 3-15; score of <8 indicative of a coma.

REFERENCE GUIDE 17

Pediatric Trauma Score

Component	Category +2	+1	−1
Size	≥20 kg	10-20 kg	<10 kg
Airway	Normal	Maintainable	Unmaintainable
Systolic BP	≥90 mm Hg	50-90 mm Hg	<50 mm Hg
CNS	Awake	Obtunded	Coma/decerebrate
Open wound	None	Minor	Major/penetrating
Skeletal	None	Closed fracture	Open/multiple fractures

Sum range is −6 to +12.
Children with a pediatric trauma score of 8 or less should be transferred to a pediatric trauma center.

From Talbert JL, Mollitt DL, et al: The pediatric trauma score as a predictor of injury severity in the injured child, *J Pediatr Surg* 22 (1):14-18, 1987.

Airway
Normal: requiring no additional supportive measures
Maintainable: partially obstructed airway requiring simple measures such as head positioning, oral airway, mask oxygen
Unmaintainable: requiring definitive management and requiring intubation, cricothyrotomy, or other invasive procedures

Systolic BP
If BP cuff size inadequate, the following can be used:
- Pulse at the wrist: +2
- Pulse at the neck or groin: +1
- Absence of palpable pulse: −1

Open wound
No evidence of external trauma: +2
Abrasions or minor cutaneous injury: +1
Any penetrating injury or major avulsion or laceration: −1

Skeletal (fractures)
None, no evidence: +2
Minor, single closed fracture or suspicion thereof: +1
Open fracture(s) or multiple closed fractures: −1

REFERENCE GUIDE 18

Pediatric Tube Size

This table is to serve as a guide. These guidelines may need to be adjusted based on the patient's individual needs.

Equipment	Premature	Neonate	6 mo	1 yr	2 yr	3 yr
Airway						
Oral airway size	Infant	Infant/small	Small	Small	Small	Small
Endotracheal tube (ETT)	2.5-3.0	3.0-3.5	3.5-4.0	4.0-4.5	4.0-4.5	4.5
ETT mark at lip (cm)	7.0-8.0	9.0	10.5	11	12	13
Laryngoscope blade s = straight c = curved	0s	1s	1s	1s	1s	1s
Suction catheter (French)	6	8	8	8	8	8
Breathing Circulation						
Chest tube (French)	10-14	10-14	14-20	14-24	14-24	14-24
Gastrointestinal/Genitourinary						
Gastric tube (French)	5	5	8	8	10	10
Urinary catheter	5 (feeding tube)	5-8 (feeding tube)	8	10	10	10

Adapted from Werner H: *University of Kentucky Children's Hospital, Division of Pediatric Critical Care Medicine, Pediatric resuscitation reference card,* 2002. Used with permission. Emergency Nurses Association: *Emergency nursing pediatric course provider manual,* ed 3, Park Ridge, Ill, 2004, the Association.

4 yr	5 yr	6 yr	7 yr	8 yr	9 yr	10 yr	11-14 yr
Medium	Medium	Medium	Medium	Medium large	Medium large	Medium large	Large
5.0-5.5	5.0-5.5	5.5-6.0	5.5-6.0	6.0-6.5	6.0-6.5	6.5	7.0-7.5
14	14.5	15	15.5	16	16.5	17	18-19
2s/c	2s/c	2s/c	2s/c	2-3s/c	2-3s/c	2-3s/c	2-3s/c
10	10	10	10	10	10-12	12	12
20-32	20-32	20-32	20-32	28-38	28-38	28-38	28-38
10	10	10	12	12	12	12	12-16
10-12	10-12	10-12	12	12	12	12	12-14

REFERENCE GUIDE 19

Pediatric Vital Signs and Weights: Normal

Age	Wt (kg)	Wt (lb)	Average Respiratory Rate	Average BP (59th Percentile)	Pulse Rate (95% range)
Term neonate	3.5	8	50	70/50	95-150
3 months	6.0	13	40	85/50	110-175
6 months	7.5	16	30	85/50	110-160
1 year	10	22	25	90/55	90-150
2 years	12	26	25	90/55	90-150
3 years	14	31	25	90/55	75-130
4 years	16	35	24	95/60	75-130
6 years	20	44	23	95/60	70/130
8 years	24	53	22	95/60	65-125
10 years	30	66	20	100/65	60-110
12 years	38	84	18	105/65	60-100
14 years	50	110	18	110/70	60-100

Adapted from Werner H: *University of Kentucky Children's Hospital, Division of Pediatric Critical Care Medicine, Pediatric resuscitation reference card,* 2002. Used with permission.

REFERENCE GUIDE 20

Safety in the Emergency Department

Patient and situational risk factors may contribute to a violent situation in the emergency department.

1. Patient risk factors:
   - History of psychiatric disorders or illness.
   - Specific psychiatric disorders may increase the risk of violence (e.g., bipolar disorder, schizophrenia, paranoia, auditory/visual hallucinations, and acute psychotic disorder).
   - Drug and/or alcohol abuse.
   - Phencyclidine (PCP), methamphetamine, ketamine, and MDMA (Ecstasy) may produce paranoia and agitation resulting in violent behavior.
   - Past history of verbal abuse and/or physical violence.
   - Combative or agitated behavior of unknown etiology (e.g., Alzheimer's disease).

2. Potential or actual high-risk situations:
   - Patient with membership or activity in a gang.
   - Gang members may present to the emergency department.
   - Angry and/or agitated patient or family member with a weapon or item that can be used as a weapon.
   - Patient with pending or actual incarceration.
   - Grieving family or friends of a patient who had a sudden unexpected death.
   - Long wait times in the emergency department.
   - Patients seeking narcotics or controlled substances.
   - Alleged perpetrator and victim of a crime in the emergency department at the same time as patients.

3. Strategies for emergency department health-care providers to reduce a violent situation:
   - Do not allow yourself to be trapped in a room with the patient between you and the only exit. Always stand closer to the door.
   - Remove items like stethoscopes, scissors, and hemostats from pockets or uniform before entering a patient's room.
   - Remove items that may be a potential weapon from patient's room. See Protocol C.
   - Place patient in hospital gown. Check and inventory all items of clothing and personal belongings (e.g., coat, purse, bags, and wallets) for harmful objects and remove such from the bedside.
   - Do not be confrontational with patient. Interactions should be carried out in a respectful and nonjudgmental manner.
   - Do not speak in a loud, aggressive, or authoritative manner.
   - Maintain open body language (i.e., keep your arms at your side; assume a relaxed posture).

- If not contraindicated, offer the patient food and drink. Eating may serve as a distracter and a comfort measure.
- Develop and implement safety protocols that follow institutional policies and comply with state regulations. (See sample protocols A-C.)

4. Recognize signs of an impending volatile situation:
   - Threatening or sudden change in body language (e.g., clenched fists, pacing, sweating, kicking at objects, or throwing objects)
   - Verbal threats
   - Auditory and/or visual hallucination
   - Increase in agitation
   - Rambling speech

5. How to protect yourself from a violent situation:
   - Remain calm.
   - Do not attempt to remove a weapon from the patient.
   - Do not turn your back to the patient.
   - Avoid direct eye contact with the patient.
   - Speak calmly to the patient.
   - Slowly back yourself out the door.
   - Have another staff member notify security or police.

6. Security mechanisms to use in the emergency department:
   - Armed or unarmed security officer station in the emergency department.
   - Metal detector
   - Assistance buttons (panic buttons) located throughout the emergency department, when activated, will alert and direct security officers to an area of threatened violence.
   - Staff education
   - Health-care workers should be educated in ways to manage a potential or actual violent situation. This should be an ongoing competency.
   - Visitor policy
   - Include how many people and who may be at the bedside (e.g., aunts, uncles, friends). The number of visitors is at the discretion of the RN.
   - Visitors should be given a pass that is clearly visible and worn at all times.
   - Security monitors/cameras should be located at key entrances, including ambulance entrance.
   - Electronic key card entry system will help limit unauthorized entry into the department.

- Lockdown system prevents entry into the emergency department but will allow egress. May need to be used in one or more of the following:
  - Hostage situation
  - Civil unrest as in a riot situation
  - Patient or visitor actively using a weapon
7. Recommendations:
   - Develop a tool to report acts of violence in the emergency department.
   - Maintain an established safety committee in the emergency department.
   - Read OSHA's guidelines on violence in the work force.
   - Speak with your local police or security department about performing a worksite analysis to identify areas that are a potential security risk.

Sources of additional information:

Workplace violence, Department of Health and Human Services (DHHS) pub no 2002-101, National Institute for Occupational Safety and Health (NIOSH).

Guidelines for preventing workplace violence for health care and social service workers, US Department of Labor, OSHA 3148.

ED Safety Protocol A

Checking personal belongings in patients with actual or potential safety risk

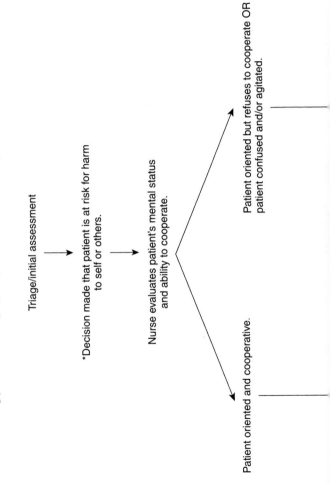

Triage/initial assessment

*Decision made that patient is at risk for harm to self or others.

Nurse evaluates patient's mental status and ability to cooperate.

Patient oriented and cooperative.

Patient oriented but refuses to cooperate OR patient confused and/or agitated.

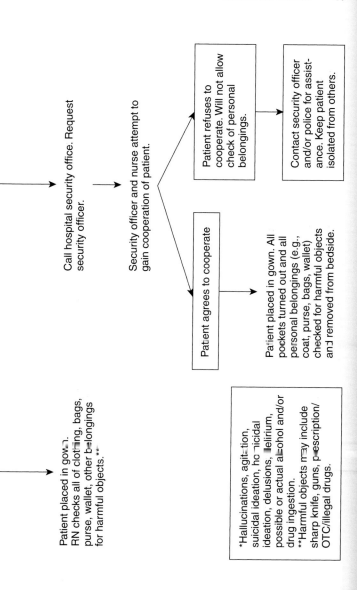

Patient placed in gown.
RN checks all of clothing, bags,
purse, wallet, other belongings
for harmful objects.**

Call hospital security office. Request
security officer.

Security officer and nurse attempt to
gain cooperation of patient.

Patient agrees to cooperate

Patient placed in gown. All
pockets turned out and all
personal belongings (e.g.,
coat, purse, bags, wallet)
checked for harmful objects
and removed from bedside.

Patient refuses to
cooperate. Will not allow
check of personal
belongings.

Contact security officer
and/or police for assist-
ance. Keep patient
isolated from others.

*Hallucinations, agitation,
suicidal ideation, homicidal
ideation, delusions, delirium,
possible or actual alcohol and/or
drug ingestion.
**Harmful objects may include
sharp knife, guns, prescription/
OTC/illegal drugs.

ED Safety Protocol B

Requesting security officer to observe/monitor patients in ED (72-hour hold)

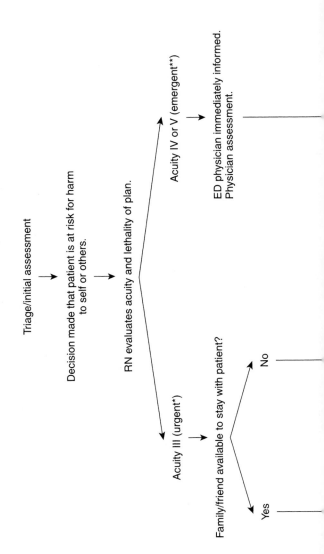

Triage/initial assessment

→

Decision made that patient is at risk for harm to self or others.

→

RN evaluates acuity and lethality of plan.

Acuity IV or V (emergent**)

→

ED physician immediately informed. Physician assessment.

Acuity III (urgent*)

→

Family/friend available to stay with patient?

No

Yes

RN requests that family member/friend stay with patient at all times and inform RN if leaving.

RN reevaluates patient every 1-2 hours to determine whether acuity is increased.

RN evaluates patient every 60 minutes to determine whether acuity is increased and need for security officer to observe/monitor patient.

- Call hospital security office and request 72-hour hold.
- RN gives brief report to security officer. Report includes patient name and reason for 72-hour hold (e.g., SI/HI***).
- Physician signs completed 72-hour hold form within 1 hour of request. Officer receives copy of face sheet.
- RN reassesses and documents patient condition every 60 minutes and prn.
- RN evaluates continued need for security officer every 2 hours and informs officer of patient status.

* Acuity III: Considering suicide but no specific plan or low-lethality plan. Agrees to no-harm contract.
** Acuity IV: Current high-lethality plan to harm self or others and the means to obtain resources to carry out plan OR previous suicide attempt with moderate to high lethality.
NOTE: Renew no-harm contract every hour.
Acuity V: Current high-lethality plan to harm self or others and immediate means to carry out plan (gun on person) OR auditory hallucinations related to killing self or others OR has attempted to carry out plan.
NOTE: Renew no-harm contract every hour or more often as needed.
*** Suicidal ideation, homicidal ideation.

ED Safety Protocol C

**Promoting a safe environment/treatment area
for potentially or actually suicidal or homicidal patients**

Triage/initial assessment

Decision made that patient is at risk for harm
to self or others AND Acuity IV or V

Attempt to place patient in treatment area
that allows direct visual observation from several areas.

Before placing patient in room, the RN or designee
removes any potentially dangerous objects, including:

- Sharp items
- Suction tubing
- Ceiling mounted and rolling IV poles
- BP cuffs and tubing
- Telephone and cord
- Chairs
- Bedside tables
- Any rolling equipment (e.g., otoscope,
  pulse oximeter)
- BVMDs
- Call light cord
- Alcohol pads
- Bottle(s) of isopropyl alcohol
- Bottle(s) of betadine
- Bottle(s) of hydrogen peroxide
- All clothing and personal belongings including
  belts, shoelaces, and other belongings.

NOTE: Any emergency equipment should be placed within easy
access outside of the room.

ED Safety Protocol D

Activation of Assistance or Panic Button

To be used when there is high risk or actual physical harm to staff, other patients, and/or visitors.

Activate in following situations/circumstances:

- Patient/visitor with weapon and verbalizing/ demonstrating intent to use.
- Patient/visitor is physically assaulting an individual(s) or body language suggestive of an impending assault (i.e., raised fist, corners or blocks staff person from leaving room).
- Hostage situation

ED staff does the following:

- Stop flow of visitors into ED.
- Direct or escort visitors in area to lobby or a safe area.
- Direct patients into their rooms and pull curtain/ close door.
- Do not allow yourself to be "blocked in" between patient/visitor and door of exam room.
- Speak to patient/visitor with a calm tone.
- Do not attempt to grab weapon from patient/visitor.
- Make every effort to remove yourself from danger.

Skin Rash Diseases

Disease	Type of Rash	Incubation	Duration	Comments
Maculopapular rashes				
Candida (Monilia) *(yeast infection)*	Oral: White patches on mucous membranes; Skin: Red lesions with serous drainage, white crust (usually in diaper rash)	N/A	Until treated	Proliferates in warm, moist environments. Predisposing conditions: diabetes, HIV, immunologic defects (depressed T-cell function), systemic antibacterial agents, chemotherapy.
Contact dermatitis *(hypersensitivity)*	Red maculopapular lesions; sharp demarcation between involved and uninvolved areas of skin; may develop into a secondary lesion (e.g., vesicles or wheals)	Lesions developing within a few hours to days after contact with allergen	Until treated; may gradually disappear without treatment	Common causes include irritating agents such as soaps, detergents, and rough sheets. If linear, suspect plant contact.
Impetigo *(bacterial)*	Rash begins as vesicular lesions, advances to thick yellow crusts (formed by exudate from vesicle or bulla) on a red base; usually seen on hands and feet, and around mouth; may cause cellulitis	4-10 days	Until treated with antibiotics	Highly contagious: transmitted by contact with fluid in blisters; usual cause *Staphylococci*, *Streptococci*, or a combination of both.
Rocky Mountain spotted	Rash consists of pink macules on peripheral extremities that become papular after 1-2 days and soon spread	2-14 days	Until treated with antibiotics	Tick-induced Rickettsia. Systemic signs for 1-3 days, consists of fever (sudden onset),

fever *(bacterial)*	to palms and soles. Petechiae and hemorrhages are common.		headache, vomiting, and myalgias; seen primarily April through September. Not transmitted person to person.
Rubella (German measles, measles) *(viral)*	May see reddish spots on soft palate initially. Macular pink to red rash. First appears on head and spreads downward. Rapidly becomes papular	14-23 days; contagious from 7 days before to 5 days after rash appears.	3-4 days	Highly communicable; rash preceded by low-grade fever, coryza, sore throat, cough, conjunctivitis, cervical lymphadenopathy. Infection can occur without rash. Infection during first trimester of pregnancy may lead to infection of fetus and produce a variety of congenital anomalies. Can cause joint pain.
Rubeola (hard measles, red measles) *(viral)*	Koplik's spots appear on buccal mucosa (pinpoint white lesions on a red base) 24-48 hours before rash appears; rash consists of reddish macules and begins on face and spreads downward; within 1-2 days, rash is confluent. Rash color fades to yellow-tan.	10-20 days; contagious from 4 days before to 5 days after rash appears.	10-15 days	Highly communicable. Preceded for 2-3 days by cough, coryza, and conjunctivitis.
Roseola *(viral)*	Maculopapular, small, pink, widely disseminated, and nonpruritic	1-2 days	1-2 days	Fever can be as high as 106° F. Rash follows 3-4 days of fever.

Continued

Disease	Type of Rash	Incubation	Duration	Comments
Scabies (*parasite*)	Initially linear, threadlike gray to brown lesions between fingers and toes and on the ankles, axilla, and elbows; advanced: pruritic red papules.	Itching begins 14-60 days after initial contact.	Until treated	Parasitic mite that burrows under the skin; severe itching, especially at night. Transmitted by direct physical contact.
Scarlet fever (Scarlatina) (*bacterial*)	Fine raised generalized maculopapular rash ("sandpaper rash"); may be absent around mouth and face; red "strawberry tongue"; bright red lines found in axilla and antecubital fossa (Pastia's lines); may peel after 5 days.	1-2 days, contagious until 1-2 days after start of antibiotics.	Resolves quickly after antibiotics given	Caused by group-A beta-hemolytic streptococcal bacteria. Accompanied by sore throat, fever, vomiting, headache, and malaise. Spread by direct contact or exhaled droplets. Rash can last up to 2-3 weeks.
Small pox (*viral*)	Rash of red, flat lesions appear in 2-3 days, first in the mouth and pharynx, on palms, soles of feet, face and forearms, spreading to the trunk. Lesions become vesicular, then pustular, and then crust.	7-17 days	Approximately 3 weeks	Most infectious during first week of illness. Preceded by high fever, fatigue, head and back ache. Use N-95 respirator for health-care worker. Place patient in room with negative pressure ventilation, notify public health authorities immediately.

Tinea corporis (ringworm) (fungal)	Reddish, round or scaly patch that has well defined margins; spreads peripherally and clears centrally	10-14 days	Until treated	Fungus through direct or indirect contact.
Varicella (chicken pox) (viral)	Rash begins as small red macules and then progresses to papules and then vesicles; after the vesicles rupture, a dry crust forms over the lesion; all types of lesions may be present at the same time.	14-21 days; contagious up to 5 days before eruption of lesions until all lesions are crusted over	5-20 days	Highly contagious; accompanied by fever, mild malaise; lesions start on scalp and trunk and then spread centrifugally to extremities; scratching may cause secondary infection.

Rashes associated with hemorrhagic lesions

Petechiae	Small, 1-mm to 2-mm, pinpoint reddish purple macular lesions that do not blanch with pressure.	N/A	N/A	Causes include platelet disorders, leukemia, meningococcemia, bacterial meningitis.
Purpura	Larger ecchymotic lesions that are macular and do not blanch with pressure.	N/A	N/A	Causes include Henoch-Schönlein purpura, idiopathic thrombocytic purpura, hemophilia, trauma, viral infections.

Macule: Circumscribed flat discoloration that may be brown, blue, red, or hypopigmented

Papule: An elevated solid lesion up to 0.5 cm in diameter; color varies; papules may become confluent and form plaques

Plaque: A circumscribed, elevated superficial solid lesion more than 0.5 cm in diameter, often formed by the confluence of papules

Vesicle: A circumscribed collection of free fluid up to 0.5 cm in diameter

Coryza: Runny nose

Bulla: A vesicle more than 0.5 cm in diameter, elevated, fluid filled

Pustule: A circumscribed collection of leukocytes and free fluid that varies in size

REFERENCE GUIDE 22

Algorithm for Suspected Stroke

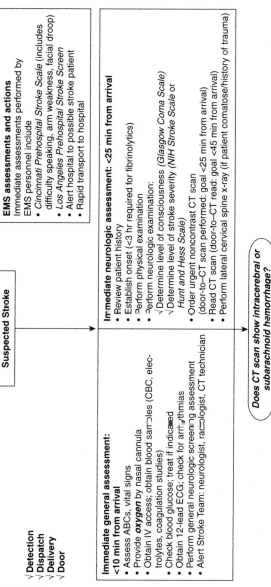

Algorithm for Suspected Stroke

√ Detection
√ Dispatch
√ Delivery
√ Door

Suspected Stroke

EMS assessments and actions
Immediate assessments performed by EMS personnel include
- *Cincinnati Prehospital Stroke Scale* (includes difficulty speaking, arm weakness, facial droop)
- *Los Angeles Prehospital Stroke Screen*
- Alert hospital to possible stroke patient
- Rapid transport to hospital

Immediate general assessment: <10 min from arrival
- Assess ABCs, vital signs
- Provide **oxygen** by nasal cannula
- Obtain IV access; obtain blood samples (CBC, electrolytes, coagulation studies)
- Check blood glucose; treat if indicated
- Obtain 12-lead ECG; check for arrhythmias
- Perform general neurologic screening assessment
- Alert Stroke Team: neurologist, radiologist, CT technician

Immediate neurologic assessment: <25 min from arrival
- Review patient history
- Establish onset (<3 hr required for fibrinolytics)
- Perform physical examination
- Perform neurologic examination:
  - √ Determine level of consciousness *(Glasgow Coma Scale)*
  - √ Determine level of stroke severity *(NIH Stroke Scale or Hunt and Hess Scale)*
- Order urgent noncontrast CT scan (door-to-CT scan performed: goal <25 min from arrival)
- Read CT scan (door-to-CT read: goal <45 min from arrival)
- Perform lateral cervical spine x-ray (if patient comatose/history of trauma)

Does CT scan show intracerebral or subarachnoid hemorrhage?

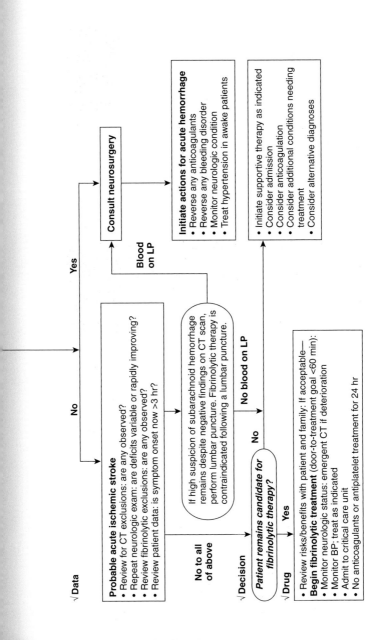

√ Data

Probable acute ischemic stroke
- Review for CT exclusions: are any observed?
- Repeat neurologic exam: are deficits variable or rapidly improving?
- Review fibrinolytic exclusions: are any observed?
- Review patient data: is symptom onset now >3 hr?

No   Yes

Consult neurosurgery

If high suspicion of subarachnoid hemorrhage remains despite negative findings on CT scan, perform lumbar puncture. Fibrinolytic therapy is contraindicated following a lumbar puncture.

Blood on LP

Initiate actions for acute hemorrhage
- Reverse any anticoagulants
- Reverse any bleeding disorder
- Monitor neurologic condition
- Treat hypertension in awake patients

No to all of above

No blood on LP

√ Decision

Patient remains candidate for fibrinolytic therapy?

No   Yes

- Initiate supportive therapy as indicated
- Consider admission
- Consider anticoagulation
- Consider additional conditions needing treatment
- Consider alternative diagnoses

√ Drug

- Review risks/benefits with patient and family: If acceptable—
Begin fibrinolytic treatment (door-to-treatment goal <60 min):
- Monitor neurologic status: emergent CT if deterioration
- Monitor BP; treat as indicated
- Admit to critical care unit
- No anticoagulants or antiplatelet treatment for 24 hr

Tetanus Immunization Guidelines

Tetanus Prophylaxis in Conjunction With Wound Care for Person 7 Years of Age or Older

History of Tetanus Immunization	Clean, Minor Wounds		All Other Wounds	
	Td indicated?	TIG indicated?	Td indicated?	TIG indicated?
Unknown or <3 doses	Yes	No	Yes	Yes
3 or more doses	No*	No	No†	No

* Yes, Td indicated if last dose was received more than 10 years ago.
† Yes, Td indicated if last dose was received more than 5 years ago.

Tetanus Prophylaxis in Conjunction With Wound Care for Children 7 Years of Age

History of Tetanus Immunization	Clean, Minor Wounds		All Other Wounds	
	DTP indicated?	TIG indicated?	DTP indicated?	TIG indicated?
Unknown or <3 doses	Yes	No	Yes	Yes
3 or more doses	No*	No	No†	No

* Yes, DTP indicated if routine immunization schedule has lapsed.
† Yes, DTP indicated if routine immunization schedule has lapsed or if last dose was received more than 5 years ago.
Td, tetanus and diphtheria toxoids; DTP, diphtheria and tetanus toxoids and pertussis vaccine.
From Centers for Disease Control: National immunization program recommendations for tetanus immunization, Atlanta, 2003.

REFERENCE GUIDE 24

Revised Trauma Score (RTS): Adult

The revised trauma score is a predictor of severity of injury. Patient parameters are taken in the following categories and added. The lower the score is, the higher the predicted mortality.

Category	Scale	Score
A. Respiratory rate per minute	10-29	4
	>29	3
	6-9	2
	1-5	1
	0	0
B. Systolic blood pressure (auscultated or palpated)	>89	4
	76-89	3
	50-75	2
	1-49	1
	no pulse	0
C. Glasgow Coma Score (Compute the Glasgow score. Use the following scale to find the score for C.)	13-15	4
	9-12	3
	6-8	2
	4-5	1
	3	0

To find the RTS, add the scores of A, B, and C.
Total score will range from 0-12.

Glasgow Coma Score*

Glasgow Coma Scale		
Category	Response	Score
Best eye-opening response	Opens eyes spontaneously	4
	Opens eyes to verbal stimuli	3
	Opens eyes to painful stimulus	2
	No eye opening	1
Best motor response	Follows commands	6
	Localizes to pain/purposeful movement	5
	Withdrawal in response to pain	4
	Abnormal flexion in response to pain	3
	Abnormal extension in response to pain	2
	No response to pain	1
Best verbal response	Oriented and converses	5
	Confused and converses	4
	Inappropriate words	3
	Incomprehensible sounds	2
	No verbal response	1
Possible point total is 3 to 15.	Total	

*See Reference Guide 10 for more detailed explanation of Glasgow Coma Score.

REFERENCE GUIDE 25

Ventilator Alarm Troubleshooting

Alarm	Possible Causes
High pressure	Secretion buildup, kinked airway tubing, bronchospasm, coughing, fighting the ventilator, decreased lung compliance, biting on endotracheal tubing, condensation in the tubing
Low exhaled volume	Disconnection from ventilator, loose ventilator fittings, leaking airway cuff
Low inspiratory pressure	Disconnection from the ventilator, loose connections, low ventilating pressure
High respiratory rate	Anxiety, pain, hypoxia, fever
Apnea alarm	No spontaneous breath within preset time interval

Modified from Stillwell SB: *Mosby's critical care nursing reference,* ed 3, St Louis, 2002, Mosby.

REFERENCE GUIDE 26

Ventilator Modes

Type	Description
Assist-control (A/C)	Patient or ventilator triggered breaths, either volume or pressure controlled.
Continuous positive airway pressure (CPAP)	Positive pressure applied during spontaneous breathing and maintained throughout the entire respiratory, cycle; decreases intrapulmonary shunting.
Continuous mandatory ventilation (CMV)	Ventilator delivers the breaths at a preset rate and volume or pressure.
Intermittent mandatory ventilation (IMV)	Ventilator delivers breaths at a set rate and volume or pressure. Patient is able to breathe spontaneously between machine breaths.
Mandatory minute ventilation (MMV)	Patient breathes spontaneously, but a minimum level of minute ventilation is ensured.
Pressure-controlled/inverse-ratio ventilation (PC/IRV)	Provides inspiratory time greater than expiratory time, thereby improving distribution of ventilation and preventing collapse of stiffer alveolar units (auto-PEEP). Patient is unable to initiate an inspiration.
Positive end-expiratory pressure (PEEP)	Positive pressure applied during machine breathing and maintained at end-expiration; decreases intrapulmonary shunting.
Pressure support ventilation (PSV)	Patient's inspiratory effort is assisted by the ventilator. PSV decreases work of breathing caused by demand flow valve, IMV circuit, and narrow inner diameter of ETT.
Synchronized IMV (SIMV)	Intermittent ventilator breaths synchronized to spontaneous breaths to reduce competition between ventilator and patient. If no inspiratory effort is sensed, the ventilator delivers the breath.

ETT, endotracheal tube.
From Stillwell SB: *Mosby's critical care nursing reference*, ed 3, St Louis, 2002, Mosby.

REFERENCE GUIDE 6a

unit two

Triage

Triage

Brigette Holleran Ganahl

Triage is one of the most important and challenging tasks of the Emergency Department (ED). The definition of triage is the screening of patients according to urgency of condition or complaint. Patients are assigned to an acuity level based on the findings from the history and triage assessment. Using a standardized triage acuity system will expedite treatment according to need. The task of rapidly obtaining adequate data while maintaining vigilance over patients who are being processed through the department is complex.

Efficient and experienced triage nurses will assess, prioritize, categorize, and monitor patients who present to the ED. They must value issues of customer service and professionalism. Facilities vary, but most institutions require one RN to lead the triage effort. Local and state legislation and boards of nursing specify which disciplines can perform triage assessments. Although this is a difficult subject to standardize, there are common elements of triage regardless of where you practice. The four basic elements of triage include:

I. An across-the-room assessment
II. Determination of chief complaint
III. Focused assessment
IV. Assigning an acuity level

In reality, these separate components often are completed simultaneously. Generally, the triage nurse must first assess the basic ABCDs (Airway, Breathing, Circulation, and Disability) and use this objective data in conjunction with the patient's subjective data to assign an acuity level. This process takes no more than 3 to 5 minutes for most patients.

I. ACROSS-THE-ROOM ASSESSMENT

This assessment begins the moment that visual contact is made with the patient. The goal is to determine whether the patient needs immediate interventions. The nurse rapidly evaluates the condition of the patient based on his or her general appearance, work of breathing, and skin color. The nurse uses her senses of vision, hearing, and smell to formulate a nursing opinion about the patient's condition. This opinion usually is formed before the first question is ever asked.

- Do you sense that the patient is ill?
- Are the patient's posture and gait appropriate?
- Do you hear abnormal breathing sounds?
- Are there obvious wounds, deformities, or bleeding?
- What color is the skin?
- Does the patient appear to be in distress?
- How is the patient interacting with the environment?
- Is the patient alert or lethargic?
- Are there any unusual odors?

Triage decision point: Does the patient need emergent interventions (Triage Box 1)? If yes, take the patient to the treatment area.

II. CHIEF COMPLAINT

This is the patient's or caregiver's own words of why the patient is seeking care in the ED. A good way to elicit this information is to ask a question such as, "What's the reason you came to the ED today?" If the condition or complaint is not new or acute, ask what has changed about the problem. Patients often have multiple complaints or describe vague symptoms that do not paint a complete picture. The nurse must sift through the information, redirecting the patient to applicable information.

TRIAGE BOX 1   FINDINGS NEEDING EMERGENT INTERVENTION

Patients with emergent conditions often have a combination of these symptoms:

Work of breathing:	Abnormal sounds
	Grunting
	Wheezing
	Stridor
	Drooling
	Inability to speak
	Ineffective respiratory pattern
Skin color:	Abnormal pallor
	Dusky
	Mottled
	Cyanotic

Patient information often will be obtained from a family member, caregiver, or emergency medical services (EMS) professional. A helpful mnemonic for obtaining information from EMS personnel is MIVT: **m**echanism of injury, **i**njuries found, **v**ital signs, and **t**reatment.

III. FOCUSED ASSESSMENT

Subjective information
Subjective Data Related to the Complaint

After identifying the chief complaint, the triage nurse should request information pertaining to the following:

- Onset of symptoms
- Precipitating events
- Mechanism of injury, if applicable
- Progression of symptoms from original onset to time of triage
- Treatment before arrival and the effect (e.g., splinting, medications, ice, heat)
- Is this problem current, past, or chronic in nature?
- PQRST pain assessment. A systematic way to evaluate the presence of pain:
  - *P (provoke):* What provokes the pain? What makes it better or worse? What are positions of comfort and discomfort?
  - *Q (quality or character):* What type of pain is it (burning, tight, crushing, tearing, pressure)?
  - *R (radiation):* Where does the pain start? Where does it go? Have the patient point with one finger to where the pain is the most uncomfortable.
  - *S (severity):* How severe is the pain on a scale of "0" to "10" ("0" representing no pain and "10" representing the worst pain)? See Reference Guide 16.
  - *T (time):* When did the pain start? How long did it last? At what time did the intensity change?

Subjective Data Related to Patient History and Demographics

- Demographic information: name, date of birth, age, gender
- Allergies to medications
- Weight: actual or stated
- Past medical history (e.g., disease, surgeries, hospitalizations, pregnancies)
- Family history
- Social history
- Last menstrual period
- Immunizations

- Current medication used (include dosages if available; include over-the-counter or herbal remedies if applicable)
- Alcohol and tobacco use
- Abusive relationships

A useful mnemonic for obtaining the history of a child or infant is CIAMPEDS (Triage Box 2)

Objective Data

The nurse collects objective data by examining the area of complaint using inspection, palpation, and auscultation. Proceed from least invasive to most invasive and from the area of chief complaint to other body systems as appropriate. Nursing judgment and experience are required to determine which physical parameters to assess and which to defer, because a complete assessment is not necessary at the triage area.

TRIAGE BOX 2   CIAMPEDS MNEMONIC FOR OBTAINING THE HISTORY OF A CHILD OR INFANT

C *(chief complaint):* Why did you bring the child to the ED?

I *(immunizations):* Are the childhood immunizations up to date?
(Isolation): What is the potential for communicable disease exposure

A *(allergies):* Is he or she allergic to any medications, foods, or latex? Describe the allergic reaction.

M *(medications):* Is the child taking any prescription or over-the-counter medications? What was the last dose and the time it was given?

P *(past medical history):* Are there any significant illnesses, hospitalizations, or injuries?
(parents' perception): What is different that concerns you?
How does he or she look to you?

E *(events surrounding the injury or illness):* What was the child doing when he or she was injured or became ill?

D *(diet):* How is the child eating or nursing? When was the last meal? How much did he or she eat or drink?
(diapers): How many wet diapers have there been in the past 24 hours, and when was the last one?

S *(symptoms associated with the illness or injury):* Are there any other symptoms?

Emergency Nursing Association: *Emergency nursing pediatric course provider manual,* ed 3, 2004, the Association.

Enough information must be obtained to allow the nurse to assign the patient an appropriate acuity level.

Obtain vital signs, including blood pressure, heart rate, respiratory rate, and temperature. The exam includes an evaluation of the airway, breathing, circulation, and disability. This is a more detailed assessment than the "across-the-room assessment."

Airway
- Patency

Red flags
- Inability to speak or difficulty speaking
- Stridor
- Drooling
- Tripod posture/sniffing position
- Obstruction: complete or partial (secretions, emesis, or foreign body)
- Edema: oropharyngeal, facial, neck

Breathing
- Rate and depth of respirations
- Breath sounds
- Chest expansion and symmetry
- Oxygen saturation
- Skin color

Red flags
- Increased work of breathing
- Inadequate chest expansion
- Nasal flaring
- Retractions or use of accessory muscles
- Expiratory grunting
- Wheezing
- Diminshed or unequal breath sounds
- Pursed-lip breathing
- Tachypnea, bradypnea, or periods of apnea
- Asymmetrical chest wall movement
- Tracheal deviation
- Distended neck veins
- Abnormal skin color
- Irregular respiratory pattern

Circulation
- Heart rate
- Quality of pulses (central and peripheral)
- Blood pressure
- Skin color and temperature
- Capillary refill

Red flags
- Abnormal skin color
  - Pallor
  - Mottling
  - Dusky
  - Petechiae
  - Purpura
- Uncontrolled bleeding
- Weak or absent pulses
- Hypotension
- Capillary refill greater than 2 seconds (this information is more useful in infants and children than adults)
- Bradycardia or tachycardia
- Diaphoresis
- Reduced skin turgor

Disability
- Level of consciousness
- AVPU:
  A: Awake
  V: Responds to verbal stimuli
  P: Responds to painful stimuli
  U: Unresponsive
  GCS: see Reference Guides 10 (adult scale) and 16 (pediatric scale)
- Interaction with environment and caregiver
- Pupillary response
- Orientation to person, place, and time (compare with baseline)
- Muscle tone

Red flags
- Altered level of consciousness
- Inability to recognize familiar people
- Unusual irritability
- Decreased or flaccid muscle tone
- Seizure activity or hyperactive muscle tone

IV. MAKING THE TRIAGE DECISION

After the data has been collected, the patient is assigned an acuity level. The most common methods currently practiced are the three-tier and five-tier acuity models.

Three-Tier Triage Model
- **Emergent:** Involves immediate threat to life, vision, or limb.
  - Requires continuous monitoring and reassessment.

- ○ Examples include cardiopulmonary arrest, compromised airway, severe respiratory distress, multisystem trauma, burns, coma, dislocation with neurovascular compromise, uncontrolled bleeding, chemical injury to eye, patient with plan to harm self/others.
- **Urgent:** Will not cause a threat to life, vision, or limb if treatment is delayed for up to 2 hours. Reassessment should occur every 30 to 60 minutes.
  - ○ Examples include abdominal pain, asthma exacerbation, renal calculi, and dyspnea with normal vital signs and oxygen saturation.
- **Non-urgent:** Condition will require evaluation, but time is not a critical factor. These patients should be reassessed every 1 to 2 hours.
  - ○ Examples include sprains, rashes, chronic headaches, STDs, wound checks, suture removal, viral symptoms without fever, respiratory distress, and productive cough.

NURSING ALERT

Patients with the following complaints should never be classified as non-urgent:
- Severe pain of any kind
- Chest or abdominal pain
- Altered mental status
- Inability to walk (acute)

Five-Tier Triage Model

This method is an expansion of the three-tier model. It includes the following levels: critical, emergent, urgent, stable, and minimal. It allows nurses to further categorize patients and provide resources based on the severity of the complaint or condition. The five-tier system adds branches to the levels of emergent and urgent found in the three-tier model. This increases uniformity among triage nurses and helps to validate parameters used to sort patients.

Level 1: Condition is critical: Requires immediate treatment and continuous monitoring and reassessment

- *Examples include:* Cardiopulmonary arrest, multiple trauma, compromised airway, severe respiratory distress, chest pain with symptoms indicative of an MI, hypotension, suicidal thoughts with a lethal plan and the means to carry out the plan, uncontrolled life-threatening hemorrhage, imminent emergency delivery, active seizures, anaphylaxis, and coma.

Level 2: Condition is unstable or emergent: Requires treatment and reassessment within 5 to 15 minutes.

- *Examples include:* Chest pain with symptoms indicative of angina, open fractures, dislocation with neurovascular compromise, dyspnea with retractions, sickle cell crisis, reported sexual assault, maltreatment, eye injury with loss of vision, acute asthma attack, severe pain, suspected CVA, pregnant with active bleeding.

Level 3: Condition is potentially unstable or urgent: requires treatment and reassessment within 30 to 60 minutes.

- *Examples include:* Closed fractures, dislocations without neurovascular compromise, renal calculi, abdominal pain, noncardiac or minor chest pain, severe emotional distress, drug ingestion.

Level 4: Condition is stable: Requires treatment and reassessment every 1 to 2 hours.

- *Examples include:* sore throat, minor burn, vaginal discharge, strains, sprains, earache, rash suggestive of contact dermatitis, minor laceration, upper respiratory infection with fever less than 101° F, urinary tract infection without fever and flank pain, constipation.

Level 5: Condition is routine: Requires treatment and reassessment every 4 hours.

- Wound checks without complications, suture removal, cold symptoms without fever or productive cough, prescription refill.

Documentation

Document all pertinent, appropriate subjective and objective information that supports the triage acuity-level decision. Actions and treatments initiated at triage should be documented as well as details that are pertinent negatives (e.g., denies pain on inspiration). When documenting a triage assessment, use as many of the patient's own words in quotation as possible, in addition to the objective data that has been collected.

Life Span Issues at Triage
Pediatric

Neonates (under 30 days old), infants, and children always should be given special consideration at triage because of their high risk for illness and rapid deterioration. Knowing the appropriate guidelines for vital signs and growth and development issues including weight and height will be important for pediatric triage. (See Reference Guide 19.) Using age-specific guidelines will assist the nurse in tailoring the assessment to get the most information out of both the child and caregiver. Ask the primary caregiver for his or her observations and impressions of the child. This can provide important information about the child's condition.

Variations in anatomy and physiology add another challenging dimension to pediatric triage:

- Infants less than 4 months are obligate nose breathers.
- The diaphragm is the major muscle of breathing.
- Ribs are more horizontal than vertical.
- The chest wall is thin with poorly developed muscles.
- Tidal volume is 10 ml/kg.
- Respiratory rate decreases with age.
- Abdominal distension will result in pressure on the diaphragm and will impede respiratory effort.
- Tachycardia is the best method of compensation for decreasing cardiac output.
- Functional murmurs may be present in infants.
- Hypotension is a late sign of hypovolemia.
- Circulating blood volume is 85 ml/kg in neonates, 80 ml/kg in infants, and 75 ml/kg in children.
- Bradycardia is an ominous sign in children.
- The anterior fontanel closes by 24 months.
- The Babinski reflex usually is present until the child begins to walk.
- Temperature regulation is not fully developed, so infants and children are predisposed to hypothermia.
- Shivering does not occur in infants because of neuromuscular immaturity.

In addition to the general guidelines for triage, the following should be considered for all pediatric patients:

- Temperature should be checked rectally under age 2, oral or axillary temperature for ages 3 and above.
- Blood pressure should be checked for ages 3 and older and in any child triaged as emergent.
- Actual weight in kilograms.
- Oxygen saturation for child with an associated respiratory complaint.
- Treat the parent and child as a unit.
- Offer simple, honest, and creative explanations based on the age and developmental level of the child.
- Protect the modesty and privacy of children.

Geriatric

Patients over the age of 75 need to be considered for placement in a higher acuity level because of their increased risk for rapid deterioration. They are also more likely to have chronic medical conditions that may alter assessment findings.

Always be respectful, and do not rush the older patient through triage. Older adults often dismiss alterations in health as "a normal part of aging." When assessing the geriatric patient, remember the following physiologic changes and considerations:

- Protective airway mechanisms may be diminished
- Decreased lung elasticity and smaller airways
- Limited chest expansion
- Increased risk for upper respiratory infection, influenza, and pneumonia
- Distant heart tones
- Decrease in cardiac reserve
- Heart does not react as quickly or efficiently to increased demands for output
- Decreased gastric motility
- Diminished short-term memory
- Depressed sense of pain
- Decreased resistance to infection
- Decreased bone and muscle mass
- Decreased joint flexibility
- Decreased temperature regulation
- Fragile skin, reduced elasticity
- Decreased urine-concentrating ability

Suspected Abuse

Pediatric and elderly populations are at an increased risk for neglect and physical, emotional, and sexual abuse. Include a high index of suspicion for abuse in cases where repeat injuries occur, unusual or apparent injuries (e.g., cigarette burns) are present, or the injury does not match the description of the event. Bruises at various stages of healing and previous untreated fractures are red flags. Delays in seeking care should be considered suspicious. A keen sense of how the child or adolescent interacts with the caregiver also should give clues to the validity of the presentation. Red flags for neglect include poor hygiene, malnutrition, and unexplained dehydration. Law mandates that a nurse must report any suspicion of abuse or neglect to the appropriate authorities (see Chapter 2).

Cultural Considerations

Cultural practices play a significant role in the perception of health care. Language barriers need to be addressed, and services of an interpreter may be required. Acknowledging cultural diversity should reduce anxiety and promote a therapeutic relationship between provider and patient.

Reassessment

Reassessment of patients in the ED waiting area becomes the responsibility of the triage nurse. The nurse must reassess the patient's condition, including vital signs, based on acuity.
If the nurse identifies a decline in patient condition during reassessment, appropriate interventions should be implemented.

Triage Pitfalls

- Don't forget to maintain confidentiality in the triage or lobby setting.
- Don't lose objectivity with patients who frequent the facility.
- Don't allow a busy ED population to influence your triage decision.
- Don't become distracted by the negative attitudes of demanding patients.

Disaster Triage

A disaster situation can produce multiple patients with injuries ranging from minor to life threatening. Disaster triage is differentiated from standard triage in that patients who have little or no chance of survival are not resuscitated, leaving the rescuer to work more aggressively on patients who may have a better chance of survival.

When a disaster occurs, the routine of the emergency department and hospital may be interrupted. Depending on the scope of the disaster, activation of the disaster plan may be required, as the number of victims who are received may be overwhelming to a facility. The facility also may continue to treat patients with illness or injury unrelated to the disaster.

Most disasters occur outside the hospital environment as a result of natural (e.g., hurricanes, tornadoes, earthquakes) or non-natural mechanisms (e.g., bus, plane, or train crashes; bombs; hazardous material spills). A disaster also may occur inside the hospital as a result of fire or a major malfunction of a system that makes the facility inoperable.

If the disaster is external, patients often have received a triage designation by the prehospital emergency services personnel and are forwarded to the appropriate level facility based on injuries.

The following color designations are used to tag patients in disaster situations:

1. *Red:* Critically injured requiring immediate care
2. *Yellow:* Urgent care is required, but conditions are not as life threatening as those in the red category
3. *Green:* Those with minor injuries that will not result in complications if treatment is delayed for several hours
4. *Black:* Injuries sustained are incompatible with life, or it is impossible to perform basic or advanced life support. This designation is used for those patients who are so critically injured that death is imminent. No efforts to resuscitate are made.

Alternate forms of registration may need to be used to track patients through the hospital system. Most disaster tags have a number associated with them that can be recorded onto a log, and the patient may be tracked with that number until the patient is registered into the system.

Legal Issues
Consent for Treatment
Medical treatment cannot be given without consent. State laws dictate the age of consent and exceptions for special circumstances.

- *Informed consent:* A patient understands and agrees to be treated
- *Implied consent:* In emergent situations, it is understood that the patient would give consent if able, to save life, vision, or limb
- *Emancipated minors:* Consent is valid if the patient is considered capable of understanding the consequences of treatment.
  - Patients under the age of 18 who are married, are pregnant, or have living children
  - Patients under the age of 18 who are self-supporting as documented by court services
  - Patients who are under 18 who have allegedly been sexually assaulted (encourage parental consent)

Confidentiality
Hospitals have a legal and ethical duty to maintain the confidentiality and the privacy of patients. Confidentiality and privacy of the patients must be maintained at triage. Triage should be performed in an area where information cannot be overheard. Information about the patient must not be available for anyone to view other than the individuals who are involved in the patient's care and approved significant others.

EMTALA

The Emergency Medical Treatment and Active Labor Act (1995) is a federal statute that imposes a duty on hospitals and physicians who are reimbursed for Medicare services. It requires that physicians and hospitals evaluate patients seeking care in the ED and include a medical screening exam by a physician or other designated advanced practitioner. This includes a complete triage assessment by the nurse. If transfer to another facility is deemed necessary, stabilization must be provided before transfer to the best of the referring facility's ability. The facility must use available ancillary services to determine whether an emergency medical condition exists. A patient can be transferred for two reasons: (1) the patient requests the transfer or (2) the hospital does not have the capabilities to provide the care needed, and the medical benefits of transfer outweigh the risks of transfer. You must have written consent from the patient, legal guardian, or person with power of attorney. The patient must be transported by a qualified team, and copies of documentation must be sent with the patient.

Leaving Without Being Seen

It is important for the triage nurse to discuss the risks of leaving the department without being evaluated by a physician, physician's assistant, or nurse practitioner. Time, date, reason for leaving, patient's condition, and any other pertinent information should be documented. Remember that most triage systems will lead to frustration for patients that have non-acute conditions and fall in the non-urgent acuity category. (Leaving without being seen is different from leaving against medical advice [AMA]. Leaving AMA occurs when the patient has been seen by the physician.)

Reportable Occurrences

Local and state law mandates the circumstances that should be reported to health departments, law enforcement, and/or social service agencies. Below are some common examples:

- Sexual assault
- Child/elder abuse and/or neglect
- Gunshot/knife wound
- Suicide attempt
- Animal bite
- Domestic violence
- Assault
- Sexually transmitted infection
- Tuberculosis

We have included in Triage Box 3 Pam's Pearls for Triage. These pearls are in memory of Pam Kidd and have come from seasoned triage nurses. This list is not inclusive; we hope to continue to add to it!

TRIAGE BOX 3   PAM'S PEARLS FOR TRIAGE

- Recheck placement of the endotracheal tube any time you move a patient, especially in children.
- Do not assume the accident caused the problem; the problem may have caused the accident.
- If a patient looks sick, he or she probably is, but patients do not have to look acutely ill to be acutely ill.
- Listen and evaluate carefully the patient who tells you he or she is going to die; intuition may be telling the patient something that is not apparent to you.
- If rapid fluid administration is the goal, the fluid will infuse only as fast as allowed by the narrowest portion of the line, catheter, or vein. So do not use tubing with a mini-drip chamber, do not use small-gauge catheters (use 16-gauge or larger), and do not piggy-back the fluid into another line—the connection will be the limiting factor in the speed of fluid flow.
- Administer thiamine before administering glucose in the unconscious person (especially if alcohol abuse is suspected) to prevent Wernicke-Korsakoff syndrome.
- Ask the patient to point to where pain is. A description may not accurately pinpoint the location.
- Rectal bleeding is dark and tarry when the source is in the upper GI tract, and it is bright red if the source is in the lower GI tract.
- Take all suicidal gestures seriously.
- Placenta previa is painless; placental abruption is very painful.
- Never minimize the complaint or ignore the patient who complains of the worst headache of his or her life.
- Overtriage is better than undertriage. When in doubt, consider placing the patient in a higher acuity level.
- Shoulder blade pain (especially left shoulder pain) may be a sign of intraabdominal bleeding.
- Triage guidelines never replace sound nursing judgment.

Continued

TRIAGE BOX 3   PAM'S PEARLS FOR TRIAGE—cont'd

- Trust your intuition.
- Obtain manual blood pressure if the automatic blood pressure is outside normal ranges for the patient.
- Listen to the parent who states that his or her child is just not acting right.
- The quietest child in the room is usually the sickest.
- A regular tampon or sanitary napkin holds approximately 30 ml.
- Honeybees can sting only once; the stinger is left in the skin.
- Jewelry or anything constrictive should be removed as soon as possible from a burn patient because of the rapid onset of edema.
- High fever associated with petechiae can be indicative of meningococcemia.
- Necrotizing fasciitis can spread so rapidly you can see it advance within moments.
- If a patient complains of the room spinning, inquire as to whether the room is spinning **around** the patient, or the patient is spinning around **in** the room. A sense of the room spinning around is usually of vestibular etiology, while the sense of spinning around in the room is of the CNS in etiology.
- Take care with chronic cocaine abusers if a nasogastric tube is ordered; the nasal septum may be damaged and easily perforated.
- The amount of atropine needed to treat organophosphate overdoses can be massive.
- Severe pain between the shoulder blades may be indicative of an acute dissecting aortic aneurysm.

unit three

Patient Conditions

1 chapter

Abdominal Conditions

Billie Jean Walters

INTRODUCTION

Abdominal pain is estimated to account for up to 10% of all ED visits. There are three types of abdominal pain: primary, somatic, and referred.

1. **Primary** or visceral pain
   - Originates in the organ itself
   - Experienced with conditions such as appendicitis, pancreatitis, and bowel obstruction
   - Described as cramping, gaslike
   - Intensifies then decreases
   - Usually periumbilical
2. **Somatic,** or secondary pain
   - Results from irritation of surrounding structures and nerve fibers
   - Experienced with conditions such as peritonitis or gastroenteritis
   - Described as sharp and localized
   - Patients often assume a knee-chest position for comfort
3. **Referred** pain
   - Located distal to the affected organ
   - Results from irritation of the dermatome of the affected organ (such as in the case of cholecystitis and renal colic)

FOCUSED NURSING ASSESSMENT

A focused assessment should briefly reassess the ABCs for changes and necessary interventions. Nursing assessment should focus on ventilation, perfusion, cognition, elimination patterns, and associated signs and symptoms.

1. Oxygenation and ventilation:
   - Assess for respiratory rate, depth, work of breathing, quality of breath sounds, and presence of adventitious breath sounds.
   - Respiratory rate may increase in the presence of pain or be depressed if the patient has received narcotic pain medication.
   - Guarding and splinting may occur secondary to abdominal pain with respiration.
   - Pleural effusion may develop secondary to diaphragmatic inflammation in pancreatitis.[1]
   - Atelectasis may result from abdominal distention and decreased movement of the diaphragm.[1]
   - Acid-base imbalances associated with vomiting, diarrhea, or cirrhosis may result in hypoxemia and/or hypercarbia.[2]

2. Perfusion:
   Heart rate and blood pressure changes:
   - Obtain apical heart rate, peripheral pulses, blood pressure, level of consciousness (LOC), skin color, temperature, and capillary refill. If hypovolemia is suspected, orthostatic vital signs should be performed.
   - Moderate to severe dehydration related to vomiting or diarrhea, or hypovolemia caused by gastrointestinal bleeding results in a weak, thready, rapid pulse and orthostatic changes in blood pressure and pulse.[3]
   - Pancreatitis is manifested by hypotension caused by third spacing. Third spacing occurs when fluid is shifted out of the intravascular compartment and sequestered in a non-functional space, such as the peritoneal space. The fluid becomes trapped in the space and is unavailable for use by the body, thus causing hypotension. Tachycardia occurs in an effort to compensate for the decrease in blood pressure.[1]

3. Cognition changes:
   - Assess LOC for any changes in mentation.
   - Shock, dehydration, and metabolic acidosis can cause a decreased LOC ranging on a continuum from mild headache to coma occurring secondary to hypoperfusion.[3]
   - Patients with fulminant hepatic failure develop encephalopathy secondary to reduced cerebral perfusion pressure associated with decreased mean arterial pressure.[4]

- Increased ammonia levels in fulminant hepatic failure may alter level of consciousness.
4. Skin changes:
   - Assess skin color, temperature, and condition. Assess mucous membranes for color and hydration status.
   - Dehydration can result in reduced skin turgor, pallor, and dry mucous membranes.[3]
   - Jaundice may result from acute cholecystitis, pancreatitis, or hepatic failure.[5]
5. Sexuality:
   - Males and females should be assessed for the presence of sexually transmitted diseases (STIs).
   - Females of childbearing age should be evaluated for the possibility of pregnancy by ascertaining the last menstrual period (LMP), number of pregnancies, births (gravida, para), and use of birth control methods.
6. Elimination:
   - Assess urinary elimination patterns and times of last void and bowel movement.
   - Assess bowel elimination patterns for changes in color, odor, or consistency. (Table 1-1)
   - Assess presence of urinary symptoms, such as frequency, dysuria, or urgency. Assess urine for color, odor, and concentration.
   - If nausea and vomiting are present, assess duration and frequency, as well as whether the patient is able to tolerate any oral liquids.

LIFE SPAN ISSUES

Pediatric

1. Children may have vague signs and symptoms of an abdominal process and are often unable to give a reliable history. A child's pain may be diffuse and may not localize to the expected area.[6] A reliable pediatric pain scale should be used to determine the level of discomfort that the child is experiencing (see Reference Guide 15).
2. Infants and children have a higher percentage of water making up their total body weight, which predisposes them to dehydration with fluid loss through hemorrhage or vomiting and diarrhea.
3. Hypothermia can occur rapidly in pediatric patients, especially when room-temperature fluids are administered intravenously or when the ambient room temperature is cool.

TABLE 1-1

Changes in Stool	Disease Process Involved
Diarrhea	Gastroenteritis
Black, tarry stool	Upper GI bleeding
Bright red, bloody stool	Lower GI bleeding
Clay-colored stool	Biliary obstruction
Fatty, frothy stool	Pancreatitis

Geriatric

1. Geriatric patients may not present with typical signs and symptoms of a disease process because of sensory loss. Their symptoms tend to be vague, and their reported pain level may not correlate with the severity of the illness.[7] Confusion or dementia also may affect the accuracy of the history given by an elderly patient.
2. A decrease in subcutaneous tissue and a decreased metabolic rate predispose the geriatric patient to hypothermia, which can be worsened by administration of room-temperature intravenous fluids.
3. Physiologic changes of the body may affect the geriatric patient's ability to absorb, metabolize, or excrete drugs from the body. The elderly have a lower percentage of body water, which contributes to a higher concentration of drugs, as the body is less able to dilute the drug. Therefore the elderly often need smaller doses of medications to reach therapeutic levels. The function of the liver and kidneys decreases, resulting in medications remaining in the system for a prolonged period of time.

Pregnancy

1. Peristalsis is decreased secondary to hormone levels, which can result in nausea, vomiting, indigestion, or constipation.[7] The risk of aspiration also is increased related to the relaxation of the gastroesophageal sphincter.
2. The gravid uterus displaces abdominal organs, which may cause pain to be more diffuse.[8]
3. Abnormal laboratory studies may not be reliable in the diagnosis and treatment of pregnant women with abdominal pain, as anemia and leukocytosis both are present in pregnancy.[8]

INITIAL INTERVENTIONS

1. Initiate and/or prepare for the following in patients with symptoms of severe fluid volume loss or active bleeding:
   - Oxygen administration
   - IV access with a large-bore catheter
   - IV administration of isotonic solutions
   - Continuous cardiac monitoring
   - Continuous pulse oximetry
   - Urinary catheter
2. Maintain NPO status. Record time and type of last oral intake.
3. Anticipate/prepare for insertion of a nasogastric tube (see Procedure 19).
4. Anticipate/prepare for rehydration via IV therapy or oral fluids in patients with dehydration (see Procedure 29).
5. Anticipate and facilitate diagnostic work-up, including laboratory tests and radiography.
6. Anticipate IV and/or PO replacement of electrolytes.
7. Provide comfort measures (e.g., positioning, access to bathroom, and an emesis basin).
8. Assess and reassess pain and provide medications as ordered.
9. Anticipate the need for administration of antiemetics.
10. Provide frequent assessment of the ABCs and a focused assessment of the abdomen.
11. Monitor lab results and notify the physician of critical values.
12. Provide information to the patient and family about the plan of care.
13. Provide preoperative teaching if the patient is to have a surgical procedure.
14. Provide discharge teaching to the patient and family if the patient is to be discharged from the ED.
15. Nursing care priorities are listed in the table on pp. 110-111.

PRIORITY DIAGNOSTIC TESTS

Laboratory Tests
Serum
Ammonia: Elevated in fulminant hepatic failure and severe hypokalemia.

Amylase and lipase: Elevated in acute pancreatitis and cholecystitis.

Beta HCG: Elevated in pregnancy.

Bilirubin: May be increased in cholecystitis, acute pancreatitis and fulminant hepatic failure.

Blood urea nitrogen (BUN): Blood urea nitrogen (BUN) will be abnormal in moderate to severe dehydration states and with fluid shifts that accompany bowel obstruction, hepatic failure, and pancreatitis.

Complete blood count (CBC) with differential: White blood cell (WBC) count may be elevated in the presence of infection or inflammation. Hemoglobin (Hgb) and hematocrit may be decreased in the presence of hemorrhage or chronic blood loss. Pregnant women may have anemia related to increased plasma volume. Fulminant hepatic failure causes a decreased platelet count.

Electrolytes: Hypokalemia can result from pancreatitis, severe gastroenteritis, and the severe vomiting and diarrhea related to fulminant hepatic failure.

Liver function tests (LFTs): Aspartate aminotransferase (AST), alanine aminotransferase (ALT), alkaline phosphatase (ALP): Elevated in hepatic failure. Liver function tests (LFTs) may be elevated in acute pancreatitis, gallbladder disease, hepatitis, or alcoholism, or related to certain types of medications.

PT/PTT and fibrinogen: May be increased in fulminant hepatic failure or in hemorrhage from esophageal varices.

Type and crossmatch: To ascertain the correct type of blood to infuse in patients who do not respond to fluid resuscitation or have severe anemia secondary to chronic blood losses.

Urine

Urinalysis: Specific gravity is higher in the presence of dehydration and liver disease.

Beta HCG urine: Elevated in pregnancy.

Radiographic Tests

Flat and upright abdominal film: To detect air, dilation, looped bowel, thickening of the bowel wall, and foreign bodies. No preparation required.

Upright chest film: To look for presence of pleural effusions. No preparation required.

Special Diagnostic Studies

Abdominal ultrasound—Gallbladder, Renal, Appendix: To detect free air, fluid levels, dilation, looped bowel, thickening or inflammation of the organ, gallstones, kidney stones, tumors, lesions, and foreign bodies. The patient must be NPO for gallbladder ultrasound.

Abdominal CT scan: To detect free air, fluid levels, dilation, looped bowel, thickening or inflammation of the organ, gallstones, kidney stones, tumors, lesions, and foreign bodies. Oral and/or IV contrast may be ordered.

N U R S I N G   A L E R T

If patients are being discharged from the ED to undergo tests at a later time, discharge instructions should include information regarding the test and the proper preparation for the test.

Clinical Conditions
Acute Pancreatitis

Acute pancreatitis is usually a result of chronic alcohol abuse or gallbladder disease and is often a result of overeating or binge drinking.[9] Pancreatic enzymes are released into the tissue of the pancreas, which causes damage to the cells of the pancreas and pancreatic inflammation.[10] The enzyme release and subsequent tissue destruction is a process called autodigestion.[10] Acute pancreatitis can have multiple complications, including pancreatic abscess, respiratory distress, sepsis, and multisystem organ failure. The mortality rate from acute pancreatitis ranges from 2% to 9%.[9]

Signs and symptoms
- Sudden onset of epigastric pain, which may radiate into the back and left upper quadrant.
- The pain may worsen in the supine position and improve when the patient assumes a fetal or upright position.[9]
- Abdominal distention and tenderness
- Fever
- Diminished bowel sounds

Diagnosis
- History and physical exam
- Elevated amylase, lipase, liver function studies, and WBC count.
- Abdominal ultrasound may be useful, but the pancreas may be obscured by gas.[9]
- CT scan that reveals inflammation or enlargement of the pancreas.[9]

Treatment
Care of the patient with acute pancreatitis focuses on reducing inflammation and pain.[10]

- Provide analgesics as ordered. Opioid analgesics are the preferred method of pain relief. Nonsteroidal antiinflammatory drugs also may be used to assist with pain control.
- Antibiotics may be administered if a bacterial source is suspected or if gut decontamination is required.[12]
- Monitor respiratory function by assessment of respiratory rate, depth, and work of breathing. Pulse oximetry is a useful adjunct to respiratory assessment. Lung sounds also should be assessed for the presence of crackles, which may indicate pleural effusion.[10]
- Administer IV fluids. Pancreatitis creates third spacing with associated loss of intravascular volume.
- Anticipate placement of a nasogastric tube.

Appendicitis
- Most common abdominal reason for surgical intervention.
- Usually occurs when the lumen of the appendix becomes blocked and bacteria enters the appendix.
- Appendicitis also can be caused by a viral infection or adhesions, which result in inflammation of the appendix.

Signs and symptoms
- Dull right-lower-quadrant or periumbilical pain localizing at McBurney's point (midway between the anterior iliac crest and umbilicus) at 2 to 12 hours after onset
- Pain is steady and severe, and increases with movement and at the time of perforation of the appendix
- Rebound tenderness at McBurney's point
- Positive psoas sign (pain with extension and elevation of the right leg)
- Anorexia, nausea, and vomiting
- Slight fever
- Tachycardia

Diagnosis
- Physical examination
- Elevated WBC count
- Helical (spiral) CT scan may be performed and is 98% accurate for identifying cecal-wall thickening present in appendicitis.[11]
- Ultrasound also may show cecal-wall thickening and is 93% to 98% accurate for identification.[11]

NURSING CARE PRIORITIES

Potential/Actual Problem	Causes	Signs and Symptoms	Interventions
1. Impaired oxygenation	• Electrolyte imbalance • Acid-base imbalance • Altered respiratory pattern secondary to pain and/or abdominal distention	• Dyspnea on exertion • Tendency to assume a three-point position (sitting, bending forward, fetal position) • Lethargy • Fatigue • Altered level of consciousness	• Continuously assess patient's respiratory rate and effort. • Monitor oxygen saturation (maintain saturation above 94%). • Administer oxygen as needed. • Replace electrolytes as ordered.
2. Pain	• Cramping • Burning • Vomiting • Diarrhea • Abdominal distention	• Complaints of pain • Crying • Moaning • Irritability • Facial grimacing • Restlessness • Hostility	• Assess/reassess pain using a pain scale. • Administer pain medications as ordered, preferably intravenously. • Monitor vital signs after pain medication. • Insert a nasogastric tube, if ordered, for protracted nausea, vomiting, or ileus.
3. Inadequate fluid volume	• Anorexia • Nausea and/or vomiting • Diarrhea	• Delayed capillary refill • Elevated heart rate • Altered mental status	• Assess/reassess for signs and symptoms of dehydration. • Monitor vital signs.

		Decreased urine output	Measure orthostatic vital signs.
		Dry mucous membranes	Monitor intake and output.
		Furrowed tongue	Assess color and concentration of urine.
		Decreased skin turgor	
		Depressed fontanel in infants	
		Pale or flushed color	
		Flat neck veins	
4. Anxiety	Hospitalization	Inability to relax	Provide a calm quiet environment.
	Invasive procedures	Nervousness	Provide reassurance and comfort.
	Potential for surgery	Increased heart rate	Explain all procedures and answer questions.
		Increased respiratory rate	Involve the family in patient teaching.
		Elevated blood pressure	
5. Knowledge deficit	Disease process	Lack of integration of treatment plan into activities	Assess current knowledge level.
	Medication treatment	Requests information	Initiate ongoing patient and family teaching congruent with knowledge level.
	Procedures		Utilize family to reinforce teaching.
	Diet		Obtain dietary consultation.
	Fluid intake		

Treatment
- Rehydration with IV fluids
- If a history and physical examination indicate suspicion for appendicitis, but it has not been "ruled in," the patient should remain NPO and undergo further observation with serial WBC counts and IV rehydration until further diagnostic procedures and a surgical consult are completed.[12]
- Maintain NPO status.
- Follow-up exam with the primary physician should be scheduled if the patient is to be discharged. The patient should be instructed to return with worsening symptoms.
- If the diagnosis of appendicitis is confirmed, surgical intervention via laparotomy or laparoscopy should be performed. Antibiotics and IV fluids should be given preoperatively to reduce the incidence of infection and to correct electrolyte imbalances.[12]

Bowel Obstruction

Bowel obstruction may result from one of many causes: adhesions, ileus, impaction, diverticulitis, volvulus, incarcerated inguinal hernia, worms, or malignancy. The obstruction may be partial or complete and is most often located in the ileum of the small bowel. A bowel obstruction is a dangerous condition with a high incidence of complications such as infection and perforation with consequent peritonitis.[13]

Signs and symptoms
- Abdominal pain that is localized and colicky.
- Changes in bowel habits. Constipation is seen with a complete obstruction, while a partial obstruction may allow for leakage of small amounts of stool.[13]
- Abdominal distention.
- Bowel sounds will be absent in a complete obstruction and hyperactive above the obstruction.
- Nausea and vomiting (may be fecal-smelling emesis).

Diagnosis
- Abdominal x-ray shows dilated, fluid-filled loops of bowel proximal to the obstruction.
- Serum electrolyte levels are abnormal because of the loss of fluid and electrolytes from accumulated abdominal contents.

Treatment
- IV rehydration
- Electrolyte replacement
- Insertion of a nasogastric tube to suction to help prevent vomiting and pulmonary complications such as aspiration.

- Antibiotics
- Surgical intervention is considered in cases of perforation and ischemic bowel.

Cholecystitis

Cholecystitis is the second-most-common cause of abdominal pain. Pain is produced primarily from obstruction of the cystic duct in the gallbladder because of gallstones or, secondarily, from staphylococcal or streptococcal infection. The incidence of cholecystitis is increased for women greater than 40 years of age and for all patients over 70 years of age.

Signs and symptoms
- Right-upper-quadrant pain
- Fever
- Nausea and vomiting

Diagnosis
- The classic presentation of right-upper-quadrant pain, fever, nausea, and vomiting create a high index of suspicion for cholecystitis.
- Ultrasound also may be utilized and may reveal a thickening of the wall of the gallbladder or the presence of gallstones.[14]
- Laboratory tests should include:
  - CBC
  - Electrolytes
  - Bilirubin

Treatment
- Keep the patient NPO and provide IV rehydration.
- Anticipate insertion of a nasogastric tube.
- Provide pain medication with opioid analgesics as ordered.
- Cholecystectomy via either laparoscopic or open procedure.

Crohn's Disease

Crohn's disease is a chronic, inflammatory process of the bowel that produces a thickened, incompressible bowel wall and is characterized by periods of acute exacerbation and remission. The disease occurs most often in Eastern European Jews between the ages of 15 and 30 years and is familial in nature.

Signs and symptoms
- Low-grade fever
- Weight loss
- Fatigue
- Right-lower-quadrant pain or cramping that may be relieved when the patient has a bowel movement
- Diarrhea

- Blood, mucus, or pus in bowel movements
- Anemia may be present secondary to blood loss.

Diagnosis
- Barium enema and/or upper GI series
- Colonoscopy with biopsy

Treatment
- The treatment goal is to reduce inflammation and exacerbation through symptom control and proper nutrition.[15]
- Antidiarrheals, antibiotics, antiinflammatories, and steroids for symptom control.
- Surgical intervention if obstruction or perforation is suspected.[15]

Dehydration

Many patients with abdominal conditions exhibit some degree of dehydration and electrolyte imbalance based on the severity of the illness. The severity of the dehydration is rated as mild (<5%), moderate (6% to 9%), and severe (>10%) based on the severity of the fluid deficit. The geriatric and pediatric patient populations are the most susceptible to dehydration. The percentage of total body water in infants and children ranges from 60% to 75%; thus a small loss of volume can cause dehydration. The percentage of total body water decreases throughout the lifespan. The percentage of total body water in the elderly ranges from 45% to 50%, which places them at in increased risk of dehydration. Weight is an important indicator of dehydration, as an acute weight loss of 1 kg is comparable to a fluid loss of 1 L.[3]

Signs and symptoms
- Dry mucous membranes
- Decreased skin turgor
- Orthostatic hypotension
- Hypotension
- Sunken eyes
- Acute weight loss
- Decreased urine output
- Mental status changes ranging from confusion to lethargy to coma

Diagnosis
ADULT
- Decrease in weight
- BUN/creatinine ratio >20%
- Decrease in urine output <1 ml/kg/hr
- Stool cultures for ova, parasites, *E. coli*

PEDIATRIC
- Decrease in weight
- Decrease in fluid intake
- Decrease in urine output. This can be identified in infants through the number of wet diapers in a 12-hour to 24-hour period. Toddlers through adolescents may be assessed by the report of the number of voids in the same time period.
- Change in mental status
- Stool cultures for ova, parasites, *E. coli*

Treatment
- Identify and correct the underlying cause of dehydration.
- Rehydration with oral or intravenous fluids, depending on the degree of dehydration.
- Instruction regarding diet should be given. Initially, a clear liquid diet is recommended. Clear liquids include: water, gelatin, broth, Pedialyte, and clear soft drinks. Sports drinks such as Gatorade are acceptable for oral rehydration; however, electrolyte solutions such as Pedialyte are preferred. Advance to "BRAT" diet: broth, rice, applesauce, toast/tea.

Esophageal Varices

Esophageal varices are dilated lower esophageal veins that result from portal hypertension. Portal hypertension is most often caused by cirrhotic changes.[16] The rupture and subsequent bleeding of these vessels constitute a life-threatening emergency, as death occurs in approximately 30% of the initial bleeding episodes.[16] Mortality within 1 year of the first episode of hemorrhage ranges from 32% to 80%.[16] The rupture of esophageal varices accounts for 10% of all upper gastrointestinal (UGI) bleeding and occurs more often in men.[16]

Signs and symptoms
- Hematemesis
- Hypotension
- Tachycardia
- Decreased hematocrit

Diagnosis
- Based on patient history
- Decreased platelet count

Treatment
- Hemodynamic support by infusion of isotonic fluids and administration of blood and blood products.
- Administration of vasopressors such as vasopressin to reduce portal pressure.[16]

- Placement of an inflatable balloon tamponade device, such as the Minnesota tube or Sengstaken-Blakemore tube is a temporary measure to stop variceal bleeding. However, bleeding often recurs when the tube is deflated, and therefore the placement of a Minnesota tube should be considered only when definitive care is immediately unavailable.[16]
- Endoscopic sclerotherapy is a definitive approach to acute variceal bleeding and stops bleeding in approximately 90% of patients.[16]
- Surgical intervention should be attempted in the presence of continued bleeding unresponsive to other therapies.

Fulminant Hepatic Failure

Fulminant hepatic failure is defined as development of jaundice that progresses to coma within 2 weeks or less in individuals who had no prior evidence of liver disease.[17] Most cases of hepatic failure are caused by an acute episode of viral hepatitis, although use of common drugs such as acetaminophen, valproate, methyldopa, tetracycline, and NSAIDs also can cause failure. Massive cellular liver necrosis and disruption of all metabolic functions of the liver occur, producing neurologic, cardio-pulmonary, renal, hematologic, and metabolic deficiencies. The prognosis for survival ranges from 30% to 40%.[17]

Signs and symptoms
- Jaundice
- Edema
- Dehydration
- Bleeding/bruising
- Fever
- Anorexia
- Encephalopathy with symptoms ranging from confusion to coma

Diagnosis
- History and physical exam
- Abnormal liver function and coagulation studies

Treatment
Treatment of fulminant hepatic failure is aimed at supportive therapy. The patient should be admitted to an intensive care unit for strict monitoring of vital signs, intake and output, and laboratory values such as blood glucose, electrolytes, lactic acid, and coagulation studies.[17] Complications of fulminant hepatic failure include gastrointestinal bleeding and infection. Prophylactic use of either H_2 blockers or proton pump inhibitors and antibiotic therapy are recommended. Fresh frozen plasma may be infused if the prothrombin time is greater than 50.[17]

Gastritis and Gastroenteritis
Gastritis occurs when food is ingested too quickly or when noxious agents (e.g., coffee or alcohol) are ingested. Gastroenteritis is classified as a sudden onset of diarrhea that may or may not have associated symptoms such as nausea and vomiting.[18] Causative organisms of gastroenteritis include bacterial, viral, and parasitic agents. Bacterial organisms include *Salmonella, Shigella,* and *Campylobacter.* Viral causes include rotovirus and Norwalk virus. Parasitic causes include *Giardia lamblia* and cryptosporidium. Contact isolation and strict handwashing are employed to help reduce transmission of gastroenteritis.

Signs and symptoms
- Diarrhea with or without nausea and vomiting
- Abdominal cramping
- Colicky abdominal pain, localized to the epigastric area in gastritis

Diagnosis
- History
- Stool culture to determine etiology

Treatment
- Identification of causative organism
- Oral or intravenous rehydration
- Antiemetics

NURSING SURVEILLANCE

1. Monitor the severity of the condition based on changes in ABCs.
2. Monitor the level and type of pain and the response to pain-management strategies.
3. Monitor intake and output and check gastric and rectal secretions for occult or gross bleeding.
4. Monitor the patient for cardiac arrhythmia.
5. Monitor the patient for signs and symptoms of decreased perfusion.
6. Assess for changes in LOC.
7. Monitor urinary output.
   - 1 to 2 ml/kg/hr in children
   - greater than 30 ml/hr in adults

EXPECTED PATIENT OUTCOMES

1. Rehydration and volume replacement to support a mean arterial pressure of 90 to 105 mm Hg.
2. Patient will have adequate pain control.

PATIENT/FAMILY DISCHARGE IMPLICATIONS AND EDUCATION

1. Check orthostatic vital signs before discharge.
   - Pulse rate should be within normal limits.
   - Patient should not become hypotensive with position changes.
2. Instruct the patient and family about dietary restrictions.
3. Instruct the patient and family about advancement of dietary intake.
4. Patient and family education regarding:
   - Signs and symptoms of dehydration
   - Potential for aspiration in pediatric and geriatric patients with recurrent vomiting
5. Instruct the patient and family about the need for follow-up care for the following:
   - Fever over 101° F
   - Vomiting more than six times in 24 hours
   - More than eight diarrhea stools in 24 hours
   - Cultures and sensitivities pending from ED laboratory work
6. Provide teaching regarding medications:
   - Purpose of prescribed medications
   - Common side effects
   - Precautions (e.g., drowsiness with narcotics, do not drive or do tasks requiring alertness)

REFERENCES

1. Cole L: Unraveling the mystery of acute pancreatitis, *Dimens Crit Care Nurs* 21 (3):86-90, 2002.
2. Fall PJ: A stepwise approach to acid-base disorders, *Postgrad Med* 107 (3):251-263, 2000.
3. Suhayda R and Walton J: Preventing and managing dehydration, *Med-Surg Nurs* 11 (6):267-278, 2002.
4. Larsen FS et al: Cerebral perfusion, cardiac output, and arterial pressure in patients with fulminant hepatic failure, *Crit Care Med* 28 (4): 996-1000, 2000.
5. Newberry L, ed: *Sheehy's emergency nursing principles and practice,* ed 5, St Louis, 2002, Elsevier Science.
6. McConnell EA: Appendicitis: what a pain, *Nursing* 31 (8):32hn1-32hn3, 2001.
7. Bickley LS and Szilagyi PG: *Bates' guide to physical examination & history taking,* ed 8, Philadelphia, 2002, Lippincott Williams & Wilkins.
8. Angelini DJ: Update on non-obstetric surgical conditions in pregnancy, *J Midwifery Womens Health* 48 (2):111-118, 2003.
9. Munoz A and Katerndahl DA: Diagnosis and management of acute pancreatitis, *Am Fam Physician* 68 (1):164-174, 2000.
10. Hale AS, Moseley MJ and Warner SC: Treating pancreatitis in the acute care setting, *Dimens Crit Care Nursing* 19 (4):15-21, 2000.

11. Nipper ML and Jacobson LK: Expanded applications of CT, *Postgrad Med* 109 (6):68-76, 2001.
12. Pisarra VH: Recognizing the various presentation of appendicitis, *Dimens Crit Care Nurs* 20(3): 24-27, 2001.
13. McConnell EA: What's behind intestinal obstruction? *Nursing* 31 (10): 58-61, 2001.
14. Lillemoe KD: Surgical treatment of biliary tract infections, *Am Surg* 66 (2):138-144, 2000.
15. Gurenlian JR: Crohn's disease, *Access* 17 (3):30-32, 2003.
16. Sharara AI and Rockey DC: Gastroesophageal variceal hemorrhage, *N Engl J Med* 345 (9):669-679, 2001.
17. Van Thiel DH, Brems J, Nadir A et al: Liver transplantation for fulminant hepatic failure, *J Gastroenterol* 36:1-4, 2000.
18. Jones S: A clinical pathway for pediatric gastroenteritis, *Gastroenterology Nursing* 26 (1):7-17, 2002.

2 chapter

Abuse

Patty Ann Sturt

CLINICAL CONDITIONS
BATTERED WOMEN
CHILD MALTREATMENT
ELDER ABUSE
SEXUAL ABUSE

INTRODUCTION

Abuse occurs among people of all ages, races, religions, socioeconomic and educational levels, and religious backgrounds. The individuals most vulnerable to abuse are children, women, and the elderly; however, abuse also can occur to men.

The emergency department (ED) nurse may be the first health care professional to interact with the patient. Individuals reporting rape, sexual assault, or abuse should not be questioned at triage. This may increase any guilt or embarrassment the person may be experiencing. If no life-threatening injuries are present, escort the patient immediately to a private treatment area to obtain the triage assessment data.

FOCUSED NURSING ASSESSMENT

Nursing assessment for all individuals of suspected abuse should focus on oxygenation and ventilation, perfusion, cognition, tissue integrity, sexuality, and safety and security.

Oxygenation and Ventilation

- Stridor and respiratory distress may be present in cases where the victim was strangled by hands or by rope or other objects. Patients with a reduced level of consciousness, such as infants with shaken impact syndrome (shaken baby syndrome), are at increased risk for airway compromise.
- Absent or decreased breath sounds may occur with inflicted blunt or penetrating injuries to the chest. Suspect rib fractures

if there is crepitus and respiratory distress. Suspect a pneumothorax or hemothorax if the patient complains of shortness of breath and you note unilateral decreased breath sounds. Breath sounds may be decreased if the patient is hypoventilating secondary to increased intracranial pressure (ICP) from a brain injury.

Perfusion
- Assess skin color, temperature, and pulses. Pale, cool skin may indicate hemorrhage from inflicted blunt or penetrating abdominal trauma involving the spleen or liver. Delayed capillary refill is a reliable indicator of decreased perfusion associated with hypovolemia or hemorrhage in infants and children. A weak or absent pulse distal to an injured extremity is indicative of impingement on vascular structures.
- Monitor the heart rate and blood pressure. Tachycardia and hypotension may indicate hypovolemia.

Cognition
- Perform a neurologic assessment. An altered level of consciousness may be seen in brain injuries caused by abuse. Some examples would include infants exhibiting shaken impact syndrome, children repeatedly hit across the head, and women who are forcibly thrown against an object and strike their heads.
- Obtain a Glasgow Coma Scale score (see Reference Guide 10 for adult scale and 16 for pediatric and infant scale) and assess pupil size and reaction.

Tissue Integrity
Ecchymosis, lacerations, abrasions, burns, or open wounds may be present in a patient who has experienced physical abuse.

Sexuality
Sexual abuse can occur in both sexes and at any age. Assess the patient for any trauma to, or discharge or drainage from, the genitals or rectum. Determine the last menstrual period. Ask the patient about the use of birth control and the possibility of pregnancy (see Sexual Assault Evidence Collection Procedure 31).

NURSING ALERT

Any patient with suspected sexual abuse should be interviewed and examined in a private area.

Safety and Security

Emergency department nurses should be aware of the factors that increase the risk of abuse.

- Assess the potential for suicide. Battered women may attempt suicide (see Chapter 3).
- Assess the potential for homicide. Battering is considered the most important precipitant for women killed by men and for men killed by women. Determine whether the partner has threatened to kill the patient. Risk factors for homicide include sexual abuse, guns in the home, the partner being addicted to drugs or intoxicated daily, the woman making plans to leave, and either partner having threatened or attempted suicide.

LIFE SPAN ISSUES

See Table 2-1 for the risk factors associated with pediatric abuse, abuse to women, and elder abuse.

Pediatric Issues

- In 2000, 3 million cases of child abuse or neglect were reported to local child protection agencies in the United States.[1]
- Between 3 million and 10 million children witness domestic violence in their lifetimes. The risk of child abuse increases if the mother is being battered.[1]
- Fractures are rare with infants less than 1 year of age and suggest abuse.

Abuse to Women

- Violence occurs even after a relationship has ended. Approximately one fifth of both fatal and nonfatal incidents involve relationships that have been terminated or estranged.[2]

Geriatric

- Studies indicate that 2% to 5% of people over the age of 65 have been abused.[3]

INITIAL INTERVENTIONS

The partner accompanying the patient may insist on staying with the patient during the visit to the emergency department and may answer any questions for the patient. The partner should remain in the lobby during the patient interview. Regardless of the victim's age or the type of suspected abuse, the following interventions must be considered:

- Place the patient in a room that is far from an exit. If the patient or family thinks you suspect abuse, they may leave if left unattended.

TABLE 2-1   Risk Factors for Child Abuse, Abuse to Women, and Elder Abuse

Risk factors for child abuse

Child Risk Factors	Parental Risk Factors
• Physical disability • Mental or psychosocial deficits • Parent's perception of the child as difficult or different • Premature birth • Product of a multiple birth • Chronic illness • Developmental delays • Infants with fussy temperaments	• Childhood history of abuse • Drug or alcohol dependency • Unmet emotional needs • Single parent • Social isolation • Low self-esteem • Inadequate social supports • Unemployment or poverty • Unrealistic expectations of child • Adolescent parent

Risk factors for abuse to women

Battered Mate	Batterer (Abusive Partner)
• Engages in excessive minimization and denial • High economic and emotional dependency on the abusive mate • Family history of abuse • Constantly seeks approval from abusive partner • Poor self-image	• Dependency on alcohol and/or drugs • Demonstrates cruelty to animals (e.g., savagely beats a dog or other pet) • Comes from a violent home environment • Poor self-image • Exhibits excessive jealousy • Rigid expectations of partner • Lack of ability to differentiate feelings—emotions such as fear are expressed as anger

Risk factors for elder abuse

Elder Victim	Elder Abuser
• Female >70 years of age • Physical or mental impairment • Tendency to internalize blame • Social isolation and belief that he or she causes the assaults • Demonstrates passivity and compliance	• Family history of abuse • Financial stressors • Displaces anger onto the elder

- Perform a primary assessment to identify all life-threatening injuries (see Chapter 21).
- Implement measures to maintain a patent airway. Always consider the possibility of a spine injury in patients with inflicted trauma to the head and upper torso.
- If the patient exhibits signs and symptoms of hypovolemic shock, initiate 100% oxygen per nonrebreather mask and two large-bore IVs of Ringer's lactate or normal saline.
- Perform a secondary survey (see Chapter 21) to identify all injuries.
- Splint and immobilize all extremities as indicated.
- Implement measures to prevent and control increased ICP for patients with a brain injury sustained from physical abuse (see Chapter 15).
- Maintain confidentiality and privacy for any patient with injuries from suspected abuse.
- Use words appropriate to the developmental level of the patient. For example, a 4-year-old will not understand the word "urine" but may understand "pee."
- Treat the abused individual with respect and empathy. Many abused individuals experience embarrassment, guilt, and shame.
- Determine the tetanus and diphtheria immunization status of any patient with impaired skin integrity as a result of suspected abuse.
- Nursing care priorities are listed in the table on pp. 126-127.

PRIORITY DIAGNOSTIC TESTS
Laboratory Tests
Coagulation Profile
- To determine whether any multiple unexplained bruises are from a bleeding disorder.
Complete Blood Count (CBC)
- To assess hemoglobin and hematocrit of patients when symptoms of hemorrhage (hypovolemic shock) are present.
- To assess the white blood cell (WBC) count in children/elderly to determine whether weight loss is related to an infectious process or malnutrition. Malnutrition increases the individual's susceptibility to an infection.
Electrolytes and Glucose
- Hypokalemia and hypoglycemia, as well as other electrolyte abnormalities, may be present in malnourished children and elderly persons.

Type and Cross-Match
- Obtain when symptoms of hypovolemic shock are present.

Radiographic Tests
Radiographs
- A complete skeletal survey is usually indicated for infants less than 2 years of age who have evidence of abuse or for infants less than 1 year of age who show evidence of significant neglect. In the absence of major identifiable trauma or intrinsic bone disease, unexplained fractures of the ribs, sternum, skull, humerus, and femur may indicate abuse. Other skeletal radiologic findings suggestive of abuse include multiple and often symmetric fractures of the limbs, multiple fractures at different stages of healing, or a spiral femur fracture in a nonambulatory child.
- With the elderly, unexplained fractures of the skull, nose, or facial bones, multiple fractures in various stages of healing, or spinal fractures are suggestive of abuse.

Computed Tomography (CT) Scan
- *Children:* may reveal skull fractures. Bilateral skull fractures or skull fractures in an infant are suggestive of abuse. Cerebral edema may occur in cases involving shaken impact syndrome.
- *Adults:* may reveal skull fractures, contusions, or intracranial bleeds from inflicted head trauma.

Sexual Abuse or Assault (Laboratory)
- Perform a Venereal Disease Research Laboratory (VDRL) test or a rapid plasma regain (RPR) test to detect syphilis.
- Perform a serum or urine pregnancy test.
- Obtain gonococcal and Chlamydia cultures of the oropharynx, rectum, or vagina, depending on the history. Obtain all three cultures in young children.
- Obtain vaginal swabs to test for spermatozoa and seminal plasma contents.
- Obtain saliva swabs to test for ABO-antigen typing. The swabs determine whether the patient secretes properties of his or her blood type in body fluids.
- HIV antibody testing of adult abuse victims in the ED is controversial, because most EDs do not provide private counseling to individuals. Patients can be referred to health departments or clinics that offer testing and specialize in sexually transmitted infections.

For more information see Procedure 31: Sexual Assault Evidence Collection.

NURSING CARE PRIORITIES

Potential/Actual Problem	Causes	Signs and Symptoms	Interventions
Airway compromise and impaired breathing/oxygenation	• Laryngeal edema from strangulation • Blunt trauma to neck or chest • Penetrating trauma to neck or chest • Decreased level of consciousness	• Stridor • Cough • Decreased breath sounds • Respiratory distress	• See Reference Guide 14, Chapter 21, and procedure 1. • Oxygen by nonrebreather mask. • Prepare for chest tube if pneumothorax or hemothorax suspected. • Anticipate need for intubation if Glasgow Coma Scale score is 8 or less.
Fluid volume deficit	• Blunt or penetrating trauma to torso • Severe malnutrition • Fluid loss from burn injury • Pelvis, femur, or multiple fractures	• Tachycardia • Hypotension • Delayed capillary refill (infants and children) • Pale, cool skin • Obvious external hemorrhage	• See Reference Guide 8, Chapter 4, and Chapter 21. • Initiate two large-bore IVs with Ringer's lactate or normal saline. • Obtain type and crossmatch for blood. • Administer blood products as ordered. • Prepare patient for surgery.
Risk for future injury	• Abusive environment	• Fear • Concern for safety of children and self	• See Chapter 3. • Report suspected abuse to appropriate authorities.

- Frequent visits to an ED for injuries
- Depression
- Suicidal ideation

- Develop a safety plan (see discharge implications).
- Provide information on spouse abuse centers.
- Initiate a social services consult.
- Give parents information on support services for children with physical, developmental, or mental disabilities.
- Provide information on community agencies that assist with child care or elder care.
- Discuss removing or disabling guns at home.

Rape trauma syndrome or posttraumatic stress disorder

Sexual assault

- Powerlessness
- Fear
- Severe anxiety
- Somatic complaints
- Inability to perform daily activities

- Contact rape crisis center.
- Facilitate referral for counseling.
- Develop trusting relationship with patient.
- Explain all procedures and plan of care.
- Provide active listening.

CLINICAL CONDITIONS

Battered Women

Battering includes physical or emotional abuse by a husband or significant other. Some characteristics often associated with battered victims include the following:

1. Denial of battering because of fear or shame
2. Self-blame for what has happened
3. Feelings of confusion, depression, and low self-esteem
4. Reluctance to take action because of emotional and financial dependence on batterer or lack of emotional and financial resources
5. Reluctance to take action because of fear of retaliation by the abuser
6. A tendency to rationalize the incident because the batterer was intoxicated

The batterer often will accompany and stay with the victim to prevent her from reporting the abuse. Ask the accompanying spouse, mate, or friend to wait in the lobby. Interview the woman in a place that affords privacy. Some women will admit that a boyfriend or spouse beat them, while others will not. Questioning should be conducted in a supportive, nonjudgmental, and nonassuming manner. The following questions may be helpful in eliciting a history:

- "It seems that the injuries you have could have been caused by someone hurting or abusing you. Did someone hurt you?"
- "Sometimes when people come to the ED with physical symptoms like yours, we find that they are having some sort of trouble at home. I am concerned that someone is hurting you. Is this happening to you?"

See Box 2-1, Injuries Commonly Seen in Battered Women.

Symptoms

Symptoms will be based on the injuries.

Diagnosis

Diagnosis is based on an examination and on a history obtained from the patient.

Treatment

- Perform a primary survey to identify and treat life-threatening injuries.
- Perform a secondary survey to identify any other injuries.
- Assess the potential for suicide and homicide (see Chapter 3).
- Battered women may stay in an abusive relationship for many reasons. Notify the appropriate adult protection agency according to your hospital policy and state laws.

BOX 2-1   INJURIES COMMONLY SEEN IN BATTERED WOMEN

Skin integrity
- Burns resulting from:
  - Splashes
  - Friction (being dragged on the ground)
  - Chemicals
  - Cigarettes or cigars
- Knife wounds
- Scalp, facial lacerations
- Oral mucosa lacerations

Musculoskeletal system
- Facial or nose contusions or fractures
- Skull fractures
- Patterned bruises
- Torso injuries
- Breast contusions
- Fractured ribs
- Abdominal contusions (especially during pregnancy)
- Back or spine injuries

Neurologic impairment
- Altered consciousness from strangulation attempts
- Intracranial hemorrhage
- Postconcussion symptoms
- Visual impairment resulting from corneal abrasion or retinal detachment

Obstetric complications
- Miscarriage
- Abruptio placentae
- Premature uterine contractions
- Intrauterine fetal demise
- Low-birth-weight infant

- Document all injuries. Photographs and body maps are helpful in delineating the locations and sizes of the injuries.
- Instruct and assist the woman in developing an emergency safety plan if she needs to leave the home immediately.

- Provide the woman with the phone number of resources such as the closest women's shelter and a crisis line.

Child Maltreatment

Child maltreatment can entail one or more of the following:

1. **Physical abuse:** Any intentionally inflicted injury to a child by a caregiver
2. **Sexual abuse:** Any sexual activity or contact between a child and adult (or older child), whether by physical force, persuasion, or coercion
3. **Emotional abuse:** Adult behaviors that are degrading, terrorizing, belittling, isolating, and threatening, or exposure to spouse abuse
4. **Neglect:** Usually involves acts of omission or failure to meet basic needs of child; basic needs include food, clothing, medical care, and safe environment

Physical abuse in children

INJURIES TO SKIN AND SUBCUTANEOUS TISSUES

Injuries to the skin and subcutaneous tissue often are seen in abused children. Children who fall and injure themselves and are not abused usually have bruises over bony prominences such as the chin, forehead, elbow, knee, and shin.

SYMPTOMS

Bruises

Often bruises will represent the configuration of the object used to cause the harm, such as the outline of fingers, belt straps, or buckles, or circumferential bruises around the ankles or wrists from cords or rope (Figures 2-1 to 2-3).

Stages and colors of bruising include purple for 1 to 5 days; green in 5 to 7 days; yellow in 7 to 10 days; and brown in >10 days. Multiple bruises in various stages of healing are suggestive of abuse. Document the size, location, and color of the bruise. Do not document the suspected age of the bruise.

DIAGNOSIS

- Diagnosis is based on an examination and history that are not consistent with the injuries.

TREATMENT

- Apply ice packs and elevate the injured extremity. Monitor the amount of swelling.
- Immobilize/splint the area.

Burns

Death rates from abuse-related burns are high, and children with inflicted burns are likely to be injured again.

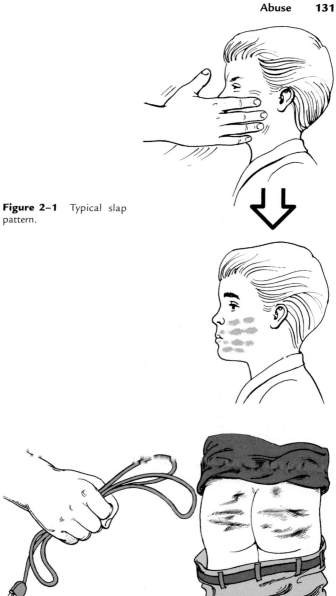

Figure 2–1   Typical slap pattern.

Figure 2–2   Loop or cord marks on buttocks.

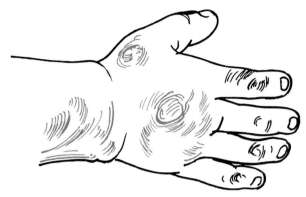

Figure 2–3   Blistering and edema in acute binding injury.

SYMPTOMS
Splash burns
Splash injuries occur when hot water, liquid, or food is thrown or poured on the victim. The burns will not be uniform in depth and will involve different body areas. The top of the head and the anterior face, chest, and abdomen are most likely to be involved if a child pulls a pot of hot liquid on himself or herself.
Immersion burns
In immersion injuries the burn depth is uniform and wound boundaries are distinct. Inflicted immersion injuries from dipping or dunking generally involve the perineum, buttocks, external genitalia, or the hands (Figure 2-4).
Cigarette burns
Circular burns to the soles of the feet and palms of the hands may be seen when cigarettes are intentionally placed on those areas.
DIAGNOSIS
• Diagnosis is based on an examination and history.
TREATMENT
See Chapter 4.
Head injuries
Brain injuries are the leading cause of death among children who are physically abused. Subdural and subarachnoid hemorrhages are common abuse-related intracranial injuries.

There may be serious intracranial injury without evidence of external injury.

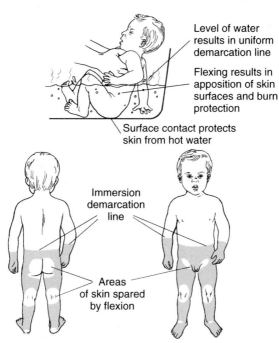

Level of water
results in uniform
demarcation line

Flexing results in
apposition of skin
surfaces and burn
protection

Surface contact protects
skin from hot water

Immersion
demarcation
line

Areas
of skin spared
by flexion

Figure 2–4   Typical immersion burn. Uniform degree of injury with interspersed protected areas.

SYMPTOMS
- Scalp bruises, subgaleal hematomas, and bald patches are common signs of abuse involving the head.
- Altered LOC
- Sluggish or dilated, nonreactive pupil(s)
- Abnormal respiratory patterns
- Seizures and other signs of increased ICP
- Bilateral periorbital ecchymosis
- Retinal hemorrhage (seen with shaken impact syndrome)

DIAGNOSIS
- Diagnosis is based on an examination, clinical findings, and history that do not correlate with the injury.

TREATMENT
- Maintain a patent airway and spinal immobilization.
- Monitor the patient for symptoms of increased ICP.

- Provide 100% oxygen.
- Intubate as necessary.
- Initiate nursing interventions to reduce ICP (see Chapter 15).
- Initiate an IV line.
- Prepare the patient for surgery.

Shaken impact syndrome

Shaken impact syndrome is a result of the vigorous shaking of an infant or small child.

SYMPTOMS

- Retinal hemorrhage
- Altered LOC (usually from increased ICP from an epidural or subdural hematoma)[4]
- Full or bulging anterior fontanel
- Seizure activity
- Dilated, nonreactive pupils
- Decerebrate posturing
- Abnormal respiratory rate and pattern
- Bruising of the upper extremities

DIAGNOSIS

- Diagnosis is based on an examination and history.

TREATMENT

- Initiate nursing interventions to reduce ICP
  (see Chapter 15).

Abdominal injuries

Bruises over the abdomen are not common in children. Children with abuse-related abdominal injuries are usually less than 2 years of age. A blow to the middle abdomen can cause a blowout rupture of the stomach or intestines. The liver and spleen may be injured by compression forces against the abdomen caused by a foot or object (see Chapter 21).

SYMPTOMS

- Distended or rigid abdomen
- Abdominal rebound tenderness
- Vomiting
- Abdominal pain
- Symptoms of hypovolemic shock

DIAGNOSIS

- Diagnosis is based on the results of a CT scan, a CBC, abdominal films, and the physical examination.

TREATMENT

- Administer 100% oxygen per nonrebreather mask.
- Start two large-bore IVs of Ringer's lactate or normal saline. For children, a large-bore IV is 22-gauge or larger.

- Obtain type and cross-match and administer blood as ordered.
- Insert a gastric tube and urinary catheter.
- Prepare the patient for surgery.

⤜ NURSING ALERT ⤛

Document all findings thoroughly but in an objective manner. Document patient/caregiver statements as direct quotes using quotation marks. Forensic (color) photographs should be obtained. Many law enforcement agencies have the ability and equipment to obtain forensic photographs of injuries. Body diagrams may be helpful in delineating the location and size of the injuries. This information may be very helpful later in court. Do not alienate the parents or caregivers. Keep them informed of the plan of care. Be nonjudgmental during your communication and interactions with the parents or caregivers. *Remember:* it is the law in every state to report suspected child maltreatment to the appropriate child protection agency. The nurse is a "mandated reporter." Know your departmental and hospital policies and the laws in your state on reporting abuse. Facilitate an emergency protection admission for protective custody to the hospital if the child is determined to be at greater risk if sent home with the caregiver.

Münchausen syndrome by proxy

Münchausen syndrome by proxy is a form of child abuse in which a parent or caregiver (usually the mother) fabricates or induces symptoms of an illness in a child. The caregiver involved is usually described as intelligent, knowledgeable, and genuinely concerned for the child.

SYMPTOMS

- The fabricated illnesses typically include histories of fever, vomiting, diarrhea, seizures, rash, blackouts, apnea, hematemesis, and hematuria.
- The caregiver may actually induce symptoms in the child by suffocation, by administration of drugs or toxic substances, or by placing her own blood in the child's urine, vomitus, or stool specimens.

DIAGNOSIS

- Symptoms are observed only by the caregiver and disappear when the child is separated from the caregiver.

- History of visits to the ED to treat illnesses for which no cause can be determined
- Treatment of the child in numerous medical facilities
- Unusual symptoms that make no clinical sense
- Discrepancies between the history and physical findings

TREATMENT

- The treatment will be based on the child's actual clinical presentation.
- Do not allow the caregiver to have access to any laboratory specimens, because he or she may attempt to alter the specimen.
- Document all physical findings and the history given by the caregiver using direct quotes.

Elder Abuse

Elder abuse can include any of the following:

1. **Physical abuse:** The willful infliction of bodily harm onto a person 60 years of age or older by a spouse, child, family member, or primary caregiver; examples include pushing, kicking, hitting, slapping, punching, rough handling, inappropriate use of physical or chemical restraints, or sexual assault
2. **Psychologic and emotional abuse:** Infliction of mental anguish caused by actions or verbal assaults against the victim's well-being; examples include name-calling, insults, attacks on the victim's self-esteem, treating the victim as a child, threats of violence against the victim, controlling the victim's activities
3. **Neglect:** Passive or active withholding of services necessary to maintain the health and welfare of the victim; includes food, clothing, medications, basic hygiene, and health-related services
4. **Exploitation:** Improper use of the victim or the victim's resources by the caregiver for purpose of financial or material gains

Elder abuse rarely occurs in isolation or as a single incident. It is usually a recurring problem that may increase in frequency and severity over time. It will be necessary to interview the caregiver and the elder patient separately. Provide a private, quiet place for the interview. Listen carefully and convey a nonjudgmental, empathetic attitude. Ask open-ended questions. The following questions may be helpful:

- "We sometimes see people with injuries like yours. Sometimes they are the result of an argument. Has this happened to you?"
- "Can you describe what happens when you and your family member (caregiver) argue or have problems? Do these behaviors include hitting or threats to harm you?"

- "Have there been threats to abandon or confine you, or to withhold medicine or food from you?"
- "Could you describe your routine day to me (activities, bathing, hygiene)?"

The following questions may be helpful in interviewing the caregiver:

- "Caring for someone who is impaired as (the patient) is can be a very difficult task. It must be frustrating at times. How do you handle it?"
- "Is it difficult to obtain the medications your (patient) needs?"
- "Who is available to help you at home? Do you ever get a break to relax?"
- "How do you cope with having to care for (the patient) all the time?"
- "During the interview we noticed bruises on (the patient's) face and arms. Do you know how he (she) got them?"

SYMPTOMS
- Symptoms depend on the injuries.

DIAGNOSIS
- Diagnosis is based on an examination and information obtained from the history.

TREATMENT
- The treatment will depend on the specific injuries.
- Notify a social worker or social agency if possible. The social worker may go into the home to assess the interactions and environment.
- Carefully document information obtained from the interview and any physical findings.
- Provide the caregiver with information regarding community resources and support groups.
- Notify the appropriate adult protective agency.

Sexual abuse in children
Explain to the child during the interview that you are there to listen. Convey interest, sincerity, and respect. Never interview the child in front of the possible abuser. Determine and use the child's own terminology for describing body parts. The following questions may help when interviewing the child:

- "Sometimes kids are asked to keep secrets. These secrets can be scary. You are safe with me. Has this happened to you? Can you tell me about the secret?"
- "Sometimes grownups do things to kids that hurt and are scary. Has someone hurt you?"

Assessment of the genitals and rectum should be done only once, if at all possible, to prevent unnecessary emotional trauma to the child. Thus the nurse and physician should do this together. To examine the genitals, place the child supine in the frogleg position. For anal examination, place the child in the lateral decubitus position. To help the child relax, a trusted family member, social worker, or nurse should be at the head of the examining table to comfort the child. The child should not be restrained for this part of the examination. If the child is very uncooperative, the examination should be stopped and the child sedated if necessary.

SYMPTOMS
- Inflammation or redness of the genitals and/or rectal area
- Drainage, discharge, or bleeding from the genitals and/or rectal area
- Tears, abrasions, or ecchymosis of the genitals and/or rectal area

---

NURSING ALERT

Victims of child abuse often will need to be seen in a pediatric or gynecology clinic that is capable of performing a colposcopy. A colposcope allows an examination of the external genitalia as well as the vagina and cervix. Vascular changes, scars, and variations are best noted with a colposcope. However, this instrument does not eliminate the need for a gross examination in the ED.

DIAGNOSIS
- Diagnosis is based on an examination and history obtained during the interview with the child (and parent).

TREATMENT
- Unless life-threatening bleeding is present, definite treatment may not be needed in the ED.
- Document the child's statements from the interview and any abnormal physical findings.
- It may be necessary to refer the child to a play therapist.
- Follow-up of culture results and treatment will be necessary.
- Report the suspected abuse to the appropriate child protection agency.

EXPECTED PATIENT OUTCOMES

1. Patent airway
2. Bilateral equal breath sounds

3. Heart rate of 60 to 100 beats/min (or age appropriate)
4. Systolic BP of >90 mm Hg (or age appropriate) or at level needed to maintain adequate perfusion (see Reference Guide 19 for vital signs in children)
5. Improvement or no further deterioration in neurologic status
6. Open and effective communication between the patient and nurse
7. Understanding of abuse and neglect as a crime against the patient
8. Understanding and verbalization of community resources and support systems

DISCHARGE IMPLICATIONS
Child Abuse
1. Instruct the parent on alternative coping mechanisms to deal with stress (e.g., leave the room immediately if ready to hit the child, or telephone a friend or relative).
2. Provide the parent with phone numbers of support groups. These may be listed in local telephone books or under city, county, or state information.

Battered Women
If a battered woman decides to return to the home, there are some things she can do to protect herself. Include these with the discharge instructions:
1. Have a room in the house that has a strong lock.
2. Keep a bag or suitcase packed.
3. Hide extra money, car keys, and important documents, such as the marriage license, Social Security card, and family birth certificates, in a safe, secure place so they can be obtained quickly.
4. Teach the children or encourage the neighbors to call the police during an attack.
5. Plan for a place to go in an emergency—a woman's shelter, a social agency, or the home of a trusted friend or relative.
6. When possible, call the police and get names and badge numbers of police officers in case there is need for a record of the attack.
7. Leave the house and take the children if an attack is imminent.
8. Go to a hospital or ask for medical attention when in a safe place. Usually domestic violence shelter programs will provide a staff member to accompany the at-risk individual to the

hospital or ED. Sometimes women are hurt more seriously than they think during a physical assault.

9. Obtain and keep a record of any injuries, including photographs, to have the strongest possible case to press charges.

Even if the woman will not admit to being battered or abused, provide her with written information of spouse abuse centers and shelters in the area (when you suspect battering).

Elder Abuse

1. Community referrals are important with elder abuse. These referrals may include the department of social services, senior citizen centers, community mental health centers, long-term care ombudsmen, agencies on aging, and national committees dealing with elder abuse.

2. Instruct caregivers on alternative methods to cope with stress.

REFERENCES

1. Meyers HP: Evaluation of physical abuse in children, *Adv Nurse Pract* August, 33-36, 2002.
2. Gerard M: Domestic violence, *RN* 63 (12):53-56, 2000.
3. Fulmer T: Elder neglect assessment in the emergency department, *J Emerg Nurs* 26 (5):436-443, 2000.
4. Fountain GK and Pierce B: Child abuse and neglect. In Newberry L, ed: *Sheehy's emergency nursing principles and practice*, ed 5, St Louis 2003, Mosby.

chapter 3

Behavioral Conditions

PSYCHIATRIC CONSIDERATIONS

Jo Anne Mathews

CLINICAL CONDITIONS

Bipolar Disorder
Homicidal Ideation/Violence Toward Others
Movement Disorders
  Extrapyramidal Symptoms (EPS)
  Neuroleptic Malignant Syndrome (NMS)
  Tardive Dyskinesia (TD)
Panic
Paranoid Schizophrenia
Psychoses
Suicidal Ideation/Self-Harm Behaviors

INTRODUCTION

Mental health emergencies result from situations in which a patient is at risk because of intense personal distress, suicidal intentions, or self-neglect, and situations in which a patient places others at risk. Some patients may behave in an aggressive manner, make threats, or act violently. Visits to the emergency department (ED) for psychiatric services peak between the hours of 6 PM and 10 PM. People with mental illness often lack a primary care physician and seek health care only in a crisis.[1]

In difficult circumstances, almost any patient may behave violently and pose a risk to his or her own safety or that of others. The immediate goal in resolving a psychiatric emergency is to reestablish inner and outer controls for the patient in the least coercive way.

FOCUSED NURSING ASSESSMENT

A holistic comprehensive physical assessment must be performed to evaluate for all possible causes of presenting psychiatric symptoms. Many medical illnesses cause or exacerbate psychiatric symptoms.

Assessment includes a mental status examination and often includes a standardized measurement tool. Despite the importance of the task, there are no concrete guidelines that identify the areas of clinical assessment on which the psychiatric emergency service should focus when making disposition decisions.[2]

Oxygenation and Ventilation
- Respiratory rate may be elevated in panic disorder, bipolar disorder, and acute psychosis.

Perfusion
- Tachycardia and elevated BP may be present related to panic attacks, fever, or neuroleptic malignant syndrome (NMS).

Cognition
Assess the neurological status, including cognition; sensation, and mobility.
- Assess for personality and behavior changes by interviewing both patient and family members or caregivers.
- Obtain history of current illness as well as prior history of mental and physical illness.
- Explore the use of alcohol or illicit drugs and patterns of drug usage. Consider using screening tools. The CAGE screening test for alcoholism is composed of four questions to assess for alcoholism. One positive answer warrants further evaluation. The Clinical Institute Withdrawal Assessment for Alcohol (CIWA) is used to assess for alcohol withdrawal.
- Assess all medications, including prescription, over-the-counter, and herbals.
- Investigate history of recent head injuries, falls, and exposures to toxins.

Neurological Status
- Orientation and reality are impaired in dementia and schizophrenia. The Mini Mental Status Examination (MMSE) is a tool that asks a series of 12 simple questions to assess mental functioning.
- Mobility is impaired in extrapyramidal symptoms (EPS) and tardive dyskinesia (TD).

Sexuality
- Changes in medications may affect sexuality.
- A decrease in sexual drive is usually noted in the presence of depression.

TABLE 3-1 Predictors of Admission/Discharge	
Significant Predictors of Admission/Discharge	**Additional Assessment Considerations**
Level of danger to self	Danger to others
Severity of psychosis	Severity of current psychopathology
Ability to care for self	Severity of substance abuse
Severity of lack of impulse control	Degree of social support
Severity of depression	Whether the patient was cooperative

- Hypersexuality or promiscuity may be present in manic episodes of bipolar disorder.

Tissue Integrity
- Self-inflicted injury may be present related to bipolar disorder or borderline personality disorder (BPD).
- Vulnerability to assault or exploitation may occur in patients with schizophrenia or in those with bipolar disorder during manic episodes.

Safety
- Verbalization of suicidal ideation may occur in patients with depression or schizophrenia, or those in a depressed episode related to bipolar disorder.
- Venting of anger
- Expression of anxiety/fears
- Self-neglect in depression or dementia
- Nihilistic delusions (the belief that nothing exists) may occur in patients with schizophrenia.
- Significant predictors of admission and discharge are found in Table 3-1.[1]

LIFE SPAN ISSUES
Pediatric
1. Children and older teenagers presenting with psychiatric emergencies differ in types of illnesses and the need for care. Twice as many older children (age 17-19) suffer from schizophrenia/psychosis.[3]
2. Pediatric patients with psychiatric emergencies have a much higher rate of admission and extended ED stays than pediatric patients with medical conditions.

3. Suicidal ideation, a feeling of being out of control, aggressive behavior, and drug-related antisocial behavior were among the complaints presented most often in the pediatric population.[4]
4. Adolescent Hispanic females have an increased prevalence of suicide attempts and are twice as likely to require medical attention resulting from the suicide attempt.[5]
5. Substance abuse is correlated highly with suicide attempts among adolescents.[5]
6. More than 50% of 13 to 19-year-olds report intermittent suicidal thoughts, and 12% to 15% have come close to attempting suicide. Adolescent females are more likely than males to attempt suicide.[5]
7. In children and adolescents, panic disorder is most often preceded by or occurs as a comorbid condition with separation anxiety disorder.

Geriatric

1. The main risk categories for mental health problems in the elderly are: individuals recently discharged from the hospital, recently widowed, living alone, or living in poverty; and the socially disadvantaged.[6]
2. Most elderly patients presenting with a psychiatric complaint have been symptomatic for more than a month; 51% to 75% of patients have a past psychiatric history; 36% to 57% have previous psychiatric hospitalizations; and 18% to 30% are in current treatment.[6]
3. In contrast to younger patients, the elderly are more likely to be diagnosed with major depression and have medical comorbidity. The elderly are less likely to have a diagnosis of schizophrenia or personality disorder and parasuicidal behavior.[6]
4. The progressive changes that occur in the aging process may have psychological implications (e.g., psychological consequences of deafness include persecutory ideation often resulting from misinterpretation, depression, social deprivation, and loneliness).[6]

INITIAL INTERVENTIONS

1. Initial interventions focus on tuning in to the patient's emotional reactions and feelings, building an alliance or trust, and showing empathy by offering to meet the patient's physical needs.

2. Provide a safe environment by
   - Dressing the patient in a patient gown.
   - Providing for one-on-one patient care.
   - Clearing the room of any potential hazards.
3. Reduce environmental stimuli and consider isolating the patient.
4. Provide comfort measures by offering food, fluids, and warmth.
5. Acknowledge the patient's affect/feelings.[7]
6. Remain calm and professional (don't take comments personally).[7]
7. Maintain a leg-length distance from the patient and allow for a ready exit if the patient becomes violent.
8. Talk with the patient and reassure the patient that the ED is a safe place.
9. Gather/validate history from family or other sources.
10. Evaluate for the presence of any medical etiology.
11. Assess for current substance use.
12. Clarify the purpose of the evaluation process; set common goals.[7]
13. Determine stressors.[7]
14. Nursing care priorities are listed in the table on pp. 146-147.
15. Medicate as ordered (see Box 3-1).[8]

PRIORITY DIAGNOSTIC TESTS

Blood glucose level: Hypoglycemia can result in confusion and combativeness, which can mimic psychosis.

Blood ethanol level: Elevated blood alcohol levels can cause patients to become verbally or physically abusive or lead to alcohol psychosis.

Complete blood count: Antipsychotic medications such as Thorazine and Navane can cause a decrease in the white blood cell count (agranulocytosis).

Creatinine kinase: May be elevated in NMS.

Drug levels: Specific drug levels, such as lithium, can be drawn to assess for therapeutic effect.

Electrolyte levels: Electrolyte imbalances can cause alteration in mental status. Hyponatremia can cause seizures. Patients on lithium are prone to hyponatremia secondary to increased thirst and subsequent water intoxication.

Nursing Care Priorities

Potential/Actual Problem	Causes	Signs and Symptoms	Interventions
1. Violence toward others	• Neurobiologic • Physiologic/general medical conditions • Substance abuse • Psychosocial influences • Adverse drug reaction	• Agitation (shouting, demanding, profanity, threatening violence, pacing, fist-clenching, intensified facial expressions) • History of violence • Paranoia • Hallucinations • Expresses a specific plan • Uncooperative • Nondirectable • Acting out by spitting or other physically threatening gestures • Possession of a weapon	• Provide safe environment. • Search patient and belongings. • Reduce stimulation. • Offer choices when possible. • Maintain safe distance (leg length) and call for security. • Show concern; offer food/drink. • Identify patient's feelings. • Allow verbal expression of anger (venting). • Identify stressors. • "Show of concern/force" • Pharmacologic or physical restraint • Diagnostic tests
2. Violence toward self	• Neurobiologic • Physiologic/general medical conditions • Substance abuse • Psychosocial influences • Adverse drug reaction	• Hopelessness • Impulsivity • History of previous attempt • Specific/lethal plan	Same interventions as for violence toward others

3. Altered thought processes	• Neurobiologic • Physiologic/general medical conditions • Substance use • Psychosocial influences • Adverse drug reaction	• Paranoia • Hallucinations • Confusion • Decreased cognitive ability	• Calm, reassuring approach emphasizing patient's safety. • Provide safe environment. • Listen for "kernel of truth" in statements.
4. Impaired movement	• EPS • TD • NMS	• Uncontrollable, purposeless movements • Related autonomic instability • Anxiety • Impaired cognition	• Obtain a thorough history and assessment. • Describe abnormal movements. • Reassure patient. • Vital signs • Provide for patient safety.
5. Anxiety	• Situational, maturational, or social stressors; separation phobias; or grief • Medical conditions • Substance induced • Psychiatric conditions (OCD, PTSD)	• Transient tachycardia • Elevated systolic BP • Decreased ability to problem solve • Decreased coping ability • Feeling of uneasiness, worry, dread, especially about the future	• Use simple, direct commands; brief statements. • Assess for level of anxiety: mild, moderate, severe, panic. • Reassure patient that he or she is safe. • Medicate prn. • Approach in a calm, non-threatening manner. • Reduce environmental stimuli.

BOX 3-1   OVERVIEW OF ACUTE PSYCHOSIS AND AGITATION WHEN RAPID TRANQUILIZATION IS NEEDED, AND ORAL MEDICATIONS ARE REFUSED

- Benzodiazepine (BZD) (e.g., lorazepam) IM alone
- IM antipsychotic alone (Haldol or ziprasidone)
- Combination of an IM BZD and IM antipsychotic (e.g., lorazepam and haloperidol or ziprasidone)
- Combination of an IM BZD, IM antipsychotic, and IM anticholinergic (e.g., lorazepam, haloperidol, and diphenhydramine)

Folate and B_{12}: Levels of folate and B_{12} may be decreased in chronic alcoholics.

Heavy metal screen: Lead poisoning can cause altered mental status leading to verbal or physical violence.

Pregnancy testing: Should be performed for women of childbearing age.

Thyroid function tests: Hypothyroidism can cause emotional lability and mood changes. Hyperthyroidism can cause emotional lability and psychosis.

Urine toxicology screen: Ingestion of illicit drugs such as marijuana, PCP, LSD, cocaine, and methamphetamine can cause hallucinations, delusions, or other psychotic or violent behaviors.

CLINICAL CONDITIONS

Bipolar Disorder

Bipolar disorder is an illness characterized by episodes of depression and mania. Mania is a symptom of the disorder characterized by a persistently elevated, expansive, or irritable mood. Labile mood swings between euphoria and irritability may occur. The mood swings exhibited by an individual with bipolar disorder are dramatic, and these patients often present to the ED with psychotic symptoms. Patients experiencing psychotic symptoms are incapable of self-care and have an increased risk of violence.

TABLE 3-2   Overview of Presenting Symptoms With Possible Psychiatric and Medical Causation[9]—cont'd

Patient's Symptoms	Possible Psychiatric Causation	Possible Medical Causation
Restlessness	Anxiety disorder	Alcohol or drug withdrawal
Irritability		Hyperinsulinism
Panic attacks		Hyperthyroidism
Decreased concentration		Coronary insufficiency
Increased or decreased sleeping	Depression	Cancer
Increased or decreased appetite		Hypothyroidism
Disinterest in activities		Hypoinsulinism
Suicidal ideation		Sleep apnea
		Liver failure
		Parkinson's disease
		Sepsis
Increased energy	Mania	Hyperthyroidism
Emotional lability		Multiple sclerosis
Hypersexuality		Brain tumor
Decreased sleeping		Reaction to steroids
Paranoid responses	Psychotic disorder	Medication induced
Delusional ideas		Toxin induced
Hallucinations		Hypothyroidism
Isolating behavior		Head trauma
Confusion	Substance abuse	Malnutrition
Unsteady gait		Liver failure
Slurred speech		Alcohol or drug withdrawal
Changes in personality		Hyperinsulinism
Loss of memory	Dementia	Cerebral vascular accident
Changes in behavior		Organic brain syndrome
Impaired intellect		Subdural hematoma
Confusion		Medication induced
Perceptual disturbances	Delirium	Head trauma
Agitation		Cancer
Intermittent confusion		Sepsis
Changes in consciousness		Hypoxia
		Sleep deprivation

Signs and Symptoms

Signs and symptoms during a manic episode include:

- Verbal expressions of increased self-esteem or grandiosity. Grandiose delusions are common and may include a special relationship to God or a famous person or ability.
- Decreased need for sleep
- Speech is pressured, loud, rapid, and difficult to interrupt. Joking, punning, amusing irrelevancies, theatrical dramatic mannerisms and singing or clanging (words that sound the same strung together with no meaning) may occur. Conversation may include loud complaints, hostile comments, and angry tirades.
- Flight of ideas may be evident, with racing thoughts and abrupt topic changes.
- Increased distractibility and psychomotor agitation.
- There may be a history of hypersexuality, reckless driving, or buying sprees.
- The threat of violence may be explicit in verbalizations or expressed intent. In other instances the risk can only be inferred from the patient's agitation and dysphoric (anxious or depressed) mood state combined with paranoid delusional thinking. When these features are combined with rapid mood cycling, the risk of violence may be high.[10]
- Hallucinations and delusions
  Signs and symptoms during a depressive episode include:
- Feelings of intense sadness or hopelessness
- Loss of interest in activities
- Decreased energy
- Restlessness
- Change in sleep pattern
- Change in appetite
- Suicidal ideation

Diagnosis

In the ED, diagnosis will focus on recognition of the presenting symptoms as well as history and physical exam.

Treatment

- Provide a calm, safe environment.
- Reduce external stimulation by providing a quiet room.
- Isolate the patient from others to promote safety of the patient and others.
- Medications such as benzodiazepines may be given in conjunction with a typical or atypical antipsychotic.

- Mood stabilizers like lithium are prescribed for long-term maintenance therapy.
- Impaired judgment and psychotic symptoms that can occur with this illness may require family support for treatment decisions. Involuntary hospitalization may be necessary.
- Rule out effects of substance use, medications, toxin exposure, general medical conditions, brain tumor, Cushing's syndrome, and multiple sclerosis. Assess for antidepressant use, light therapy, or recent electroconvulsive therapy (ECT).

Homicidal Ideation/Violence/Violent Behavior

Nurses may be subjected to verbal or physical assault. Assaults are perpetrated most often by patients with some form of cognitive dysfunction or patients with substance abuse issues. Family members and visitors often become angry because of the enforcement of hospital policies or because of the patient's condition or situation. Anger also can result from long wait times and can be directed toward the health-care system in general (46.5%).[11] Substance use disorders are associated with greater-than-average risk for violence. There is also a high risk of violence in bipolar disorder if agitation, dysphoria (unpleasant mental state), and paranoid delusions are combined with rapid mood cycling.

Signs and Symptoms

- Anxiety
- Irritability
- Increased aggressiveness
- Impaired impulse control
- Impaired reality testing may be due to substance use of alcohol, hallucinogens, PCP, or cocaine, or withdrawal from alcohol, opioids, or hypnotic sedatives. A person abusing marijuana or hallucinogens may commit violence related to increased anxiety, paranoia, and false perception of reality.

Diagnosis

Diagnosis in the ED is focused on the presentation of the patient.

Treatment

Interventions focus on patient and staff safety.

- Increase staff availability; call security; consider show of "concern" (force).
- Maintain constant/close monitoring.

- Remove any objects from the immediate environment that may be used as weapons.
- Differentiate between patient venting as release and coping mechanism versus real threats, which are specific and very directed.
- Consider restraint/seclusion.
- Medicate with benzodiazepines.

Motor Disorders
Extrapyramidal Symptoms (EPS)

Acute EPS occur in the first days or weeks of taking an antipsychotic medication[10] (60% of patients on antipsychotic medications develop clinically significant EPS).[10] EPS are usually dose-dependent and reversible.[10]

Signs and Symptoms

EPS are often characterized by:

- *Parkinsonism:* Muscle rigidity, shaking, tremors, gait disturbance, muscle aches.
- *Dystonia:* Side effect of antipsychotic medications resulting in muscle spasms of the face, tongue, neck, or occasionally the entire body.
- *Akathisia:* Motor restlessness characterized by fidgety movements like swinging of legs, rocking from foot to foot while standing, pacing to relieve restlessness, or inability to sit or stand still for several minutes. May be confused with psychomotor agitation of psychosis.[10]

Treatment

- *Parkinsonism:* Treat with anticholinergic and consider discontinuing the medication.
- *Dystonia:* Treat with antihistamine; most dangerous effect is laryngospasm; rule out head trauma, viral encephalitis, stroke, brain tumor, wasp stings, toxic levels of manganese or carbon disulfide. May treat with anticholinergic drugs such as Cogentin.
- *Akathisia:* Treat with benzodiazepines or beta blockers such as propranolol and slow reduction of antipsychotic medications.

Neuroleptic Malignant Syndrome (NMS)

NMS is a sudden, unpredictable condition occurring early in the course of antipsychotic treatment. The rate of occurrence is approximately 1% to 2% in persons taking antipsychotic medications and can be life-threatening. If left untreated, NMS is fatal in 5% to 20% of these patients.[10]

Signs and Symptoms
- Symptom triad of rigidity, hyperthermia, and autonomic instability (i.e., hypertension and tachycardia)
- Often associated with elevated serum creatinine kinase

Treatment
- Discontinuation of antipsychotic medication
- Supportive therapy
- Reversal agents may be used (e.g., bromocriptine, pergolide, or lisuride with dantrolene sodium or azumolene).

Tardive Dyskinesia (TD)

Tardive dyskinesia (TD) appears as slow, rhythmical, automatic, stereotypical movements, either generalized or in single muscle groups, resulting as a side effect of antipsychotic medications.[10]

Signs and Symptoms
- Involuntary movements of tongue, jaw, trunk; may be rapid, jerky, non-repetitive, slow, sinuous, continual, or rhythmic.

Treatment
- TD may be treated by a reduction in antipsychotic medications.

Panic Attack

Panic attack is a discrete period of intense fear or discomfort, in which four (or more) of the symptoms below develop abruptly and reach a peak within 10 minutes, often accompanied by a sense of imminent danger or impending doom and an urge to escape. Studies show that panic and other anxiety disorders are more common in medically ill patients than the population at large. Conditions specifically associated with panic disorder are irritable bowel syndrome, migraines, and pulmonary disease. Panic attacks may be a symptom of several anxiety disorders, including panic disorder. The patient should be assessed for increased suicidal ideation, comorbidity of substance use, mood disorders, other anxiety disorders, and personality disorders. All are at a higher rate in persons with panic disorder.[12]

Signs and Symptoms
- Palpitations, pounding heart, or accelerated heart rate
- Sweating
- Trembling or shaking
- Sensations of shortness of breath or smothering
- Feeling of choking

- Chest pain or discomfort
- Nausea or abdominal distress
- Dizziness, unsteadiness, lightheadedness, or faintness
- Derealization (feelings of unreality) or depersonalization (feeling of being detached from oneself)
- Fear of losing control or going crazy
- Fear of dying
- Paresthesias (numbness or tingling sensations)
- Chills or hot flashes

Diagnosis
- It is important to rule out general medical conditions (e.g., hyperthyroidism) or effects of a substance (e.g., caffeine intoxication) first.

Treatment
- Symptoms often improve when treated with selective serotonin reuptake inhibitors (SSRIs), even in the absence of a full-blown panic attack.
- Identify and validate the symptoms that the patient is experiencing while reassuring the safety of the patient.
- Medicate as ordered with SSRIs, benzodiazepines, tricyclic antidepressants (TCAs), or monoamine oxidase inhibitors (MAOIs).
- Supportive therapy
- Treatment of comorbid illnesses

Paranoid Schizophrenia

Paranoid schizophrenia is characterized by the presence of hallucinations or delusions that may be grandiose or persecutory in nature and are usually centered on a central theme. This form of schizophrenia predisposes the patient to violence toward himself or herself or others.

Signs and Symptoms
- Auditory or visual hallucinations
- Paranoid behavior or statements
- Anxiety
- Aggression

Diagnosis

As with most psychiatric illnesses, exacerbation of the existing illness is often the reason for being evaluated. The diagnosis is based on presenting symptoms and history.

Treatment
- Maintain safety of patient and staff.
- Medicate with antipsychotics as needed.

Psychosis
The broadest definition of psychosis includes symptoms of delusions, hallucinations, disorganized speech, and grossly disorganized or catatonic behavior. In some psychotic states, other symptoms may be present as well (e.g., as in schizophrenia) and include affective flattening, alogia (inability to engage in an active, normal flow of conversation), and avolition (inability to initiate or complete tasks). A variety of medical conditions may cause psychotic symptoms, including neurological conditions (e.g., neoplasms, CVD, Huntington's disease, epilepsy, auditory nerve injury, deafness, migraine, CNS infections), endocrine conditions (e.g., hyperparathyroidism and hypoparathyroidism), metabolic conditions (e.g., hypoxia, hypoglycemia), fluid or electrolyte imbalances, hepatic or renal disease, and autoimmune disorders with CNS involvement (e.g., systemic lupus erythematosus).[12] Psychotic symptoms may occur in depression, schizophrenia, mania, and substance use.

Signs and Symptoms
- Hallucinations may occur in any sensory modality, including auditory, visual, olfactory, gustatory, and tactile.
- Delusions, erroneous beliefs that usually involve a misinterpretation of perceptions or experiences. Common themes include:
  - Persecutory (the feeling that someone is "out to get them")
  - Referential (the sense that something is meant specifically for them)
  - Somatic (the belief that they have a medical illness or defect)
  - Grandiose (exaggerated sense of power or importance)

Diagnosis
- Physical exam and history.
- Differential diagnosis for the psychotic/violent patient[13,14]:
  - Acute psychosis: schizophrenia, bipolar affective disorder, manic and depressive states
  - Alcohol withdrawal: delirium tremens
  - Central anticholinergic syndrome
  - Drug intoxication: cocaine, amphetamines, hallucinogens, corticosteroids, ethanol, lithium, LSD, mescaline, mushrooms, PCP, salicylates
  - Dementia
  - Infections: encephalitis. meningitis, sepsis

- ○ Head trauma
- ○ Metabolic: hepatic encephalopathy, hypertensive encephalopathy, hypoglycemia, hyperglycemia, hyponatremia, uremia, hypoxia
- ○ CVA
- ○ Seizures
- ○ Vasculitis
- ○ Intracranial hemorrhage, tumor, or mass
- ○ Consider "dip dope" intoxication[13]: smoking cigarettes or marijuana after soaking them in embalming fluid, which contains formaldehyde and methanol. Also sold as: "illy," "fry," "hydro" or "wet." The cigarette may be "dipped" in PCP.

Treatment
- Provide for patient and staff safety.
- Medicate with antipsychotics and/or benzodiazepines (see Table 3-3).

NURSING ALERT

Antipsychotics are divided into two categories: atypical and typical. Atypical antipsychotics differ from typical antipsychotics in their pharmacologic structure. Atypical antipsychotic medications such as clozapine (Clozaril) and risperidone (Risperdal) are the current preferred treatment of choice. Typical antipsychotics such as chlorpromazine (Thorazine) and thiothixene (Navane) cause more side effects and have an increased risk of extrapyramidal symptoms.

- Treat underlying physiologic problem.
- If delusions are present, it is important to look for the "kernel of truth," the one word or thought on which the delusion may be based. This will help you to connect with the person experiencing the delusion.[15]

Suicidal Ideation

The frequency of both suicide attempts and completed suicides is substantially higher among patients with substance use disorders than in the general population (three to four times higher rate of completed suicides and lifetime mortality rate of 15%). The presence of major depressive disorder substantially increases the suicide risk of these patients.[10]

TABLE 3-3   Treatment of Acute Psychosis

Etiology	Parenteral Medication
Unknown etiology	Benzodiazepine, antipsychotic
Alcohol intoxication	Benzodiazepine
Hallucinogen intoxication	Benzodiazepine, antipsychotic
Schizophrenia	Benzodiazepine, antipsychotic
Mania	Antipsychotic
Psychotic depression	Benzodiazepine
Personality disorder	Benzodiazepine, antipsychotic
Posttraumatic stress disorder	Benzodiazepine, antipsychotic

Data from: Alan MH, Currier GW, Hughes et al: Expert consensus guidelines series: treatment of behavioral emergencies, *Postgrad Med Suppl*, May, 2001, pp 1-88.

- Some of the greatest risk factors contributing to the risk for suicide include:
  - History of and seriousness of previous suicide attempt
  - Suicidal or homicidal intent with a specific plan
  - Access to means for suicide and lethality of means
  - Concurrent substance or alcohol use
  - Presence of psychotic symptoms such as command hallucinations
  - Severe anxiety
  - Bipolar illness with rapid mood swings
  - Family history of or recent exposure to suicide
- Among patients with psychiatric disorders, patients with bipolar illness are among highest risk for suicide.
- Suicide occurs in up to 10% of patients with schizophrenia.

Diagnosis

- A suicide risk assessment, such as the SAD PERSONS Scale, should be performed. This scale is helpful in identifying those who are at risk for committing suicide. Each item is given a value of one point, and a score of greater than 2 indicates a need to follow up with a mental health professional. A score of 5 or greater indicates an urgent need for treatment, and a score of 7 to 10 indicates the need for hospitalization.[16]
  - *Sex:* Females attempt more often, but males are more likely to have a completed suicide, as men usually choose more lethal means.
  - *Age:* Greater risk at ages less than 25 or greater than 45.

- ○ *Depression:* Suicide usually occurs during an episode of acute depression.
- ○ *Previous attempt:* Previous attempt increases the likelihood of future attempts.
- ○ *Ethanol abuse:* Alcohol abuse increases the risk of suicide.
- ○ *Rational thought loss:* Inability to logically think through problems increases the risk of suicide.
- ○ *Social supports lacking:* Absence of or recent loss of social support such as family or close friends increases the risk of suicide.
- ○ *Organized plan:* A person with an organized plan is more likely to commit suicide.
- ○ *No spouse:* Lack of or recent loss of an intimate partner relationship can increase the risk of suicide.
- ○ *Sickness:* Physical illness or a comorbid mental illness increases the risk of suicide.

Treatment

- Provide for a safe environment by placing patient in a hospital gown, clearing area of any harmful objects.
- Initiate constant observation with frequent interaction.
- Reassure patient that you will help keep him or her safe.
- Initiate a no–self-harm contract.

NURSING SURVEILLANCE

1. Monitor the trend of behaviors, environmental factors affecting the patient's behavior, and implement various intervention strategies.
2. Assess for the presence of biochemical imbalances and overdoses.
3. Follow organizational guidelines regarding physical and chemical restraints.
4. Reevaluate the patient's risks of harm to himself or herself or others.
5. Evaluate the patient's response to medications and other interventions.
6. Assess the patient's level of consciousness.
7. Monitor the patient's vital signs as indicated.

EXPECTED PATIENT OUTCOMES

The patient will:

- Exhibit behaviors congruent with a no-self-harm contract: cooperative, calm, and directable, with no specific plan or means of suicide available upon discharge. Availability of a social support system is a plus.

- Articulate specific coping strategies and resources if symptoms recur or if suicidal or homicidal ideation returns.
- Verbalize signs and symptoms of escalating anxiety and techniques for interrupting the progression of the anxiety.
- List steps in a relapse prevention plan (recognizing relapse symptoms, who to call for immediate help, what specific interventions to initiate).

PATIENT/FAMILY DISCHARGE IMPLICATIONS AND EDUCATION

1. Teach the patient and family or significant others about the need for follow-up treatments and appointments.
2. Provide the patient with information about community resources.
3. Instruct the family or significant others in recognizing signs of increased anxiety and agitation, in strategies to reduce anxiety and agitation, and in when to seek treatment in the ED or other facilities.
4. Help the patient/family/significant other evaluate the level of need for psychiatric follow-up care (e.g., nursing-home care, intensive outpatient care).
5. Make appointments for follow-up counseling.
6. Perform medication teaching.
7. Teach the patient how to recognize relapse triggers and explore coping strategies.

REFERENCES

1. Lamberg L: Psychiatric emergencies call for comprehensive assessment and treatment, *JAMA* 288:686-687, 2002.
2. Way B and Banks S: Clinical factors related to admission and release decisions in psychiatric emergency services, *Psychiatr Serv* 52:214-218, 2001.
3. Peterson D, Roy A, Miller SZ, et al: Children with psychiatric emergencies have unique issues that require new strategies for treatment, study at Children's Hospital of New York-Presbyterian to be presented at Pediatric Academic Societies Meeting, New York-Presbyterian, 2002.
4. Falsafi N: Pediatric psychiatric emergencies, *J Child Adolesc Psychiatr Nurs* 14:81-94, 2001.
5. Zayas L and Kaplan C: Understanding suicide attempts by adolescent Hispanic females, *Social Work,* 45:53-64, 2000.
6. Melding P and Draper B: *Geriatric consultation liaison psychiatry,* New York, 2001, Oxford University Press.
7. Kahn M: Emergency psychiatry: Tools of engagement: avoiding pitfalls in collaborating with patients, *Psychiatr Serv* 52:1571-1572, December, 2001.
8. Allen M, Currier G, Hughes D, et al: The Expert Consensus Guideline Series: treatment of behavioral emergencies. A Postgraduate Medicine Special Report, May, 1-90, 2001; www.psychguides.com.

9. Pestka E, Billman R, Alexander J, et al: Acute medical crises masquerading as psychiatric illness, *J Emerg Nurs* 28:531-535, 2002.
10. American Psychiatric Association: *APA practice guidelines for the treatment of psychiatric disorders compendium 2000*, Washington, DC, American Psychiatric Association.
11. May D and Grubbs L: The extent, nature, and precipitating factors of nurse assault among three groups of registered nurses in a regional medical center, *J Emerg Nurs* 11:11-17, 2002.
12. American Psychiatric Association: *Diagnostic and statistical manual of mental disorders*, ed 4, Washington, DC, 1996, American Psychiatric Association.
13. Mendyk S and Fields D: Acute psychotic reactions: consider "dip dope" intoxication, *J Emerg Nurs* 28:432-435, 2002.
14. Giorgi-Guarnieri D, Rose SR, and Ward K: Face-to-face with psychosis in emergency medicine, *J Crit Ill* 17:397-400, 2002.
15. Moller M and Murphy M: *Three R's psychiatric wellness approach*, www.PsychiatricWellness.com.
16. Patterson WM, Dohn HH, Bird J, et al: Evaluation of suicidal patients: the SADPERSONS scale, *Psychosomatics* 24 (4):343-349, 1983.

chapter 4

Burns

Julia Fultz

The goals of burn management in the emergency department (ED) are to stop the burning process; maintain oxygenation, ventilation, and perfusion; preserve viable tissue; and prevent infection.

FOCUSED NURSING ASSESSMENT

The first priority in caring for the burn patient is to stop the burning process. After that goal has been achieved, the burn patient is treated as a trauma patient, and the nursing assessment follows the primary and secondary assessment outlined in Chapter 21, with the following modifications and additions. The burn injury itself is evaluated after the initial assessment and interventions have been performed.

Oxygenation and Ventilation
- Inspect the face, mouth, and nose for soot, burns, blisters, edema, carbonaceous sputum, and singed nasal and facial hairs. If such signs are present, maintain a high index of suspicion for an inhalation injury.
- Assess for altered voice or hoarseness.
- Monitor breathing for abnormal inspiratory sounds (e.g., stridor, hoarseness) indicating partial occlusion of the pharynx or larynx potentially from burn edema.
- Evaluate level of consciousness. Consider hypoxia from inhalation injury as a cause for agitation or a change in level of consciousness.

> ⋙ **N U R S I N G   A L E R T** ⋘
>
> Suspect inhalation injury if the patient was in a confined
> burning environment (e.g., closet) or has an altered level of
> consciousness. Inhalation injuries may not manifest themselves
> for several hours after injury. Epithelial sloughing from inhalation
> injuries can occur from 6 to 72 hours after injury. After the
> onset of signs and symptoms of inhalation injury, rapid progression
> to airway obstruction can occur. Prepare for prophylactic
> endotracheal intubation in any patient who exhibits questionable
> respiratory mechanics or has clinical indications of an inhalation
> injury.

- Evaluate respiratory rate, use of accessory muscles, chest wall
  symmetry, and excursion. Circumferential full-thickness burns
  to the chest may impair chest expansion because of eschar
  formation. An escharotomy may be needed to facilitate chest
  expansion. (See Initial Interventions, p. 169, for a description of
  an escharotomy.)
- Auscultate the lungs for bilateral air movement and
  adventitious sounds such as crackles, wheezing, and
  rhonchi.

Perfusion
- Evaluate for signs of hypovolemia (tachycardia, tachypnea, dry
  mucous membranes, decreased urine output, pale color, cool
  skin temperature, altered level of consciousness, delayed
  capillary refill, and hypotension). Burn shock may develop in
  hypovolemic patients who are not adequately treated.
- Assess capillary refill, torso and extremity temperature, and
  skin color.
- Palpate pulses for presence, quality, and equality, especially
  those distal to the burn. Nonpalpable pulses should be
  evaluated with a Doppler ultrasound. Circumferential eschar
  formation or edema to an extremity may interfere with
  perfusion. Monitor the trend of pulses by serial examinations.
  Progressive weakening of pulses or absence of pulses is an
  indication for escharotomy.
- The swelling of a burned limb invalidates the readings from
  a noninvasive blood pressure (BP) cuff placed on that limb.
  Edema caused by a burn will reach its peak during the second
  24-hour period after burn injury.

- Note color and clarity of the urine. Dark urine may be indicative of decreased renal perfusion caused by hypovolemia, myoglobin, or hemoglobin.

Cognition
- Assess cerebral perfusion by evaluating the patient's LOC. Signs and symptoms of inadequate cerebral perfusion may indicate carbon monoxide poisoning (see section Carbon Monoxide Poisoning), hypovolemia, or a head injury.

Sensation and Mobility
Comfort
Pain
- Symptoms include hyperventilation and increased heart rate.
- Note signs of discomfort (e.g., restlessness, frowning, decreased attention span, grimacing, groaning, crying, rocking).
- Document patient's pain using self-reporting pain-scoring system (Reference Guide 15).
- Full-thickness burns are insensate, but the outer margins of the burn may be partial-thickness burns and therefore painful.

Anxiety
- Note patient's anxiety level.

Hypothermia
- Document temperature: Skin with either partial-thickness or full-thickness burns has lost its ability to function. Monitor temperature closely.

Tissue Integrity
Extent of Burn
The extent of the burn is calculated after the initial assessment and interventions. It is calculated as a percentage of the total body surface area (TBSA) injured with partial-thickness or full-thickness burns (see thermal injury under clinical conditions). Superficial burns are not included in the estimates of the percentage of TBSA burned because the skin does not lose its ability to function.

- The rule of nines (Figure 4-1) can be used to estimate the percentage of TBSA involved. The rule must be adapted for accurate assessment of infants and toddlers, because their body proportions are different from those of adults.
- A modified rule of nines used for the child proposes that for each year of life after 2 years of age (head is 18% of the TBSA), 1% is subtracted from the head and 0.5% is added to each leg.[1]

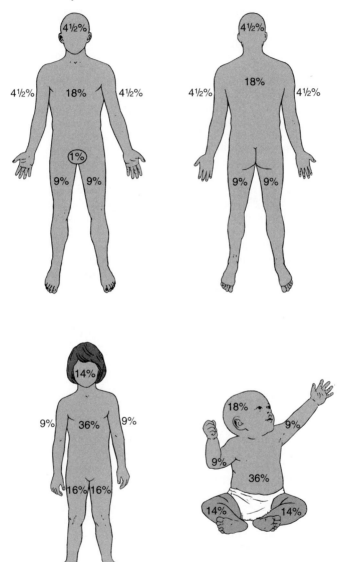

Figure 4–1 Rule of nines.

- For estimating the percentage of patchy burns, use the size of the size of the patient's hand (including the fingers), which represents approximately 1% of the body surface area.[2]
- Age-related charts, such as the Lund and Browder chart (Figure 4-2), may allow a more accurate determination of the extent of injury in children.
- Burn depth is difficult to determine during the initial evaluation, especially the superficial partial-thickness and the deep partial-thickness burns.
- For a classification of burn severity as minor, moderate, or major, see Box 4-1.

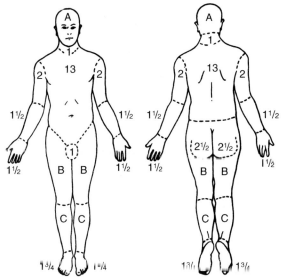

Relative percentage of areas affected by growth

	Age in years					
	0	1	5	10	15	Adult
A—½ of head	9½	8½	6½	5½	4½	3½
B—½ of one thigh	2¾	3¼	4	4¼	4½	4¾
C—½ of one leg	2½	2½	2¾	3	3¼	3½

Figure 4–2   Lund and Browder chart. (From Griglak M: Thermal injury, *Emerg Med Clin North Am* 10 (2):374, 1992.)

BOX 4-1   CLASSIFICATION OF BURN SEVERITY

Minor burn
- 15% TBSA or less in adults
- 10% TBSA or less in children and the elderly
- 2% TBSA or less full-thickness burn in children or adults without cosmetic or functional risk to eyes, ears, face, hands, feet, or perineum

Moderate burn
- 15% to 25% TBSA in adults with less than 10% full-thickness burn
- 10% to 20% TBSA partial-thickness burn in children under 10 and adults over 40 years of age with less than 10% full-thickness burn
- 10% TBSA or less full-thickness burn in children or adults without cosmetic or functional risk to eyes, ears, face, hands, feet, or perineum

Major burn
- 25% TBSA or greater
- 20% TBSA or greater in children under 10 and adults over 40 years of age
- 10% TBSA or greater full-thickness burn
- All burns involving eyes, ears, face, hands, feet, or perineum that are likely to result in cosmetic functional impairment
- All high-voltage electrical burns
- All burn injuries complicated by major trauma or inhalation injury
- All poor-risk patients with burn injury

TBSA, total body surface area.
From: Guidelines for service standards and severity classification in the treatment of burn injury. Appendix B to Hospital Resources Document, *ACS Bulletin* 69:25-28, 1984.

Elimination
- Check bowel sounds for quality and for the presence of abdominal distention. An ileus often will accompany burns of greater than 20% of TBSA.[2]
- Nausea and vomiting

LIFE SPAN ISSUES
Pediatric Patients
1. The most common burn injury in children under 3 is a scald injury.[2]

2. Young children do not have the motor dexterity to quickly remove themselves from the heat source and have thinner skin. Burns are more severe than those an adult would sustain given the same exposure.
3. Airway compromise occurs more rapidly because of the smaller size of the airway.
4. Lack of bone ossification and increased bone pliability result in early exhaustion of a child with constrictive chest burns and the associated edema.[2]
5. Children are further compromised by a higher metabolic rate, which causes increased oxygen consumption. The hypermetabolic state produced by a burn injury coupled with the normally higher metabolic rate of children may result in an increased temperature without ongoing signs of infection.[3]
6. Volume status in children is reflected in the following assessment parameters: level of consciousness, pulse pressures, arterial blood gases, distal extremity color, capillary refill, temperature, and urine output.[4]
7. BP is not a reliable indicator of shock. Compensation from vasoconstriction will maintain the BP in an acceptable range until cardiovascular decompensation occurs.[4]
8. Special attention should be given to preserving body heat. Children have a larger ratio of body surface area to weight in comparison with adults and will have a greater degree of heat and evaporative water loss.
9. Children may sustain electrical burns to the mouth by chewing on electrical cords. Children also may sustain electrical burns by inserting objects into electrical outlets.
10. Children are predisposed to hypoglycemia because of low glycogen stores. To avoid hypoglycemia, maintenance fluids containing glucose should be given in addition to the Ringer's lactate that is given for burn resuscitation. The volume of a glucose-containing maintenance fluid can be calculated with the formula in Box 4-2. The formula is weight based and adds volume to be delivered over 24 hours for each kilogram of the child's weight.

Pregnancy

1. A spontaneous termination of pregnancy usually occurs with TBSA burns of 60% or more.[2]
2. The fetal well-being depends on the hemodynamic stability of the mother.

BOX 4-2 MAINTENANCE FLUID REQUIREMENTS FOR CHILDREN[2,3]

1 kg to 10 kg = 100 ml/kg/24 hr
11 kg to 20 kg = 1000 ml (from above formula for first 10 kg)
   + 50 ml/for each kg between 11 and 20 kg/24 hr
Over 20 kg = 1500 ml (from the above formula for 20 kg)
   + 20 ml per kg for each kg above 20 kg/24 hours
Example: 21-kg child
1000 ml for the first 10 kg (100 ml × 10 kg)
+ 500 ml for 11 kg to 20 kg (50 ml × 10 kg)
+ 20 ml for 1 kg above 20 kg (20 ml × 6 kg)
= 1520/24 hr, or 66.3 ml per hr

NURSING ALERT

Plasma volume increases in pregnancy. As a result of this volume increase, a large amount of blood volume may be displaced before signs of hypovolemia are seen. The placenta is sensitive to catecholamine release and has little autoregulatory capability; thus it cannot compensate for the resulting vasoconstriction and hypoperfusion. Anticipation of shock in the pregnant patient is of the utmost importance to fetal survival.

---

3. Large amounts of supplemental oxygen are required to ensure adequate fetal oxygenation. Maternal hypoxia results in vasoconstriction of the placental and uterine blood flow, thereby causing hypoxia in the fetus, which is poorly tolerated.
4. Patients beyond 20 weeks' gestation (uterus at the level of the umbilicus) may need to be placed on either their right or left side to prevent uterine compression of the vena cava, which can result in hypotension.
5. Fetal monitoring is essential. Patients should be transferred to a burn center.

Geriatric Patients

1. Geriatric patients have a diminished sensory capacity and are sometimes cognitively impaired. A reduced reaction time coupled with frequently impaired mobility and declining physical strength increases their risk for injury. The skin is thinner, resulting in burns that are more severe.

2. Preexisting cardiopulmonary disease reduces the ability to tolerate pulmonary stressors such as inhalation burns.

3. Preexisting disease (e.g., chronic obstructive pulmonary disease, coronary artery disease, hypertension, renal compromise, or diabetes) results in a reduced reserve capacity of the body system affected by the disease. Thus the elderly are predisposed to organ dysfunction with increased morbidity and mortality.

4. Fluid resuscitation necessitates close monitoring to prevent complications from underresuscitation or overresuscitation.

5. Medication may impair cognitive ability.

INITIAL INTERVENTIONS

1. Make sure burns have been cooled and chemical burns flushed adequately (see p. 176) to prevent further tissue damage. All clothing and jewelry, which can retain heat and chemicals, should already have been removed.

2. Prevent further contamination of the burns. Use sterile gloves for all contact with burn wounds, and use gowns, gloves, masks, and head covers for moderate or major burns.

3. Oxygenation and ventilation management
   - Provide 100% oxygen by nonrebreather mask. Patients with a possible inhalation injury should be positioned with the head of the bed elevated to reduce dependent edema of the upper airway unless a potential cervical injury precludes doing so.
   - Assist inadequate respiratory effort: Use a bag-valve device attached to a 100% oxygen source. Take precautions to prevent aspiration in the unconscious patient. Have functioning suction equipment at hand.
   - Tracheal intubation: Prepare to intubate patients who are unresponsive, have inadequate respiratory mechanics, have an ineffective gag reflex, have burns of the head or neck in which edema may cause airway obstruction, or have signs of impending airway obstruction (stridor, hoarseness, dyspnea, or tachypnea).
   - Transnasal tracheal intubation is the preferred route for the burn patient if it is possible[2] (see Procedure 1). A tracheal tube at least 7.5 mm in diameter is recommended for use with adult patients to facilitate pulmonary toilet and bronchoscopy. Document the tube size and depth.
   - A well-secured endotracheal tube is of paramount importance in the initial resuscitation phase; a tracheal tube that is dislodged may be impossible to replace because of

airway edema. Avoid undue pressure against burned skin and ears when securing a tracheal tube, particularly during fluid resuscitation, when edema formation is greatest (see Figure 4-3 for an example). One can also secure endotracheal tubes by looping umbilical tape around the nasal septum and then tying the tube in place.

4. Fluid replacement: The goal of fluid replacement in the first 48 hours is to preserve vital organ perfusion, avoiding both overresuscitation and underresuscitation.

- The American Burn Association (ABA) Task Force Guidelines recommend fluid replacement in adults with >20% TBSA burns and in children (less than 5 years of age) with >15% TBSA burns.[5]

- Warmed Ringer's lactate is the replacement fluid of choice and is infused through two large-bore IV catheters, preferably placed through unburned skin. Calculate the amount using Baxter's (Parkland's) formula[5]:

Administer 4 ml/kg/% TBSA burn in the first 24 hours from the time of the injury. Give one half of the total 24-hour volume in the first 8 hours (burned tissue is most permeable during the first 8 hours after injury), one fourth during the second 8 hours, and one fourth during the third 8 hours.[5] (Literature varies regarding

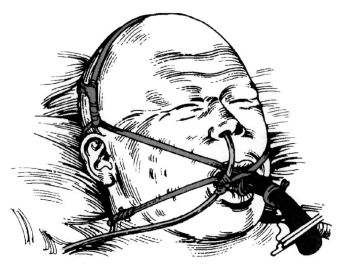

Figure 4–3   Cloth ties used to secure gastric and endotracheal tubes are kept away from the ears.

the percentage of burn for which fluid resuscitation is recommended, as does the recommended amount of fluid to be initially delivered in the first 24 hours after injury. The above guidelines for fluid resuscitation have been taken from the ABA task force guidelines.)

- Use of colloid solutions has little advantage over crystalloids during the initial hours of resuscitation because increased capillary permeability causes a loss of plasma proteins interstitially.[2] Colloids may be used 24 hours post burn when capillary seal has occurred.

NURSING ALERT

Fluid resuscitation formulas are only a guide for the initiation of fluid resuscitation. The volume required for a patient will be affected by age, severity of burn, concomitant trauma, and physiologic status. Amounts predicted by formulas often will have to be adjusted according to the patient's physiologic response to the initiation of fluid resuscitation. Box 4-3 lists certain concurrent injuries that will increase the amount of fluid needed during resuscitation.

BOX 4-3   INDICATIONS FOR INCREASED FLUID RESUSCITATION REQUIREMENTS

- Inhalation injury
- Delay in resuscitation
- Associated trauma
- Extensive depth and surface area burn
- Circumferential burns requiring escharotomy release
- High-voltage electrical injury
- Extensive muscle damage
- Preexisting medical conditions
- Extreme age-groups (infants and geriatric patients)
- Patients with prior dehydration
- Patients with drug or alcohol dependencies

Information from American Burn Association: *Advanced burn life support providers manual*, Chicago, 2001, the association; and Gordon MD and Winfree JH: Fluid resuscitation after a major burn. In Carrougher GJ: *Burn care and therapy*, St Louis, 1998, Mosby.

1. *Monitors:* Cardiac monitor, oxygen saturation monitor, and automatic BP cuff
   - Electrical injuries can result in an alteration of the cardiac conduction pathways, resulting in arrhythmias. Patients should be continuously monitored for 24 hours for arrhythmias.
   - Pulse rates of 100 to 120 beats/min after the initial resuscitation phase (a few hours after injury) can be a normal response in adults with large burn areas.[2] Heart rates in children will vary according to age. A reflex tachycardia in children may be present despite adequate volume replacement.[2,4]
   - The patient's BP is not a reliable indicator of the adequacy of fluid resuscitation.

≥⃒   N U R S I N G   A L E R T   ⃒≤

Standard pulse oximetry does not differentiate between hemoglobin saturated with carbon monoxide and hemoglobin saturated with oxygen. An acceptable oxygen saturation reading may not indicate adequate oxygenation in the presence of carbon monoxide poisoning.

---

2. *Gastric tube:* Adynamic ileus usually accompanies burn injuries involving more than 20% TBSA.[2] Patients should have gastric decompression until bowel function returns.
3. *Urinary catheter:* Urine output serves as a guide for judging the effectiveness of fluid resuscitation. Placement of a urinary catheter is essential when fluid resuscitation is initiated. Fluid replacement generally should be sufficient to maintain a urine output of 30 to 50 ml/hr in adults (~0.5 ml/kg/hr) and 1 ml/kg/hr in children weighing ≤30 kg.[2,4] One may alter fluid administration if the urine output falls below or exceeds the above limits by increasing or decreasing the infusion amount by one third for 2 to 3 hours.[2]
4. *Escharotomy:* Indicated for circumferential burns that constrict the chest or extremities and cause circulatory or respiratory compromise. The procedure is performed at the patient's bedside with sterile technique. Incisions must extend through the entire length and depth (down to, but not into, the subcutaneous fat) of the eschar, allowing for separation and expansion of tissue as the edema develops. Bleeding from

the sites must be controlled by one or more of the following: the physician using a disposable cautery, packing of the sites, pressure dressings, and elevation of the extremities. Incisions are made along the entire full-thickness burn. The preferred incision sites are[6]:

- *Extremities:* Initial incision is made along the midlateral line of the limb, including the joint. If extremity pulses do not improve, a second incision is made in the midmedial line, again including the joints.
- *Chest:* Bilateral incisions in the anterior axillary lines from the clavicle to the costal margins.
- *Abdomen:* Extend the bilateral chest incisions onto the abdomen, along the costal margin.

If an extremity remains pulseless after an escharotomy, a fasciotomy may be required.

5. Prevent hypothermia
   - Remove wet bedding after burns have been cooled.
   - Administer warmed IV fluids.
   - Cover burns with clean, dry sheets until definitive wound care can be initiated.
   - Cover patient's head to prevent heat loss.
   - Close door to room to prevent drafts.
   - Increase the temperature of the room to 29° C (85° F).

6. Elevate the head of the bed 30 degrees if not contraindicated by trauma to minimize the potential for cerebral and facial edema.

7. Eye care involves flushing with copious amounts of water or saline solution after inverting the eyelid and removing any particles (see Procedure 17).

8. Obtain an accurate preinjury patient weight. Initial resuscitation is weight based.

9. Tetanus toxoid: Necrotic tissue is an ideal medium for the growth of *Clostridium tetani*. Administer tetanus toxoid to previously immunized patients. Administer tetanus immunoglobulin for those not previously immunized or for whom the immunization status is unknown. (See Reference Guide 23 for tetanus toxoid guidelines.)

10. Administer intravenous (IV) morphine sulfate for pain control.[2] IV administration is preferred because medication absorption from muscle tissue is inconsistent. Because of the rapid elimination of morphine sulfate in the burn patient, dosing requirements may be increased from what is expected in the non-burn patient.[2] Pain medication should be

administered on a schedule rather than as needed. Patients with inadequate pain control during the initial phases of burn injury may develop long-term pain-management issues.[7]

11. Administer anxiolytics to treat anxiety. The patient's level of pain will be perceived as greater if anxiety is present.

12. Administer nonpharmacologic interventions for pain control.

13. Administer antibiotics as ordered.

14. Initiate the transfer of patients requiring treatment in a burn center (see Box 4-4).

15. Nursing care priorities are listed in the table on pp. 170-174.

BOX 4-4   AMERICAN BURN ASSOCIATION BURN CENTER REFERRAL CRITERIA[2]

1. Partial-thickness burns greater than 10% total body surface area (TBSA)
2. Burns that involve the face, hands, feet, genitalia, perineum, or major joints
3. Third-degree burns in any age-group
4. Electrical burns, including lightning injury
5. Chemical burns
6. Inhalation injury
7. Burn injury in patients with preexisting medical disorders that could complicate management, prolong recovery, or affect mortality
8. Any patients with burns and concomitant trauma (such as fractures) in which the burn injury poses the greatest risk of morbidity or mortality. In such cases, if the trauma poses the greater immediate risk, the patient may be initially stabilized in a trauma center before being transferred to a burn unit. Physician judgment will be necessary in such situations and should be in concert with the regional medical control plan and triage protocols.
9. Burned children in hospitals without qualified personnel or equipment for the care of children
10. Burn injury in patients who will require special social, emotional, or long-term rehabilitative intervention

PRIORITY DIAGNOSTIC TESTS

Laboratory

Albumin: serum: The level may be low because plasma proteins, principally albumin, are lost into injured tissue secondary to increased capillary permeability.

Arterial blood gas: The PO_2 may initially be normal with inhalation injuries. It is especially important to document a baseline pH with patients who sustain electrical burns, because acidosis is common. Patients with large burns will have a mild metabolic acidosis that will resolve with adequate resuscitation.

BUN and creatinine: serum: Blood urea nitrogen (BUN) and creatinine levels may be elevated related to fluid deficits.

Carboxyhemoglobin: serum: Screening should be done for patients with suspected inhalation injuries. Signs and symptoms appear if the level is elevated greater than 10%.

Cardiac enzymes: If an electrical injury is involved. Caution should be used in interpreting an elevated CK-MB fraction as myocardial damage. Skeletal muscle injury resulting from electrical current can contain up to 25% CK-MB fraction (normally 2% to 3%).[8]

Complete blood count: Initially, the hemoglobin and hematocrit may be elevated as losses from the intravascular volume cause hemoconcentration. Hemoglobin may be decreased because of hemolysis.

Drug screens: Serum and urine screens (including alcohol): These are especially important if the patient is unconscious or obtunded.

Electrolyte levels: serum: Levels may be normal initially, but they will change during the early course of treatment (decreased sodium because of fluid shift, elevated potassium because of fluid shifts and cell lysis).

Glucose: serum: The level may be elevated as a result of the stress response. Hypoglycemia may occur in children because of limited glycogen stores.

Lactate: serum: Indicative of the effectiveness of resuscitation. (Elevated levels directly reflect anaerobic metabolism as a consequence of hypoperfusion.)

Myoglobin: urine: Obtained on patients with electrical burns, major burns, and concurrent trauma involving crush-type injuries.

Urine analysis: Under resuscitation will cause an increased specific gravity.

NURSING CARE PRIORITIES

Potential/Actual Problem	Causes	Signs and Symptoms	Interventions
Airway obstruction	• Airway edema • Secretions • Impaired cough	• Stridor/crowing sound • Adventitious breath sounds • Increased pulmonary secretions • Hypoxemia • Alteration in level of consciousness	• Provide aggressive pulmonary toilet. • Prepare for intubation with patients suspected of having airway involvement and those with signs of respiratory distress. • Elevate head of bed 30 degrees to help reduce edema unless concurrent trauma precludes doing so.
Inadequate gas exchange	• Alveolar injury from smoke inhalation • Decreased hemoglobin • Carboxyhemoglobin	• Carbonaceous sputum • Hoarse voice • Singed nasal hairs • Burns to the face • Tachypnea • Decreased PaO_2 <80 • Increased $PaCO_2$ >45 • Decreased oxygen saturations <95% • Adventitious breath sounds • Decreased level of consciousness • Increased respiratory rate	• Provide 100% oxygen by nonrebreather mask. • Monitor respiratory rate and depth. • Assist ventilations with a bag-valve device for an inadequate respiratory effort. • Prepare to intubate patients with signs of potential airway obstruction. • Elevate the head of the bed for patients with a potential inhalation injury unless concurrent trauma precludes doing so. • Monitor oxygen saturation by pulse oximetry (pulse oximetry may not differentiate between carbon monoxide and oxygen saturated hemoglobin).

Inadequate fluid volume	• Increased capillary permeability • Plasma loss from vascular space (fluid shift) • Hemorrhage from associated trauma	• Edema • Decreased urine output • Decreased central venous pressure • Decreased pulmonary capillary wedge pressure • Hypotension on	• Prepare for an escharotomy in the case of circumferential burns of the chest that compromise chest expansion and the patient's ability to breathe. • Monitor hemoglobin. • Monitor carboxyhemoglobin levels for patients with elevated levels of carbon monoxide. • Monitor ABGs for decreasing PaO_2 and increasing $PaCO_2$ indicating worsening hypoxemia. • Monitor vital signs for tachycardia and hypotension. An adequate blood pressure is not reflective of an adequate fluid status. • Place two large-bore intravenous catheters for fluid resuscitation. Fluid replacement should be initiated with Ringer's lactate using Baxter's formula (see pp 164-165).

Continued

NURSING CARE PRIORITIES—cont'd

Potential/Actual Problem	Causes	Signs and Symptoms	Interventions
	• Insensible fluid loss	• Tachycardia • Elevated urine specific gravity • Concentrated urine	• Maintain urine output 30-50 ml/hr (~0.5 ml/kg/hr) in patients weighing greater than 30 kg, and 1 mg/kg/hr for patients under 30 kg. For patients with myoglobinuria, urine output should be maintained at 75-100 ml/hr (1.0-1.5 ml/kg/hr).[2,12] Place a Foley catheter for accurate urine output measurement.
Inadequate tissue perfusion	• Generalized edema • Avascular tissue • Decreased cardiac output • Hypovolemia	• Diminished peripheral pulses • Loss of sensory function • Cool extremities	• Remove jewelry and constrictive clothing. • Administer Ringer's lactate for fluid resuscitation. • Evaluate peripheral pulses, sensory function, skin temperature, and capillary refill. • Place BP cuff on the unaffected limb if possible. • Prepare to assist with an escharotomy for a patient with a circumferential burn of an extremity associated with perfusion deficits.

| Pain | • Stimulation of exposed pain sensors | • Moaning or crying
• Hostility
• Clenched teeth
• Facial grimacing
• Complaints of pain
• Irritability
• Increased heart rate and BP
• Restlessness
• Self-reporting pain scale | • Cool burns with tepid compresses, taking care to avoid hypothermia.
• Cover cooled burns with a clean dry sheet to prevent irritation of exposed nerve endings from air currents.
• Administer pain medications and anxiolytics as ordered.
• Advise the patient of all procedures to be performed and what to expect during the procedure.
• Utilize nonpharmacologic pain-relieving measures (e.g., breathing exercises, relaxation measures, music, television). |
| Impaired skin integrity | • Burns
• Edema
• Impaired physical mobility | • Destruction of dermis, epidermis, and underlying structures
• Fluid-filled blisters
• Mottled, waxy, white, cherry-red, or blackened skin color | • Eliminate the source of burning.
• Flush chemical burns with water for 20-30 min or more.
• Secure endotracheal and gastric tubes away from the ears if the ears are burned.
• Use water to cool tar, asphalt, and plastic that adheres to the skin.
• Turn the patient every 2 hr.
• Elevate limbs above the level of the heart to reduce edema. |

Continued

NURSING CARE PRIORITIES—cont'd

Potential/Actual Problem	Causes	Signs and Symptoms	Interventions
Hypothermia	• Loss of skin function	• Temperature less than 36.5° C (97.7° F)	• Maintain room temperature of 29° C (85° F). • Remove wet bedding. • Warm IV fluids. • Cover patient with sheet and blanket. • Cover patient's head to maintain temperature and prevent further heat loss. • Close doors to prevent drafts.
Risk of infection	• Altered integumentary system • Invasive lines	• Destruction of the dermis and epidermis	• Use sterile gloves for all wound contact. • Use sterile gowns, masks, and shoe and head covers for moderate or major burns. • Use strict aseptic technique. • Use sterile linens for patients with moderate to severe burns. • Administer antibiotics and tetanus toxoid as ordered. • Use good hand washing technique.

Chest Radiograph

Chest radiographic changes due to inhalation injury usually are seen at approximately 48 hours after an inhalation injury. An admission chest x-ray examination will provide a baseline for comparison with later films.

Electrocardiogram

An electrocardiogram (ECG) is particularly important in electrical burns because of the potential damage to the cardiac conduction system.

Laryngoscopy/Bronchoscopy

These are diagnostic measures for identifying inhalation injury and assisting in determining the severity.

Xenon-133 Ventilation Perfusion Scan

Allows identification of airway obstruction caused by inhalation injury. Xenon-133 is cleared from uninjured lung tissue and delayed in injured tissue.

CT Scan

Use this tool to rule out an intracranial hemorrhage in patients with a neurologic deterioration who have suffered an electrical injury.

CLINICAL CONDITIONS

Chemical Burns

Injury occurs when a chemical compound reacts with the skin, causing a chemical reaction. Severity of injury and outcome are related to the type of chemical (acid, alkali, or organic compound), the duration of exposure, the concentration of the substance, and the amount of the substance. The chemical reaction and subsequent tissue injury continue until the chemical is removed from the skin.

- Acid burns cause coagulation necrosis and protein precipitation. An impermeable barrier develops, which limits the extent of the tissue damage.
- Alkali burns tend to cause more damage than acid burns because they produce a tissue liquefaction necrosis; protein is denatured, and tissue planes are loosened. Tissues are dissolved, allowing a deeper spread of the chemical and thus a more severe burn.
- Organic compounds tend to disrupt the cell wall integrity, causing cutaneous damage. Organic compounds can be

absorbed, leading to systemic problems, including liver and kidney damage. Certain chemicals such as hydrofluoric acid can penetrate into the subcutaneous tissues and cause damage for several days after exposure.

Symptoms
- Pain
- The patient has skin damage resembling that of a thermal injury, with erythema, blistering, or full-thickness loss.

⇒ NURSING ALERT ⇐

The extent of the tissue injury may be deceptive. Extensive necrosis, fluid loss, and systemic toxicity may occur during the first 24 to 36 hours after the injury.

Diagnosis
- Diagnosis is determined by a history and assessment of the skin.
- Identification of the chemical agent is appropriate but is secondary to the removal of contaminated clothing and immediate irrigation of the affected area.

Treatment
- Observe strict universal precautions to avoid contaminating caregiver eyes, skin, and lungs. One should remove and dispose of the patient's contaminated clothing according to hospital policy. (See Decontamination of a Patient, Procedure 10.)
- One should brush off dry powder residue before irrigation.
- Irrigation of the area with water should be performed immediately for a **minimum** of 20 to 30 minutes. With few exceptions, neutralizing solutions have no advantage over water. Irrigation should continue until the patient voices a significant decrease in pain or the pain stops.
- Irrigation of the eye should begin with at least 1 to 2 L of normal saline and should continue until the eye's pH is 7.4.[9] If only one eye is involved in the chemical exposure, make sure the irrigation fluid runoff does not contaminate the uninvolved eye. Topical anesthetics will reduce patient discomfort caused by the irrigation.
- Treatment for a tissue injury is the same as for a thermal burn. Conventional burn resuscitation formulas can guide initial fluid resuscitation.

- Frequent assessments should be performed to evaluate for cardiopulmonary or pulmonary involvement. Airway involvement may range from mild tracheal irritation to adult respiratory distress syndrome. Cardiac involvement may range from tachycardia to profound shock.
- Identification of the offending agent will be helpful in anticipating additional side effects of the agent.
- Monitor pH because of potential systemic disturbances.
- Monitor for hypothermia.

Table 4-1 provides a list of chemical burns that require special treatment modalities or antidotes.

Electrical Burns

Contact with electricity has the potential to cause injury in three different ways[10]:

- A true electrical injury resulting from current flow. Cell damage can occur in two ways: by the effect the current has on the cell itself, such as the electrical cells in the heart, and by the production of heat as electrical energy is converted into heat energy, resulting in burns.
- An arc injury resulting from the current passing from the source to an object. Arcs produce extremely high temperatures and may produce very deep thermal burns or a flash-type burn as the current passes around the body.
- A flame injury as clothing ignites.

  The severity of electrical injuries depends on the voltage of the source, the type of current, the duration of contact, the path taken through the body, and the resistance of the tissues.[10,11]

- The strength of current is divided into two categories: high voltage, 1000 volts or greater, and low voltage, below 1000 volts. High voltage usually causes more tissue destruction.
- Types of current include "alternating current" (AC) found in households (voltage of 110 or 220) and "direct current" (DC) found in car batteries and electrosurgical devices. Lightning is also a form of DC current. Contact with AC current tends to cause muscle contraction, making it difficult for the victim to let go of the electrical source. Contact with DC current tends to cause a single violent muscle contraction, often resulting in the victim being thrown from the electrical source. A high index of suspicion must be maintained for concurrent trauma.
- The path taken by the electrical current as it passes through the body will determine the tissues affected. Predicting the extent of injury is difficult.

TABLE 4-1   Treatment of Specific Chemical Burns

Alkalis (hydroxides, carbonates, caustic sodas of sodium, potassium, ammonium, lithium, barium and calcium).
Alkalis are commonly found in fertilizers and oven and drain cleaners, and are formed when dry cement is mixed with water.

Action	Treatment
• Produces liquefaction necrosis • Combines with proteins and fats to form a soap, which allows for deeper penetration of hydroxyl ions • Dehydrates cells	• Brush away any powder residue. • Begin copious irrigation with large volumes of water under low pressure. • Strong alkalis require prolonged (may take up to 12 hr for the pH to return to normal) irrigation to limit the severity of the injury. • Certain chemicals contacting water produce heat; however, the large volumes of water used to irrigate the injury tend to limit this exothermic reaction. • Eye irrigation for alkali exposure requires copious amounts of either water or saline. Take care to avoid contamination of an unaffected eye by irrigation runoff.

Anhydrous ammonia

Used to manufacture explosives, petroleum, cyanide, plastic, and synthetic fibers; a cleaning agent; an agricultural fertilizer; and a coolant in refrigerator units.

Action	Treatment
• Very low temperature, freezes tissues • Ammonia vapors readily dissolve in moisture of skin, eyes, mouth, and	• Irrigation of the eyes and skin. • Intubate for respiratory distress using a large endotracheal tube to allow for aggressive pulmonary toilet.

lungs, then form hydroxyl ions, causing chemical burns.

- Utilize PEEP.

Elemental metals (sodium and potassium)

Action	Treatment
• Harmless until activated with water • Tissue damage because of thermal and chemical injury	• **Do not use water.** • Use a class "D" fire extinguisher or sand in the prehospital setting to extinguish flames; the patient is then transported, with metal covered with oil (mineral oil or cooking oil) to separate it from water. • Remove small pieces of metal from the skin and then debride and cleanse the thermal injury.

Formic Acid

A caustic organic acid used in industry and agriculture

Actions	Treatments
• Cutaneous injury by coagulation necrosis • Systemic toxicity: acidosis, hemolysis, hemoglobinuria	• Lavage wound with copious amounts of water. • Administer sodium bicarbonate for acidosis. • Administer mannitol to promote diuresis in patients with hemolysis. • Prepare for hemodialysis in severe cases.

Continued

TABLE 4-1   Treatment of Specific Chemical Burns—cont'd

Hydrocarbons

Gasoline, turpentine, kerosene, propane, butane, toluene, freon

Actions	Treatments
• Targets lungs, CNS, and heart. • *Pulmonary:* injury from aspiration. Hydrocarbons (HCs) are poorly water soluble and can penetrate to lower airway, causing bronchospasm, inflammatory response, hypoxia, direct parenchymal injury, and alveolar collapse from effect on surfactant. Onset of symptoms may be delayed. • *CNS:* Some HCs cause depression, have a narcotic-like effect, and may cause euphoria, confusion, obtundation, or disinhibition. • *Heart:* ventricular arrhythmias, myocardial dysfunction • *Skin:* HCs cause cell-membrane injury	• Remove from exposure site. • Remove clothing, provide copious irrigation of skin for dermal exposure. • Use ECG and pulse oximeter monitoring. • Prepare for early intubation for severe aspiration. • Provide burn wound care. • Routine decontamination (ipecac or gastric lavage) of the GI tract is not recommended because of the risk of aspiration, for which the consequences are much more severe in comparison with the relatively low risk of systemic toxicity from absorption from the GI tract. Small amounts of HCs are very toxic to the lungs. • Monitor for signs and symptoms of toxicity. Patients who have had accidental exposures and are asymptomatic should be monitored for a period of time and discharged with follow-up care.

and dissolution of lipids, causing skin necrosis, severe burns. When skin has been broken down, HCs can produce systemic toxicity: hepatic necrosis and renal failure.

Hydrofluoric acid

Hydrofluoric acid is used in aluminum cleaning products, paint removers, and rust removers, and in the computer chip industry.

Actions	Treatments
• Penetrates the skin and mucous membranes of the respiratory tract.	• Aggressively lavage with water or, if available, a solution of benzalkonium chloride for 15-30 min immediately after contact.
• Causes deep burns and intense pain.	• Remove blisters because they may harbor fluoride ions.
• Onset of symptoms may be delayed for hours if exposure was to a weaker (10%-20%) solution.	• Treat mild burns with topical calcium gluconate gel, 3.5 g of calcium gluconate powder in 150 ml of a water-soluble lubricant applied with a gloved hand, then cover with an occlusive dressing. Deeper burns may require subcutaneous infiltration at the injury site or an intra-arterial infusion of 10% calcium gluconate into the appropriate artery supplying the injured site.
• Binds calcium and magnesium.	
• Can cause fluoride toxicity, arrhythmias, and hypocalcemia.	• Irrigation of eyes with copious amounts of normal saline is required for at least 30 min.
• Prolonged QT interval is a reliable indicator of calcium hypocalcemia.	• Treat inhalation injury with high-flow oxygen and possibly with nebulizer treatments of gluconate. Evaluate patient for laryngeal edema, pulmonary edema, pneumonitis, and pulmonary hemorrhage.

Continued

TABLE 4-1   Treatment of Specific Chemical Burns—cont'd

- Treat hypocalcemia with 10% calcium gluconate IV.
- Monitor cardiac rhythm for 24-48 hr if exposure was significant.

Phenol (carbolic acid)

Phenols are found in chemical disinfectants and commercially available germicidal solutions and are used in industrial, agricultural, cosmetic (face peels), and medical fields.

Actions	Treatments
• Causes severe skin burns, coagulation necrosis.	• Irrigate with large volumes of water under low pressure. Small amounts of water are detrimental.
• Binds irreversibly to albumin.	• Removal and dilution are best accomplished by wiping the skin with undiluted 200-400 molecular weight polyethylene glycol (PEG) if available or isopropanol (isopropyl alcohol). Phenol is poorly soluble in water. Decontamination with water is appropriate until a PEG solution can be obtained.
• Absorbed phenol may cause profound CNS depression, coma, respiratory failure, hypotension, hypothermia, arrhythmias, and a metabolic acidosis.	• Remove contaminated hair as soon as possible. Phenols may become trapped in hair.
• May induce fatal systemic toxicity by affecting the liver and kidneys.	
• Dilute solutions are more rapidly absorbed than concentrated ones.	

White phosphorus

White phosphorus is commonly found in fireworks and weaponry and is used in the manufacture of insecticides, rodent poisons, and fertilizers.

Actions	Treatments
• Danger of spontaneous combustion when exposed to air; when it ignites, it will burn until the entire agent is oxidized or the oxygen has been consumed. • Tissue injury is caused primarily by heat production. • It forms acids with the addition of water. • Metabolic abnormalities (hypocalcemia and elevated phosphorus level). • ECG changes: prolonged QT interval, bradycardia, ST-T wave changes.	• Remove the patient's clothing and the chemical particles from the skin. • Submerse the affected area in cool water to isolate the chemical from the air (white phosphorus becomes a liquid at warmer temperatures [44° C, 111.2° F]). • Wash the skin with a suspension of 5% sodium bicarbonate and 3% copper sulfate in 1% hydroxyethyl cellulose as soon as available (made by hospital pharmacy). Phosphorus will turn black, allowing for easier identification of particles. Oxidation rate is reduced by the copper sulfate. Copper sulfate is toxic if absorbed systemically, so treatment with the suspension is limited to 30 min, then the suspension is thoroughly washed from the skin. • Use a fluorescent light (Wood's lamp), as it illuminates the phosphorus and may aid in removal. • Treat burn according to burn protocols.

Data from: American Burn Association Advanced burn life support provider manual, 2001, Chicago, the association; Edlich RF, Bailey TL, and Bill T]: Chemical injuries. In Marx J, Hockberger R, and Walls R, eds: Rosen's emergency medicine concepts and clinical practice, ed 5, St Louis, 2002, Mosby; Lee DC: hydrocarbons. In Marx J, Hockberger R, and Walls R, eds: Rosen's emergency medicine, concepts and clinical practice, ed 5, St. Louis, 2002, Mosby; and Sanford AP and Herndon DN: Chemical burns. In Herndon DN, ed: Total burn care, ed 2, St Louis, 2002, Saunders.

- Tissue resistance varies.[12] Electrical current passes through tissue with lower resistance more rapidly than it does through tissues with high resistance. As it takes longer for the current to pass through an area of high resistance, the potential is present for more electrical energy to be converted into thermal energy and produce greater damage. Moisture substantially lowers tissue resistance.

High resistance	Tendon, fat, bone
Moderate resistance	Dry skin
Low resistance	Nerves, blood, mucous membranes, muscle

NURSING ALERT

As a result of the implosive and explosive effects of lightning, the victim can be thrown. Maintain a high index of suspicion for life-threatening blunt, traumatic injuries.

Symptoms

Electrical injuries produce a wide variety of injuries to body systems internally and externally. Initially, the extent of damage may be difficult to determine.

Cardiac

Cardiac symptoms are due to either direct myocardial cell damage or damage to the conduction system.

- Ventricular fibrillation (more common with AC exposure)
- Asystole (more common with high voltage and lightning exposure)
- Additional ECG changes may include sinus tachycardia, nonspecific ST and T wave changes, QT segment prolongation, ventricular ectopy, various heart blocks, atrial fibrillation, and bundle branch blocks.[11,12]
- Myocardial cell damage may produce signs of a myocardial contusion.
- Acute hypertension may occur, especially with lightning injuries.
- Lightning produces a massive countershock, which stuns the myocardium, producing asystole. Automaticity may reestablish a rhythm.

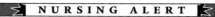

NURSING ALERT
Patients in cardiopulmonary arrest caused by electrical injury respond exceedingly well to CPR and should receive aggressive resuscitation.

Respiratory
- Respiratory arrest may occur as a result of:
  - Electrical current passing through the respiratory centers in the brain
  - Tetanic contraction of the diaphragm and chest wall muscles, preventing lung expansion and resulting in suffocation
- Pulmonary contusions: primarily if a lightning strike occurred
- Chest wall damage from trauma caused by explosion or fall

Integument
- Externally, the thermal injuries range in depth from superficial to full thickness, with possible destruction and necrosis of underlying structures and organs. Significant internal damage may exist with little external damage evident.
- Contact points are often the hands and the skull. Ground points are most often the heels.[12] Identification of contact and ground points may help determine the path of the current.
- Oral burns may be seen in children who have been exposed by chewing on electrical cords.
- Lightning strikes often cause a flashover phenomenon, in which the electrical current passes over the body instead of through it. This results either in superficial burns that are linear or punctate in form, or alterations in the skin (which are not actually thermal injuries) such as feathering, which produces a red branching pattern on the skin, described as spidery or featherlike in appearance.[12]

Neurologic
- Transient loss of consciousness, confusion, amnesia, or short-term memory loss.
- Headaches, skull fractures, intracranial hemorrhage, and seizures, especially if the electrical current entered through the head.
- Spinal cord injuries from high-voltage contact, potential for paraplegia.
- Lightning strike victims may have a temporary paralysis from vascular spasm and neurologic system effects.
- Neurologic damage may be immediate or delayed.

Vascular
- Thrombosis from the heating of the blood vessels, more so in smaller vessels because there is less blood flow to help dissipate the heat.
- Vascular spasms, especially with lightning injuries. Extremities will be cold, blue, mottled, and pulseless. This usually resolves within a few hours without treatment. If it does not, consider compartment syndrome or thrombosis of the vessels.
- Hemorrhage from damaged vessel walls, may be immediate or delayed.

Musculoskeletal
- Fractures or dislocations from violent muscle contractions or falls.
- Compartment syndrome may develop as a result of vascular injury.
- Release of myoglobin from damaged muscle cells.

Renal
- Light red to reddish brown or tea-colored discoloration of the urine. The urine may contain hemoglobin and/or myoglobin. Myoglobin is released when muscle tissue breaks down. The urine will be light red to reddish brown or tea colored, but there will be few if any red blood cells present on microscopic evaluation. Myoglobin molecules are large and can block the renal tubules, resulting in acute tubular necrosis if the kidneys are not well flushed. A urine reagent strip dipped in urine with myoglobin will read positive for hemoglobin because reagent strips cannot distinguish between myoglobin and hemoglobin.

Sensory
- Visual disturbances from eye damage
- Rupture of the tympanic membrane
- Hearing loss

Diagnosis
- Based on history: can be difficult to diagnose if adequate history is not available
- Assessment of the wounds

Treatment
- Manage any airway, oxygenation, and circulation problems first.
- Provide spinal immobilization if the potential for fractures from falls is present.
- Monitor cardiac rhythm and obtain an ECG. Treat arrhythmias with standard advanced life-support measures.

- Minimal fluid requirements when surface burns are present is based on the formula 2 to 4 ml/kg/percent of thermal burn.[2] Patients experiencing lightning injuries seldom require massive fluid resuscitation,[12] but if significant deep-tissue burns are present, this volume may be inadequate.[2]
- Urine output should be 30 to 50 ml/hr (0.5 to 1.0 ml/kg/hr) unless urine is pigmented (myoglobin), then urine output should be 75 to 100 ml/hr (1.0 to 1.5 ml/kg/hr) until pigment clears. Maintaining an alkaline urine pH (pH >6.0) will increase the solubility of myoglobin in the urine and improve the rate of clearance. Adding sodium bicarbonate to intravenous fluids and maintaining slight alkalinity of the blood (pH at least 7.45) also ensures the urine pH is alkaline.[2,12]
- If myglobinuria is present, an osmotic diuretic such as mannitol may be used initially to promote renal perfusion and prevent obstruction from myoglobin casts, but is seldom needed. If a diuretic is administered, the rate of fluid administration will need to be increased to compensate for the diuresis and prevent hypovolemia. Urine output can no longer be used as the major determinant of adequate fluid resuscitation.
- Perform frequent vascular checks of extremities. If vascular compromise is present, an escharotomy or fasciotomy must be performed.
- Frequently orient those who are confused.
- Maintain pain and anxiety control.

Inhalation Injury

An inhalation injury can be caused by the inhalation of chemicals, gases, or heat. The severity is related to the amount and composition of the inhaled substances. Morbidity and mortality of burn-injured patients significantly increases when the burn is accompanied by an inhalation injury.[5] There are three types of inhalation injuries: carbon monoxide inhalation, upper-airway injury (above the glottis), and lower-airway injury (below the glottis).[2]

Carbon Monoxide Inhalation

Carbon monoxide (CO) is a byproduct of the combustion of organic material. It is a colorless, odorless gas with an affinity for hemoglobin that is over 200 times that of oxygen. CO binds to hemoglobin, forming carboxyhemoglobin, blocking the uptake and transport of oxygen, and resulting in cellular hypoxia. CO also enters tissues, binding with other hemoproteins and interfering with cellular function.[13] Patients who were in an enclosed area during a fire are predisposed to CO poisoning.

Symptoms

Organs first affected are those with high oxygen needs, such as the brain and the heart. Symptoms result from tissue hypoxia, not from parenchymal injury. Carbon dioxide removal is not affected, so patients are usually not tachypneic nor cyanotic.[2] Oxygen saturation levels detected by pulse oximetry usually are normal.

- Mild symptoms include a headache, confusion, and weakness.
- More severe symptoms include vomiting, tachycardia, tachypnea, hallucinations, seizures, arrhythmias, and eventual coma and death.
- Symptoms often are related to the amount of hemoglobin saturated with CO. However, as the patient is treated with oxygen, serum CO levels will decrease faster than the level of CO bound in tissues[14]; thus symptoms may appear worse than expected given the resulting level of carboxyhemoglobin. See Table 4-2 for signs and symptoms of carbon monoxide poisoning.

TABLE 4-2   Signs and Symptoms of Carbon Monoxide Poisoning

% CD Saturation	Signs and Symptoms
0%-10%	Normal, smokers, and those living in urban areas
10%-20%	Slight headache, confusion, and dyspnea on exertion
20%-30%	Headache, throbbing in the temples
30%-40%	Fatigue, severe headache, visual disturbances, dizziness, nausea and vomiting, and chest pains in individuals with coronary artery disease
40%-50%	As above, except more pronounced symptoms
50%-60%	Syncope, tachycardia, tachypnea, combativeness, respiratory failure, shock, convulsions, coma, cherry-red skin color (present in only 50% of patients), and death
60%-70%	Shock, coma, seizures, depressed cardiac and respiratory function; may result in death
70%-100%	Often results in death

Data from Traber DL, Nerndon DN, and Soejima K: The pathophysiology of inhalation injury. In Herndon D, ed: *Total burn care*, ed 2, St Louis, 2002, Saunders; pp. 221-231; and American Burn Association: *Advanced burn life support providers manual*, Chicago, 2001, the association.

Diagnosis
- History and duration of exposure to products of combustion, especially in an enclosed area
- Carboxyhemoglobin level

Treatment
- Warmed and humidified 100% oxygen by nonrebreather mask. Oxygen assists in removing the CO from the hemoglobin.
- Intubation if the patient cannot maintain and protect his or her own airway as indicated by a decreased LOC.
- The half-life of carboxyhemoglobin is approximately 4 hours for patients without supplemental oxygen and approximately 1 hour for patients on 100% oxygen.[2,14]
- Monitor carboxyhemoglobin levels. Patients should remain on 100% oxygen until carboxyhemoglobin levels are less than 10%.
- In severe cases with a very high carboxyhemoglobin level associated with severe clinical symptoms, hyperbaric oxygen therapy may be suggested, although it is controversial. Hyperbaric therapy speeds up the removal of CO from hemoglobin and reduces the short-term and long-term effects of CO poisoning.[15]

Upper-Airway Injury (Supraglottic)

An upper-airway injury may result from a thermal injury or inhaled chemicals or gases that have a high water solubility and are rapidly absorbed on the moist surfaces of the mouth, nose, and upper airway (e.g., chlorine, ammonia, and sulfur oxides and dioxides).

Symptoms
- Related to the thermal injury and may be absent initially. Edema peaks at 24 to 48 hours after injury.
- Symptoms include erythema, edema, hoarseness, blisters, or ulcerations of the oropharynx and larynx.
- Symptoms also may include a mechanical obstruction of the airway secondary to edema (e.g., stridor, tachypnea, dyspnea, and crowing respirations). Hypovolemia may initially delay the development of edema.

Diagnosis
- There is a history of heat or hot liquids entering the airway.
- Direct visualization of damage to the larynx, pharynx, and vocal cords.

Treatment
- Elevate the head of the bed if not contraindicated by concurrent trauma.

- Provide warm, humidified oxygen.
- Administer aerosolized epinephrine.
- Prepare for early intubation of patients who have the potential for airway obstruction.

Lower-Airway Injury (Infraglottic)

The ability of the supraglottic area to cool hot air usually prevents thermal injury to the infraglottic structures. Inhalation injuries to the infraglottic structures are usually a result of inhaled toxic fumes, gases, mists, and very small particles that have a low water solubility and therefore are not absorbed in the upper airway. Injury is sustained primarily to the upper and small airways. Exposure to a fine mist containing such particles will affect the smaller airways and the lung parenchyma.

Symptoms

Onset is unpredictable. Patient is often asymptomatic on initial presentation, with the onset of symptoms delayed.

- The patient may have sooty sputum (generally a reliable symptom), burns to the face, singed nasal hairs, and inflammation of oropharyngeal mucosa. Inhalation injuries to the lower airway may occur without evidence of external signs.
- Cough, hoarseness, dyspnea, wheezing, stridor, bronchorrhea, chest tightness.
- Hypoxemia
- In severe cases: pulmonary edema, acute respiratory distress syndrome

Diagnosis

- The patient has a history of exposure to products of combustion, especially in a small area.
- Physical examination
- A bronchoscopy is the standard definitive diagnostic measure.[5] It will reveal tracheobronchial injuries such as mucosal inflammation, ulcerations, necrosis, soot, foreign particles, and edema. These clinical findings often are present before obvious respiratory compromise and alterations in arterial blood gases occur.[16]
- A xenon-133 ventilation perfusion scan identifies injury to small airways and parenchymal injury. The scan usually is performed within 24 to 48 hours after the injury. A delay in the clearance of xenon from the lungs is indicative of parenchymal injury.[16]

Treatment

Treatment is supportive.

MINIMAL TO MILD INJURY

- Provide warm, humidified oxygen per nonrebreather mask.
- Elevate the head of the bed unless contraindicated by suspected spinal cord injury.
- Use bronchodilators for bronchospasms and wheezing.
- Monitor arterial blood gases and pulse oximetry, and for changes in assessment indicating a delayed airway obstruction.
- Implement incentive spirometry to prevent atelectasis.
- Observe closely for 24 hours those who are asymptomatic but have a history of significant exposure because of the unpredictable course of inhalation injuries.

MORE SEVERE INJURY

- Provide humidification of inspired oxygen.
- Begin aggressive pulmonary toilet to mobilize and remove secretions, taking care not to further damage lung mucosa when suctioning.
- Use beta 2–agonist nebulizer treatments or IV bronchodilators for bronchospasms and wheezing. Administer IV aminophylline if wheezing persists.[16]
- Obtain an arterial blood gas analysis (nonspecific indicator of inhalation injury; however, with progression of pulmonary dysfunction, arterial oxygen desaturation and retention of carbon dioxide may occur).
- Closely monitor fluid status. Patients with inhalation injuries may require a greater amount of fluid during the resuscitative phase of the injury, as much as 5.7 ml/kg/% TBSA burn.[17]
- Perform tracheal intubation and implement mechanical ventilation for respiratory failure (tachypnea >30 breaths per minute and use of accessory muscles, hypoxemia [Pao_2 <70 mm Hg], and hypercapnia [$Paco_2$ >50 mm Hg]). Intubated patients with inhalation injuries will require greater airway pressures to adequately ventilate because of the narrowed air passages. However, high airway pressures reduce mucosal capillary blood flow, which can result in mucosal ischemia. To adequately ventilate a patient and reduce the effect of high airway pressures, one should provide the patient a higher rate (15 to 20 breaths per minute and a lower tidal volume [6 ml/kg] with a PEEP of 5).[17]

Thermal Burns

The extent of the injury is a result of the intensity of the heat (temperature) and the duration of exposure. Burn injury results in a redistribution of fluid. An increase in capillary permeability occurs in the burned areas and in tissue immediately surrounding the burn by way of a complex chain of events. Plasma shifts from the intravascular space into the interstitial fluid space, producing edema and resulting in a decrease in circulating intravascular volume. When the TBSA of burn involvement exceeds 25%, there is an increased capillary permeability (capillary leak) and edema formation in non-injured tissues and organs. If not treated, a life-threatening hypovolemia, called burn shock, occurs.

Symptoms

Burns are classified by the degree to which the epidermis and the dermis are damaged. Determination of the depth of the wound is based on appearance and presence or absence of sensation.

Superficial (first-degree) burns

Superficial burns involve only the epidermis and are characterized by pain, edema, and erythema that blanches (e.g., sunburn). First-degree burns are not included in the estimation of burn injuries because the skin does not lose its protective function.

Partial-thickness (second-degree) burns

Partial-thickness burns involve the epidermis and varying portions of the dermis. This classification of burns has been further divided into superficial partial-thickness burns and deep partial-thickness burns according to the depth of damage to the dermis.

Superficial partial-thickness burns

Superficial partial-thickness burns involve the epidermis and the upper portion of the dermis. The skin is erythematous and moist with thin-walled, fluid-filled blisters. Nerve endings are intact and irritated, causing extreme pain. The burned areas blanch when pressure is applied. Healing takes 2 to 3 weeks, and there is usually no scarring.

Deep partial-thickness burns

Deep partial-thickness burns involve the epidermis and deep layers of the dermis. The skin is pale to waxy-white in color with blisters like tissue paper that contain little if any fluid. The skin does not blanch with pressure. The wound has a reduced pinprick sensation that can make it difficult to differentiate from full-thickness burns. However, pressure applied to the burn can be felt. These burns heal in 2 to 3 weeks but have a greater potential for hypertrophic scar formation.

Full-thickness (third-degree) burns

Full-thickness burns involve the epidermis and the entire dermis and can extend into the underlying subcutaneous tissues (Figure 4-4). The surface is dry, hard, inelastic, and insensate. The burn may

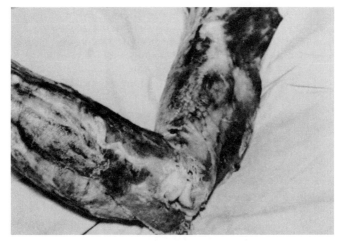

Figure 4–4 Full-thickness burn exposing elbow joint. (From Dressler DP, Hozid JL, and Nathan P: *Thermal injuries,* St Louis, 1988, Mosby.)

appear waxy, white, cherry red, yellow, brown, or black. Nerve endings have been destroyed, although some sensation may be intact at the edges of the burn and cause discomfort. Unless the burn is very small, skin grafting will be needed. Burns that extend into underlying structures such as fascia, muscle, or bone may be termed fourth-degree burns.

Diagnosis
- Diagnosis is based on history and on assessment of the skin.

Treatment
Initial treatment is focused on stopping the burning process and on oxygenation, ventilation, and fluid resuscitation.
- Cool burned areas with tepid to cool moist compresses for 5 minutes, taking care to avoid hypothermia. When the burn has cooled, remove all wet bedding and dressings.
- Avoid overresuscitation and underresuscitation by titration of the amount of fluid being given and reassessment for effectiveness. The amount of fluid used during the resuscitation phase should be enough to maintain adequate organ perfusion.
- Assess for vascular compromise from swelling or compartment syndrome.

- Evaluate circumferential burns for circulatory compromise and prepare for an escharotomy if compromise occurs.
- Maintain the body temperature. Hypothermia results in vasoconstriction that will further compromise circulation to the injured area. Cover the patient with a clean sheet and a blanket for comfort. Maintain the room temperature above 89° F (29° C).[18]
- Cover the patient with a clean, dry sheet and blanket if the patient is to be transferred to a burn center. It is not necessary to debride the burn or dress it with topical ointments.[2] If admission to the hospital or transfer to a burn center will be delayed beyond 24 hours, wound care should be initiated after consultation with the receiving physician.[2]
- Ensure adequate pain and anxiety control, especially before cleansing the injury.
- Cleanse the wound gently with a mild soap and rinse with warm water.
- Remove pieces of clothing, foreign matter, and charred skin by soaking, rinsing, or gentle cleansing with wet gauze. Sloughed or necrotic skin will need to be debrided according to hospital protocol if the patient is not to be transferred. The debridement of burn blisters is a controversial issue; options are to leave the blisters undisturbed, drain them and leave the injured epithelium in place, or remove the injured epithelium completely.[19] The physician treating the patient will determine the care. The wound should be cleansed before the dressing is applied regardless of the method that is chosen for dealing with the blisters.
- Any tar or asphalt that remains on the skin should be cooled immediately to stop the burning process. Tar should then be covered with a petroleum-based ointment (e.g., mineral oil or bacitracin, Neosporin, neomycin) or commercially prepared solvents. Butter will emulsify tar, and sunflower oil has been known to remove both tar and asphalt. Cover the area with a dressing. Ointment will need to be removed and reapplied every 1 to 2 hours until the tar is removed.[20] When the tar has been removed, the burn can be assessed.

Special Precautions With Burns

Ears: Rupture of the tympanic membrane is common with patients struck by lightning. Cartilage has a poor blood supply, which means the healing process is slow. With thermal burns, pressure must be kept off the ears; therefore the use of pillows must be avoided. Cloth ties used to secure endotracheal tubes and nasogastric tubes must be kept away from the ears (Figure 4-3).

Lips: Position oral endotracheal tubes to prevent pressure on the lips. Use bacitracin to prevent drying and cracking.

Eyes: The single most important treatment is copious irrigation with normal saline within seconds of the injury. Invert the eyelid and remove any particles before irrigating. Irrigate for 30 minutes. Assess for eyelash inversion, which will cause corneal abrasions. The cornea must be kept moist (see Chapter 12). If only one eye is injured, prevent contamination of the unaffected eye from irrigation fluid runoff. Topical anesthetics may help reduce the pain and aid in irrigation.

Hands and feet: Preserving function is of the utmost importance. Elevate the extremity above the heart to prevent dependent edema that will delay healing. If fingers and toes are wrapped, they are wrapped individually; do not "mitten" them. If the patient cannot maintain the fingers in a position of function independently, the hand should be splinted.

Perineum: A urinary catheter must be placed until the edema resolves. Massive swelling occurs in the scrotum as a result of dependent edema. If the patient is on bed rest, the area must be cleansed thoroughly and ointment applied after voiding or defecation.

Joints: Exposed bones or tendons should be kept moist with saline-moistened sterile gauze.

NURSING SURVEILLANCE

1. Conduct repeated primary and secondary examinations of the affected body systems and injuries.
2. Monitor the urine for myoglobin (identified by reddish brown or tea-colored urine and urinalysis results negative for red blood cells).
3. Evaluate the effectiveness of measures to control pain and anxiety.
4. Ensure infection control and aseptic techniques.
5. Monitor serum electrolyte levels.
6. Evaluate for hypothermia/maintain normothermia.
7. Evaluate hydration status:
   Underhydration: complaints of thirst, poor skin turgor, increased heart rate, decreased urine output, decreased capillary refill, change in level of consciousness, persistent metabolic acidosis, base deficit.

Overhydration: bounding pulses, crackles, edema, shortness of breath, cough, increased urine output.
8. ECG monitoring for arrhythmias.

EXPECTED PATIENT OUTCOMES

1. Maintained Glasgow Coma Scale score of 15
2. Adequate oxygenation and ventilation: $PaCO_2$ of 35 to 45, PaO_2 of 80 to 100, O_2 saturations >95%.
3. Stable vital signs: Heart rate less than 100 beats/min (less than 120 beats/min in patient with extensive burns as a result of hypermetabolic state); respiratory rate, BP, and cardiac rhythm within normal limits for patient's age.
4. Palpable pulses in all extremities
5. Urine output of 30 to 50 ml/hr for an adult (~0.5 ml/kg/hr), 1 ml/kg/hr for children under 30 kg, and 75 to 100 ml/hr, or 1.0 to 1.5 ml/kg/hr, for adult patients with myoglobinuria.[2,12]
6. Urine negative for myoglobin
7. Urine specific gravity 1.005 to 1.030
8. Adequate pain and anxiety control as evaluated by self-scoring pain scale
9. Decreasing carboxyhemoglobin level
10. Core temperature remains 37° C (98.6° F) or higher.
11. Transfer to a burn center when indicated (see Box 4-4, ABA Transfer Criteria).

REFERENCES

1. Helvig E: Pediatric burn injuries, *AACN Clin Issues* 4 (2):433-442, 1993.
2. American Burn Association. *Advanced burn life support providers manual*, Chicago, 2001, the association.
3. Hockenberry MJ: *Wong's nursing care of infants and children*, ed 7, St Louis, 2003, Mosby.
4. Benjamin D and Herndon DN: Special considerations of age: the pediatric burned patient. In Herndon DN, ed: *Total burn care*, ed 2, St Louis, 2002, Saunders, pp 427-438.
5. American Burn Association. Practice guidelines for burn care, *J Burn Care Rehabil*, April, 2001 (suppl).
6. Mozingo DW: Surgical management. In Carrougher GJ, ed. *Burn care and therapy*, St Louis, 1998, Mosby.
7. Marvin JA: Management of pain and anxiety. In Carrougher GJ, ed: *Burn care and therapy*, St Louis, 1998, Mosby.
8. McBride JW: Is serum creatinine kinase-MB in electrically injured patients predictive of myocardial injury? *JAMA* 255:764-767, 1986.
9. Edlich RF, Bailey TL, and Bill TJ: Chemical injuries. In Marx J, Hockenberger R, and Walls R, eds: *Rosen's emergency medicine, concepts and clinical practice*, ed 5, St Louis, 2002, Mosby.

10. Perdue GF and Hunt JL: Electrical injuries. In Herndon DN, ed: *Total burn care*, ed 2, St Louis, 2002, Saunders.
11. Koumbourlis AC: Electrical injuries, *Crit Care Med* 30(11 suppl)S: 424-430, 2002.
12. Price TG and Cooper MA: Electrical and lightning injuries. In Marx J, Hockenberger R, and Walls R, eds: *Rosen's emergency medicine, concepts and clinical practice*, ed 5, St Louis, 2002, Mosby.
13. Piantadosi CA: Carbon monoxide poisoning, *N Engl J Med* 347 (14): 1054-1055, 2002.
14. Traber DL, Herndon DN, and Soejima K: The pathophysiology of inhalation injury. In Herndon DN, ed: *Total burn care*, ed 2, St Louis, 2002, Saunders.
15. Weaver LK, Hopkins RO, Chan KJ, et al: Hyperbaric oxygen for acute carbon monoxide poisoning, *N Engl J Med* 347 (14):1057-1067, 2002.
16. Fitzpatrick JC and Cioffi WG: Diagnosis and treatment of inhalation injury. In Herndon DN, ed: *Total burn care*, ed 2, St Louis, 2002, Saunders.
17. Warden GD: Fluid resuscitation and early management. In Herndon DN, ed: *Total burn care*, ed 2, St Louis, 2002, Saunders.
18. Gordon M and Marvin J: Burn nursing. In Herndon DN, ed: *Total burn care*, ed 2, St Louis, 2002, Saunders.
19. Flanagan M and Graham J: Should burn blisters be left intact or debrided? *J Wound Care* 10 (1) 41-45, 2001.
20. Edlich RF, Bailey TL, and Bill TJ: Thermal burns. In Marx J, Hockenberger R, and Walls R, eds: *Rosen's emergency medicine, concepts and clinical practice*, ed 5, St Louis, 2002, Mosby.

5 chapter

Cardiovascular Conditions

Theresa M. Glessner

INTRODUCTION

Many cardiovascular conditions have similar initial presentations, so it is important to do a carefully focused survey. If the cardiovascular system is involved, the patient will need to be closely monitored. Assuming that life-threatening conditions will be treated according to ACLS protocol, information must be gathered based on the patient's chief complaint. Many patients presenting with cardiovascular conditions have pain, so pain assessment is of paramount importance when the patient presents to the emergency department (ED) for care.

FOCUSED NURSING ASSESSMENT

Ventilation
Breathing Patterns
- Assess the patient's breathing pattern.
- Low cardiac output and congestive heart failure (CHF) produce respiratory distress secondary to pulmonary congestion caused by fluid volume overload in the ventricle.
- The patient with fluid overload may appear short of breath and have crackles on auscultation.

Perfusion
Nursing assessment focuses mainly on perfusion.

Heart Sounds
- The presence of an S_3 or S_4 may indicate heart failure.
- The presence of a murmur may indicate valvular or septal insufficiency.

Breath Sounds
- Crackles that do not clear with coughing may indicate CHF.

Color
- Pale or cyanotic color may indicate poor cardiac output secondary to an MI or problems related to a great vessel, such as exsanguinating hemorrhage.
- Pale or cyanotic extremities that are cool or pulseless indicate an arterial or venous occlusion.

Peripheral Pulses
- Weak or absent pulses may indicate an acute arterial or venous occlusion.
- Weak pulses also may indicate low cardiac output secondary to an acute MI, CHF, or great-vessel problem.

Edema
- Peripheral edema may be associated with congestive heart failure.

Capillary Refill
- Delayed capillary refill indicates low cardiac output, a vessel occlusion, hypothermia, fluid volume deficit, or shock.

Skin Temperature
- Cool extremities may indicate vessel occlusion or low cardiac output.
- Skin also should be assessed for diaphoresis, which may indicate pain, anxiety, or low cardiac output.

Blood Pressure and Heart Rate
- Obtain blood pressure (BP) and heart rate.
- A rise in heart rate may indicate an anxiety, fluid volume depletion, or low cardiac output.
- A fall in heart rate may indicate an arrhythmia or cardiovascular insufficiency.
- A rise in BP may indicate anxiety, pain, vasoconstriction, or noncompliance with medications.
- A fall in BP is indicative of vasodilation, dehydration, or cardiovascular collapse.

- Prescribed medications such as beta-blockers and calcium channel blockers affect heart rate and BP as well as compensatory mechanisms.

Cardiovascular Risk Factors
- Refer to Table 5-1 for risk factors.

LIFE SPAN ISSUES
Pediatric Patients
- Cardiovascular conditions in pediatric patients may be diagnosed or undiagnosed congenital anomalies and complications related to their treatment.
- CHF may occur as a result of inadequate pumping and may be related to anomalies such as a ventricular septal defect.
- An MI in children is always an ischemic event, not an atherosclerotic event, and may be secondary to an anomaly.
- Bradycardia can be caused by hypoxemia, conduction disturbance, or a congenital anomaly, or may occur postoperatively after repair of a congenital anomaly.

Women
- More women than men report loss of appetite, paroxysmal nocturnal dyspnea, and back pain as the first symptoms noted in relationship to the onset of an MI.
- Women are also less likely to report symptoms and less likely to seek or receive treatment for symptoms of an MI.[1]

NURSING ALERT
- *Always* carefully evaluate chest pain during pregnancy.

Pregnancy
- Hemodynamic changes during pregnancy include a marked increase in blood volume and cardiac output.
- Peripheral vascular dilation causes an increased heart rate and decreased BP.
- During the postpartum period, deep venous thrombosis and pulmonary emboli may develop from amniotic emboli.
- Other conditions that may interfere with the cardiovascular system during pregnancy include pregnancy-induced hypertension, gestational diabetes, vaginal bleeding, spontaneous abortion, placenta previa, abruptio placentae, and postpartum hemorrhage (see Chapter 15).
- Pregnancy-induced cardiomyopathy and pulmonary embolism are potentially life threatening to the mother and the fetus.

TABLE 5-1   Cardiovascular Risk Factors

Risk Factor	Explanation
Tobacco abuse	Cigarette smokers and those inhaling second-hand smoke develop blood vessel changes, which places them at risk for cardiovascular disease.
Hypertension	Uncontrolled or poorly controlled hypertension increase the risk for an MI as a result of increased afterload and preload.
Diabetes	Related to blood vessel changes and predisposition to vasoconstriction.
High cholesterol	Hypercholesterolemia increases risk for an MI as a result of increased risk for plaque formation leading to coronary artery occlusion.
Heredity	Patients with a family history of cardiac or vascular disease are at increased risk for these conditions.
Sedentary lifestyle	Sedentary lifestyle increases the risk for an MI and for vascular occlusion related to the development of pooled blood leading to blood clots in the small vessels.
Age	As age increases beyond the third decade, the risk of cardiovascular disease increases because of blood vessel changes associated with aging.
Obesity	Obese patients are at higher risk of vascular occlusion and an MI secondary to a sedentary lifestyle and an increased load on the heart.
Ethnic and racial origin	Blacks are more likely than whites to develop cardiovascular disease. Blacks also are more likely to develop cardiovascular disease at an early age.
Gender	Men are at increased risk for heart disease. Hormonal and stress factors have a part in the development of heart disease in men and postmenopausal women.
Stress and anxiety	Stress, anxiety and a "type A" personality increase the risk of an MI.
Medication history	Females who smoke and use contraceptives experience an increased incidence of vascular disease and have been shown to develop blood clots more readily.
Social history	Cocaine users are at risk for developing tachyarrhythmias and myocardial ischemia leading to cardiovascular insufficiency and collapse.

American Heart Association: Risk factors of cardiovascular disease, www.americanheart.org. Accessed Nov. 16, 2004.

Geriatric Patients
- There is an increased incidence of cardiovascular disease in the geriatric patient related to the development of arteriosclerosis causing increased peripheral vascular resistance.
- The heart loses elasticity with age and thus is less responsive to demands.
- The geriatric heart takes much longer to increase its rate in response to increased myocardial demands.
- Silent myocardial infarctions are more common in the geriatric population because of decreased nerve innervation to the heart.
- Symptoms are not always well described by the geriatric patient because of communication problems, neuropathies, and other physiologic changes associated with aging.[2]

INITIAL INTERVENTIONS

Assess airway and breathing and implement measures to facilitate breathing:
- Elevate the head of the bed.
- Decrease sensory stimulation.
- Allow the patient to assume a position of comfort.
- Prepare for endotracheal intubation if there is evidence of severe respiratory distress with airway compromise and no evidence of compensation.
- If the patient is apneic, open the airway, ventilate, administer oxygen at 100% per bag-valve mask, and prepare to intubate.
- Administer oxygen to maintain an SpO_2 of greater than 95%. Oxygen should be administered to all patients with cardiovascular compromise to optimize oxygenation to all cells.
- Administer oxygen at 2 L/min per nasal cannula if there is no respiratory distress. If respiratory distress is present, administer oxygen at 100% per nonrebreather mask.

Assess circulation:
- If no pulse is present, administer CPR.
- If a pulse is present, assess pulses and capillary refill.
- Establish peripheral intravenous (IV) access, preferably with an 18-gauge or larger IV, and administer normal saline at a keep-vein-open rate.
- If the patient is hypotensive (SBP <90), establish two large-bore IVs and administer a bolus of Ringer's lactate or normal saline and then reassess. If hypotension continues, repeat the procedure and prepare to insert a central venous access line for further fluid administration as well as medication administration.

- Initiate continuous ECG, blood pressure, and pulse oximetry monitoring as soon as possible.
- Obtain a 12-lead ECG.
- Obtain blood specimen for anticipated laboratory studies as ordered by the physician.
- Assess chest pain, and if the pain appears to be indicative of cardiac ischemia:
  ○ Administer one nitroglycerin 0.4 mg sublingual or nitrospray every 3 to 5 minutes for three doses, as ordered.
  ○ Maintain a systolic blood pressure of at least 90 mm Hg.
  ○ Prepare to initiate a nitroglycerin drip as ordered.
  ○ Nitropaste 1 to 2 inches to the chest wall may be applied for relief of pain and to reduce afterload.
  ○ Continuously monitor the patient's pain level, BP, and ECG during nitroglycerin administration.
- Assess localized extremity pain, which could possibly be related to vascular insufficiency.
- Monitor color, pulses, pain, movement, and edema in the affected extremity.
- Anticipate venous or arterial studies.
- Anticipate aortogram or CT scan of the chest or abdomen if aortic disruption is suspected.
- Monitor BP closely and administer IV sodium nitroprusside or IV labetalol if hypertension develops.
- Hypotension is considered an ominous sign and should be treated with volume resuscitation (Ringer's lactate or normal saline), dopamine, Levophed, or epinephrine drips.
- Nursing care priorities are listed in the table on pp. 210-212.

PRIORITY DIAGNOSTIC TESTS
Cardiac Conditions
   ECG: An electrocardiogram (ECG) determines areas of cardiac injury, myocardial infarction, or conduction disturbance (see Reference Guide 7). Obtaining a preoperative baseline is necessary. Repeat ECGs may be ordered to monitor for changes in response to treatment.

Vascular Conditions
   Angiography: Angiography directly images an artery through a percutaneously inserted sheath to visualize any narrowing, occlusion, or rupture.[12] Percutaneous angioplasty and stent placement can be performed at the time of this procedure to relieve any occlusion or stenosis that may be causing poor perfusion.

NURSING CARE PRIORITIES

Potential/Actual Problem	Causes	Signs and Symptoms	Interventions
Decreased cardiac output	• Inability of the damaged myocardium to pump effectively	• Increased capillary refill time • Altered level of consciousness • Urinary output less than 30 ml/hr	• Administer medications to increase cardiac contractility as ordered. • Administer medications to decrease myocardial oxygen demand (diuretics, vasodilators) as ordered.
Altered tissue perfusion	• Decreased cardiac contractility • Obstruction of blood flow to vital tissues • Decreased blood volume	• Peripheral cyanosis • Diminished peripheral pulses • Altered level of consciousness • Urinary output less than 30 ml/hr • Chest pain • Shortness of breath • Cardiac arrhythmias • Increased afterload • Increased PAP, CVP, PAWP	• Monitor vital signs. • Increase cardiac contractility with medications. • Increase circulating blood volume with intravenous fluid. • Relieve blood vessel obstruction with vasodilators, anticoagulants. • Prepare the patient for possible therapies (thrombolytic therapy, percutaneous angioplasty, or operative intervention). • Prepare for and assist with invasive hemodynamic monitoring.

Impaired gas exchange	• Diminished contractility of the heart • Increased myocardial afterload	• Shortness of breath • Decreased oxygen saturation • Poor arterial gas exchange	• Administer oxygen to maintain oxygen saturation of greater than 95%. • Continuously monitor oxygen saturation. • Position the patient for comfort. • Prepare for intubation. • Administer diuretics as ordered to relieve fluid overload.
Fluid volume excess	• Decreased contractility of the heart • Increased myocardial afterload • Decreased renal perfusion	• Urinary output less than 30 ml/hr • Increased peripheral edema • Increased pulmonary secretions • Decreased cardiac output • Increased PAWP	• Monitor I & O. • Afterload reduction with medications. • Diuretics
Fluid volume deficit	• Hemorrhage • Nausea and vomiting	• Delayed capillary refill • Elevated heart rate • Altered mental status • Urinary output less than 30 ml/hr	• Monitor I & O. • Monitor vital signs. • Administer IV fluids and/or blood products as ordered.

Continued

NURSING CARE PRIORITIES—cont'd

Potential/Actual Problem	Causes	Signs and Symptoms	Interventions
		• Pale skin • Decreased blood pressure	
Pain	• Poor tissue perfusion or ischemia • Obstruction of blood flow	• Complaints of pain • Crying • Moaning • Grimacing • Restlessness	• Assess pain using a pain scale; reassess after any intervention. • Position the patient for comfort. • Administer pain medication as ordered.
Anxiety	• Pain • Poor mentation	• Behavior changes • Restlessness • Repetitive questioning about condition	• Offer reassurance and support to the patient and family. • Provide a quiet, calm environment. • Explain all procedures to the patient and family, using nonmedical terms. • Administer anti-anxiety medication as ordered.

Duplex examination: A duplex examination is a combination of Doppler flow and direct ultrasound color-flow imaging through a blood vessel. This may be performed to image an artery or vein to identify an occlusion.[3]

Laboratory Tests

Arterial blood gases: ABGs are used to assess acid–base status and oxygenation. Refer to Reference Guide 2.

Brain natriuretic peptide (BNP): BNP is a hormone that is secreted primarily from the ventricles. The level is elevated in congestive heart failure (CHF) and is a useful tool along with clinical correlation to confirm the diagnosis of CHF.

Cardiac enzymes: Cardiac markers are enzymes or proteins that are released into the bloodstream during an ischemic cardiac event. Refer to Reference Guide 7 for cardiac marker elevations.

Complete blood count: CBC can be utilized to assess for the presence of blood loss or an infectious or inflammatory process. The white blood cell (WBC) count is elevated in an inflammatory process, which can be a cause of chest or cardiac pain. Decreased hematocrit may indicate bleeding or chronic anemia.

Electrolytes: Increased or decreased levels of potassium or sodium can cause arrhythmias. Potassium, sodium, and chloride can be depleted with diuretics.

Liver function tests: The liver metabolizes many cardiac drugs, and elevated liver function tests indicate liver damage that could affect drug administration or blood clotting.

Magnesium: Decreased magnesium can cause ventricular arrhythmias.

PT/PTT: Prolonged PT/PTT can cause bleeding. A baseline and continuous monitoring are necessary, especially if anticoagulants are administered.

Serum creatinine and BUN: Serum creatinine and blood urea nitrogen (BUN) provide an indication of renal function. One or both of these values will be elevated in renal failure or in states of hypoperfusion.

Serum, phosphorus, and calcium: Low levels of serum phosphorus and calcium can reduce the pumping ability of the heart.

Type and crossmatch: Obtaining a type and crossmatch allows for blood and blood products to be available if bleeding starts or if operative management of the condition is required.

Radiographic Tests

Acute abdominal series: An acute abdominal series aids in ruling out a problem or disruption of the abdominal aorta. Aneurysms will occasionally be seen on x-ray films.

Chest x-ray: A chest x-ray examination rules out any radiographically visible cause of chest pain and gives an indication of the presence of pulmonary disease and edema, as well as the size of the heart and other structures. Widening of the mediastinum may be detected and is indicative of aortic dissection. Chest x-ray also is performed for preoperative evaluation in the event of surgical intervention.

CT scan of the chest or abdomen: A CT scan will show a transverse view of the large blood vessels and give a measurement of an aneurysm or dissection and may rule out other pathologic processes in the chest or abdomen.

Other Tests

Doppler flow studies: These studies are noninvasive and give an indication of arterial and venous flow and pressure measurement in the extremities. Prolongation of the systolic wave indicates a probable occlusion.

Echocardiogram: An echocardiogram gives an indication of myocardial damage by looking at wall motion and giving an indication of ejection fraction. The transthoracic approach is helpful in determining valve function.

Pericardiocentesis: Pericardiocentesis is performed when fluid is suspected in the pericardial sac. Fluid removal will allow the heart to contract more efficiently. Asystole and pulseless electrical activity are possible indications for pericardiocentesis.

Diagnostic cardiac catheterization: A diagnostic cardiac catheterization provides direct visualization of the coronary arteries and valves. Ventricular ejection fraction can be measured. If lesions are identified, percutaneous intervention such as angioplasty or stent placement may be performed.

Stress test: Stress testing may be indicated to assess for the presence of ischemia. Exercise or pharmacologic stress testing may be performed and may be paired with nuclear imaging to assess myocardial perfusion. ST segment depression (>1 mm) during exercise indicates ischemia. If this test is ordered on an outpatient basis, the patient should receive appropriate discharge instructions.

Venogram: A venogram provides direct visualization of the vein after contrast has been injected, allowing visualization of an occlusion.

Clinical Conditions
Acute Aortic Dissection

Aortic dissection is a condition in which the intimal layer of the aorta tears, exposing the diseased medial layer. With each systolic pulsation, pressure in the aorta forces blood between the two layers, creating a false lumen. Stretching and enlargement of the false lumen can eventually weaken the structures, and the vessel may rupture. As the dissection enlarges, vessels branching from the aorta can dissect or become occluded. Aortic dissections occur most often in the ascending aorta but also can occur around the aortic arch, in the descending aorta, and in the abdominal aorta. Hypertension, aortic valve disease, chest trauma, congenital heart disease, and connective tissue disorders such as Marfan's syndrome are the most common causes of aortic dissection.

Symptoms
- Anterior chest, back, periscapular, abdominal, and lumbar pain are the most common presenting symptoms, usually acute in onset and described as severe and "tearing" or "knife-like" in nature. Pain can migrate as the dissection progresses.
- Systolic and diastolic murmurs if the ascending arch is involved.
- Dizziness or an altered level of consciousness if the aortic arch is involved.
- If either subclavian artery is involved, unequal peripheral pulses or a blood pressure variation may be noted between the right and left arms.
- Significant differences in the blood pressure between the upper and lower extremities.
- Peripheral pulses may be diminished or absent.
- Decreasing hematocrit and hypovolemic shock may indicate profound blood loss.
- Decreased urine output if the renal arteries are involved.

Diagnosis
- Widening of the aorta in the area of the dissection will appear on chest or abdominal x-ray films.
- Transesophageal echocardiography (TEE) will reveal the location of the tear.
- CT scan (conventional or helical) of the chest and abdomen, with contrast, will reveal the area of dissection.
- A definitive diagnosis is made with an aortogram.

Treatment
- Controlling the arterial BP to maintain systolic pressure between 90 and 100 mm Hg and mean arterial pressures

between 60 and 80 mm Hg or at the lowest level to maintain adequate perfusion of the brain, heart, and kidneys. Sodium nitroprusside is the drug of choice for BP control; however, beta-blockers also may be used. Maintain a quiet environment.
- If the patient is in shock associated with leaking or rupture, fluid resuscitation is indicated.
- Replacement of blood loss with packed red blood cells may be necessary.
- Pain and anxiety relief
- Surgical intervention is necessary, and most often occurs on an emergent basis.

Acute Arterial Occlusion

Acute arterial occlusion results from compression or obstruction of an artery. An embolus is the most common cause, followed by thrombus and traumatic injury. Acute arterial occlusion occurs most often in patients with a history of peripheral atherosclerotic disease.

Symptoms
- Sudden onset of extremity pain and numbness
- Pale, cool, cyanotic extremity
- Absence of peripheral pulses

Diagnosis
- Doppler flow studies may show the area of arterial occlusion.
- Invasive studies such as an arteriogram will reveal arterial occlusion. Arteriogram gives the surgeon a "road map" with which to plan an operative or nonoperative intervention.

Treatment
- Initiation of an anticoagulant, such as heparin, or a fibrinolytic drug, such as tPA.
- If the occlusion is severe, the patient may require an embolectomy, thrombectomy, bypass, or angioplasty.
- Nonoperative intervention includes anticoagulation with agents such as heparin, Coumadin, aspirin, and clopidogrel, as well as pain control with opioid analgesics.

Angina

Angina results when there is a decrease in myocardial oxygen supply to the heart. This is usually related to narrowing of a coronary artery secondary to atherosclerosis or coronary vasospasm. Angina is more common in patients who have a history of angina, CAD, previous MI, hypertension, or diabetes. There are three types of angina:
- Stable angina occurs with activity, emotional duress, or extreme temperature exposure and ceases with rest or administration of nitroglycerin.

- Unstable angina occurs both at rest and with exertion and usually lasts more than 20 minutes. Episodes typically occur more often, are longer in duration, and are more severe. Unstable angina belongs to a disease continuum known as "acute coronary syndromes," because symptoms of unstable angina initially are difficult to distinguish from those of acute MI.
- Prinzmetal's or variant angina usually results from coronary vasospasm and is cyclic, occurring at the same time daily and while the person is at rest. This type of angina usually occurs in younger age-groups.

Symptoms
- Substernal or epigastric pain occurring with activity or at rest, sometimes precipitated by emotional stress.
- Pain usually lasts 3 to 5 minutes but may last up to 20 minutes.
- Pain varies in severity and may be described as heaviness, tightness, fullness, squeezing, or crushing in nature.
- Angina also may present with atypical symptoms such as:
  - Shortness of breath
  - Fatigue
  - Severe weakness
  - Presyncope or syncope
  - Palpitations
  - Pain in the neck, jaw, ear, arm, or epigastric area

Diagnosis
- If the patient is having pain at the time the ECG is performed, ischemia will be evident on the ECG as evidenced by ST-segment depression. The ST depression will return to baseline when the pain resolves.
- Cardiac enzymes will not be elevated unless muscle damage has occurred.

Treatment
- Provide oxygen, nitroglycerin for pain relief, beta-blockers, and calcium channel blockers.
- Reducing stress, assisting the patient in finding a position of comfort, reducing environmental stimuli, and maintaining a calm manner while caring for the patient also may alleviate anginal symptoms.

Cardiac Arrest/Sudden Cardiac Death
Cardiac arrest results from a lethal arrhythmia. Most often, it presents as ventricular tachycardia and ventricular fibrillation;

however, the arrhythmia may present as, or deteriorate to, asystole, or pulseless electrical activity (PEA). Cardiac arrest may occur secondary to a variety of disease processes. Palpitations, dizziness, chest pain, or shortness of breath may precede sudden cardiac death, but often there is no warning. If the patient has lived through multiple episodes of sudden death, there may be an aura that the patient can relay.

Symptoms
- Respiration, pulse, and blood pressure are absent.
- The patient is unresponsive and cyanotic, and pupils do not react to light.

Diagnosis
- Ventricular fibrillation or tachycardia, pulseless electrical activity or asystole on ECG.
- ABGs may show metabolic and respiratory acidosis if the patient has been in cardiac arrest for a prolonged period.

Treatment
- Initiate ABCs and ACLS protocol.
- Assess for the underlying cause of the arrest, such as cardiac tamponade, hypovolemia, hypoxemia, tension pneumothorax, or acidosis, and treat if possible.
- Epinephrine will be the first and most frequently used drug and may be given intravenously as well as through the endotracheal tube.
- If asystole is present, ensure that the ECG leads are properly applied. **Always** confirm asystole by checking the rhythm in two leads.
- Antiarrhythmics such as amiodarone, lidocaine, or procainamide will be administered if the rhythm is ventricular tachycardia or ventricular fibrillation.
- If the patient survives sudden death, evaluation for an automatic implantable cardioverter-defibrillator (AICD) should be initiated.
- If the patient has an AICD in place, ACLS protocol should be followed. An individual touching a patient when the AICD fires can receive up to a 2-joule shock.[4]

Cardiogenic Shock
Cardiogenic shock is a complication of an acute MI in those with severely impaired pumping function of the heart. Other causes include valvular dysfunction, ventricular septum rupture, papillary muscle rupture, arrhythmias, chest trauma, and end-stage cardiomyopathy.

Symptoms
- Symptoms are similar to those of an acute MI but are much more severe, with signs of reduced cardiac output, such as:
  - Expressions of a feeling of impending doom ("I'm going to die")
  - Confusion
  - Restlessness
  - Decreased urine output
  - Poor peripheral perfusion
  - Diaphoresis
  - Hypotension
- Signs of pulmonary congestion:
  - Crackles
  - Tachypnea
  - Orthopnea
  - Tachycardia

Diagnosis
- An electrocardiogram (ECG) to assess for cardiac arrhythmias and ST segment changes, which may indicate ischemia or infarction.
- Arterial blood gas studies show hypoxia and metabolic acidosis.

Treatment
- Provide oxygen and prepare for endotracheal intubation.
- Establish IV access.
- Anticipate administration of medications, such as:
  - Furosemide and nitrates, to reduce preload
  - Dopamine and dobutamine to increase contractility
  - Nitroprusside to decrease afterload
- If cardiac output and tissue perfusion continue to be inadequate, intraaortic balloon pump therapy may be initiated.
- ACLS protocol should be initiated if cardiopulmonary arrest occurs.

Congestive Heart Failure (CHF)

CHF occurs when the heart muscle is unable to pump adequately, resulting in vascular congestion, decreased cardiac output, and decreased tissue perfusion. CHF is often associated with pulmonary edema.

Symptoms
- Peripheral edema
- Cough
- Crackles
- Tachypnea
- Orthopnea

- Shortness of breath
- Fatigue
- Weight gain
- S_3 gallop
- Later symptoms include pink, frothy sputum, tachycardia, and cyanosis.

Diagnosis
- A chest x-ray may reveal pulmonary infiltrates and an enlarged heart.
- Hypoxemia and acidosis will be present on arterial blood gases.
- Ventricular hypertrophy and possible myocardial ischemia may be present on an ECG in the acute phase.

Treatment
- Provide oxygen (may require higher concentration of oxygen to keep saturation >95%).
- Assist the patient in maintaining a position of comfort.
- Obtain IV access for administration of furosemide, inotropic agents such as digoxin or dobutamine, or morphine to reduce anxiety and decrease the work of breathing.
- Anticipate the use of vasodilators such as nitroglycerin, nitroprusside, or hydralazine to reduce BP as well as afterload.
- Reduce anxiety as much as possible.

Endocarditis
Endocarditis is an infection of the endocardium (inner layer) and often the valves of the heart. Endocarditis can be classified as either acute or subacute. Subacute bacterial endocarditis (SBE) occurs over weeks to months, usually in those with underlying congenital heart disease or valvular heart disease. Because of the insidious onset, the clinical presentation is less acute. Acute bacterial endocarditis (ABE) has a more rapid onset, occurring over days to weeks, and the patients appear much more acutely ill. ABE also occurs in patients with no known congenital or valvular history. Risk factors for endocarditis include a history of cardiac surgery or other invasive procedure, IV drug use, congenital heart disease, or rheumatic heart disease.

Symptoms
- Fever (SBE demonstrates a low-grade fever, while ABE demonstrates a fever of greater than 102° F and has an abrupt onset.)
- Chills
- Fatigue

- Myalgia
- Weight loss
- Anorexia
- Night sweats
- Tachycardia
- New onset cardiac murmur
- Petechiae
- Signs of cardiac failure, such as peripheral edema

Diagnosis
- Elevated WBC count
- Blood cultures will be drawn to aid in identification of the causative organism.
- The serum glucose level may be increased secondary to the infectious process.
- A chest x-ray examination may show cardiomegaly.
- The erythrocyte sedimentation rate (ESR) will be elevated secondary to the ongoing inflammatory process.
- Definitive diagnosis is made by an echocardiogram that shows valvular incompetence or vegetation.

Treatment
- Administer antibiotics that are specific to the presumed causative organism.
- Provide palliative treatment for fever, such as Tylenol or ibuprofen.
- Provide symptomatic treatment of heart failure.

Myocardial Infarction

Myocardial infarction (MI) occurs when a complete or near-complete occlusion of a coronary artery produces a relative or absolute lack of blood supply to the myocardial tissue. The resulting cellular hypoxia produces ischemia, injury, and necrosis of myocardial tissue. This type of occlusion is most often related to atherosclerotic plaque formation that results in a progressive narrowing of the coronary artery. The atherosclerotic plaque ruptures, producing an uneven surface with subsequent thrombus formation and platelet aggregation, resulting in occlusion of the coronary artery. Coronary occlusion also can be caused by arterial spasm. Like unstable angina, MI is grouped into the disease continuum known as "acute coronary syndromes." Myocardial infarction can be further classified as Q-wave MI or non–Q-wave MI.

Symptoms
- Chest pain with or without radiation to the left arm, neck, or jaw. Pain may be described as sharp, heavy, tight, crushing,

burning, or squeezing in nature. The discomfort may be severe or vague and may occur at rest or during activity.

- Associated symptoms include: nausea, vomiting, diaphoresis, pallor, or shortness of breath.

Diagnosis

- A 12-lead ECG may show changes consistent with injury (see Reference Guide 7); however, changes may not be evident on the initial ECG; therefore history and risk factors should be considered.
- Cardiac serum markers (myoglobin, Troponin I, Troponin T, creatinine kinase [CK]) are released into circulation when myocardial tissue damage occurs. The markers have elevations at different times, and therefore serial testing should be performed. See Reference Guide 7 for cardiac marker elevations associated with MI.
- The creatinine kinase isoenzyme MB is specific to cardiac muscle and will be elevated in MI, but the elevation does not occur until approximately 6 hours after infarction.
- An echocardiogram may be ordered to assess cardiac wall motion and valvular function.
- Cardiac catheterization and intervention such as percutaneous transluminal coronary angioplasty (PTCA) may be performed if a coronary occlusion is detected.

Treatment

- Provide continuous cardiac monitoring.
- Administer oxygen therapy (2 L/min per nasal cannula if not in respiratory distress).
- Administer nitroglycerin titrated to pain relief and BP. If pain is not relieved by nitroglycerin, morphine sulfate IV should be administered. Morphine is the drug of choice for relief of pain associated with an acute MI.[5]
- Begin fibrinolytic therapy (tPA, retaplase, or streptokinase) or prepare for cardiac catheterization with possible percutaneous catheter-based intervention such as PTCA and/or stent placement. The earlier that fibrinolytic therapy or catheter-based intervention is initiated, the greater is the chance of survival.[5]
- Anticoagulation with heparin or a glycoprotein (IIb/IIIa) inhibitor, such as Integrilin, may be initiated.[5]
- Aspirin should be administered unless the patient has known hypersensitivity and can be administered orally, rectally, or per nasogastric tube.

- Beta-blockers such as Lopressor may be administered intravenously to reduce heart rate and blood pressure, thereby decreasing the workload of the heart.
- An intraaortic balloon pump (IABP) may be inserted to increase coronary artery perfusion, reduce afterload, and relieve continuing pain.

Pericarditis

Pericarditis is a condition in which the pericardial sac becomes inflamed by conditions such as MI, trauma, or infections. Pericarditis also can result from radiation therapy or after open-heart surgery.

Symptoms
- Sudden, severe, sharp chest pain that may radiate to the back or shoulders and increases with movement or inspiration. Pain may diminish with sitting up and leaning forward.
- A pericardial friction rub is audible along the left lower sternal border and is intensified when the patient leans forward.
- Tachycardia and hypotension may result from decreasing cardiac output associated with cardiac compression secondary to the accumulated fluid in the pericardial sac.
- Malaise
- Dyspnea

Diagnosis
- A chest x-ray examination may show cardiomegaly or evidence of a pericardial effusion.
- An ECG will show ST elevation in the limb leads and in the precordial leads but no QRS changes.
- An echocardiogram will reveal an accumulation of fluid in the pericardial sac.

Treatment
- Pericardiocentesis may be needed in the presence of cardiac tamponade or to relieve a large effusion to prevent tamponade and cardiac failure.
- Antiinflammatory drugs or analgesics will help relieve the associated pain.
- Treatment of any underlying condition such as an MI, infection, or rheumatic fever is paramount.
- Surgical interventions such as a pericardial window or pericardiectomy will reduce discomfort and accumulation of fluid.

Venous Thrombosis

Venous thrombosis is a condition in which a vein is occluded by a blood clot. The risk factors for development of blood clots arise from a triad of symptoms known as Virchow's triad: venous stasis, hypercoagulability, and intimal vessel injury. The most common cause of venous thrombosis is immobility, which occurs most often after a period of bed rest or prolonged sedentary activity such as a long airline flight. Other causes include oral contraceptive use, cancer, chemotherapy, and hypercoagulable states such as polycythemia. Venous thrombosis usually occurs in the lower extremities below the knee.

Symptoms
- Pain, tenderness, swelling, and warmth of the affected extremity.
- A positive Homan's sign (pain with dorsiflexion of the foot) may be elicited; however, it will not appear in all patients with venous thrombosis.

Diagnosis
- A venogram is a definitive indicator of a deep venous thrombosis.[6]
- Venous duplex examination is the standard diagnostic test used to diagnose a DVT.
- Serial calf measurements will show a difference from right to left and may be helpful.

Treatment
- Intravenous heparinization is the gold standard of treatment for DVT.
- Follow-up treatment includes anticoagulation with drugs such as warfarin sodium (Coumadin) or a low-molecular-weight heparin, such as Lovenox. The therapy usually will continue for 6 months to 1 year after deep venous thrombosis.
- For uncomplicated DVT, low-molecular-weight heparin may be used on an inpatient or outpatient basis.

NURSING SURVEILLANCE
- Monitor vital signs, including oxygen saturation.
- Monitor for level of pain (see Reference Guide 15).
- Administer pain medications and monitor for relief of pain.
- Monitor I & O and continually assess fluid balance.
- Monitor the ECG for any changes or arrhythmias.
- Monitor mentation, an indicator of perfusion.
- Monitor peripheral perfusion and peripheral pulses.

EXPECTED PATIENT OUTCOMES
- Pain decreases in severity as documented on the "1-to-10" pain scale.
- Systolic BP is maintained above 90 mm Hg.

- Heart rate is maintained above 60 beats/min and below 100 beats/min.
- Urine output is >30 ml/hr.
- Mental status is at baseline; the patient is awake and alert.
- Oxygen saturations are >95%.
- Peripheral perfusion is restored or maintained.

DISCHARGE IMPLICATIONS

Cardiac

- Instruct the patient and family in the signs of an MI and when medical assistance is needed for symptoms.
- Instruct the patient and family to use 911.
- Instruct the patient and family on appropriate use of sublingual nitroglycerin or nitropaste.
- Instruct the patient and family about the correct use of discharge medications and give medication information sheets to the patient or family for reference.
- Discuss the importance of CPR training in the event of a cardiac arrest.
- Provide information to the patient and family about the importance of follow-up care and risk-factor modification.

Vascular

- Instruct the patient and family in the importance of having coagulation studies checked frequently if the patient is on an anticoagulant.
- Instruct the patient in what to do in the event of reocclusion.
- Instruct patients with suspected or documented aortic aneurysms in the signs of rupture and impending rupture. Emphasize the importance of follow-up care.
- Instruct patients with peripheral vascular disease in palliative measures for pain, such as the use of support hose and elevation of the extremity.

REFERENCES

1. Giardina EG: Heart disease in women, *Int J Fertil Womens Med* 45(6):350-7; 2000.
2. Mozaffarian D, Kumanyika SK, Lemaitre RN, et al: Cereal, fruit, and vegetable fiber intake and the risk of cardiovascular disease in elderly individuals; *JAMA* 289 (13):1659-1666, 2003.
3. Halperin JL: Evaluation of patients with peripheral arterial disease, *Thromb Res* 106(6):v303-311, 2002.

4. Stillwell SB: *Mosby's critical care nursing reference*, ed 3, St. Louis, 2002, Mosby.

5. Antman EM, Anbe DT, Armstrong PW, et al: *ACC/AHA guidelines for the management of patients* with ST elevation myocardial infarction, 2004. Available at www/acc.org/clinical/guidelines/stemi/index.pdf.

chapter 6

Communicable Diseases

Deborah M. Anderson

CLINICAL CONDITIONS

Cellulitis and Skin and Soft-Tissue
    Infection
Diphtheria
Hepatitis
Human Immunodeficiency Virus
Measles
Meningococcal Infection
Mononucleosis
Mumps
Parotitis
Pertussis
Rheumatic Fever—Acute
Rubella (German measles)
Severe Acute Respiratory Syndrome (SARS)
Smallpox
Streptococcal Infection—Acute
Tetanus
Tuberculosis
Varicella (Chickenpox)

INTRODUCTION

The first step in controlling the spread of any communicable
disease is prompt identification. The next step is application
of appropriate infection-control procedures to protect
the patient, caregivers, and visitors. Communication
among caregivers, infection-control personnel, and public
health authorities is paramount in preventing disease
transmission.

FOCUSED NURSING ASSESSEMENT

Nursing assessment should focus on ventilation, perfusion,
mobility, mental status, and neurovascular status.

Ventilation
Airway
- Maintain patency of the airway.
- Patients with a stiff jaw and dysphagia are at risk of aspiration and laryngospasm. Suction equipment should be at the bedside, and the staff should be prepared to assist with intubation and to administer a neuromuscular blocking agent.

Breath Sounds
- Consolidation may be present in pneumonia associated with human immunodeficiency virus (HIV) infection and in tuberculosis (TB).
- Wheezing may be present in pertussis.

Perfusion
Apical Heart Rate
- The auscultation of a murmur may indicate acute rheumatic fever.
- A systolic mitral regurgitation murmur is best auscultated at the apex, using the diaphragm of the stethoscope while the patient holds his or her breath after exhaling.
- A diastolic aortic regurgitation murmur is best auscultated in the third left intercostal space.
- Diminished heart sounds may indicate pericardial effusion (associated with carditis induced by acute rheumatic fever).
- Palpitations and syncope may occur because of conduction defects associated with disseminated Lyme disease.

Neck Veins
- Congestive heart failure (CHF) may be a complication of acute rheumatic fever. Patients exhibit jugular venous distention and facial edema.
- Neck veins may be flat and urine output decreased in cases of hypovolemia as a result of fluid loss from vomiting and diarrhea that are caused by food poisoning.

Mobility
- Red, swollen joints that are warm to the touch may be present in cases of acute rheumatic fever.

Mental Status
- Assess the patient's level of responsiveness and record a Glasgow Coma Scale score. Some infections may produce central nervous system changes (e.g., cytomegalovirus, meningitis, or encephalitis).

Neurovascular Integrity

- Assess the neurovascular status of all extremities. Several skin and soft-tissue diseases have vascular implications (e.g., necrotizing fascitis, cellulitis, and Kaposi's sarcoma).
- Assess the vascular status of extremities by noting the level at which the skin loses its hair and becomes shiny.
- Note the transition zone from warm to cold when palpating.
- Crepitus will be present on palpation in cases of necrotizing fascitis. Because of the speed at which this disease progresses, patients with crepitus should be triaged immediately to the treatment area.
- Assess sensation using a pinprick or pinwheel. The point at which the patient begins to feel the prick and the point where the sensation turns to pain should be noted.

LIFE SPAN ISSUES

Pediatric

1. Children with TB have fewer pulmonary symptoms. They have fever, malaise, and weight loss. They have a higher incidence of extrapulmonary TB involving the brain (meningitis), hematologic system (miliary TB), and bones (arthritis).
2. Infants between 1 and 2 months of age are at the greatest risk for pertussis and its complications (seizures, encephalopathy, and pneumonia). There is a higher rate among females than among males.
3. Acute rheumatic fever rarely occurs initially with adults. School-age children are at greatest risk.
4. The older the child is when developing acute rheumatic fever; the less likelihood there is of carditis developing as a complication.
5. Children with HIV infections may exhibit enlarged lymph glands, low platelet counts, and a history of recurrent otitis media or pneumonia.
6. Hepatitis A and E are usually milder with children and have a shorter course of disease. Fever may be absent. Hepatitis B, C, and D progress to chronic liver disease more often with infants than with adults.

Adulthood

1. Mumps is more serious for an adult because complications of meningitis and epididymoorchitis (infection of the epididymis and testicles) are more common.

Geriatric Patients

1. The geriatric population is at the greatest risk of contracting tetanus. They may not be adequately immunized.
2. The geriatric population is at risk for TB because most were exposed to TB early in the century when prevalence was high (reactivation of previously acquired disease). They may have outlived their initial infecting organism and are now susceptible to reinfection. TB may present as a pleural effusion in the geriatric population and initially be misdiagnosed as CHF.

Women and Pregnancy

1. Most vaccines are contraindicated during pregnancy because they contain live virus or organism. Several communicable diseases (e.g., rubella), when contracted during the first trimester, result in a high incidence of fetal anomalies and death.
2. Hepatitis E that is transmitted by a fecal-oral route, mainly in developing countries, has a high mortality rate in pregnant women. Hepatitis caused by the hepatitis E virus is clinically indistinguishable from hepatitis A disease. Symptoms include malaise, anorexia, abdominal pain, arthralgia, and fever.
3. Women with cervical cancer, abnormal Pap smears, genital warts, recurrent pelvic inflammatory disease, and vaginal candidiasis have a higher rate of HIV infection.

INITIAL INTERVENTIONS

- Be prepared to provide an airway in cases of partial or complete airway obstruction.
- Initiate intravenous (IV) access in anticipation of fluid and medication administration for cases of hypovolemia or infection.
- Initiate cardiac monitoring when extra heart sounds are auscultated or hypotension, hypertension, or tachycardia is present.
- Initiate pulse oximetry in cases of dysphagia, dyspnea, persistent coughing, or sputum production.
- Obtain a wound or rash culture (sometimes a punch biopsy may be needed by the physician) before cleansing the wound or rash site.
- Measure and document the rash using a total body drawing, or photograph the rash (with the patient's permission).
- Administer the appropriate vaccine to provide active or passive immunity. Table 6-1 lists treatments for communicable and infectious diseases. Table 6-2 lists precautions with

Text continued on p. 249

TABLE 6-1[1,3,7,8,10-12] Comparison of Communicable Diseases

Disease	Adult Symptoms	Pediatric Symptoms	High-Risk Group	Diagnosis	Treatment	Incubation Period	Transmission Route	Peak Period	Complications
Hepatitis A	• Anorexia • Nausea and vomiting • Right-upper-quadrant abdominal pain • Diarrhea • Aversion to cigarettes • Malaise • Headache • Fever • Jaundice, dark urine, clay-colored stools	Same symptoms as adult but less severe.	• Contact with family member who is infected • Day-care centers • Foreign travel • Sexual contact with infected person • Drug users	Anti-HAV IgM antibody confirms active hepatitis A, or previous.	Supportive immunoglobulin given for anticipated exposure (0.02 ml/kg IM)	15-50 days	Fecal-oral transmission spread by saliva, contaminated food, and water.	Variable	No chronic complications; confers lifelong immunity

Continued

TABLE 6-1[1,3,7,8,10-12] Comparison of Communicable Diseases—cont'd

Disease	Adult Symptoms	Pediatric Symptoms	High-Risk Group	Diagnosis	Treatment	Incubation Period	Transmission Route	Peak Period	Complications
Hepatitis B	• Anorexia • Nausea and vomiting • Right-upper-quadrant abdominal pain • Diarrhea • Aversion to cigarettes • Malaise • Headache • Fever • Arthralgia • Jaundice, dark urine, clay-	Children often have no symptoms, but if symptoms are present will be the same symptoms as adult but less severe.	• Sexual contact with an infected person • IV drug users who share needles • Babies born to mothers with the virus • People who live with a hepatitis B carrier	• HBsAg: presence of hepatitis B surface antigen • HBeAg: "e" antigen indicates high infectivity	Hepatitis B immune globulin (0.06 ml/kg IM) and hepatitis B vaccine given after exposure (0, 1, 6 mo)	45-180 days	Parenteral or sexual transmission via blood, blood products, saliva, cerebrospinal fluid; peritoneal, pleural, pericardial fluid; synovial fluid, amniotic fluid, semen, vaginal secretions, unfixed tissues/organs,	Variable	• Chronic hepatitis • Liver cancer • Cirrhosis

			Health-care workers				and any other body fluid containing blood.	Variable	• Chronic hepatitis • Cirrhosis • Liver cancer
	colored stools								
Hepatitis C	• Insidious onset • Anorexia • Nausea and vomiting • Right-upper-quadrant abdominal pain • Malaise • Headache • Fever • Jaundice, dark urine, clay-colored stools	Same symptoms as adult but less severe	• Health-care workers • IV drug abusers • Hemophiliacs • Renal patients	• Serology/anti-HCV (EIA) • PCR and TMA amplification can detect low levels of HCV RNA in serum. • HCV RNA is a reliable indicator for demonstrating that hepatitis C	• Symptomatic treatment • Corticosteroids may be used • Immunoglobulin (0.06 ml/kg within first 2 weeks of exposure)	• 2 weeks to 6 months • Chronic infection up to 20 years before cirrhosis or hepatoma	• Percutaneous transmission through blood transfusions, pooled plasma products, IV drug abuse, hemodialysis • Body tattooing and piercing		

Continued

TABLE 6-1[1,3,7,8,10-12] Comparison of Communicable Diseases—cont'd

Disease	Adult Symptoms	Pediatric Symptoms	High-Risk Group	Diagnosis	Treatment	Incubation Period	Transmission Route	Peak Period	Complications
	• Blood dyscrasia • Arthritis • Hepatomegaly			infection is present and is the most specific test for infection.					
Hepatitis D (coinfection with hepatitis B)	• Symptoms similar to those of hepatitis B • Hepatomegaly • Jaundice is more severe symptoms than seen with		• IV drug abusers • Hemophiliacs	Anti–hepatitis D antibodies in serum (RIA or EIA)	Hepatitis B immune globulin and hepatitis B vaccine given after exposure	2-8 weeks	Parenteral or sexual transmission	Variable	Chronic hepatitis

	Signs and Symptoms		Populations at Risk	Diagnosis	Treatment	Incubation	Transmission	Prognosis	Comments
		hepatitis B alone.							
Hepatitis E	• Anorexia • Nausea and vomiting • Right-upper-quadrant abdominal pain • Jaundice	Occurs rarely in children	• Visitors to developing countries • Rare in United States	• Depends on clinical presentation • Serologic test • For antibody to HEV available only in research labs	Symptomatic	15-64 days	Fecal-oral; spread by contaminated water	Variable	High mortality rate in pregnant women
Human immunodeficiency virus	• Flu-like symptoms • Lymphadenitis • Vaginal candidiasis • Recurrent shingles • Oral candidiasis	• Flu-like symptoms • Lymphadenitis • Vaginal candidiasis • Recurrent shingles • Oral candidiasis	• Homosexuals, predominantly male • IV drug abusers • Hispanics • Blacks • Sex	Rapid ELISA used to screen for infection. If positive, it is confirmed with Western blot test or the IFA test.	• A variety of combination drug therapies are used to reduce HIV RNA levels, maintain	• Variable • Time from HIV infection to AIDS: range 1-15 yr • Most adults	Parenteral or sexual transmission	Variable	May present first with hepatitis B, syphilis, and tuberculosis

Continued

TABLE 6-1[1,3,7,8,10-12] Comparison of Communicable Diseases—cont'd

Disease	Adult Symptoms	Pediatric Symptoms	High-Risk Group	Diagnosis	Treatment	Incubation Period	Transmission Route	Peak Period	Complications
	• Skin condition • Fatigue • Visual changes • Fever • Sore throat	• Skin condition • Fatigue • Visual changes • Fever • Sore throat	workers (prostitutes) • Hemophiliacs		or raise CD4+ T cell counts, and delay the development of HIV-related symptoms. • Treatment of opportunistic infections (e.g., *Pneumocystis, Candida*)	develop AIDS within 10 years. • Mean incubation period in infants is shorter.			
Lyme disease	• Bull's-eye rash	• Bull's-eye rash	• People with	• Clinical findings	Doxycycline, ampicillin,	3-32 days	Bite of tick infected	Summer and	• Carditis • Encephalitis

• Fever • Headache • Neck pain • Myalgia	• Fever • Headache • Neck pain • Myalgia • Joint and tendon pain • Malaise • Cardiac anomalies	outdoor occupations such as farming or forestry • Hikers in New England, mid-Atlantic, north central U.S. regions	• Serologic test: • IFA, ELISA • Western blot • Punch biopsy of rash shows spirochetes with antibodies to *Borrelia burgdorferi*	or Ceftin	with *B. burgdorferi*	early fall	• Arthritis
Mumps	• Epididymo-orchitis • Testicular atrophy • Meningitis	• Low-grade fever • Headache • Vomiting • Sore throat • Unilateral or bilateral	15-19-yr-olds (not vaccinated or infected)	Complement fixation, hemagglutination inhibition, and enzyme-linked	• Symptomatic • Adult males are placed on bed rest • Analgesics • Immunization	• 15-18 days average • Range 14-25	• Droplet, oral contact • Contact with articles recently contaminated with saliva	Winter and early spring	• Orchitis • Oophoritis • Meningo-encephalitis • Pancreatitis

Continued

TABLE 6-1[1,3,7,8,10-12] Comparison of Communicable Diseases—cont'd

Disease	Adult Symptoms	Pediatric Symptoms	High-Risk Group	Diagnosis	Treatment	Incubation Period	Transmission Route	Peak Period	Complications
		parotid swelling		immunosorbent assay tests	of contacts				
Pertussis	Persistent cough lasting >7 days	• Paroxysmal cough • Whoop • Cough-induced vomiting • Leukocytosis	• Infants 1-2 mo old • Females > males • < 3 doses of DTP vaccine	• Antipertussis toxin 1 g G-antibody measured by enzyme-linked immunosorbent assay • Culture of nasopharyngeal secretions	Erythromycin	7-20 days	• Direct contact with respiratory secretions • Airborne route by droplets • Respiratory isolation for known cases	Every 3-4 yr	• Pneumonia • Seizures • Cranial nerve abnormalities

Disease									
Rheumatic fever—acute	Appears rarely as primary disease in adults	• Fever • Malaise • Weight loss • Arthralgia • Carditis • Chorea • Subcutaneous nodules	• Ethnic groups • Group aged 3-15 yr • Military • School populations	• Presence of streptococcal antibodies • Positive throat culture for group A *Streptococcus*	• Salicylates • Supportive treatment • Steroids may be given for carditis	2-3 weeks	Initial infection with group A *Streptococcus* (usually strep throat or fever)	Variable	• Carditis/valve disease • Polyarthritis • Chorea
Rubella	• Rash • Low-grade fever • Malaise • Conjunctivitis • Sore throat	Pink papular rash on face and neck that spreads to extremities	7 mo to 40 yr	Rubella antibody assay tests	• Symptomatic • Antipyretics (no aspirin) • Immunization of contacts	14-21 days	Airborne transmission and/or direct contact with saliva	Winter and early spring	• Arthralgia • Arthritis • Congenital rubella syndrome for infants born to females who acquire rubella in first trimester of pregnancy

Continued

239

TABLE 6-1 [1,3,7,8,10-12] Comparison of Communicable Diseases—cont'd

Disease	Adult Symptoms	Pediatric Symptoms	High-Risk Group	Diagnosis	Treatment	Incubation Period	Transmission Route	Peak Period	Complications
Rubeola (typical)	• Fever • Macular rash progressing head to toe • Koplik's spots • Photophobia • Leukopenia	• Fever • Macular rash progressing head to toe • Koplik's spots • Photophobia • Leukopenia	• Persons in late teens and early 20s • Children with vitamin A deficiency	Hemagglutination inhibition and complement-fixation tests	• Symptomatic • Antipyretics • Fluids • Dark room • Measles vaccine within 72 hours of exposure	• Average 10 days • 7-18 days from exposure to onset of fever • 14 days until rash appears	• Airborne by droplet spread • Direct contact with secretions	Winter and spring	• Pneumonia • Encephalitis
Rubeola (atypical) occurs in persons previously immunized with original	• Abrupt onset • Headache • Arthralgia • Abdominal pain • Macular rash start-	• Headache • Arthralgia • Abdominal pain • Macular rash starting with extremities	Adults born between 1957 and 1967	Hemagglutination inhibition and complement-fixation tests	Symptomatic	10-14 days	Droplets from nasopharyngeal tract	Winter and spring	• Rare • Encephalitis • Acute thrombocytopenic purpura

killed-virus measles vaccines.	ing with extremities and moving central	and moving central							
Tetanus	• Pain • Stiffness in the jaw, abdomen, or back • Dysphagia • Reflex spasms	• Pain • Stiffness in the jaw, abdomen, or back • Dysphagia • Reflex spasms	• Occupational groups (wounds obtained in farming, forestry activities) • Persons over age 50	• Cultured from wound swab • Negative culture results do not always mean tetanus is not present.	• 500-6000 units IM of human tetanus immunoglobulin • Benzodiazepines to treat spasms • Neuromuscular blocking agents (e.g., pancuronium)	• 2 hr • 5 to 10 days after infection, or as late as 50 days after infection	Contact between an open wound and spores in the soil	Variable, based on contact with soil, especially where horses are present	Respiratory failure
Tuberculosis	• Changes in mental status	• Children may have more extra-	• Foreign-born persons	• Presence of acid-fast bacilli on	Respiratory isolation	2-10 weeks, although can be	• Airborne route Isolation:	Variable	• Meningitis • Hematologic

Continued

TABLE 6-1 [1,3,7,8,10-12] Comparison of Communicable Diseases—cont'd

Disease	Adult Symptoms	Pediatric Symptoms	High-Risk Group	Diagnosis	Treatment	Incubation Period	Transmission Route	Peak Period	Complications
	• Weight loss • Fever • Night sweats • Cough • Hemoptysis • Chest pain (treatment for adults is 6 months)	pulmonary symptoms (e.g., abdominal pain) (treatment for children is 9 months)	from India, China, Philippines • Alcoholics, IV drug abusers • Institutionalized individuals (prisons, nursing homes)	sputum smear • Lesions on chest x-ray • Positive tuberculin skin test		latent for more than 50 yr (immunosuppressed individuals usually will develop active TB within 4-8 weeks)	• Strict respiratory isolation • Negative pressure room • PPE: N95 respiratory • If patient out of room: mask		abnormalities • Pleural effusion
Multidrug-resistant	• Cough • Weight loss	• Cough • Weight loss	Immuno-compro-	Anergy testing comparing	Treatment: four drugs	2-10 weeks, although	• Exposure by airborne	Variable	• Meningitis • Hematologic

| tuberculosis | • Diarrhea
• Abdominal pain | • Diarrhea
• Abdominal pain
• Changes in mental status | mised individuals (HIV positive) | reaction to purified protein derivative with other antigen reactions | are necessary in the initial phase for the 6-month regimen to be maximally effective. Thus, in most circumstances, the treatment regimen for all adults with previously untreated tuberculosis should consist | can be latent for more than 50 yr (immunosuppressed individuals usually will develop active TB within 4-8 weeks) | droplet nuclei when patient laughs, talks, coughs, sneezes, sings Isolation:
• Strict respiratory
• NPV
• PPE: N95 respirator for staff
• If patient out of room: mask | abnormalities
• Pleural effusion |

Continued

TABLE 6-1 [1,3,7,8,10-12] Comparison of Communicable Diseases—cont'd

Disease	Adult Symptoms	Pediatric Symptoms	High-Risk Group	Diagnosis	Treatment	Incubation Period	Transmission Route	Peak Period	Complications
					of a 2-month initial phase of ionized (INH), rifampin (RIF), pyrazinamide (PZA), and ethambutol (EMB) until drug susceptibility is determined.				
Varicella (chicken-pox)	• Low-grade fever • Lesions in several	• Low-grade fever • Lesions in several	Immuno-compromised individuals	Immuno-fluorescent detection of viral	Antihista-mines; 125-625 units of	10-21 days	Direct contact with vesicle discharge or mucous	Winter and spring	• Encephalitis • Pneumonia • May precede

stages (macules, papules, vesicles, crusted lesions) • Rash appears on trunk, then face and scalp. • Lesions in mouth, throat, and conjunctiva	stages (macules, papules, vesicles, crusted lesions) • Rash appears on trunk, th⬛n face and scalp. • Lesions ⬛ mouth, throat, a⬛d conjunc⬛va	antigen ir lesions, culture, cr serologic findings confirms the diagnosis.	varicella immuno-globulin within 96 hr of exposure; use in pregnant women, immuno-compromised	membranes
				Reye's syndrome

TABLE 6-2[3,9-12] **Vaccine Precautions**

Vaccine	Side Effects	Dose	Special Considerations
Measles, mumps, and rubella (MMR)	Rash, low-grade fever, seizures, arthritis	• 0.5 ml Sub-Q • Pediatric: first dose at 15-18 mo, second dose at 4-6 yr	Contraindicated in pregnancy, persons allergic to eggs or who have hypersensitivity reaction to neomycin
Diphtheria, tetanus, pertussis (DTP)	Fever, crying, irritability, seizures	0.5 ml IM	• Persons with known seizure history are at greater risk of experiencing seizure after administration • Persons with ≥105° F temperature or persistent crying after previous administration should not receive another dose
Tetanus toxoid (Td) diphtheria	Local redness and tenderness, headache, malaise	• 0.5 ml IM or Sub-Q • Adult booster every 10 years	Contraindicated in persons with a known allergy to gamma globulin or thimerosal
Tuberculin skin test	Local redness at injection site	0.1 ml of 5 tuberculin units of purified protein derivative ID	• Induration (degree to which tissue is hard or firm), not erythema, is significant • Test should be read within 48-72 hr

Continued

Varicella vaccine	Rash, low-grade fever, malaise	• Adults: 2 doses of 0.5 ml Sub-Q, 4-8 weeks between doses. • Pediatric: give at age 12 mo or older, one dose of 0.5 ml Sub-Q.	• Caution: wait 5 wk if immune globulin has been given. • Do not give to immunocompromised or pregnant patient, active TB or febrile illness.[8]
Rabies	• Local pain • Low-grade fever	Dose dependent on formulation	• For known hypersensitivity to vaccine, if revaccination necessary, give antihistamines. • Corticosteroids, immunosuppressive agents interfere with development of active immunity.
Vaccinia	Fever	Multiple puncture technique with bifurcated needle in deltoid or posterior aspect of triceps	Severe reaction: eczema vaccinatum localized or systemic
Influenza	Local soreness	0.5 ml	• Most influenza vaccine distributed in the United States contains thimerosal, a mercury-containing compound, as a

TABLE 6-2[3,9-12] **Vaccine Precautions—cont'd**

Vaccine	Side Effects	Dose	Special Considerations
			preservative, but influenza vaccine with reduced thimerosal content is available in limited quantities (see Inactivated Influenza Vaccine).
			• Because of the increased risk of influenza-related complications, women who will be beyond the first trimester of pregnancy (>14 weeks' gestation) during the influenza season should be vaccinated.
Pneumococcal Conjugate (pediatric) Polysaccharide (adult)	• Local pain • Erythema	0.5 ml	• Febrile seizures more common in PCV7. • Check if also received Dew vaccine concurrently if seizure. • Safety of polysaccharide vaccine during the first trimester of pregnancy has not been evaluated.

BOX 6-1   VACCINATION PEARLS OF WISDOM

1. Cellular pertussis vaccines have been developed that provide protective immunity with fewer side effects (fever, crying, irritability, seizures, and encephalopathy).
2. The combination antigen vaccine DTP (diphtheria, tetanus, and pertussis) is used for children less than 7 years of age. Tetanus and diphtheria (Td) is recommended for individuals 7 years of age and older because side effects from the pertussis vaccine are more severe in this age-group.
3. If a series of immunizations is started but is interrupted, it is not necessary to restart the series or to give extra doses.
4. Patients who served in the armed forces since 1941 can be assumed to have received at least one dose of tetanus vaccine.
5. An episode of tetanus does not provide immunity, so a complete series of immunizations is indicated.
6. Persons who received the measles vaccine from 1957 to 1967 should receive additional vaccination or have a measles antibody titer drawn to confirm immunity.

selective vaccines. Box 6-1, Vaccination Pearls of Wisdom, discusses misperceptions about vaccination to provide a resource for answering patient and parent questions.

- Nursing care priorities are listed in the table on pp. 250-251.

PRIORITY DIAGNOSTIC TESTS

Laboratory Tests

Alanine transaminase (SGPT): This level may be elevated in hepatitis.

Anergy testing: Anergy testing is performed to identify a reduction or lack of an immune response to a specific antigen. Anergy testing may be initiated in the emergency department (ED) for geriatric and immunocompromised patients because these individuals may have a fading immune response to organisms to which they have been previously exposed.

Antibody tests: These tests can detect exposure to a particular organism if the patient is able to mobilize an immune response to the organism. The development of antibodies against a particular organism is a positive test result. Antibody tests are used to detect exposure to hepatitis, *Streptococcus,* mumps, and several other diseases.

NURSING CARE PRIORITIES

Potential/Actual Problem	Causes	Signs and Symptoms	Interventions
Potential for ineffective airway clearance	• Excessive sputum production • Inability to control secretions • Laryngospasm • Nasopharyngeal edema	• Dyspnea • Anxiety • Cyanosis • Decreased oxygen saturation • Increased respiratory rate • Cough • Upper airway rhonchi	• Monitor oxygen saturation. • Administer humidified oxygen. • Suction to remove accumulated secretions. • Ensure adequate hydration.
Inadequate fluid volume	• Dehydration • Nausea resulting in a decreased intake • Vomiting • Diarrhea	• Decreased blood pressure • Thirst • Delayed capillary refill • Elevated heart rate • Altered mental status • Decreased urine output • Dry mucous membranes • Pale color	• Initiate intravenous access for fluid administration. • Monitor vital signs, including orthostatic vital signs. • Monitor intake and output.

| Decreased cardiac output | • Pericardial effusion
• Valve disease | • Altered level of consciousness
• Decreased urinary output
• Increased heart and respiratory rates
• Diminished pulse quality
• Dependent edema
• Rales
• Pale, cool extremities | • Administer oxygen.
• Minimize activity to reduce oxygen demands.
• Administer diuretics as ordered.
• Anticipate the need for surgical repair. |
| Pain | • Vomiting
• Diarrhea
• Skin lesions | • Complaints of pain
• Blood pressure and heart rate changes
• Crying/moaning
• Irritability
• Facial grimacing
• Restlessness | • Pain medications as ordered, preferably intravenously
• Nonpharmacological interventions such as relaxation therapy, guided imagery, music therapy
• Monitor oxygen saturation with pulse oximetry (maintain saturation above 94%).
• Monitor vital signs after pain medication.
• Patient to reassess pain using a pain scale. |

NURSING ALERT

Occasionally a patient wants his or her TB test read in the ED. Reactions should be read within 48 to 72 hours after administration. Induration (the degree to which the tissue is hard on palpation), not erythema, is significant. The following parameters should be used:

- 5 mm of induration is positive in a person with recent TB exposure, an HIV-positive individual, and a person with a chest film indicative of TB lesions.
- 10 mm of induration is positive in increased-risk groups.
- 15 mm of induration is positive in all groups.

Aspartate transaminase (SGOT): This level may be elevated in hepatitis.

Bilirubin: Serum bilirubin levels are elevated in hepatitis.

CD4 count: This is a measurement of the number of helper-T lymphocytes in the blood that bear the CD4 surface molecule, which is the cellular receptor for HIV.

CD8 count: This is a measurement of the number of suppressor lymphocytes. People who are not infected with HIV tend to have more CD4 than CD8 lymphocytes.

C-reactive protein: This value may be elevated in Lyme disease.

Complete blood count (CBC): Leukocytosis may be present, with an increased lymphocyte count for children who have pertussis or measles.

Culture and sensitivity testing: Wounds may be cultured for the presence of spirochetes (Lyme disease) and tetanus. Vesicles may be aspirated after cleansing with povidone-iodine solution and rinsing with alcohol, using a small-gauge needle attached to a tuberculin syringe. Sputum cultures may be performed to test for acid-fast bacilli (tuberculosis). Nasopharyngeal cultures may be performed to detect *Streptococcus* and pertussis infections. Stool cultures may be obtained to identify the causative organism in suspected cases of food poisoning.

Erythrocyte sedimentation rate: This value may be elevated in Lyme disease.

Immunofluorescence assay (IFA): A test used to identify HIV in infected cells.

Monospot: This heterophil agglutination test detects antibodies to the Epstein-Barr virus (the usual causal agent for mononucleosis).

Rapid antigen tests: These tests detect cell wall antigen of dead or viable bacteria and viruses by means of latex agglutination or enzyme-linked immunosorbent assay (ELISA). A positive test result indicates a current or previous infection.

Western blot test: This test is used to confirm the presence of certain antibodies as a follow-up to enzyme-linked immunosorbent assay testing. Viral proteins (e.g., HIV) are readily visualized.

Radiographic Tests

Chest x-rays: A chest film may be ordered to detect lesions in tuberculosis. Cardiac enlargement and pericardial effusion may be detected in cases of carditis with acute rheumatic fever.

Extremity x-rays: These may be ordered in cases of skin and soft-tissue infection to rule out osteomyelitis or the presence of a foreign body or pathologic fracture.

Radionuclide scans: These may be used to confirm osteomyelitis. Increased radionuclide uptake in any area is a positive result for that area.

Other Tests

Echocardiogram: An echocardiogram may be obtained to document pericardial effusion and valve disease associated with acute rheumatic fever.

Electrocardiogram: The P-R interval may be prolonged in carditis (associated with acute rheumatic fever), producing a first-degree or second-degree heart block.

Lumbar puncture with cerebrospinal fluid (CSF) analysis: Certain communicable diseases may result in encephalopathy and meningitis. CSF is examined for antibodies to specific organisms, to confirm that neurologic complications are related to progression of a specific disease.

Clinical Conditions
Cellulitis and Skin and Soft-Tissue Infection

Cellulitis is a bacterial infection of the connective tissue of the skin seen most often in the face and lower legs, although it can occur elsewhere.

Symptoms
- Erythema, tenderness, edema, and increased warmth
- Possible fever, chills, muscle aches, malaise
- Enlargement of regional lymph nodes
- Blisters may be present.

- In children, facial cellulitis may result from *Haemophilus influenzae* infection. The skin becomes dusky and purplish with facial edema.
- Ludwig's angina is a type of cellulitis that results from infection of the second and third lower molar. It is a rare but life-threatening illness characterized by tongue swelling, dysphagia, and drooling.

Diagnosis

- A skin biopsy may be performed, but diagnosis in the ED setting often is based on clinical presentation.

Treatment

- Antibiotics are initiated.
- Surgical drainage may be used for abscesses.
- Analgesics will be administered before drainage.
- Assess the tetanus status and administer Td or Hyper-Tet as indicated.
- Cultures of the drainage should be obtained before starting antibiotic therapy.
- Heat application may facilitate drainage and earlier healing.
- Elevation of the affected part reduces edema and pain.
- Bleeding wounds should be dressed in dry gauze until the bleeding stops.
- A wet-to-dry saline dressing can be applied to draining wounds.
- In Ludwig's angina, treatment focuses on airway maintenance, IV antibiotic therapy, pain control, and nutritional support.

Diphtheria

Diphtheria is a highly contagious, acute bacterial infection of the upper respiratory tract or sometimes the skin. A gray or white, adherent exudate forms over the tonsils and pharynx, which can cause obstruction of the airway. Virulent strains or untreated cases of the disease produce a toxin that can affect other organs, causing organ dysfunction including myocarditis and neuritis 2 to 6 weeks after onset. It is passed from person to person by airborne or droplet transmission. Diphtheria infections of the skin result in painful, swollen, reddened lesions that are also contagious. For more information, please refer to a communicable disease textbook, call the Centers for Disease Control and Prevention (CDC), or visit the CDC web site at www.cdc.gov.

Symptoms

- Sore throat
- Slight fever and chills

- Cold symptoms: runny nose, congestion
- Gray, adherent exudate in nose, mouth, or throat that bleeds when scraped
- Difficulty breathing if the exudate covers the glottic opening
- Systemic symptoms include those of heart failure or paralysis.

Diagnosis
- Diagnosis is determined by clinical presentation.

Treatment
- Diphtheria toxoid
- Penicillin and erythromycin may be ordered to kill the bacteria producing the toxin.
- Treatment is supportive, by artificially maintaining organ function until the toxin clears.

Isolation
Strict (non-AFB) respiratory isolation for pharyngeal exudate and contact precautions for cutaneous lesions

Hepatitis
Hepatitis is an acute inflammation of the liver. It may be produced by a virus, a chemical or drug reaction, or alcohol abuse. A viral infection is the most common cause of hepatitis, and it is typically transmitted by a fecal-oral route (hepatitis A and E) or by a blood or sexual transmission route (hepatitis B, C, D, and G).

Symptoms
Many people with hepatitis are asymptomatic. For those who experience symptoms, regardless of the origin, the symptoms are similar and include fever, malaise, anorexia, arthralgia, vomiting, diarrhea, right upper-quadrant pain, and color changes in the stool (clay), urine (dark), and skin (jaundice).

Diagnosis
- Elevation of the level of liver enzymes
- Hepatomegaly and hepatic tenderness
- Antibody testing (except in hepatitis E and G, where no test is available), and a liver biopsy. HIV and syphilis testing should be initiated.

Treatment
- General care of the patient with hepatitis includes rest, fluids, antiemetics, avoidance of alcohol, and adequate nutrition.
- Treatment of hepatitis A is supportive, consisting of rest and fluids. Immune globulin is administered to all patient contacts and to the patient. Patients usually recover with no long-term effects.
- Hepatitis B is treated symptomatically and with rest and fluids. Patients may develop a chronic infection, and hepatitis B can cause death. Medications include adefovir dipivoxil, alpha

interferon, and lamivudine. Hepatitis B testing is recommended yearly to determine the antibody level for personnel repeatedly exposed to blood. A booster vaccine should be administered if the antibody levels fall below 10 international milliunit/ml.[1]

- Hepatitis C is treated with alpha interferon and ribavirin.
- A hepatitis D infection can occur only if the patient has a hepatitis B infection; therefore prevention of hepatitis B is the best prevention for hepatitis D. Treatment for both D and E is symptomatic. Patients usually recover from hepatitis E without long-term problems. Hepatitis D, although rare, can cause death.
- Hepatitis G, the most recently identified hepatitis virus, often is found with hepatitis C. Chronic liver disease is not associated with hepatitis G.

Human Immunodeficiency Virus (HIV)

Patients may arrive at the ED with a known HIV infection or with symptoms and an unconfirmed suspicion of the disease. The goals of the ED visit should be to improve the immune status and to prevent or treat opportunistic infections.

HIV has been divided into four stages:

1. *Acute retroviral syndrome:* development of HIV-specific antibodies 1 to 3 weeks after exposure
2. *Early infection:* also called the asymptomatic phase. T cell counts remain close to normal. This stage can last for years.
3. *Early symptomatic disease:* occurs at the end of the asymptomatic phase but before a diagnosis of AIDS
4. *Acquired immune deficiency syndrome (AIDS):* This stage is diagnosed when the patient meets the defined criteria established by the Centers for Disease Control and Prevention (CDC). This usually occurs when the patient's immune system becomes severely compromised.

Symptoms

- 1-3 weeks after exposure the patient complains of flu-like symptoms that last for 1-2 weeks. CD4+ T cell counts fall initially and then return to normal.
- Swollen glands are often the first symptom of the third stage. CD4+ T cell count drops below 500-600 cells/mcl, and symptoms begin to appear, such as persistent fever, headaches, diarrhea, night sweats, malaise, weight loss, and localized infections (thrush is the most common; others include shingles, herpes outbreaks, and neurologic manifestations).
- The immune system becomes severely compromised as the disease progresses into the fourth stage, AIDS. The patient may

present with a variety of opportunistic diseases, including fungal, viral, bacterial, and protozoal infections, cancers, wasting syndrome, and dementia. A specific discussion of all opportunistic infections to which a patient with HIV and AIDS is susceptible is beyond the scope of this book.

Diagnosis

- HIV is confirmed by a positive result on the ELISA and Western blot test or the immunofluorescence assay (IFA) tests.
- Syphilis, hepatitis B, and TB testing may be performed because these diseases often occur in tandem.
- Decreased CD4+ T cell count and WBC count are predictive of opportunistic infections (see Box 6-2, CD4+ T Cell Counts and Opportunistic Infection Susceptibility).

Treatment

- There are four general classes of antiretroviral agents. Treatment usually consists of a combination of drugs.[2]
  1. Nucleoside reverse transcriptase inhibitor (zidovudine, didanosine, stavudine, lamivudine)
  2. Non-nucleoside reverse transcriptase inhibitor (nevirapine, delavirdine, efavirenza)
  3. Protease inhibitor (saquinavir, indinavir, ritonavir, nelfinavir, amprenavir). These drugs may produce anemia and thrombocytopenia.
  4. Fusion inhibitors: (enfuvirtide) reserved for patients who have failed initial regimens.
- Periodic updates of HIV/AIDS treatment guidelines are available from the CDC National AIDS Clearinghouse (800-458-5231) and posted at www.cdcnpin.org.
- Suppression and treatment of the opportunistic diseases will vary according to the specific disease.

BOX 6-2   CD4+ T CELL COUNTS AND OPPORTUNISTIC INFECTION SUSCEPTIBILITY

- T helper cell count 200-500/mm^3 = tuberculosis, Kaposi's sarcoma, thrush, and oral hairy leukoplakia
- T helper cell count 200-250/mm^3 = *Pneumocystis carinii* pneumonia, toxoplasmosis
- T helper cell count below 50/mm^3 = cytomegalovirus, lymphoma, meningitis

>   ⩹ **N U R S I N G   A L E R T** ⩺
>
> To prevent the development of viral resistance to the drugs
> being taken, it is imperative for the patient to be very
> conscientious in taking medications as scheduled and to
> avoid missing doses.

Measles (Rubeola)

Symptoms

- A dry cough, headache, low-grade fever, sore throat, Koplik's spots (small, grain-of-sand-size, irregular, bright red spots with blue-white centers, occurring on the inside of the cheek), and a nonblanching, diffuse rash.
- A hacking cough, conjunctival irritation, and photophobia may occur before the appearance of Koplik's spots.
- Atypical measles is a form of the disease that strikes individuals who received measles vaccine containing the killed measles virus instead of live attenuated virus. Persons immunized between 1957 and 1967 are at risk for atypical measles.
- Symptoms of atypical measles include a high-grade fever, edema of the feet and lips, and a rash that begins on the extremities and migrates to the head (see Figure 6-1).

Diagnosis

- Diagnosis usually is based on clinical presentation, exposure, and vaccination history.
- The WBC may be low, with lymphocytosis present.

Treatment

Treatment is symptomatic.

- Administer antipyretics and fluids.
- Rest in a darkened room may be suggested if photophobia is present.
- Administer postexposure prophylaxis to all exposed, susceptible persons such as other members of the household, preferably within 72 hours but up to 6 days after exposure, with immune globulin (0.25 mg/kg, maximum dose 15 ml; immunocompromised patients should receive 0.5 mg/kg).[3]

ISOLATION

Strict respiratory isolation is indicated for 4 days after the onset of rash. In immunocompromised patients, isolation should be for the duration of the illness.

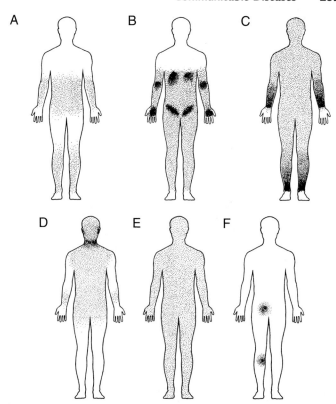

Figure 6-1 **A,** Meningococcemia. Meningococcemia begins as macules, progresses to petechiae, then forms purpura. It is located on extremities and trunk. **B,** Atypical measles. This type of measles is manifested as a maculopapular rash along skin creases. **C,** Rocky Mountain spotted fever. This fever produces a diffuse rash with heavier concentration at distal extremities. **D,** Typical measles. Typical measles starts behind the ears and moves first to the face and neck, then downward over the rest of the body; the measles appear as discrete spots on the patient's extremities. **E,** Rubella. Rubella begins on the face and progresses to the neck, trunk, and extremities, respectively. **F,** Lyme disease. Lyme disease produces a centrifugal rash that varies in diameter with a red outer border and a clearer center. The rash is seen in higher frequency in the popliteal and groin regions. The patient with Lyme disease may have multiple or singular lesions.

Meningococcal Infection

Meningococcal disease, caused by the bacteria *Neisseria meningitidis*, is transmitted by nasopharyngeal droplets. The organism can produce acute meningitis or fulminant meningococcemia characterized by disseminated intravascular coagulation (DIC) and septic shock.

Symptoms

- If the organism produces bacterial meningitis, the classic symptoms are fever, nuchal rigidity, severe headache, nausea, and vomiting. Patients also may experience photophobia, seizures, a decreased level of consciousness, and in severe cases coma.
- Petechiae and purpura are common with both the meningitis and meningococcemia forms.
- A skin rash produces lesions on the extremities and trunk (Figure 6-1).
- Lesions may be macules before becoming petechiae.
- Malaise, hypotension, and pulmonary edema with CHF may occur in sepsis.

Diagnosis

- Diagnosis is determined by clinical presentation and examination of the cerebrospinal fluid.
- CSF in bacterial cases is usually purulent.
- A Gram stain of CSF should be performed immediately and examined microscopically.
- Cultures of the cerebrospinal fluid reveal meningococci.
- Cultures of the blood, nasopharyngeal secretions, and sputum are performed.
- Send the CSF for WBC count (elevated), WBC differential (predominant white blood cell will be polymorphonuclear cells), total protein content (elevated), and glucose level (decreased).[1]
- Send additional tests as indicated for ruling out other diagnoses.
- The intracranial pressure may be elevated.

Treatment

- Droplet isolation: should wear mask when within 3 feet of patient
- Intravenous antibiotic therapy should be started as soon as cultures are obtained. Penicillin, ampicillin, and a cephalosporin (third generation) are the drugs of choice.
- Volume replacement and vasopressors may be required.
- Pain medication for headache
- Antipyretics

- Low lighting
- Consider the need for antibiotic treatment for those who have been in close or prolonged contact with the patient.

Mononucleosis

Mononucleosis is caused by the Epstein-Barr virus, a type of herpes virus. Adolescents, college students, and military recruits are most susceptible to this disease. Transmission of the virus is by nasopharyngeal droplets, primarily by kissing, coughing, sneezing, and sharing of a glass, cup, or straw.

Symptoms
- A fever, enlarged and painful lymph nodes, a sore throat, loss of appetite, and lethargy are common.
- The spleen is enlarged in some cases, with pain in the left upper quadrant of the abdomen.
- Testicular pain

Diagnosis
- A positive monospot test result confirms the diagnosis.
- Liver enzymes may be elevated if there is liver involvement.
- Lymphocytosis and leukocytosis may be present in the WBCs.

Treatment
- Supportive treatment with fluids, soft foods, and rest is recommended.
- Contact sports and aspirin products should be avoided for up to 8 weeks to help prevent splenic rupture and bleeding.

Mumps Parotitis

Mumps is an acute viral disease characterized by fever and swelling and tenderness of one or more of the salivary glands.

Symptoms
- The major symptom of mumps is nonsuppurative swelling and tenderness of the salivary glands.
- A fever often is present.
- Males may have unilateral swelling of the genitalia. Females may have mastitis.

Diagnosis
- Diagnosis is based on clinical presentation and antigen testing.
- A mumps infection confers lifelong immunity.

Treatment
- Treatment is supportive, as there is no cure.
- Antipyretics and analgesics may be ordered.
- Topical warm or cold compresses may relieve discomfort.
- Patients should be placed on bed rest until their temperatures return to normal. This appears to limit the severity of the disease.

- Scrotal support should be used in cases of orchitis and epididymitis.
- Avoid sour foods, because these foods cause pain secondary to stimulation of salivary flow.
- Isolation: strict respiratory isolation is indicated for the hospitalized patient. School children should be secluded for 9 days after the onset of swelling.[1]

Rheumatic Fever, Acute

Acute rheumatic fever is an inflammatory disease that develops only after a streptococcus bacterial infection (e.g., scarlet fever, strep throat). It affects primarily school-age children.

Symptoms
- Fever
- Arthritis in the knees, elbows, ankles, and wrists
- Joint swelling
- Chest pain and shortness of breath. Cardiac involvement can range from minor arrhythmias to severe CHF.
- Mitral and aortic valve disease may be present.
- A non-pruritic pink-red rash with a sharp outer edge (erythema marginatum) may appear on the trunk, upper arms, and legs.
- Chorea (involuntary purposeless movements of the extremities and face) may occur in conjunction with heart problems.

Diagnosis

Diagnosis is based on the revised Jones' criteria[4] (Box 6-3).

Treatment

Treatment is supportive.
- Antiinflammatory medication: salicylates (arthritis) and corticosteroids (severe carditis and congestive heart failure)
- Individuals with positive cultures for strep throat also should be treated with antibiotics.
- Continuous low-dose antibiotics (such as penicillin, sulfadiazine, or erythromycin) can be given to prevent recurrence. The amount of time low-dose antibiotics should be administered is controversial. Suggestions range from until the individual reaches 18 years of age to lifetime administration.
- Patients with valve disease will require additional antibiotic preparation before dental and surgical procedures.
- Acute rheumatic fever can be prevented by adequately treating the initial streptococcal infection. After acute rheumatic fever

BOX 6-3   REVISED JONES' CRITERIA FOR ACUTE RHEUMATIC FEVER

The patient must have evidence of a previous group-A streptococcal infection and either the presence of two major criteria or the presence of one major criterion and two minor criteria.

Major criteria
- Carditis
- Polyarthritis
- Chorea
- Erythema marginatum (skin rash)
- Subcutaneous nodules

Minor criteria
- Arthralgia
- Fever
- Prolonged P-R interval on electrocardiograph
- Elevated erythrocyte sedimentation rate
- Elevated C-reactive protein

occurs, it can reappear, and secondary prophylaxis is then indicated. Recurrences are less likely after puberty.

Pertussis (Whooping Cough)

Symptoms
- Typically two to three coughs, then a high-pitched inspiratory sound (whoop) resulting from spasm
- Pertussis begins with a low-grade fever, nasal congestion, and a mild cough. After 2 weeks, the cough worsens. Also may experience vomiting with severe coughing.
- Thick respiratory secretions
- In adults, leukocytosis and lymphocytosis may be absent, while it is often present in children with pertussis.
- Children have a greater incidence of protracted paroxysmal coughing that is worse at night.

Diagnosis

Diagnosis is confirmed by the antipertussis toxin antibody production.

Treatment
- Treatment is supportive, using fluids and antipyretics. Use humidifier to moisten secretions. May need IV fluids and oxygen support.

- Antibiotics may be ordered to prevent a bacterial respiratory infection and pneumonia.
- Monitor for signs of impending respiratory failure.

ISOLATION

Respiratory isolation for known cases. Suspected cases should be removed from the presence of young children and infants, especially unimmunized infants, until the patients have received at least 5 days of a minimum 14-day course of antibiotics.

Rubella (German Measles)

Rubella can be difficult to distinguish because it presents similarly to measles and scarlet fever. It can be passed from mother to fetus and can cause birth defects if the infection occurs in early pregnancy.

Symptoms

- A low-grade fever
- A sore throat
- A pink papular rash on the face and neck that spreads to the trunk and extremities is characteristic.
- Postauricular and suboccipital lymph nodes are enlarged and usually tender.
- The WBC count is normal.

Diagnosis

- Diagnosis is determined by rubella antibody assay tests.

Treatment

- Antipyretics and antipruritic medications may be ordered.

ISOLATION

Admitted patients suspected of having rubella should be managed under contact isolation precautions and placed in a private room; attempts should be made to prevent exposure of nonimmune pregnant women. Exclude children from school and adults from work for 7 days after onset of rash.[1]

Severe Acute Respiratory Syndrome (SARS)

SARS is a viral respiratory illness that was initially defined in November 2003. The severity of illness may be highly variable, ranging from mild illness to death.

Symptoms

- Initial presentation after exposure:
  - Fever (>100.4° F [>38.0° C])
  - Headache
  - Malaise
  - Myalgia
  - Diarrhea
- Days 3 to 7:
  - Dry, nonproductive cough

- Chest x-ray initially normal; 3 days after exposure, infiltrates are present
- Dyspnea, which may cause hypoxemia (10% to 20% of these cases will require intubation and ventilation)
- Leukopenia
- Thrombocytopenia
- Low platelets

Diagnosis

- Diagnosis is based on clinical presentation.
- If SARS is suspected, notify your local health authority, CDC, or the World Health Organization (WHO) for specific instructions on specimen collection, specimen packaging, and specimen destination instructions.

Treatment

Treatment is symptomatic. The most efficacious treatment regimen, if any, currently is unknown.[5] Treatment regimens have included several antibiotics to presumptively treat known bacterial agents of atypical pneumonia. In several locations, therapy also has included antiviral agents such as oseltamivir or ribavirin. Steroids also have been administered orally or intravenously to patients in combination with ribavirin and other antimicrobials.

> **NURSING ALERT**
>
> Wear full protective attire as required for contact and airborne precautions (disposable gown, utility gloves, and N95 respirator) plus eye protection (goggles or face shield) as long as the patient is in the room. After the patient has been transferred or discharged, wear gown and gloves for postdischarge cleaning. Postpone initiation of cleaning to allow time for the ventilation system to remove any residual airborne viral particles. Check with facility's engineering director.

In the United States, the CDC requests that reports of suspected cases be directed to the SARS Investigative Team at the CDC Emergency Operations Center, telephone (770) 488-7100. Outside the United States, clinicians who suspect cases of SARS are requested to report such cases to their local public health authorities. Additional information about SARS (e.g., infection-control guidance and procedures for reporting suspected cases) is available at www.cdc.gov/ncidod/sars.[4]

Smallpox

There are two clinical forms of smallpox, variola major and variola minor. Variola major is the severe and most common form of smallpox, with a more extensive rash and higher fever. There are four types of variola major smallpox: ordinary (the most common type, accounting for 90% or more of cases), modified (mild and occurring in previously vaccinated persons), flat, and hemorrhagic. Both of the latter types are rare and very severe. Variola major has a historic overall fatality rate of about 30%, but flat and hemorrhagic smallpox usually is fatal. Variola minor is a less common presentation of smallpox and a much less severe disease, with historic death rates of 1% or less.[6]

Transmission

- Direct and fairly prolonged face-to-face contact generally is required to spread smallpox from one person to another. Smallpox also can be spread through direct contact with infected bodily fluids or contaminated objects such as bedding or clothing.
- The infected person is contagious until the last smallpox scab falls off.

Symptoms[6]

The symptoms of the most common type of smallpox, ordinary smallpox, vary depending on the number of days since exposure.

Incubation period: Duration 7 to 17 days: not contagious

- No symptoms during this period

Prodrome phase: Duration 2 to 4 days: sometimes contagious

- Fever (101° to 104° F), malaise, aching, vomiting (sometimes)
- Patient feels poorly

Early rash: Duration about 4 days: highly contagious

- A macular rash first develops on the tongue and in the mouth as small red spots. These spots become sores that break open and deposit large amounts of the virus into the mouth and throat. The patient is most contagious during this phase. Simultaneously, as the sores are breaking open, the fever declines and a macular rash develops on the face, spreading to the arms and legs, then to the hands and feet. Within 24 hours the rash covers the entire body.
- After 3 days, the rash transforms into papular lesions, which will fill with a thick, opaque fluid. A depression in the center of the papule produces one of the major distinguishing characteristics of smallpox: The lesions often are described as looking like a belly button.

- Fever may rise again (may remain high until the lesions scab).

Pustular rash: Duration about 5 days: contagious

- The lesions become pustules that are round and firm to the touch.

Pustules and scabs: Duration about 5 days: contagious

- The pustules form a crust and then a scab. By 2 weeks after the rash appeared, most of the sores have scabbed over.

Resolving scabs: Duration about 6 days: contagious

- Scabs are falling off, leaving marks on the skin that will become pitted scars.

Scabs resolved: No longer contagious

Diagnosis

- History and physical exam, especially if an outbreak is documented
- Microscopic identification of the virus in the vesicle fluid
- Polymerase chain reaction (PCR) will identify the virus in vesicle fluid or blood within a few hours.
- If the risk for smallpox is high, clinicians who suspect cases of smallpox are asked to immediately contact the local or state health departments. Outside the United States, clinicians who suspect cases of smallpox are requested to report such cases to their local public health authorities.

Treatment

Treatment is largely supportive.

- Isolation until all pox scabs fall off (3 to 4 weeks)
- The smallpox vaccine, if administered within 3 days of exposure, may reduce the severity of symptoms the patient experiences.
- Adequate fluid intake
- Pain and fever control
- Prevention of bacterial superinfection by keeping lesions clean

Additional information about smallpox (e.g., infection-control guidance and procedures for reporting suspected cases) is available at www.cdc.gov.

Isolation

- Place patient in a private, negative-airflow room (airborne infection isolation) if available. If not available, place patient in private room and keep door closed. Keep doors closed at all times, except when patient or staff must enter or exit.
- Staff and visitors should wear N95 or higher quality respirators, gloves, and gowns.
- Patients should wear a surgical mask when outside the negative-pressure isolation room and must be gowned or wrapped in a sheet so that their rash is fully covered.

Streptococcal Infection, Acute

Acute streptococcal infection usually presents as a sore throat. However, children may have only fever and rash.

Symptoms

- The patient may have a high fever (>38.5° C or 101.5° F), headache, nausea, and vomiting.
- Pharyngeal edema, exudative tonsillitis, and enlarged and tender cervical lymph glands may be present. Coincident otitis media may be present.
- The rash of scarlet fever (red, diffuse macules) may be present.

Diagnosis

- A throat culture positive for group-A beta-hemolytic *Streptococcus* remains the criterion standard for the diagnosis of streptococcal pharyngitis. Culture results will be available in 24 to 48 hours. The patient also may have an increased serum level of antistreptolysin O or other antibodies to *Streptococcus*.
- A rapid strep test may be performed, with results available within 10 to 20 minutes. If the rapid strep test result comes back positive, appropriate antibiotic therapy should be initiated. A negative rapid test does not exclude the diagnosis of an acute strep infection; therefore, if the rapid strep test results are negative, a culture can be performed.

Treatment

- Antibiotic therapy is indicated for at least 10 days to prevent complications from strep infection, such as acute rheumatic fever.
- Amoxicillin is the drug of choice for treating children.
- Cephalosporin or erythromycin is recommended for penicillin-allergic individuals. Beware of potential for cross-sensitivity in patients who are allergic to penicillin.

Tetanus

Tetanus is caused by a spore-forming rod found in contaminated soil. It most often follows an acute injury, but it also can infect chronic wounds (e.g., decubiti and skin abscesses). The disease symptoms result from a potent neurotoxin released from the spores, which affects the function of the reflex arc in the spinal cord and brainstem. The spores can live in the body for months or years, producing disease at a time removed from the initial injury.

Symptoms

Tetanus produces rigidity and spasms of skeletal muscle. The toxin spreads by way of the circulation.

- Nerves with the shortest axons are affected first.
- Symptoms begin in the facial muscles and jaw, progressing to the neck, trunk, and extremities. The muscles become

progressively rigid. Apnea and hypoxia can result from spasms of the respiratory muscles and the larynx.

- Dyspnea and dysphagia are common.
- Generalized spasms occur, often induced by sensory stimuli. The spasms resemble epileptic seizures and are very painful. Spasms can be severe enough to cause fractures and muscle injury.
- The autonomic nervous system may malfunction, causing severe hypertension, arrhythmias, and cardiac arrest.
- Urinary retention may occur.

Diagnosis
- Diagnosis usually is based on clinical presentation. Attempts for laboratory confirmation are of little help. The organism rarely is recovered from sites of infection, and usually there is no detectable antibody response.

Treatment
- Place the patient in a quiet, darkened room to reduce sensory input.
- Rapid deterioration is expected; therefore the patient is intubated and given neuromuscular blocking agents (e.g., pancuronium).
- Tetanus toxoid booster and tetanus immune globulin are administered to prevent further absorption of the toxin. (See Reference Guide 23, Tetanus Immunization Guide.)
- Wounds should be cleaned and debrided.

Tuberculosis
Tuberculosis is an infectious disease caused by the *Mycobacterium tuberculosis* bacteria and most often affects the lungs but can affect the kidneys, bones, adrenal glands, lymph nodes, and meninges. It is spread by airborne droplets and usually is transmitted when there is frequent, close exposure.

Symptoms
- Initially person is symptom free.
- Fatigue, night sweats, anorexia, and weight loss are the predominant symptoms.
- Cough with purulent sputum
- Dull chest pain or chest tightness
- It is possible to have active disease without symptoms.

Diagnosis
- Diagnosis usually is based on a positive tuberculin skin test result and lesions appearing on a chest film. (A patient may take from 3 to 10 weeks after exposure to develop the immune response that will result in a positive tuberculin skin test.)

- Immunocompromised patients may not be able to mount an immune response; diagnosis may be based on clinical presentation alone.
- Microscopic analysis of sputum samples for the acid-fast bacilli.
- Culture of the mycobacterium is the most accurate test, but results may take 6 to 8 weeks.

Treatment

- Because of the relatively high proportion of adult patients with tuberculosis caused by organisms that are resistant to isoniazid, four drugs are necessary in the initial phase for the 4-month to 7-month regimen to be maximally effective. Thus, in most circumstances, the treatment regimen for all adults with previously untreated tuberculosis should consist of a 2-month initial phase of isoniazid (INH), rifampin (RIF), pyrazinamide (PZA), and ethambutol (EMB) until drug susceptibility is determined.[8]
- Baseline liver function should be assessed before any TB medication is started because of the potential for hepatitis. Liver enzymes should be monitored during therapy because of the risk of drug-induced hepatitis.
- Visual acuity must be examined before and during ethambutol therapy.

Isolation

TB precautions in the ambulatory-care setting should include:

1. Placing these patients in a separate area apart from other patients and not in open waiting areas
2. Giving these patients surgical masks to wear and instructing them to keep their masks on
3. Giving these patients tissues and instructing them to cover their mouths and noses with the tissues when coughing or sneezing[7,8]

All persons who enter an isolation room should wear respiratory protection. Visitors should wear respirators while in the isolation room and should be given general instructions on how to use them. To prevent the escape of droplet nuclei, the TB isolation room should be maintained under negative pressure. Doors to the isolation room should be kept closed except when patients or personnel must enter or exit the room so that negative pressure can be maintained.

- All staff caring for patient should wear fit-tested N95 respirators.[1,7,8]

> ### NURSING ALERT
>
> Both ED and prehospital personnel should receive tuberculin skin testing every 6 months because of their high potential for exposure. Personnel should wear N95 respirators when suctioning the airway of high-risk individuals.[1,8]

Varicella (Chickenpox)
Symptoms
- The rash associated with chickenpox is extremely pruritic and ranges from macules to papules to vesicles, with crusted lesions simultaneously.
- A low-grade fever may be present.
- Reactivation of the varicella virus may occur in the form of herpes zoster (shingles).
- Vesicles are gray in appearance and are located along a dermatome (nerve fiber). They arise from an erythematous base and contain clear fluid. Common sites include the thoracic area (50%), lumbosacral and cervical region (10% to 20%), and trigeminal nerve (10% to 20%).[8,3,9]

> ### NURSING ALERT
>
> Beware of vesicles on the side or tip of the nose. This is highly associated with trigeminal nerve involvement. An immediate ophthalmic consultation is warranted because of the high incidence of complications, including, but not limited to, optic neuritis and glaucoma. Perform a visual acuity check. (See Procedure 36.)

Diagnosis
- Diagnosis usually is determined by clinical presentation, although antibody testing may be performed.
Treatment
- Acetaminophen, lotions (calamine), soothing baths (oatmeal and/or baking soda to reduce itching), analgesics, antihistamines, and steroids may be given to provide relief from symptoms.
- Trim fingernails to prevent scratching of vesicles and scabs.
- Acyclovir may be used if initiated within 24 to 48 hours of the onset of rash. Intravenous acyclovir can be used if the patient is immunocompromised.

⋙ **N U R S I N G   A L E R T** ⋘

Remember to warn patients and parents not to use aspirin or aspirin products if the patient is younger than 21 years of age because of the association between Reye's syndrome and aspirin use.

NURSING SURVEILLANCE

1. Monitor the cardiac pattern and treat potentially lethal arrhythmias (second-degree and third-degree heart block may occur in acute rheumatic fever).
2. Monitor the trend of the patient's temperature. An elevated temperature may further dehydrate a patient with fluid volume deficit.
3. Monitor urine output and color to assess core perfusion and liver function.
4. Monitor the trend of oxygen saturation. Desaturation may occur in a patient who is not responding to drug therapy or who requires artificial ventilation because of respiratory paralysis or spasm.
5. Monitor the patient's level of consciousness.
6. Ensure that appropriate isolation precautions are taken.

EXPECTED OUTCOMES

1. The fever decreases or is absent.
2. The airway remains patent.
3. The breathing pattern is adequate (whether maintained by patient or artificially) as demonstrated by SpO_2 greater than 94% and arterial blood gases normal for condition.
4. Appropriate isolation precautions are taken.

PATIENT/FAMILY DISCHARGE IMPLICATIONS AND EDUCATION

Discharge instructions should be based on the clinical diagnosis of the patient. Refer to Table 6-1 for specific information about transmission routes, incubation periods, and complications associated with diseases. Some diseases require greater detail in discharge instruction and are discussed below.

1. *Acute rheumatic fever:* Patients should be examined daily for the first weeks of the disease to detect carditis early, before valve damage. The seriousness of this disease and the need

for long-term antibiotic therapy must be explained to the patient.

2. *Hepatitis:* Patients discharged with hepatitis should be instructed to rest and to anticipate low energy levels for up to 6 months. Alcoholic beverages should be avoided for 6 to 12 months. Instruct the patient that immunity to one type of hepatitis does not confer immunity to another type.

3. *HIV:* If HIV testing has been performed (with written informed consent of the patient), certain counseling must be provided. Patients must be informed about the medical significance of the test; whether the test result is negative or positive; test limitations; how HIV is spread; the availability of medical and psychosocial care; and social consequences of testing.[2] HIV-infected individuals should be referred to support groups and instructed on the prevention of disease transmission to others.

4. *Lyme disease:* Patients should be instructed to wear light-colored clothes, long sleeves, and pants with wrist and ankle bands before entering tick-infested areas. Insect repellent should contain DEET.

5. *Mumps:* The patient is contagious until the swelling subsides. The patient should remain home from work and school.

6. *Rubella:* The patient should remain home from work and school for 7 days after the onset of the rash. After receiving the MMR vaccine, the female, postpubertal patient should be warned not to become pregnant for at least 3 months. All pregnant first-trimester patients should be referred to an obstetrician.

7. *Skin conditions:* Encourage all family members to wash with antibacterial soap and not to share razors or towels and washcloths.

8. *Tuberculosis:* If active disease is suspected, patient should be given masks and instructed to wear them at all times whether outside or at home. Patients should be taught to report early signs of hepatitis because of the toxic effects of TB medications on the liver. Anorexia, nausea, weakness, jaundice, clay-colored stools, and dark urine should be reported promptly to the patient's primary health-care provider.

9. *Varicella and herpes zoster:* Active lesions are potentially infectious. Inform the patient to avoid neonates, pregnant women, and immunosuppressed patients.

REFERENCES

1. Benenson AS, Chin J, and Ascher MS: *Control of communicable disease manual,* ed 17, Washington, DC, 2000, American Public Health Association.

2. *Treatment guidelines,* CDC National AIDS Clearinghouse, www.cdcnpin.org.

3. Centers for Disease Control and Prevention. Measles, mumps, and rubella-vaccine use and strategies for elimination of measles, rubella, and congenital rubella syndrome and control of mumps. Recommendations of the Advisory Committee on Immunization Practices (ACIP), *MMWR* 47 (RR-8):1-58, 1998.

4. American Heart Association: Special writing group of the committee on rheumatic fever, endocarditis, and Kawasaki disease of the council on cardiovascular disease in the young: guidelines for the diagnosis of rheumatic fever, *JAMA* 268:2069-2073, 1992.

5. *Severe acute respiratory syndrome, SARS,* Centers for Disease Control, www.cdc.gov.

6. *Smallpox information,* Centers for Disease Control, www.cdc.gov.

7. Centers for Disease Control and Prevention: National plan to combat multidrug resistant tuberculosis recommendations and reports, *MMWR* 41 (RR-11):1-48, 1992.

8. Centers for Disease Control and Prevention: *Treatment of tuberculosis, American Thoracic Society, CDC, and Infectious Disease Society of America recommendations and report,* June 20, 52 (RR11):1-77, 2003.

9. Centers for Disease Control and Prevention: Prevention of varicella update recommendation of the Advisory Committee on Immunization Practices (ACIP), *MMWR* 48 (RR06):1-5, 1999.

10. Centers for Disease Control and Prevention: Diphtheria, tetanus, and pertussis: recommendations of the Advisory Committee on Immunization Practices (ACIP), *MMWR* 40 (RR10):1-18, 1991.

11. Centers for Disease Control and Prevention: Vaccinia (smallpox) vaccine recommendations of the Advisory Committee on Immunization Practices (ACIP), *MMWR* 50 (RR10):1-25, 2001.

12. Orenstein WA, Wharton M, Bart KJ, et al: Immunization varicella-zoster virus. In Mandell GL, Bennett JE, and Dolin R, eds: *Principles and practice of infectious diseases,* Philadelphia, 2000, Churchill Livingstone; pp 211-230.

chapter 7

Ear, Nose, Throat, and Facial/Dental Conditions

Mark B. Parshall

INTRODUCTION

Dental, facial, and ear, nose, and throat (ENT) emergencies range from relatively minor to life threatening. Emergency priority is given to:

- Upper airway injuries or obstructions resulting from bleeding, swelling, infection, burns, or foreign bodies
- Uncontrolled bleeding or hemodynamic instability
- Mixed presentations involving alterations in consciousness

High-energy blunt facial or soft-tissue neck injuries (e.g., motor vehicle collisions, especially if not restrained; bicycle or motorcycle collisions, especially if not helmeted; "clothesline" injuries; and impact to the face or neck with a blunt instrument) carry a risk for airway compromise or cervical spine injury. In less pressing situations, attention is directed toward preservation or restoration of structural and functional integrity, to pain reduction, and to addressing psychosocial responses to potential disfigurement or disability.

FOCUSED NURSING ASSESSMENT

Airway

- Cardinal signs of acute airway compromise include an impaired ability to speak or swallow, stridor, crowing, retractions, cyanosis, and, generally, obvious distress. Not all of these signs will be present in every instance.
- If the patient assumes a "tripod" position or is deliberately quiet in an effort to improve air movement, suspect epiglottitis.[1-4]
- Classic signs of epiglottitis have been termed the "four D's"—dysphagia, drooling, dysphonia (muffled voice), and distress.[2] Drooling is not always present. The complaint of "difficulty swallowing" often is used by patients to describe painful swallowing; thus clarification of such complaints is important.[4]
- Muffled speech, tongue protrusion, trismus (inability to open the mouth), or torticollis (neck spasm that causes the head to tilt to one side) may be associated with pharyngeal wall abscess or cellulitis of the floor of the mouth or soft tissues of the neck and may threaten the upper airway.
- Corrosive ingestions, such as battery acid or lye, may cause substantial upper airway injury and swelling. Immediate triage to, and initial treatment in, a resuscitation area are indicated.

Breathing

- Abnormalities in rate, depth, or symmetry of breathing in conjunction with a high-energy mechanism of injury above the clavicles may indicate an airway injury or an associated intrathoracic injury.
- An altered breathing pattern when the airway is clear may be a sign of a central nervous system (CNS) problem (e.g., a head or spinal cord injury).

Circulation

- Bleeding from the face, nose, or scalp may be profuse; nevertheless, depending on the history and mechanism of injury, the presence of hemodynamic instability or shock may be due to less obvious injuries (e.g., concomitant abdominal or thoracic injuries).
- In otherwise healthy patients, bleeding from anterior epistaxis is rarely severe enough to cause significant hemodynamic compromise. Therefore a finding of tachycardia and moderate to severe hypotension in epistaxis should heighten the examiner's index of suspicion for posterior bleeding.

Alterations in Consciousness

- Vasovagal syncope is a potential response to blood loss, pain, or emotional distress.

Sensation and Mobility

- Sudden loss of vision, whether traumatic or spontaneous, warrants ophthalmological consultation at the earliest opportunity. Concurrent serious ocular injury, such as hyphema, diplopia, ptosis, or enophthalmos, may exist in facial, head, or neck injury. Delay in obtaining an ophthalmological consultation can lead to suboptimal outcomes.[5]
- In facial trauma, localized areas of sensory loss (e.g., numbness, anesthesia) often are associated with fractures overlying or close to the canals or foramina through which branches of the trigeminal nerves pass (CN V: ophthalmic, maxillary, and mandibular divisions). Infraorbital anesthesia associated with fractures of the orbital rim or floor, and numbness of the upper lip, are associated with maxillary alveolar fracture; sensory loss in the lower lip or chin is associated with fractures of the mandible.[6]
- Sensory or motor abnormalities also may be associated with severe facial infections secondary to swelling and nerve compression.
- Unilateral impairment of facial motion (forehead, eyelids, mouth) is indicative of a facial nerve (CN VII) palsy and may be idiopathic (Bell's palsy) or secondary to trauma, herpes zoster infection, or tumor. Although Bell's palsy is more common than other etiologies, it is a diagnosis of exclusion.[7]
- Impaired mobility of the mandible is common in mandibular fracture. Inability to close the mouth fully may be associated with injury to the temporomandibular joint(s) or mandibular condyle(s).

Sexuality
- Herpetic or chancre-like perioral or intraoral lesions in children may be a sign of sexual abuse.

Tissue Integrity
- Soft-tissue facial trauma is most often related to falls. Facial fractures are most often related to vehicular collisions and interpersonal violence.[8]
- The most common mechanisms for ocular injuries are vehicular collisions, falls, battery, and sports injuries.[5] Midfacial fractures (e.g., orbital blowout and LeFort II and III fractures) increase the risk of permanent eye injury.[9]
- Intraoral lacerations, step-offs, and malocclusion may be signs of mandibular or maxillary alveolar fracture.
- Complex facial lacerations and those that disrupt the vermilion border of either lip, the margins or tarsal plate of one or more eyelids, or the auricle often require the attention of an appropriate specialty consultant (e.g., in areas of plastic or oral surgery, ophthalmology, ENT).
- Avulsed teeth are accorded a higher triage priority than most other dental complaints (e.g., odontalgia) because of the limited window for replantation (30 minutes or less).[10-12] To avoid damaging the periodontal ligament, which can adversely affect outcomes of replantation, the root of an avulsed tooth should not be handled or grasped.[13]

Safety
- Victims of domestic violence often present with facial injuries.
- Facial trauma resulting from interpersonal violence often is associated with alcohol or drugs and possible ongoing belligerence.[8] It may be necessary to triage a patient to a secure area and have security personnel immediately on hand, even in cases where the injuries themselves may not be emergent.

LIFE SPAN ISSUES
Infants and Children
1. Airway structures are less rigid in children than in adults and thus more likely to be compromised by swelling, infection, or trauma.
2. Infants less than 4 months of age are obligate nose breathers, so nasal congestion or swelling can lead to significant respiratory distress. Nasal flaring with infants is often a sign of significant respiratory compromise or distress.

3. Retractions in any age-group are a potentially serious sign; for children, supraclavicular retractions are usually most indicative of severe effort.

4. Epiglottitis can occur in any age-group. Although, it has been most common among children between 3 and 6 years of age,[1,2,4,14] the incidence in children is decreasing, most likely because of vaccination against *Haemophilus influenzae*. Thus the overall incidence may be expected to decline, while the relative prevalence in adults compared with children may be increasing.[7,15] Adult epiglottitis usually presents as a severe sore throat; stridor, drooling, and respiratory distress are less common in adults with epiglottitis than in children.[7]

5. Croup is most common from 3 months to 3 years of age,[4,14] but may be seen in children as old as 6 with a peak incidence around 1-2 years of age.[16-18]

6. Aspiration of a foreign body should be considered in the case of a child with a sudden onset of wheezing or stridor and retractions, or in the case of a child with chronic wheezing that is unrelieved by aerosolized bronchodilators.

7. Falls are the most common cause of facial injuries to children.[8] The nurse should be alert to injuries that appear inconsistent with the mechanism reported or allegedly resulting from activities beyond the developmental abilities of the child.

8. Midfacial fractures are relatively uncommon among school age and younger children. When present, they suggest a high-energy mechanism of injury with an increased risk of intracranial injury.

9. Nasal foreign bodies occur most often in childhood, especially with toddlers. Foreign bodies of the ear also are common in childhood but are found in individuals of any age, often related to using various small objects to "clean" the ear canals.

10. Avulsed primary (deciduous) teeth generally are not replanted to avoid injury to nonerupted permanent teeth.[13]

11. A child who is lethargic, "too quiet," or apathetic should be triaged for emergency examination.

Adults

1. The most common cause of facial fractures to young adults is interpersonal violence. With males, this tends to arise from altercations with strangers in settings where alcohol has been ingested. In cases involving females, assailants are more often known to the victim and often are domestic partners.[8]

2. The initial onset of Ménière's disease generally occurs between 30 and 50 years of age.

Geriatric Patients

1. Falls are the most common cause of facial and head injuries for the geriatric population.[8] The nurse must be alert to an alleged mechanism of injury inconsistent with the injuries seen.

2. It is important in cases of geriatric patients who have sustained falls to determine whether there was a loss of consciousness either before or after the fall. Of particular concern is a history of falls or increasing confusion over a span of several weeks, because this could indicate a subacute or chronic subdural hematoma.

3. Older adults also are more prone to posterior epistaxis[19,20] and profuse bleeding from facial and scalp wounds.

4. Ludwig's angina, a severe cellulitis of the oral cavity, is most common among geriatric patients who have some degree of immune compromise.[10]

5. Verbal communication with hearing-impaired elderly can be improved by standing directly in the patient's view and speaking slowly or, in some cases, by having the patient put on a stethoscope and speaking into the bell. Either of these approaches is apt to be more successful and less frustrating to all concerned.[7]

Pregnancy and Lactation

1. Because facial injuries often require multiple radiological views, assessment of pregnancy status in all female patients of childbearing age is essential.

2. For women who are pregnant or lactating, appropriate cautions should be employed when prescribing and administering medications.

3. Pediatric dental abnormalities associated with maternal tetracycline use are less common because of the increase in the number of classes of broad-spectrum antibiotics.

INITIAL INTERVENTIONS

1. A patient with actual or potential airway compromise should be triaged directly to a treatment area where suction and intubation equipment are readily available.

2. Cardiac and continuous pulse oximetry monitoring should be initiated if signs of airway compromise are present. (Epiglottitis in children may be an exception so as to avoid agitating the child.)

3. When possible, elevate the head of the bed to facilitate air movement.

4. Bleeding should be controlled with direct pressure.

5. Large-bore IV access should be established if the patient is hemodynamically unstable or may become unstable.
6. A patient with epistaxis should be triaged to an examination chair unless he or she is hypotensive or syncopal.
7. Nursing care priorities are listed in the table on pp. 282-285.

PRIORITY DIAGNOSTIC TESTS

Laboratory Tests

Arterial blood gas: An ABG is useful in cases of partial airway obstruction or trauma. Avoid the test in cases of suspected pediatric epiglottitis.

Blood studies: Trauma (per trauma protocol or as indicated): CBC, ethanol, chemistry panel, and blood bank (type and screen or crossmatch and coagulation studies).

In posterior epistaxis, a baseline CBC, PT and PTT, and type and screen often are ordered in the ED. They are rarely necessary in cases of anterior epistaxis.

Cultures: Obtain blood cultures in cases of orbital or pharyngeal cellulitis or peritonsillar abscess. Obtain a pharyngeal culture. Rapid streptococcal screens (latex agglutination, enzyme-linked immunoassay [ELISA], or optical immunoassay) have high specificity (~97%, i.e., a false-positive rate of ~3%); therefore, if positive, they warrant treatment without further culturing.[21] Rapid cultures (i.e., 24 hours) have a lower false-negative rate (i.e., higher sensitivity) than strep antibody screens and should be obtained if the strep screen is negative; empirical antibiotic treatment may be initiated while culture is pending.[21] If epiglottitis is suspected, no attempt should be made to swab the throat before the airway is secure.

Radiographic Tests

Barium (Ba++) swallow: Barium swallow may be ordered to assess for the presence of an esophageal foreign body, particularly food. Alternatively, a cotton pledget soaked in contrast may be swallowed.[4]

CT scans: CT scans are useful in cases of facial injuries in multiple trauma or head injury, in cases of penetrating trauma or impalement, or in cases of orbital cellulitis or severe sinusitis.

Panoramic radiographs: Panorex films may be obtained for mandible injuries, multiple dental avulsions, and periodontal abscess. C-spine must be clear to obtain. (A patient must be able to sit up in a special chair for this study. If the c-spine has not been cleared or the patient cannot tolerate sitting up, other

NURSING CARE PRIORITIES

Potential/Actual Problem	Causes	Signs and Symptoms	Interventions
1. Ineffective airway clearance	• Trauma • Foreign bodies • Infection	• Stridor, crowing • Cyanosis • Retractions • Diminished level of consciousness • Sniffing or tripod position • Muffled voice • Severe swelling of oropharynx or neck • Intraoral or nasal bleeding • Avulsed teeth • Dyspnea • Choking/gagging • Fear • Chronic cough or chronic sinus drainage	• Protect airway (suction/removal of intraoral debris, positioning, adjuncts, or intubation as indicated). • Oxygen, oximetry if indicated. • Control bleeding. • Frequent assessment of level of consciousness if indicated (e.g., high-velocity trauma) • In trauma, clearing the C-spine, if possible, facilitates positioning for airway protection. • Prompt radiologic evaluation during which patient should be continuously attended; suction should be set up and resuscitation supplies (crash cart) readily available.
2. Impaired gas exchange	Same as above	• Decreased O_2 saturation • Hypoxemia, hypercapnia	• Rule out airway obstruction or secure airway.

		• Restlessness/agitation • Cyanosis • Diminished level of consciousness • Dyspnea • Fear/anxiety/apprehension	• Oxygen and oximetry as indicated. • Aerosolized bronchodilator if indicated. • Close attendance and frequent reassurance.
3. Risk for cervical spine injury	Blunt or penetrating trauma above clavicles or other mechanism of injury	• Mechanism of injury consistent with possible c-spine injury • Peripheral sensory or motor impairment • Hypotension without tachycardia • Neck pain	• C-spine precautions until cleared.
4. Fluid volume deficit	Hemorrhage, dehydration	• Tachycardia • Narrowing pulse pressure • Hypotension • Delayed capillary refill • Diminished level of consciousness • Abnormal H&H • Sunken eyes • Dry mucous membranes	• Control bleeding. • IV fluid resuscitation. • Blood replacement as indicated. • Monitor I/O. • Oral comfort care if feasible and indicated.

Continued

NURSING CARE PRIORITIES—cont'd

Potential/Actual Problem	Causes	Signs and Symptoms	Interventions
		• Abnormal skin turgor • Listlessness • Thirst	
5. Pain	Trauma or infection	• Pain at rest or with movement or swallowing	• Ice, elevation if C-spine cleared. • Document location, quality, intensity (e.g., 0-10 rating), and other pain characteristics. • Pharmacologic pain interventions depend on underlying condition and level of consciousness, but may include opioid or NSAID analgesics or, in some cases, topical anesthesia.
6. Sensory-perceptual alteration or mobility defect	Trauma or infection	• Facial swelling • Periorbital ecchymosis • Malocclusion or trismus • Intraoral lacerations	• Monitor/protect airway, oxygenation. • Prompt radiologic evaluation. • Prompt specialty consultation as indicated.

		• Pain	
		• Numbness or anesthesia of infraorbital, upper lip, lower lip, or chin	
7. Impaired skin or mucous membrane integrity	Trauma or infection	• Lacerations	• Ice, elevation if C-spine cleared
		• Abrasions	• Laceration repair (lacerations of lid margins, tarsal plate, auricular cartilage; complex oral or facial lacerations may require specialty consultation and repair)
		• Contusions of face or mucous membranes	
		• Avulsed or luxated teeth	• Antibiotics as indicated and prescribed
		• Nasal deformity	• Appropriate reassurance about condition and prognosis and potential cosmetic consequences
		• Abscess formation	
		• CSF rhinorrhea	
		• Halitosis or purulent oral or nasal discharge	• Appropriate referral for follow-up care if discharged
		• Guarding or avoiding movement of head or neck; muffled voice	
		• Pain	
		• Localized sensory deficit	
		• Anxiety	

studies, such as an AP face, reverse Waters' view, and plain mandible films, may be ordered.)

Plain radiographs: Obtain a cervical spine series (according to mechanism of injury and trauma protocols); a lateral soft-tissue neck film (foreign bodies and often in epiglottitis); facial films (choice of views depends on what should be visualized and whether the cervical spine has been cleared); a chest x-ray film; a KUB; a soft-tissue neck film; or a "babygram" (to localize a radiopaque foreign body).

Other Tests

Continuous pulse oximetry: Continuous pulse oximetry is useful in cases of suspected airway compromise and to monitor response to oxygen therapy. A patient may have a "normal" SpO_2 and still require oxygen (e.g., if hemoglobin is low); therefore SpO_2 is more useful for establishing a trend. It should not be the sole criterion on which a decision to initiate oxygen therapy is made.

Fiberoptic endoscopic procedures (laryngoscopy, bronchoscopy, and esophagoscopy): These are diagnostic, as well as definitive, treatments for some foreign bodies. Fiberoptic laryngoscopy may be helpful in diagnosing epiglottitis in older patients.[3]

CLINICAL CONDITIONS

Acute Necrotizing Ulcerative Gingivitis

Acute necrotizing ulcerative gingivitis (ANUG) is a mixed anaerobic gingival infection, often called trench mouth or Vincent's angina.

Signs and symptoms
- Painful gingivostomatitis
- Headache
- Sore throat
- Anorexia
- Halitosis

Diagnosis
- Diagnosis is determined by the characteristic appearance of the oral cavity.

Treatment
- Oral penicillin and bicarbonate or peroxide mouth rinses.[4,11]
- Follow-up dental referral is recommended.
- Recurrences are common. And gingival debridement by a dentist occasionally may be necessary.[11]

Airway Foreign Bodies

Airway foreign bodies can occur in the pediatric and adult patient population, and may result from food, toys, or other objects.

The most common foreign body in adults is a food bolus. In cases involving children, small toys, buttons, coins, and nuts are common.

Signs and symptoms
- Moderate to severe respiratory distress with stridor, wheezing, or impaired phonation.
- An occult foreign body (e.g., one that was aspirated at some previous time and not recognized) may present with signs and symptoms of chronic cough, unequal breath sounds, and localized wheezing on forced expiration.[22]
- Breath sounds may be diminished unilaterally or diffusely.

Diagnosis
- Foreign bodies of the airway may be diagnosed by means of a history of sudden onset of distress, by radiograph (lateral neck or chest x-ray), or by fiberoptic laryngoscopy or bronchoscopy.
- An occult foreign body may be suspected with an individual who has suffered recurrent bouts of pneumonia.[22]

Treatment
- Allow the patient to remain in the position in which breathing is most comfortable and least fatiguing, usually sitting up.
- Obtain a baseline O_2 saturation and administer cool-mist oxygen per mask or blow-by as needed to maintain acceptable saturation.
- Removal is generally performed with a fiberoptic laryngoscope and forceps or via bronchoscopy.

Auricular and Nasal Septal Hematomas

A hematoma of the auricle or nasal septum threatens the viability of the underlying cartilage because the extravasated blood is between the cartilage and the perichondrium (fibrous membrane of connective tissue). This can cause avascular necrosis of the cartilage that leads to either a "cauliflower ear" or a saddle-nose deformity.[20,23] An auricular hematoma can result after a blunt blow to the external ear. A septal hematoma can occur after facial trauma.

Signs and symptoms
- The auricular hematoma is an obvious injury, characterized by swelling and ecchymosis.
- A nasal septal hematoma is not obvious to gross inspection but is a risk when the patient has a fractured nose.

Diagnosis
- An auricular hematoma is diagnosed by direct observation.
- A nasal septal hematoma is diagnosed by direct inspection of the septum, using a nasal speculum.

Treatment

- Cartilage is avascular and receives its blood supply from the perichondrium.
- The treatment for either an auricular or a nasal septal hematoma is an incision and drainage (I & D) of the hematoma.[20,23]
- After an I & D of the auricle, the convolutions of the auricle are packed with petrolatum gauze. Several gauze sponges are laced between the auricle and the scalp to hold it in a neutral position, and then the entire area is padded with fluff gauze and secured with a roll gauze bandage that covers the dressed ear.[20]
- In the case of the septal hematoma, after the I & D a small drain (e.g., a sterile rubber band) is placed and an anterior pack is inserted as with anterior epistaxis.[20] In either case, the packing and dressing must be changed daily and the respective structures inspected for evidence of reaccumulation or infection.

Cerumen Impaction

For all age-groups, impacted cerumen is generally related to attempts to remove cerumen, usually with cotton swabs that tend to tamp it further into the ear canal. At times, patients hold a mistaken belief that cerumen is a pathologic secretion, a belief that may contribute to inappropriately zealous removal attempts. Patients should be instructed not to attempt to remove wax with swabs, matchsticks, paper clips, or other small objects.

Signs and symptoms

- Unilateral or bilateral feeling of the ear feeling plugged or full, or some degree of diminished auditory acuity.[43,53]

Diagnosis

- Impaction is easily noted on an otoscopic examination.

Treatment

- Removal may be by curet (particularly in small children) or, more often, by ceruminolytics, irrigation, or a combination of the two[26-29] (see Procedure 13).
- Irrigation should not be performed if there is suspicion of tympanic membrane rupture. A ruptured tympanic membrane will not ordinarily lead to hearing loss, but it may be associated with vertigo.[24,29,30]
- Patients often have mild discomfort during irrigation but should not experience vertigo, nausea, or severe pain. If a patient becomes increasingly symptomatic during irrigation, the procedure should be discontinued, and the physician should be notified.

- Ceruminolytic agents may be recommended to prevent recurrence or to precede irrigation. In addition to conventional ceruminolytics (OTC or prescription), *liquid* docusate sodium (Colace liquid, 1% solution, 10 mg/ml) may be used. (NOTE: Docusate sodium *syrup* never should be used for this purpose).[28,29,31]
- ENT follow-up generally is not indicated unless a tympanic membrane rupture is found.

Croup (Laryngotracheitis; Laryngotracheobronchitis)

Croup is a viral illness that can cause severe airway compromise. Croup most often occurs in infants and children from ages 6 months to 6 years during the cool weather in spring and fall. The airway becomes edematous, and airway secretions are increased. The hallmark symptom of croup is stridor, a sound produced by the inspiration of air through edematous airways. Older children often present with intermittent coughing with relatively normal breathing between coughs.

Signs and symptoms
- Frequent paroxysms of the characteristic barking cough, inspiratory stridor, and retractions.
- Fever is often present, but usually is not as high as in epiglottitis.
- The symptoms often worsen at night, and the parents often report that the child sounded worse at home than on arrival in the ED (possibly because of the soothing effect of cooler, moister air outside).

Diagnosis
- Diagnosis is based on clinical presentation, as the cough is characteristic of croup. Progression of symptoms also is useful in diagnosis.
- In contrast to epiglottitis, the typical history is a respiratory infection of more insidious onset that has worsened, often over 1 to 2 days.[18]
- A number of clinical rating scales for croup severity have been published.[32]
- Membranous croup is a rare but potentially life-threatening condition. Symptoms are similar to those of viral croup, but membranous croup tends to occur with a slightly older age group (around 5 years of age), and the child appears to be in a more toxic condition than the child with viral croup.

Treatment
- Continuous oxygen saturation monitoring should be initiated. If SpO_2 is <95% on ambient air or symptoms are severe, an

appropriate flow-rate of oxygen should be started by whatever means the child will tolerate (e.g., blow-by).

- Treatment with cool mist (i.e., humidified air) is traditional, but few randomized controlled trials (vs. no mist) have been reported, and results conflict, but there is no evidence of harm in the practice.[16,33]

- Many studies of epinephrines or steroids have demonstrated their efficacy versus standard care (typically cool mist) or standard care plus placebo.

- Corticosteroids, most often oral or IM dexamethasone or nebulized budesonide, have become mainstays of treatment.[17,18,32,34,35] Steroids have a slower onset but much longer duration of action than epinephrine. Therefore they may reduce the total number of doses of epinephrine over the ED course, but nebulized epinephrine may still be necessary.

- The most common dosage of dexamethasone in published studies has been 0.6 mg/kg (maximum 10 mg), regardless of route. However, several studies indicate that lower dosages (0.3 mg/kg to 0.15 mg/kg) may be equally efficacious. Oral and IM routes of dexamethasone are equally efficacious.[32]

- Nebulized budesonide (Pulmicort) is an alternative to dexamethasone but is no more efficacious and is more expensive per dose.[32]

- Nebulized epinephrine (racemic or L-isomer) often is very helpful for more severe cases of croup. A typical dosage is 5 mg, but concentrations differ between racemic epinephrine (0.5 ml of a 2.25% solution = 5 mg) and L-epinephrine (1:1000 = 1 mg/ml; 5 ml = 5 mg).

- Patients who require epinephrine traditionally have been admitted or at least placed on holding or observation status for several hours because of the short duration of action.[17]

- Humidified heliox (an 80:20 or 70:30 mixture of helium and oxygen that is less dense and has lower viscosity than atmospheric air) has been studied in at least one small, randomized, controlled trial (vs. racemic epinephrine). Results suggested efficacy comparable with racemic epinephrine, but heliox in this setting is still investigational.[26]

- It may be appropriate to discharge patients who have received steroids in addition to racemic epinephrine, provided that: (1) they have been observed closely for several hours, during which time they have remained free of signs of respiratory distress (e.g., retractions and stridor), and (2) the parent or caregiver is responsible, understands signs and symptoms of a worsening condition, and can easily return or access appropriate follow-up.[7]

- Antibiotics are generally reserved for cases serious enough to warrant admission and are not usually part of emergency treatment. An exception is membranous croup, which probably involves some degree of bacterial superinfection. Unlike viral croup, membranous croup necessitates parenteral antibiotics.[17] The child with membranous croup requires admission to an intensive care unit and may require endotracheal intubation.

Dental Avulsions

Avulsion and displacement of teeth may occur as a result of trauma from altercations, motor vehicle crashes, or sports injuries.

Signs and symptoms

- A completely avulsed tooth is generally obvious. Luxation is displacement or incomplete avulsion of a tooth.
- Intraoral bleeding or a bloody socket often is present.

Diagnosis

- A luxation can be identified by manual examination. A lateral luxation is a displacement of a tooth in a mesial, distal, lingual, or buccal direction, and may be associated with fracture of the underlying alveolar process. In contrast, intrusive luxation means the tooth has been driven in an apical direction and is associated with crushing or fracture of the alveolus around the apex (distal root) of the tooth.[13]
- The best salvage rate for replantation occurs when extraoral time is ≤30 minutes.[11,12] Therefore it is important to establish the time of injury and how the tooth has been handled.

Treatment

- While awaiting replantation or while en route to the hospital, it is best to keep the tooth in a container with milk or saline as a transport medium.[11] Plain water should not be used because of its hypotonicity.[11,12]
- If the patient is alert and a suitable transport medium is unavailable, the tooth may be placed in the sublingual or buccal sulcus for transport.[11] (Saliva is hypotonic and highly contaminated with bacteria.) Tooth preservation sets are commercially available that use Hank's solution, a buffered solution that contains glucose, Mg^{++}, and Ca^{++} in a small jar with a basket inside for holding the tooth.[12]
- The root of the tooth should not be handled so as to avoid injury to the periodontal ligament. Before replantation the root of the tooth should be gently flushed with sterile saline.
- Early dental consultation is indicated.

- Dental fractures are less urgent and have variable prognoses, depending on what part of the tooth is involved (incisal/coronal, midroot, or apical).[13]
- Higher priority should be accorded broken teeth that have exposed pulp. This may appear as a vascular core or at times as a pink-tinged pulsation visible through a dentinal surface.[11]

Epiglottitis (Supraglottitis)

Epiglottitis is a bacterial infection usually caused by *Haemophilus influenzae* and characterized by rapid edema of the epiglottis. Symptom onset is rapid and associated with severe respiratory compromise. Epiglottitis occurs most often in children, although it can affect adults as well.

Signs and symptoms

- Rapid onset of high fever ($\geq 39°$ C) and a toxic appearance.
- In addition to the classic signs previously discussed, open-mouth breathing with tongue protrusion, a "sniffing" position, or a tripod position may be seen.[3,4]
- Cyanosis or pallor may be present and is a sign of poor prognosis because it tends to occur late in the clinical course.[1,2,4]
- In adults, epiglottitis may have a more indolent onset than in children. The chief complaint often is of the worst sore throat of the patient's life and may not be associated with high fever, stridor, or drooling.[4,7]

Diagnosis

- With children, epiglottitis is diagnosed primarily by clinical presentation and rapidity of onset; x-rays may not be necessary.
- Lateral soft-tissue neck films may be helpful in ambiguous presentations but are not always necessary for the diagnosis. A portable upright lateral neck film in the ED may suffice.
- If a child is sent to the x-ray department, a parent should be allowed to remain with the child, a crash cart should be immediately available, and an emergency nurse or physician should attend the child.
- With adults, indirect laryngoscopy (e.g., with a mirror)[14] or fiberoptic laryngoscopy can be performed, and lateral soft-tissue neck films may be more helpful than in children.[3,7]

Treatment

- Children:
  - The child and parent should be triaged immediately to a resuscitation area, and the child should be allowed to remain in whatever position facilitates breathing.[2]
  - As soon as epiglottitis is suspected, an emergency nurse or physician should continuously observe the child.[2]

- ○ The child will not tolerate lying down and should not be made to do so.[2,11]
- ○ Because of the child's tenuous airway, the nurse should avoid performing, and protect the child from, intrusive procedures.
- ○ Blow-by humidified oxygen and a cardiac monitor may be used if the child will tolerate them without increased distress, but no attempt should be made to secure a mask or nasal cannula to the child's face.[1,3]
- ○ The airway usually will be secured under direct visualization (by an otolaryngologist or anesthesiologist) in the operating room in case an emergency tracheostomy is required.[2-4,14]
- ○ In crash situations in the field or ED, a cricothyrotomy may be necessary.[2-4,14]
- ○ When the airway has been secured, attention then can be directed toward obtaining cultures or other laboratory studies, initiating IV fluids, and administering antibiotics—usually second-generation or third-generation cephalosporin.[3,36]
- Adults:
  - ○ Adults are less likely than children to need emergency intubation.
  - ○ Although less common in adults than children, development of stridor is a strong predictor of the need for intubation or tracheostomy for the adult.[37]
  - ○ Corticosteroids sometimes are ordered; evidence of efficacy in this setting is lacking, and their use is controversial.[3]

Epistaxis

The vast majority of epistaxis is anterior, most often from the mucosa of the anterior (cartilaginous) nasal septum (known as Kiesselbach's area or Little's area).[27,38]

Posterior bleeds usually are from a branch of the ethmoid artery and can be profuse or intermittent.[19]

Signs and symptoms

- Active epistaxis is obvious. Even in cases where the patient appears to be bleeding from both nares, epistaxis almost always is unilateral.
- It is helpful at triage to have the patient identify the side on which bleeding was first evident and whether the direction in which bleeding was first noted was from the naris or in the pharynx.[19,20]
- Unless syncopal, the patient should be triaged to an ENT examination chair.

Diagnosis

- The basic diagnostic question in epistaxis is the location of bleeding.

- Identification of an anterior bleeding site is diagnostic. Anterior bleeds rarely require hematologic and coagulation studies unless the patient is receiving anticoagulants or is uremic.[14]
- Posterior epistaxis is more profuse and more difficult to control.
- Epistaxis unresponsive to pressure over Little's area suggests a posterior site, as does bleeding around or behind a preexisting anterior nasal pack.

Treatment

ANTERIOR EPISTAXIS

- Have the patient sit upright and apply firm, continuous, bilateral pressure to the septal cartilage just above the nasal alae with the thumb and forefinger for about 10 minutes. Often it is helpful for the nurse to apply the pressure initially so the patient can acquire the "feel" for the location and amount of pressure.
- If the patient is unable to maintain the pressure, the nurse should maintain it.
- The patient should be supplied with a basin or suction for oral secretions but should be instructed not to expectorate forcefully or blow the nose until immediately before the nasal examination.
- Typical supplies for a nasal examination include a head lamp, nasal speculum, bayonet forceps, a Frazier suction tip, silver nitrate applicators, and bacitracin ointment.
- Cocaine diluted to a 4% or 5% solution is usually used as a topical anesthetic and vasoconstrictor. Alternatively, a mixture of tetracaine (Pontocaine) or 4% lidocaine with phenylephrine or epinephrine can be used.[14,19,20]
- At the beginning of the examination, the patient is instructed to blow out any clots from the nares. Suction with a Frazier tip should be set up and readily available.
- The physician may use bayonet forceps to place cotton pledgets moistened with anesthetic in the nasal vestibule. The pledgets should be left in place for 5 to 10 minutes, after which any localized bleeding sources can be cauterized.[19,20]
- Silver nitrate cautery is preferred over electrocautery because it is less likely to damage the septum.[20] Silver nitrate causes a crust to form at the site. This may be softened by application of an antibiotic ointment to the site. Septal perforation is a complication of cautery.
- After hemostasis has been achieved, an anterior pack with a cellulose (Merocel) tampon, Oxycel packing, or a long ribbon of petrolatum gauze can be placed.[14,19,38]

- Petrolatum gauze or Merocel packing should be removed in 1 to 2 days, either in the ED or by the patient's private physician.
- Oxycel does not have to be removed; it dries up and can be blown out by the patient in a few days.

POSTERIOR EPISTAXIS

- If an anterior site cannot be identified, or if bleeding continues in spite of packing or resumes after an anterior pack is in place, a posterior bleed is suspected.[19,20] If a posterior pack is placed, the patient should be admitted.
- A posterior bleed generally necessitates an ENT consultation.
- Geriatric patients or those with chronic obstructive pulmonary disease may require ICU admission because of a risk of hypoxemia or hypercapnia with a posterior pack in place.[14,20]
- The most common means of tamponading a posterior bleed is a double-balloon catheter (Naso-Stat or Epi-Stat).[14,20] The proximal balloon fills up the nasal cavity, and the distal balloon is inflated in the nasopharynx to block retrograde bleeding and keep the larger, nasal balloon in place. The balloons may be inflated with sterile water or normal saline.[7] A combination of petrolatum gauze or Oxycel anterior packing may be used in conjunction with balloon tamponade.[38]
- Ultimately, the patient may require surgical ligation.
- Posterior gauze packs rarely are used because they are extremely uncomfortable; however, they are occasionally needed if balloon tamponade is ineffective. A posterior gauze pack consists of a wad of tightly folded gauze sponges that are firmly tied together by a minimum of three ties that are at least 6 inches long. A Robinson catheter is passed through to the nasopharynx and brought out through the mouth. Two of the ties are tied through the eyelet of the catheter, and the third is taped to the cheek. The catheter is pulled back out the nose, and traction is applied to the two ties until the pack lodges firmly in the nasopharynx. The two nasal ties are taped to the outside of the nose or the cheek. Systemic analgesics usually are needed for pain; some physicians may order a sedative as well. On occasion, patients will have a vasovagal episode resulting from the pain and stimulation of the pack.

Esophageal Foreign Body

Esophageal foreign bodies, although less serious than airway foreign bodies, are extremely uncomfortable, and often it is difficult to be certain that a foreign body "in the throat" is in fact esophageal. If there is any doubt about the location of the foreign body (e.g., trachea versus esophagus), it is safest to triage immediately to a treatment area.

Signs and symptoms
- Sensation of a foreign body.
- Phonation is generally not impaired, and stridor should not be present.
- The patient may be retching without nausea.
- Esophageal foreign bodies often occur while eating and may be associated with stricture, especially in older adults.

Diagnosis
- Plain radiographs may identify esophageal foreign bodies if the object is radiopaque.
- Food and radiolucent objects may require a barium swallow.

Treatment
- An esophageal foreign body often will gradually pass.
- IV glucagon occasionally is helpful in relaxing the distal (smooth muscle) segment of the esophagus.
- Esophagoscopy may be necessary.
- Depending on the size, nature, and location of the foreign body, it may be removed or pushed into the stomach by means of the endoscope.

Facial Fractures

The treatment of facial bone fractures varies with the location and the amount of bony displacement. Nasal and mandibular fractures are the most common. Ice should be applied acutely to any areas of facial swelling as soon as the patient has been triaged. Because most of the facial bones are not mobile and it is difficult to assess the degree of deformity while acute swelling is present, many patients with facial fractures may be discharged with instructions to follow up with a plastic surgeon or ENT specialist after the swelling has gone down. Surgical intervention, if indicated, often is elective.

LeFort Fractures

LeFort II and III fractures are high-energy injuries from direct blows to the midface, and they should be considered based on mechanism of injury. The patient may be obtunded because of a concomitant head injury. See Figure 7-1 for the location of LeFort fractures.

Signs and symptoms
- See Table 7-1.

Diagnosis
- See Table 7-1 for differentiation of LeFort fractures.
- The fractures often are complex and may be mixed (e.g., a LeFort II pattern on one side with a III pattern on the other).

Lateral view   Frontal view

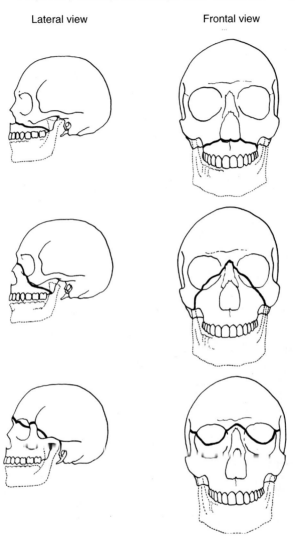

Figure 7-1 A, LeFort I facial fracture. **B,** LeFort II facial fracture. **C,** LeFort III facial fracture.

TABLE 7-1 LeFort Fractures

Fracture Type	Fracture Area	Signs and Symptoms
LeFort I	Linear maxillary alveolar fracture	• Upper jaw pain • Malocclusion • Anesthesia or numbness of the upper lip[6] • Edema • Ecchymosis • Mobility of maxillary teeth
LeFort II	Pyramid shape involving the maxilla, nasal bones, palate, and inferior or medial orbit	• Facial elongation • Infraorbital anesthesia[6] • Edema • Ecchymosis
LeFort III	Craniofacial separation with the fracture extending across the upper maxilla and nasal bones through the orbit and zygoma	• Infraorbital anesthesia[6] • Nasal and pharyngeal bleeding • Massive swelling and ecchymosis around the eyes, nose, maxilla, and upper oral cavity. • Abnormal approximation of the teeth[6] • Cerebrospinal fluid (CSF) rhinorrhea may be present but may be obscured by bleeding. A "halo" test on a piece of filter paper is helpful.

- Instability of the facial architecture is present and often can be detected by palpation.
- A definitive diagnosis is radiographic; a computed tomography (CT) scan usually is necessary.

Treatment

- LeFort fractures require surgical repair, often on a delayed basis.
- Based on the mechanism of injury, the patient initially will require spinal precautions that increase the risk of aspiration.
- Yankauer or larger-bore suction should be immediately at hand. Intubation may be required in the presence of severe airway compromise (e.g., due to intraoral bleeding or foreign bodies such as avulsed teeth).
- Prophylactic intravenous (IV) antibiotics may be ordered.
- If a CSF leak is present, the patient will require neurosurgical consultation.

Mandibular Fractures

The most common fracture sites are the mandibular angle, body, and symphysis.[10,39] Because of its shape, the mandible often is fractured in more than one location.

Signs and symptoms

- Malocclusion
- Inability to open the mouth completely (trismus)
- Crepitus
- Forcible displacement of two or more adjacent lower teeth toward the tongue is another sign of a probable mandibular fracture.[10]
- Preauricular pain suggests fracture of the mandibular condyle or subcondylar region.[6]
- Numbness of the lower lip or chin suggests fracture along the course of the ipsilateral inferior alveolar nerve (i.e., mandibular angle or body).[6]

Diagnosis

- Panoramic tomographic (Panorex) radiographs, show the entire mandible in the same plane.[10,39] This may be of some advantage in detecting multiple fractures, but overall, pantomography is no more sensitive or specific in diagnosing mandible fractures than a plain four-view mandible series.[40]
- The patient should be assessed for swelling or asymmetry, the presence and location of pain, whether pain increases with jaw opening, and whether the bite feels normal to the patient.[6]

- If clinical signs of a mandibular fracture are evident, one should assume that any intraoral laceration in the mandibular region is an open fracture.[10]

Treatment
- Suction may be necessary in the presence of blood and oral secretions, especially if spinal precautions are in place.
- Allow the patient to sit in Fowler's position after the cervical spine has been cleared.
- Oral saline rinse may reduce the formation of blood clots in the mouth.
- Increasingly, open reduction and internal fixation (ORIF) is gaining favor over intermaxillary fixation.[39] In patients with mandibular condylar fracture, ORIF has shown a lower incidence of postoperative malocclusion.[41]
- Treatment with parenteral penicillin G or ceftriaxone is equally efficacious; the latter has the advantage of less frequent administration (i.e., daily vs. every 4 to 6 hr).[42] Clindamycin is an alternative for patients with a history of penicillin sensitivity.[6]

Nasal Fractures
Nasal fractures are the most common facial bone fracture and usually result from blunt trauma.

Signs and symptoms
- Pain
- Swelling
- Possible deformity
- Epistaxis or clotted blood in the nares

Diagnosis
- Diagnosis of nasal fractures is generally made on clinical grounds.
- The patient will need a nasal speculum examination to rule out a septal hematoma.
- Radiographs are generally unnecessary, and even when positive they rarely influence treatment.[23,43]

Treatment
- A fractured nose generally is not urgent unless the fracture is open or a septal hematoma is present.
- A cold pack should be applied while the patient is awaiting treatment.
- As with facial bone fractures, the necessity of surgical repair for nasal fractures is generally evaluated after swelling has gone down, 1 to 2 weeks after the injury.

Ludwig's Angina
Ludwig's angina is a diffuse cellulitis of the sublingual, submental, and submandibular tissues of the mandible, which usually occurs

as a result of an untreated dental infection. Airway compromise can occur because of a swollen tongue or can spread to involve lateral and retropharyngeal spaces, which also threatens the airway.[44] If the retropharyngeal space is involved, the infection can extend to the mediastinum, resulting in mediastinitis.

Signs and symptoms
- High fever[10,44]
- Tense brawny edema of the submandibular area[10,44]
- Elevation or compression of the tongue to the palate because of swelling[10,44]

Diagnosis
- This condition usually is seen with older adults, often with some degree of immune compromise.[10]
- Diagnosis is based on the location and appearance of cellulitis.
- A complete blood count (CBC) and blood cultures generally are ordered as a baseline septic workup.
- Lateral soft-tissue neck and chest x-rays also may be needed.

Treatment
- Admission and IV antibiotics, usually penicillin G or Clindamycin plus metronidazole if spread to parapharyngeal spaces is suspected; a variety of alternatives are available in cases of sensitivity or documented microbial resistance.[36]

Ménière's Disease and Acute Labyrinthitis (Vestibular Dysfunction)

Ménière's disease is an inner ear disorder characterized by vertigo, tinnitus, and hearing loss. The patient may have frequent exacerbations of the disease lasting from a few minutes to a few days. Permanent hearing loss may result from multiple acute exacerbations of the disease.

Labyrinthitis is an inflammation of the inner ear, which results from a viral or bacterial infection.

Signs and symptoms
- Tinnitus
- Rotational vertigo
- Unilateral, progressive sensorineural hearing loss
- During recurrent, acute episodes, the vertigo and tinnitus become profound and may be associated with severe nausea and vomiting that can be sufficiently severe to cause dehydration and weakness
- Acute labyrinthitis has a similar presentation but is not characterized by chronic tinnitus or a progressive hearing loss.

Diagnosis
- Definitive diagnosis for Ménière's disease requires tests that are not performed on an emergency basis (e.g., audiometry and electronystagmography).
- Patients who give a history of multiple episodes of severe vertigo should be referred to an ENT specialist for a workup.

Treatment
- Treatment of an exacerbation of Ménière's disease is aimed at correcting fluid and electrolyte imbalances and relieving vertigo, nausea, and vomiting.
- Antiemetic drugs such as promethazine or droperidol may be necessary.
- Treatment for acute labyrinthitis is supportive and aimed at relieving symptoms.
- Oral meclizine is usually prescribed in the ED setting to relieve vertigo, often in conjunction with a benzodiazepine such as diazepam that helps stabilize vestibular function.[45]
- Patients need to be counseled to change positions gradually and to avoid sudden head movements.
- ENT referral is advisable, but specialty consultation in the ED and admission are rare.

Nasal and Ear Foreign Bodies

Foreign bodies inserted into the nose and ear usually involve children. Presentations of foreign bodies often are delayed and mimic signs and symptoms of infections such as sinusitis or suppurative otitis.

Signs and symptoms
- Foreign bodies of the ear often present as a conductive hearing loss.
- Occasionally an insect crawls into the ear canal and can be extremely painful and distressing at any age.

Diagnosis
- Foreign bodies of the nose may be visible on direct examination, but an index of suspicion must be maintained in cases of foul, purulent drainage.
- A foreign body of the ear can be seen via otoscopy, but if some time has elapsed since its introduction into the ear canal, cerumen or purulent drainage may obscure it.

Treatment
- In the cases of nasal foreign bodies, there is some degree of risk that the foreign body might be converted to an airway foreign body if pushed during a removal attempt.

- With ear foreign bodies there is a risk of a tympanic membrane rupture or laceration of the external auditory canal during removal.[46]

- Because of these risks, foreign body removals in the ED generally are performed by or under the supervision of a physician. It is best to set a time limit before undertaking a removal because more harm can be caused by determined removal attempts than has been caused by the foreign body itself. If the time limit has been reached without success, it is best to involve an ENT specialist.[20,24,46]

- Vegetable matter, such as a bean or wood, is difficult to remove because it swells and becomes too soft to be grasped with a forceps. Hard, spherical foreign bodies, such as beads, also are difficult to grasp.

- Foreign bodies of the ear may be removed by means of alligator forceps or suction tip, or by passing an ear curet or Fogarty catheter beyond the foreign body and gently pulling it out. Nursing responsibilities during removal consist primarily of assisting with the examination and removal. Small children will be frightened and often will need to be secured with a sheet or on a papoose board. On occasion, conscious sedation may be ordered for a child before removal.

- Insects in the ear canal can be killed by means of filling the ear canal with microscope immersion oil (highly refined mineral oil),[47] vegetable oil,[47] or 4% topical lidocaine solution.[20] Microscope immersion oil is more rapid and effective in immobilizing and killing cockroaches in vitro.[47] The killed insect can be removed by irrigation or suction or with forceps.[20,47]

- Nasal foreign-body removal can be performed with alligator forceps, with a suction tip, or by passing a Fogarty catheter past the foreign body, in much the same manner and with the same nursing responsibilities as with ear foreign bodies (see preceding entry). It is helpful to instill a topical vasoconstrictor before any removal attempts.

- Alternatively, a "positive pressure" removal technique has been described for nasal foreign bodies in children.[7,48,49] A topical vasoconstrictor is instilled into the naris. While waiting for the vasoconstrictor to take effect, the parent or caregiver is instructed to occlude the noninvolved naris manually and "give a puff of 'mouth-to-mouth'" to the child by making an airtight seal and blowing briefly (but sharply) into the child's mouth. The child is positioned supine and asked to open his or her mouth so the parent or caregiver can bestow "a big kiss."[48]

Compared with instrumentation, the procedure is relatively atraumatic and less stressful to the parent and child, and theoretically it poses less risk of conversion to an airway foreign body.[48] If it is unsuccessful, more-invasive techniques can be used.

Odontalgia

Patients with dental pain often arrive believing they must be seen by a dentist immediately to have an emergency extraction; however, this is rarely necessary. Patients complaining of severe dental pain usually come to the ED at night or on weekends when they may have difficulty accessing a dentist. It is helpful in triage to adjust the patient's expectations for the visit to: diagnosis of the problem, pain relief, determination of whether an antibiotic is indicated, and facilitation of prompt follow-up care.

Signs and symptoms
- Complaints of dental pain
- If an abscess is present, the patient's jaw or cheek may be swollen on the affected side.
- The patient may be febrile.

Diagnosis
- Odontalgia is a symptom. Diagnosis is directed toward establishing the underlying cause and initiating appropriate treatment.
- Dental or Panorex radiographs may be needed.
- Common causes of odontalgia are apical abscesses or broken teeth with exposed dentin or pulp.[11,13]

Treatment
- An I & D of an abscess by the physician may be necessary.
- Nursing care is directed toward pain relief.
- The patient generally will be sent home with antibiotics and systemic analgesics.
- Patients with chipped or broken teeth may have them temporarily sealed with calcium hydroxide paste by the emergency physician if there is exposure of dentin or pulp.[13]
- In facilities that do not have dentists on staff, it is helpful for the ED to have some arrangement with area dentists for follow-up of ED visits.

Otitis Externa (Swimmer's Ear)

Otitis externa is an infection of the external auditory canal and can be quite painful. It is often related to swimming or diving and is most common in adults and older children.

Signs and symptoms
- Pain that is worse with chewing and when the ear is moved
- Redness

- Purulent drainage from the ear
- Cellulitis may be present.

Diagnosis

- Diagnosis is made by otoscopy. The external auditory canal may be inflamed or contain exudative debris.

Treatment

- Treatment consists of gentle debridement of the ear canal with a curet or calcium alginate swab and instillation of polymyxin B–neomycin–hydrocortisone drops.[20,24]
- On occasion, a "wick" (an antibiotic-soaked strip of packing gauze) may be placed in the ear canal to help distribute the medication more evenly and prevent it from coming out of the canal.
- The patient should be instructed to avoid swimming or getting the ear canals wet for a period of about 2 weeks.
- At times, analgesic drops may be helpful.
- Older diabetic patients may develop malignant *(Pseudomonas)* otitis externa and may need to be hospitalized and given parenteral antibiotics.[24,36]

Otitis Media

Otitis media (OM) is an infection of the middle ear that usually occurs in infants and children because of their short, relatively flat Eustachian canals. There may be a recent history of an upper respiratory infection.

Signs and symptoms

- Pain that may be unilateral or bilateral
- Increasing fussiness
- Fever
- Emotional distress of the child and parent alike

Diagnosis

- Diagnosis is made by otoscopic examination. The tympanic membrane is red and does not move normally with air insufflation.
- Small children often are frightened by ear examinations and may need to be held securely. Initially, the parent should hold the child seated in his or her lap with the parent's arms crossed over the child's arms. If the child is too restless or uncooperative, the child can be positioned supine, with the arms extended upward.
- The nurse should hold the child's upper arms at either side of the head, and a second person (staff or parent) should hold the child's thighs just above the knees. This permits the examiner to gently hold the head still with one hand while using the otoscope with the other.

- If the tympanic membrane cannot be visualized because of cerumen, the physician generally clears the ear canal with a curet.

Treatment

- Traditional ED treatment has involved prescription of oral antibiotics and possibly antihistamines and decongestants, with referral for re-examination in 1 to 2 weeks after completion of a course of treatment. However, in most cases, signs and symptoms resolve spontaneously, with less than a quarter of untreated patients demonstrating signs and symptoms of persistent OM 2 weeks after diagnsosis.[50]
- There is limited benefit to antibiotic therapy, and benefits (e.g., pain relief, concerns about loss to follow-up) must be weighed in lights of risks (e.g., potential for adverse reactions).[51] In less-developed countries, mastoiditis is more common than in developed countries, and antibiotic treatment is advisable.[52]
- Amoxicillin is generally appropriate as a first-line antibiotic agent for children or adults; trimethoprim-sulfamethoxazole is an acceptable first-line alternative if the patient is allergic to amoxicillin; for cases in which first-line therapy has failed, amoxicillin-clavulanic acid, any of several second-generation or third-generation cephalosporins, or a single IM dose of ceftriaxone at 50 mg/kg are alternatives.[7,36,45,53]
- Benefits of antihistamines, decongestants, or a combination are small at best.
- Acetaminophen or ibuprofen may be ordered for pain relief.
- In general, a child with otitis media should be reexamined 1 to 2 weeks after completing a course of antibiotics (or 2 to 3 weeks after diagnosis in uncomplicated cases in which antibiotic treatment was not ordered) to make sure the infection is resolved or resolving. This is especially important for younger children (< 2 years of age) or those with persistent symptoms or a history of recurrent otitis media.[7]

Parapharyngeal, Retropharyngeal, and Peritonsillar Abscess

A parapharyngeal abscess usually extends down into the tissue planes of the neck and is more serious, although less common than a peritonsillar abscess.

A retropharyngeal abscess may be a sequel to peritonsillar infection, lateral pharyngeal abscess, or a puncture of the posterior pharyngeal wall by a foreign body (e.g., a bone shard) or iatrogenic instrumentation (e.g., endotracheal intubation or endoscopy).[44,54] It also may occur as a complication of diabetes or a compromised immune response (e.g., alcoholism, malignancy, or an HIV-related disease).[54] Untreated retropharyngeal abscess may progress to mediastinitis, but this outcome is less likely in lateral pharyngeal abscess.[44]

A peritonsillar abscess is more localized. The patient usually is symptomatic for 48 hours before the abscess becomes apparent.[14]

Signs and symptoms
- Fever
- Complaint of moderate to severe neck or pharyngeal pain, odynophagia (painful swallowing), and dysphagia (difficulty swallowing).
- Patients also may exhibit dysphonia (muffled, "hot potato" voice) or signs of airway compromise (e.g., stridor).
- Peritonsillar and parapharyngeal abscesses are unilateral and cause uvular displacement. Trismus also may be present.[4]
- A parapharyngeal abscess often presents with torticollis.[4]

Diagnosis
- Diagnosis is determined by clinical symptoms.
- Lateral parapharyngeal abscess may cause ipsilateral deficits of cranial nerves (notably glossopharyngeal [IX], vagus [X], or hypoglossal [XII]). They also may involve the cervical sympathetic chain, causing signs of Horner's syndrome (e.g., ipsilateral ptosis, miosis, and decreased lacrimation).[44]
- In cases of retropharyngeal abscess, swelling of the posterior pharyngeal wall may not be visible on physical examination.[54]
- Lateral soft-tissue neck radiographs or a CT scan may be necessary to confirm or differentiate among diagnoses.[14,54]
- Leukocytosis, high fever, and toxic appearance are common clinical findings in these conditions. A baseline septic workup may be ordered.

Treatment
- Patients with a parapharyngeal abscess are admitted, and high-dose parenteral antibiotic therapy is initiated.
- For peritonsillar abscesses, an aspiration or I & D may be performed in the ED and the patient may be discharged from the ED. However, patients usually are admitted for a short stay and IV antibiotics.
- Patients with a retropharyngeal abscess may require emergency examination in an operating room under general anesthesia.

Common treatment includes an operative I & D and admission for high-dose parenteral antibiotic therapy.

Sinusitis

Sinusitis is an inflammation of the lining of the paranasal sinuses caused by bacterial overgrowth. This condition may be acute or chronic. Chronic sinusitis occurs when chronic inflammation causes thickening of the lining of the sinuses.

Signs and symptoms

- Complaints of "sinus" congestion or headaches are extremely common.
- Sensation of pressure in the affected region and a purulent nasal discharge
- Fever

Diagnosis

- Definitive diagnosis can be made by an x-ray examination or a CT scan but often is presumptive and based on clinical presentation.
- Transillumination may be used as a diagnostic adjunct.

Treatment

- Untreated sinusitis can progress and lead to cavernous sinus thrombosis or other intracranial infections.[55]
- Treatment usually consists of penicillin or amoxicillin. Estimates of the number of treatments needed for cure or improvement range from five to seven days for penicillin or amoxicillin.[56] It is important to emphasize the importance of completing the course of antibiotics, even if symptoms improve.[50]
- OTC decongestants may afford some symptomatic relief but do not accelerate cure.
- To avoid thickening of mucus, antihistamines should be avoided unless allergy is deemed a significant etiologic factor.[20]

NURSING SURVEILLANCE

1. Airway maintenance
2. Oxygen saturation monitoring and oxygen administration as indicated
3. Control of bleeding and monitoring of fluid and blood replacement as indicated
4. Vital signs as appropriate to condition and departmental policy
5. Fever control and seizure prevention
6. Adequacy of pain relief and evaluation of responses to other interventions

EXPECTED PATIENT OUTCOMES

1. The airway is spontaneously maintainable, or an artificial airway is in place.
2. Oxygen saturation should have remained above 94% throughout stabilization, and vital signs should not have deteriorated.
3. In cases of epistaxis, bleeding should be controlled and vital signs should be within the normal range at the time of disposition. For the patient with a posterior pack, oxygen saturation monitoring and adequate IV access to permit administration of blood products, if needed, should be instituted.
4. For febrile children, a reduction in fever should be documented before discharge.
5. Nausea and vertigo should be improved at the time of discharge. The patient should be tolerating clear liquids PO.
6. Certain types of pain, particularly from otitis media and odontalgia, may not be completely controllable in the course of a brief visit but should at least be reduced.
7. After disimpaction of cerumen, auditory acuity often is subjectively improved, and this is helpful to document.

DISCHARGE IMPLICATIONS

1. The patient and family must understand the plan of care, expected self-care, medications, and expected time frames for symptom resolution and follow-up.
2. For children with croup who are well enough to be discharged from the ED, clear criteria that would warrant a return to the ED should be discussed as well. Although the efficacy of mist, per se, is unclear, it is usually recommended as a simple symptomatic treatment but should not delay a return to the ED if symptoms are severe or rapidly worsening.
3. Patients with anterior nasal packs should understand what to do if bleeding recurs and when to follow up for packing removal.
4. Instruct the parents of children with otitis media or other febrile conditions on the appropriate method to measure a child's temperature, administer antipyretics and antibiotics, if ordered, and recognize signs and symptoms of deterioration.
5. A patient with a nasal fracture should be instructed to follow up with an ENT or plastic surgeon after the swelling has gone down if it is difficult to breathe out of one naris or if the patient is not satisfied with the appearance of the nose.

6. Patients who have had an auricular or nasal septal hematoma incised and drained should be given follow-up instructions about dressing or packing changes and drain removal.
7. Patients with dental complaints should be instructed on the importance of follow-up with a dentist or oral surgeon.
8. Patients with anterior epistaxis should receive the following instructions:
   - Avoid drinking beverages that are either very hot or very cold while packing is in place.
   - Avoid aspirin and nonsteroidal antiinflammatory drugs for at least several days.
   - Do not lift heavy objects or strain while a pack is in place.
   - Patients may be more comfortable at home resting in an orthopneic position (e.g., with enough pillows to elevate the head and upper torso to the equivalent of a semi-Fowler's position).

REFERENCES

1. Neff JA: Epiglottitis, *J Emerg Nurs* 13:184, 1987.
2. Nemes J, Schmidt E, and Kelly L: Epiglottitis: ED nursing management, *J Emerg Nurs* 14:70, 1988.
3. Muñiz A: *Epiglottitis*, 2002, online review, www.emedicine.com. Retrieved June 14, 2003 from www.emedicine.com/PED/topic700.htm.
4. Kimmitz TP and Defries HO: Pharyngeal emergencies, *Top Emerg Med* 6 (3):66, 1984.
5. Pelletier CR, Jordan DR, Braga R, et al: Assessment of ocular trauma associated with head and neck injuries, *J Trauma-Injury Infect Crit Care* 44 (2):350-354, 1998.
6. Ellis E III and Scott K: Assessment of patients with facial fractures, *Emerg Med Clin North Am* 18 (3):411-448, 2000.
7. Pfaff JA and Moore GP: Eye, ear, nose, and throat, *Emerg Med Clin North Am* 15:327, 1997.
8. Hussain K, Wijetunge DB, Grubnic S, et al: A comprehensive analysis of craniofacial trauma, *J Trauma* 36:34, 1994.
9. Joseph E, Zak R, Smith S, et al: Predictors of blinding or serious eye injury in blunt trauma, *J Trauma* 33:19, 1992.
10. Shesser R and Smith M: Oral emergencies, *Top Emerg Med* 6 (3):48, 1984.
11. Klokkevold P: Common dental emergencies: evaluation and management for emergency physicians, *Emerg Med Clin North Am* 7:29, 1989.
12. Krasner PR: Treatment of tooth avulsion by nurses, *J Emerg Nurs* 16:29-35, 1990.
13. Dale RA: Dentoalveolar trauma, *Emerg Med Clin North Am* 18 (3):521-538, 2000.
14. Weimert TA: Common ENT emergencies part 2: the acute nose and throat, *Emerg Med* 24 (6):26, 1992.
15. Barkin RM: Pediatrics. A potpourri of clinical pearls, *Emerg Med Clin North Am* 15 (2):381-388, 1997.

16. Neto GM, Kentab O, Klassen TP, et al: A randomized controlled trial of mist in the acute treatment of moderate croup, *Acad Emerg Med* 9 (9):873-879, 2002.

17. Cressman WR and Myer CM III: Diagnosis and management of croup and epiglottitis, *Pediatr Clin North Am* 41:265, 1994.

18. Wright RB, Pomerantz WJ, and Luria JW: New approaches to respiratory infections in children. Bronchiolitis and croup, *Emerg Med Clin North Am* 20 (1):93-114, 2002.

19. Josephson GD, Godley FA, and Stierna P: Practical management of epistaxis, *Emerg Med Clin North Am* 75:1311, 1991.

20. Votey S and Dudley JP: Emergency ear nose and throat procedures, *Emerg Med Clin North Am* 7:117, 1989.

21. Stewart MH, Siff JE, and Cydulka RK: Evaluation of the patient with sore throat, earache, and sinusitis: an evidence based approach, *Emerg Med Clin North Am* 17 (1):153-187, 1999.

22. Wolkove N, Kreisman H, Cohen C, et al: Occult foreign-body aspiration in adults, *JAMA* 248:1350, 1982.

23. Sharp JF and Denholm S: Routine x-rays in nasal trauma: the influence of audit on clinical practice, *J R Soc Med* 87 (3):153, March, 1994.

24. Reich JJ and Turbiak TW: Otic emergencies, *Top Emerg Med* 6 (3):19, 1984.

25. Zivic RC and King S: Cerumen impaction management for clients of all ages, *Nurs Pract* 18 (3):33, 1993.

26. Weber JE, Chudnofsky CR, Younger JG, et al: A randomized comparison of helium-oxygen mixture (Heliox) and racemic epinephrine for the treatment of moderate to severe croup, *Pediatrics* 107 (6):e96 (pp 1-4), 2001. Retrieved June 7, 2003 from www.pediatrics.org/cgi/content/full/ 107/6/e96.

27. McGarry GW and Moulton C: The first aid management of epistaxis by accident and emergency medicine staff, *Arch Emerg Med* 10 (4):298, 1993.

28. Singer AJ, Sauris E, and Viccellio AW: Ceruminolytic effects of docusate sodium: a randomized, controlled trial, *Ann Emerg Med* 36:228-232, 2000.

29. Grossan M: Safe, effective techniques for cerumen removal, *Geriatrics* 55:80, 2000.

30. Ming T and Mullor GP: Removal of ear wax, *Br Med J* 325:27, 2002.

31. Chen DA and Caparosa RJ: A nonprescription ceruminolytic, *Am J Otol* 12:475, 1991.

32. Brown JC: The management of croup, *Br Med Bull* 61:189-202, 2002.

33. Jamshidi PB, Kemp JS, Peter JR, et al: The effect of humidified air in mild to moderate croup: evaluation using croup scores and respiratory inductance plethysmography (abstract), *Acad Emerg Med* 8 (5):417, 2001.

34. Ausejo M, Saenz A, Pham B, et al: The effectiveness of glucocorticoids in treating croup: meta-analysis, *Br Med J* 319 (7210):595-600, 1999.

35. Ausejo Segura M, Saenz A, Pham B, et al: Glucocorticoids for croup. In: *The Cochrane Library*, issue 2, Oxford, 2003, Update Software.

36. Gilbert DN, Moellering RC, and Sande MA, eds: *Sanford guide to antimicrobial therapy*, ed 33, Hyde Park, VT, 2003, Antimicrobial Therapy.

37. Kass EG, McFadden EA, Jacobson S, et al: Acute epiglottitis in the adult: experience with a seasonal presentation, *Laryngoscope* 103:841, 1993.

38. Jacobs EE, Ota HG, and Turner PA: Control of epistaxis. In May HL et al, eds: *Emergency medicine*, ed 2, Boston, 1992, Little, Brown.

39. Chu L, Gussack GS, and Muller T: A treatment protocol for mandible fractures, *J Trauma* 36:48, 1994.

40. Guss DA, Clark RF, Peitz T, et al: Pantomography vs mandibular series for the detection of mandibular fractures, *Acad Emerg Med* 7 (2):141-145, 2000.

41. Ellis E III, Simon P, and Throckmorton GS: Occlusal results after open or closed treatment of fractures of the mandibular condylar process, *J Oral Maxillofac Surg* 58 (3):260-268, 2000.

42. Heit JM, Stevens MR, and Jeffords K: Comparison of ceftriaxone with penicillin for antibiotic prophylaxis for compound mandible fractures, Oral Surg, Oral Med, Oral Pathol, Oral Radiol, Endodont 83 (4):423-426, 1997.

43. Nigam A, Goni A, Benjamin A, et al: The value of radiographs in the management of the fractured nose, *Arch Emerg Med* 10 (4):293, 1993.

44. Flynn TR: The swollen face. Severe odontogenic infections, *Emerg Med Clin North Am* 18 (3):481-519, 2000.

45. Weimert TA: Common ENT emergencies part 1: the acute ear, *Emerg Med* 24 (5):134, 1992.

46. Bressler K and Shelton C: Ear foreign-body removal: a review of 98 consecutive cases, *Laryngoscope* 103 (4):367, 1993.

47. Leffler S, Cheney P, and Tandberg D: Chemical immobilization and killing of intra-aural roaches: an in vitro comparative study, *Ann Emerg Med* 22:1795, 1993.

48. Backlin SA: Positive pressure technique for nasal foreign body removal in children, *Ann Emerg Med* 25:554, 1995.

49. Shapiro RS: Foreign bodies of the nose. In Bluestone CD, Stool SE, and Scheetz MD, eds: *Pediatric otolaryngology*, ed 2, Philadelphia, 1990, WB Saunders.

50. Flynn CA, Griffin G, and Tudiver F: Decongestants and antihistamines for acute otitis media in children. In: *The Cochrane Library*, issue 2, Oxford, 2003, Update Software.

51. Damoiseaux RA, van Balen FA, Hoes AW, et al: Primary care based randomised, double blind trial of amoxicillin versus placebo for acute otitis media in children aged under 2 years, *Br Med J* 320 (7231):350-354, 2000.

52. Glasziou PP, Del Mar CB, Sanders SL, et al: Antibiotics for acute otitis media in children. In: *The Cochrane Library*, issue 2, Oxford, 2003, Update Software.

53. Celin SE, Bluestone CD, Stephenson J, et al: Bacteriology of acute otitis media in adults, *JAMA* 266:2249, 1991.

54. Tannebaum RD: Adult retropharyngeal abscess: a case report and review of the literature, *J Emerg Med* 14:147, 1996.

55. Clayman, Adams GL, Paugh DE, et al: Intracranial complications of paranasal sinusitis: a combined institutional review, *Laryngoscope* 101:234, 1991.

56. Williams JW, Aguilar C, Makela M, et al. Antibiotics for acute maxillary sinusitis. In: *The Cochrane Library*, issue 2, Oxford, 2003, Update Software.

chapter 8

Endocrine Conditions

Amy Herrington

CLINICAL CONDITIONS

Acute Adrenal Insufficiency and Addison's Disease
Cushing's Syndrome
Diabetic Ketoacidosis (DKA)
Hyperosmolar, Hyperglycemic State (HHS)
Hypoglycemia
Myxedema
Syndrome of Inappropriate Antidiuretic Hormone
    Secretion (SIADH)
Thyrotoxicosis and Thyroid Storm

INTRODUCTION

Other than diabetes, endocrine emergencies are extremely rare; however, acute endocrine crises are life threatening and require rapid interventions. Patients may be aware that they have an endocrine disorder, or the diagnosis may be made or suspected for the first time in the emergency department (ED).

FOCUSED NURSING ASSESSMENT

The areas of ventilation, perfusion, cognition, and sexuality should be assessed in greater detail than other areas.

General Appearance
- Quickly assess the general appearance to obtain valuable information about the patient's status.
- Obtain an overall impression about the weight and stature of your patient. Weight loss is common in hyperthyroidism and acute adrenal insufficiency (Addison's disease). Obesity is a symptom of Cushing's syndrome and is usually manifested by round, plump facial features and neck and upper back weight gain (buffalo hump).
- Goiter is associated with thyroid syndrome.
- Muscle wasting is associated with endocrine disorders.

- Determine level of consciousness, respiratory status, and circulatory status.
- Exophthalmos (bulging eyeballs) may be present in hyperthyroidism.
- Initial interventions can begin before the more thorough assessment is conducted.

Oxygenation and Ventilation

- Ensure a patent airway. Severe cases of endocrine emergencies are associated with an altered level of consciousness. If an altered level of consciousness is present, airway management becomes the primary concern. Follow the American Heart Association guidelines for airway management and prepare for intubation.
- Endocrine disorders affect metabolism, and oxygen administration promotes oxygen availability in both overproduction and underproduction of hormones.
- Stridor is associated with large goiter in thyroid disease. Respiratory distress can occur if the goiter is large enough to compress the trachea.
- Undress the patient and assess the breathing pattern for symmetry and depth of excursion. Kussmaul respirations, described as deep, accelerated, sighing respirations, often are noted in diabetic ketoacidosis (DKA) patients.
- Auscultate breath sounds. Pulmonary edema, characterized by crackles, may occur in hypothyroidism. Diminished breath sounds may indicate infiltrates and possible infection as a precipitating cause of DKA; hyperosmolar, hyperglycemic syndrome (HHS); and thyroid disorders.
- Pulse oximetry may be useful and can provide clues regarding oxygenation.

Perfusion

- Auscultate heart sounds. A systolic murmur may be present in high-flow or hyperdynamic (e.g., hyperthyroidism) states.
- Assess skin color and temperature. Hot, dry skin is associated with DKA or adrenal crisis. Warm, moist skin is associated with hyperthyroidism. Cool, pale skin is associated with hypothyroidism.
- Assess the hydration status by examining skin turgor, mucous membranes, and orbits. Flushed, dry skin indicates dehydration. Dehydration is associated with adrenal insufficiency, HHS, and ketoacidosis.

- Assess peripheral pulses. Vasoconstriction is present in Cushing's syndrome. Diminished pulses may be present in instances of dehydration.
- Assess blood pressure: Hypotension is associated with dehydration and decreased circulating blood volume. Orthostatic changes in both blood pressure and pulse may be present. Diastolic hypertension is present in patients with chronic hypothyroidism (myxedema) caused by peripheral vasoconstriction as an effort to maintain body core temperature. Systolic hypertension is associated with Cushing's syndrome related to fluid retention and oversecretion of catecholamines.
- Assess heart rate: Bradycardia is present in hypothyroidism. Tachycardia and palpitations occur in hyperthyroidism.
- Endocrine disorders may produce arrhythmias, conduction defects, and congestive heart failure (CHF).
- Generalized edema may be present in hypothyroidism and syndrome of inappropriate antidiuretic hormone (SIADH) secretion.
- Note skin temperature. Fever may be present in hyperthyroidism or in the presence of infection, which can increase insulin requirements and may precipitate hyperglycemia and hyperosmolality in the diabetic patient.

Cognition
- Perform a neurologic assessment and document a Glasgow Coma Scale (GCS) score (see Reference Guide 10 [adults] and Reference Guide 16 [infants and children]).
- Disorientation may be a manifestation of cerebral edema secondary to hyperosmolality. Cognition is almost always impaired in HHS and DKA. Forgetfulness is seen in patients with hypothyroid disease.
- Mood changes and insomnia are characteristic of hyperthyroidism.

Sensation and Mobility
- Assess and compare the mobility, sensation, and strength of all extremities.
- Fatigue is associated with myxedema, adrenal insufficiency, and diabetes.
- Assess for reflexes and tremors. Tremors and hyperreflexia occur often in hyperthyroidism.
- Assess for pain and if present, describe the quality, duration, location, and rating on 0 to 10 scale. Headaches often are

associated with hypoglycemia. Abdominal pain is associated with DKA and acute adrenal insufficiency.

Sexuality

- Impotence and abnormal menses are associated with Cushing's disease. The date of the last menstrual period and date of onset of pubescent findings should be assessed. Central precocious puberty and other pituitary etiologies are associated with the early onset on puberty.
- Menorrhagia, or painful menstruation, is associated with hypothyroidism.
- Secondary sexual characteristics may be overpronounced (e.g., gynecomastia and breast development with males) in Cushing's disease.
- There is a decrease in body and pubic hair among females with Addison's disease. Hirsutism is associated with Cushing's syndrome. This is characterized by the growth of hair in unusual places, especially in females.

Tissue Integrity

- Assess the skin for rashes, darkening in pigmentation, or bruising. Darkly colored (hyperpigmented) skin in Caucasian patients suggests Addison's disease. Hyperpigmentation may be most visible on the back of the hands, elbows, and knees.
- Assess skin texture. Ruddy complexion is associated with Cushing's syndrome.

Safety

- Endocrine illnesses can be associated with altered thought processes. Therefore, it is important for the nurse to assess the patient for depression, mania, and suicidal thoughts. If any or all of these symptoms are present, take appropriate safety interventions to ensure that injury does not occur to the patient or others.
- Mania is most often associated with hyperthyroidism.
- Depression or psychosis can be seen with Cushing syndrome.
- Many drugs can precipitate endocrine problems; therefore a thorough medication history should be obtained (Table 8-1).

Elimination/Hydration

- Assess and palpate the abdomen for discomfort.
- Assess bowel pattern and date of last bowel movement. Constipation is associated with hypothyroidism.

TABLE 8-1 Drugs That May Precipitate
Endocrine Problems

Drug	Effect	Condition
Hydrochloro-thiazide	Decreases insulin secretion and increases insulin resistance	DKA, HHS
Beta-blocking agents (e.g., propranolol)	Decreases insulin secretion	DKA
Dilantin	Decreases insulin secretion	DKA
Alcohol	Decreases insulin secretion	DKA
Calcium channel blockers (e.g., nifedipine)	Decreases insulin secretion	DKA
Cortisol	Increases insulin resistance	DKA, HHS
Terbutaline	Increases insulin resistance	DKA
Sedatives	Decreases oxygen consumption	Hypothyroidism
Tranquilizers	Decreases oxygen consumption	Hypothyroidism
Diuretics	Decreases circulating blood volume	Hypothyroidism
Ketoconazole	Decreases steroid synthesis	Addison's disease
Rifampin	Decreases steroid synthesis	Addison's disease

DKA, Diabetic ketoacidosis; *HHS,* hyperosmolar, nonketotic state

- Determine whether the patient has been vomiting, having diarrhea, urinating excessively, or not drinking fluids in a hot, humid environment. Vomiting is associated with DKA. All of these factors promote dehydration, which can precipitate DKA and HHS.
- Vomiting and diarrhea are associated with hyperthyroidism.

LIFE SPAN ISSUES

Children
- The peak onset of insulin-dependent diabetes mellitus (IDDM) occurs from 11 to 13 years of age.[1]
- The onset of puberty and the increase of growth harmone may lead to ketoacidosis.

Pregnancy
- Pregnancy may potentiate DKA.
- Thyrotoxicosis or hypothyroidism may occur in the postpartum period.

- Gestational diabetes is more common among noncaucasian and older women.

Adults

- The risk of non–insulin-dependent diabetes mellitus (NIDDM) increases after the age of 40.[1]
- Thyroid crisis or storm occurs more often among females from 30 to 50 years of age.[2]
- Addison's disease is more common among adults 30 to 50 years old.[3]

Geriatric Patients

- HHS is more common in older individuals with NIDDM.
- Hypothyroidism causes decreased oxygen consumption and decreased heat generation. In the geriatric population, oxygen consumption and heat generation decline as part of aging.
- Myxedema is diagnosed more often in the geriatric population because the symptoms are more pronounced as a result of the lower compensatory reserve.

INITIAL INTERVENTIONS

1. Administer oxygen as needed.
2. Initiate continuous pulse oximetry monitoring.
3. Initiate cardiac monitoring.
4. Initiate serial NIBP monitoring.
5. Insert an IV catheter and obtain blood for anticipated laboratory tests. Fluid administration should be approached judiciously, as overhydration may be a problem in some endocrine disorders.
6. Nursing care priorities are listed in the table on pp. 320-321.

PRIORITY DIAGNOSTIC TESTS

Laboratory Tests

NOTE: Collect laboratory samples before administration of medication so that the baseline hormone levels may be determined. Anticipate drug administration before the return of laboratory data because of serious consequences from many endocrine disorders.

Reference Guide 6 has a table comparing the diagnostic lab values for DKA and HHS.

Serum Laboratory Tests

Adrenocorticotropic (ACTH): Elevated in Cushing's disease
Aldosterone level: Decreased in Addison's disease

Anion gap: Anion gap will be greater than 12 in DKA and will be variable in HHS. (Normal value is 8 to 12 mEq/L)

Arterial blood gases: pH value will be below 7.30 in DKA and above 7.30 in HHS. Bicarbonate levels will be less than 15 mEq/L in DKA. Bicarbonate levels will be greater than 15 mEq/L in HHS.

Complete blood count (CBC): WBC count is normally elevated without infection in diabetic patients. Levels of 40,000 cells/mm^3 have been noted in DKA without infection. An increased neutrophil count may indicate infection in diabetic patients. Hypothyroid patients may be unable to elevate the WBC count in infection because of depressed bone marrow activity. An elevated band count on the differential indicates infection in these patients.

Cortisol: Decreased in Addison's disease

Free Triiodothyronine (T$_3$): Elevated in hyperthyroidism and decreased in hypothyroidism

Free Thyroxine (T$_4$): Elevated in hyperthyroidism and decreased in hypothyroidism

Glucose: Decreased in hypoglycemia, acute adrenal insufficiency, Addison's disease, and hypothyroidism. Elevated in ketoacidosis, HHS, and Cushing's disease.

Osmolality: Decreased in DKA and elevated in HHS

Potassium: Increased in Addison's disease and untreated hyperosmolar states. The level may decrease as potassium moves back into the cell.

Rapid synthetic corticotropin stimulation test: Used to determine whether adrenal dysfunction is causing Addison's disease. Synthetic ACTH is administered IV, and cortisol levels are measured at baseline and 30-minute and 60-minute intervals after administration. Failure of cortisol levels to increase indicates a primary adrenal problem

Sodium: Hyponatremia may be present in Addison's disease and myxedema.

Thyroid stimulating hormone: Decreased in secondary hypothyroidism (pituitary tumor) and in hyperthyroidism. Elevated in primary hypothyroidism (loss of functioning thyroid tissue).

Total triiodothyronine (T$_3$) level: Elevated in hyperthyroidism. Decreased in acute illness or starvation. The level also can be reduced by Inderal, steroids, and amiodarone.

Total thyroxine (T$_4$) level: Elevated in hyperthyroidism and liver disease, and with estrogen use. Decreased in severe illness and with androgen or steroid use.

NURSING CARE PRIORITIES

Potential/Actual Problem	Causes	Signs and Symptoms	Interventions
1. Airway compromise	• Decreased level of consciousness • Goiter	• Dyspnea • Decreased respiratory rate • Altered level of consciousness • Stridor	• Open airway and support with adjunct as needed • Intubation as required • Provide suction prn. • Monitor oxygen saturation. • Preparation for intubation.
2. Impaired breathing	• Fatigue • Acidosis • Electrolyte abnormality	• Tachypnea • Dyspnea • Bradypnea • Altered level of consciousness	• Administer oxygen. • Monitor respiratory rate and effort. • Monitor oxygen saturation. • Prepare for endotracheal intubation, neuromuscular blockade, and mechanical ventilation.
3. Decreased cardiac output	• Dehydration • Decreased contractility resulting from chronic left	• Increased HR • Decreased blood pressure • Poor skin turgor	• Administer volume or diuretics as ordered. • Decrease metabolic needs by treating fever, pain, and infection.

	ventricle overdistention	• Decreased urine output • Vomiting/diarrhea • Volume overload • Crackles present in lung fields • Edema • Shortness of breath, especially with exertion	• Prepare for and assist with invasive hemodynamic monitoring. • Monitor intake and output.
4. Safety	• Electrolyte disturbances • Psychological changes related to the endocrine disorder	• Seizures (with severe hyponatremia) • Ventricular ectopy with hypokalemia • Confusion • Combativeness • Flight of ideas	• Replace electrolytes as ordered. • Monitor intake and output. • Perform frequent neurologic assessments. • Provide safe environment with constant supervision.
5. Knowledge	• Diet • Fluid intake • Medication	• Requests information • Required lifestyle changes	• Initiate teaching to the patient and family. • Provide resources for home review. • Dietary consult/nutritionist visit • Provide appropriate follow-up information.

Urine Laboratory Tests

Urine-free cortisol test: 24-hour test detects cortisol excretion in the urine, commonly seen in Cushing's disease. If the test result is positive for cortisol, ACTH tests are conducted to determine the etiology of the disease.

Urine ketones: Ketones will be present in DKA but absent in HHNC.

A quick bedside calculation of laboratory tests used in DKA and HHS is located in Table 8-2.

Radiographic Tests

CT scan: Scans of the adrenal and thyroid glands may be performed to identify gland enlargement, atrophy, and tumors.

MRI: Scans of the pituitary to assess for tumor. This scan is done with and without IV contrast.

Other Tests

ECG: T-wave changes during fluid resuscitation for dehydration may indicate impending CHF. Sinus bradycardia, a prolonged QT interval, and low voltage are seen on the ECG in hypothyroidism.

Clinical Conditions
Acute Adrenal Insufficiency (Addison's Disease)/ Adrenal Crisis

Adrenal insufficiency is a devastating disease related to the effects of decreased production or lack of glucocorticoid and mineralocorticoid hormones. These hormones are responsible for maintaining blood pressure and blood volume and for glucose regulation. The disease may be caused by a primary adrenal problem or induced secondary to a hypothalamic or pituitary problem. It also can be triggered by an acute stressor such as trauma, burns, infection, hypothermia, or surgery.

Symptoms
- Fatigue
- Weakness
- Weight loss
- Dehydration related to nausea and vomiting
- Diarrhea
- Hypotension
- Abdominal pain
- Increased skin pigmentation
- Depression

TABLE 8-2 Bedside Calculation of Laboratory Tests in DKA and HHS

Type	Rationale	Formula
Sodium correction	Serum sodium levels appear lower than they actually are in the presence of hyperglycemia.	Add 1.6 mg/dl to the patient's reported sodium level for every 100 mg/dl increase in blood glucose above normal; normal considered 100 mg/dl (example: if blood glucose is 500 mg/dl, multiply $4 \times 1.6 = 6.4$; add 6.4 mg/dl to actual reported serum sodium value).
Serum osmolality	Measured osmolality by laboratory includes all molecules. Calculating the effective plasma osmolality allows you to examine only molecules that contribute to hydration; if calculated osmolality is less than measured and patient is comatose, there is another cause other than dehydration for coma.	Effective osmolality = 2 × (measured Na in mEq/L) + blood glucose in mg/dl divided by 18. Normal = 275-295 mOsm/kg.
Anion gap	Indicates an acidotic state but does not reveal the kinds of acids that have produced the state (e.g., lactic acid vs. ketones). Remains normal in a metabolic acidosis resulting from bicarbonate loss.	Sodium − (chloride + bicarbonate). Normal range = 8-12 mEq/L.

- Females may have decreased body hair
- Tachycardia
- Salt craving

Diagnosis
- History of prior illness, injury, surgery, or medication change
- High index of suspicion with unexplained hypotension
- Hyponatremia
- Hyperkalemia
- Hypoglycemia
- Hypercalcemia
- Elevated BUN
- Low serum cortisol level

Treatment
- Correct fluid and electrolyte imbalances.
- Administer IV hydrocortisone to replace glucocorticoids.
- Administer fludrocortisone to replace mineralocorticoids.

Cushing's Syndrome

Cushing's disease is the overproduction of cortisol as a result of overactivity of ACTH. Immune suppression caused by cortisol overproduction increases the patient's risk for early death and masks signs of existing infection.

Symptoms
- Hypertension
- Fatigue
- Neuromuscular complaints
- Growth of hair in unusual places
- Abdominal pain
- Osteoporosis
- Obesity with round plump facial features, neck and upper back weight gain (buffalo hump)
- Menstrual disorders
- Unexplained hypokalemia
- Hyperglycemia
- Anxiety
- Depression

Diagnosis
- History and physical examination; elicit information about pituitary or adrenal tumors
- 24-hour urine for free cortisol
- Measurement of the ACTH level

Treatment
- Correct hypertension, hyperglycemia, and hypokalemia.

- Multiple medications are used in treating Cushing's disease. These medications have undesirable side effects and interfere with compliance.
- Surgery and pituitary irradiation may be used in some cases.

Diabetic Ketoacidosis

Diabetic ketoacidosis (DKA) is a potentially life-threatening diabetic complication occurring most often in those with type I diabetes mellitus. Most often, there is a precipitating event such as illness, infection, trauma, surgery, or a psychological stressor. DKA is caused by a deficiency of circulating insulin. The body normally utilizes glucose for energy. However, in diabetic patients there is an inability of the body to utilize glucose, as cells are unable to transport glucose without the presence of insulin. This leads to increased production of fatty acids in an effort to deliver energy to the body. The use of free fatty acids for energy versus glucose produces ketoacids and ultimately metabolic acidosis.

Symptoms

- Hyperglycemia induces diuresis, so the patient complains of polyuria, thirst, and fatigue.
- Abdominal pain related to gastric dilation
- Vomiting
- Weight loss
- Weakness
- Tachycardia
- Hypotension
- Rapid respiratory rate with deep breaths (Kussmaul's respirations)
- Mental status may range from full alertness to lethargy and coma
- Acetone odor on breath

Diagnosis

- Ketones will be present in the urine.
- Arterial blood gases will reveal a pH below 7.30.[4]
- Blood glucose levels will be elevated (>250 mg/dl).[4]
- The serum bicarbonate level may be low (<15 mEq/L).[4]

Treatment

- Successful treatment includes treatment of dehydration, hyperglycemia, and electrolyte imbalances.
- For treatment of adult patients in DKA, see Reference Guide 6 for table listing diagnostic criteria and treatment algorithm.
- In patients with renal or cardiac compromise, monitor serum osmolality and frequently assess cardiac, renal, and mental status to avoid fluid overload.

- Pediatric patients[4]:

REHYDRATION AND POTASSIUM

- ○ First hour, 0.9% NS at 10 to 20 ml/kg. May need to repeat if patient severely dehydrated. Do not exceed 50 ml/kg over first 4 hours.
- ○ After the first hour, 0.45% NS or 0.9% (depending on the serum sodium) should be infused at a rate 1.5 times the 24-hour maintenance requirements.
- ○ When renal function is assured and serum potassium known, add 20-40 mEq/L potassium. When serum glucose reaches 250 mg/dl, change fluid to 5% dextrose and 0.45% to 0.75% NS with potassium.

INSULIN

- ○ IV infusion of regular insulin at 0.1 units/kg/hr should be maintained until the pH is greater than 7.30 and the bicarbonate is greater than 15 mEq/L. Then reduce infusion to 0.05 units/kg/hr until subcutaneous insulin is initiated.

BICARBONATE

- ○ Replace bicarbonate (2 mEq/kg over 1 hour) if the patient remains profoundly acidotic (pH <7.0) after 1 hour of fluid replacement.

PHOSPHATE

- ○ Phosphate levels often are normal or increased on presentation but will decrease with insulin therapy. Although rarely done, phosphate can be replaced to avoid cardiac and skeletal muscle weakness and respiratory depression due to hypophosphatemia. Replacement must be done with caution to prevent hypocalcemia.

Hyperosmolar, Hyperglycemic State (also known as Hyperosmolar, Hyperglycemic Nonketotic Coma, or HHNK)

Patients who have HHS may not have been diagnosed with diabetes or may have type II diabetes. Often, HHS is the first indicator of a chronic problem. Almost all cases are precipitated by infection. Symptoms of DKA and HHS are similar. Both are associated with glycosuria, resulting in osmotic diuresis, with loss of water, sodium, potassium, and other electrolytes.[4] DKA and HHS differ in magnitude of dehydration and degree of ketosis and acidosis; refer to Table 8-3 for diagnostic criteria.

Symptoms

- Massive diuresis
- Polyuria, thirst, and fatigue related to calcium, potassium, and magnesium losses

TABLE 8-3   Diagnostic Criteria for DKA and HHS

	Blood Glucose	Arterial pH	Bicarbonate	Ketonemia	Effective Serum Osmolality
DKA	Greater than 250 mg/dl	Less than 7.3	Less than 15 mEq/L	Moderate	
HHS	Greater than 600 mg/dl	Greater than 7.3	Greater than 15 mEq/L	Mild	Greater than 320 mOsm/kg H_2O

- CNS symptoms are common as a result of a high serum osmolality level
- Patients complain of visual changes
- Aphasia, stupor, seizures, and hallucinations are possible

Diagnosis
- Serum glucose greater than 600 mg/dl.[4]
- Effective serum osmolality greater than 320 mOsm/kg H_2O.[4]
- Mild ketonuria or ketonemia.[4]
- The arterial pH will be greater than 7.3.[4]
- Bicarbonate greater than 15 mEq/L.[4]
- The result of a urine test may be positive for a urinary tract infection.
- A chest film may indicate pneumonia.

Treatment
- For treatment of adult patients in HHS, see Reference Guide 6 for table listing diagnostic criteria and treatment algorithm.

NURSING ALERT

When the nurse is treating both DKA and HHS, it is crucial to reassess the patient's breath sounds and neurologic status frequently to detect impending fluid overload; overaggressive rehydration will cause cerebral and pulmonary edema.

Hypoglycemia
- Hypoglycemia may occur with a diabetic patient because of inadequate food intake in relation to insulin dosage. Exercise, infection, and emotional stress also may alter blood glucose levels. Nondiabetic patients also are susceptible

to hypoglycemia. The symptoms of hypoglycemia will occur suddenly. For a comparison of the different types of insulin, see Table 8-4.

Symptoms
- Headache
- Dizziness
- Confusion
- Diaphoresis
- Tachycardia
- Palpitations

Diagnosis
- The blood glucose level usually will be below 50 to 60 mg/dl.

Treatment
- Hypoglycemia is rapidly reversed with administration of IV glucose (50 ml of dextrose 50% solution) or oral glucose if the patient is alert enough to prevent aspiration.
- Glucagon 1 mg IM may be given as an alternative.

Myxedema

Myxedema coma is an acute manifestation of hypothyroidism. A precipitating illness or event usually stimulates a hypothyroid crisis. Common precipitating conditions are stroke, infection, and traumatic injury.

Symptoms
- Altered mental status ranging from disorientation to psychosis
- Hypothermia
- Hyporeflexia
- CHF is a common complication
- Hypotension
- Hypoventilation
- Bradycardia

Diagnosis
- Diagnosis is based on the symptoms and presentation.

Treatment
- Respiratory depression may occur secondary to carbon dioxide retention. A definitive airway should be obtained. Intubation and mechanical ventilation may be initiated prophylactically because cardiovascular collapse occurs quickly with respiratory depression.
- Treat hypotension with crystalloids and/or vasopressor agents.
- IV levothyroxine is administered on suspicion of myxedema coma.

TABLE 8-4 Table of Insulin

Type of Insulin	Onset	Peak	Duration
Rapid-acting • Humalog • Novolog	15 minutes 15 minutes	30-90 minutes 40-50 minutes	3-5 hours 3-5 hours
Short-acting • Humulin R • Novolin R	30-60 minutes	50-120 minutes	5-8 hours
Intermediate-acting • Heumulin N • Novolin N	1-3 hours	8 hours	20 hours
Intermediate and short-acting mixtures • Humulin 50/50 • Novolin 70/30 • Humalog Mix 75/25 • Humalog Mix 50/50 • Novolin 70/30 • Novolin Mix 70/30	The onset, peak, and duration will vary according to the percentage of the components in the mixture.		
Long-acting • Ultralente • Lantus	4-8 hours 1 hour	8-12 hours None	36 hours 24 hours

Modified from: *US Food and Drug Administration Consumer Magazine*, January/February, 2002.

- Diuretics and digoxin are used to treat CHF.
- Hypothermia is treated via core rewarming (e.g., warmed IV fluid, nasogastric fluids, and dialysis).

➤ NURSING ALERT ➤

Avoid external warming in patients diagnosed with hypothyroidism. Peripheral vasodilation may produce cardiovascular collapse.

Syndrome of Inappropriate Secretion of ADH (SIADH)

This is a condition in which excess antidiuretic hormone is produced. SIADH is associated with lung cancer, CNS disorders, and chemotherapy.

Symptoms
- Headache
- Muscle cramps
- Generalized water retention without signs of edema
- Decreased urine output
- Tachycardia, bounding pulses
- CHF and changes in the level of consciousness (LOC) are later signs.

Diagnosis
- Simultaneous measurement of urine and serum osmolality. Serum osmolality much lower than the urine osmolality is indicative of the excretion of concentrated urine in the presence of dilute serum.
- Hyponatremia

Treatment
- Fluid restriction is initiated (500 to 750 ml/24 hr).
- Demeclocycline is administered. This drug blocks the action of ADH.
- Chemotherapy aimed at obliterating tumors may be indicated.
- Furosemide 1 mg/kg is administered to promote diuresis.

Thyrotoxicosis and Thyroid Storm

Thyroid storm is a life-threatening illness caused by the excessive release of thyroid hormones, usually precipitated by infection, injury, or the beginning of treatment for hyperthyroidism. There is debate concerning when thyrotoxicosis becomes thyroid storm. The presence of mental status changes usually signals progression of the hyperthyroid state.

Symptoms
- Elevated metabolism

- Tachycardia
- Diaphoresis
- Tremors
- Hyperthermia: >102.2° F (39° C)

Diagnosis
- Decreased TSH
- Elevated T_3 and T_4 levels
- Hyperglycemia
- Liver enzymes may be elevated.
- Tachycardia (greater than 140 beats/min)
- Atrial fibrillation
- Systolic flow murmurs
- Fever (>106° F) indicates thyroid storm.

Treatment
- Restore hemodynamic stability.
- Administer antithyroid medication (e.g., propylthiouracil or methimazole).
- Administer steroids.
- Administer acetaminophen for hyperthermia.
- Implement measures to reduce hyperthermia.
- Beta-blocking agents (e.g., propranolol) may be given to reduce the cardiac response to thyroid hormone.

NURSING SURVEILLANCE

1. Monitor the cardiac rhythm and treat potentially lethal arrhythmias (e.g., tall peak T-waves indicating hyperkalemia, severe bradycardia, and severe tachycardia).
2. Monitor the patient's temperature. Administer acetaminophen as needed.
3. Provide supportive central warming in hypothyroidism. Beware of rapid rewarming and subsequent hypotension.
4. Monitor intake and output to determine renal response to volume replacement or diuresis.
5. Monitor the LOC because of susceptibility for cerebral edema from a rapid reversal of hyperosmolar state.

EXPECTED PATIENT OUTCOMES

1. The temperature returns to baseline.
2. Blood pressure and heart rate stabilize.
3. Adequate perfusion status
4. Urine output is age appropriate.
5. No further deterioration in neurologic status.
6. Electrolytes are within normal limits.

7. Patient is adequately hydrated.
8. Serum glucose levels are within normal limits.

Patient/Family Discharge Implications and Education

1. Patients on hormone replacement should be instructed to pay attention to signs of infection. Drug doses may need to be increased in fever and diarrhea.
2. Dramatic changes in weight, advancing age, and the addition of medications for other health problems can alter the required medication dosages. Changes should be reported to the primary care provider.
3. The dosage routines for hormone replacement can be modified to fit patient response and comfort (e.g., twice daily vs. three times daily dosage). Encourage the patient to discuss dosage routines with the primary care provider. If a dose of hormone supplement is missed, patient should contact the primary care physician regarding directions. At no time should a patient double a dose without first speaking with a physician.
4. Patients taking steroids should be told to inform other physicians, dentists, and other appropriate health-care workers of steroid use before undergoing a procedure.
5. Patients should wear a "Medic Alert" bracelet because changes in the level of consciousness can occur with endocrine disorders.

REFERENCES

1. Guthrie RA, Guthrie DW: Pathophysiology of diabetes mellitus, *Crit Care Nurs Q* 27(2):113-12, 2004.
2. Manifold CA : Hyperthyroidism, thyroid storm and Graves disease. 2004. Available from www.emedicine.com/emerg/topic269.htm.
3. Odeke S, Nagelberg SB: Addison disease. 2003. Available from www.emedicine.com/med/topic42.htm.

chapter 9

Environmental Conditions

Patty Ann Sturt

INTRODUCTION

Many people participate in outdoor activities for work or recreational purposes. Individuals with altered cognition may be involuntarily exposed to inclement weather. Environmental emergencies should be considered based on the patient's symptoms and the events surrounding the illness or injury. The emergency department (ED) nurse should consider factors such as weather, submersion in water, high altitude, and contact with insects or animals when obtaining the history.

FOCUSED NURSING ASSESSMENT

A focused nursing assessment should be performed to address oxygenation and ventilation, perfusion, cognition, and skin/tissue integrity.

Oxygenation and Ventilation

- Stridor related to laryngeal edema secondary to anaphylaxis from envenomation
- Wheezing related to bronchospasm secondary to anaphylaxis from envenomation or secondary to near drowning. Wheezing also may occur in high-altitude pulmonary edema.
- Crackles/rhonchi related to pulmonary edema secondary to near drowning or high altitude
- Ineffective ventilation related to a decreased level of consciousness secondary to hypoxia from:
  - Near drowning
  - Heat stroke
  - Severe hypothermia
  - High-altitude cerebral edema
  - High-altitude pulmonary edema
  - Envenomation
  - Arterial gas embolism (diving emergency)

Perfusion

- Inadequate perfusion related to:
  - Diaphoresis or fever secondary to heat-related emergencies or stimulation of the sympathetic nervous system secondary to anaphylaxis
  - Diuresis secondary to hypothermia
  - Vasodilation secondary to envenomation or anaphylaxis

Cognition

- Decreased level of consciousness related to:
  - Increased intracranial pressure secondary to cerebral edema caused by heat stroke or high-altitude cerebral edema
  - Hypoxia secondary to near drowning
  - High-altitude pulmonary edema
  - Arterial gas embolism

Skin/Tissue Integrity
- Altered skin/tissue integrity
  - Localized erythema, ecchymosis, pain, puncture mark, or swelling (suspect bite or sting)
  - Yellow waxy skin areas (suspect frostbite)

Environmental Considerations
Consider the following factors when obtaining the history from the patient, caregiver, or prehospital personnel.
- Temperature, humidity, and wind conditions
- Temperature of water in submersion cases
- Duration of the submersion
- Altitude
  See Table 9-1 for heat/cold risk factors.

LIFE SPAN ISSUES

Pediatric
- Toddlers have the highest death rate from drowning.[1] The 15- to 24-year-old age-group has the highest risk of near drowning.[1]
- Child abuse or neglect should be considered in any bathtub child drowning.
- Children are at least risk of developing anaphylaxis because they have not been exposed to as many allergens.[2]
- Thermoregulation is not as efficient in children, making them susceptible to heat and cold illnesses.
- Children are more susceptible to cold-related illnesses because they have less subcutaneous fat.
- Infants are not able to produce heat from shivering, making them more susceptible to cold-related illnesses.

Geriatric
- Persons over the age of 65 are at lowest risk for drowning.
- The elderly are most at risk of developing anaphylaxis because of their increased exposure to potential allergens throughout life.
- Circulatory system abnormalities, diabetes, renal disease, multiple medications, pulmonary disease, and other conditions make the elderly more susceptible to heat-related and cold-related illnesses and altitude illnesses.[3]

INITIAL INTERVENTIONS

Regardless of the environmental condition, the following interventions should be considered:
1. Implement measures to maintain and protect the airway:
   - Chin lift (if spinal trauma is not suspected) or jaw thrust

TABLE 9-1 Risk Factors for Heat/Cold Injury

Risk Factor	Heat-Related Emergencies	Hypothermia
Age	Geriatric: • Decreased functioning of sweat glands, producing less evaporation to help control body temperature • Diminished cardiac reserve Pediatric: • Infants unable to increase sweat gland activity	Geriatric: • Neuropathy may decrease sense of cold. • Decreased vasoconstriction response Pediatric: • Greater body surface area for weight results in greater heat loss. • Smaller amount of fat stores • Immature temperature-regulating mechanisms in infants
Activity	Amateur athletes, military recruits, laborers	Campers, hikers, homeless, submersion in water
Environmental conditions	High heat, high humidity, low wind, closed work space, occlusive clothing	Increased wind speed, cool temperature, submersion in cold water
Medications	Phenothiazines, antihistamines, tricyclic antidepressants, beta-blockers, cocaine, amphetamines, lithium, diuretics	Phenothiazines, barbiturates
Medical history, current illness or injury	Alcohol abuse, obesity, hyperthyroidism	Hypothyroidism, hypoglycemia, alcohol abuse

- Suction oropharynx to prevent aspiration
- Nasopharyngeal airway
- Oropharyngeal airway if the patient is unresponsive or has no gag reflex
- Prepare to assist with intubation.
2. Place the patient on a pulse oximeter to monitor oxygen saturation.
3. Initiate oxygen administration immediately if hypotension, tachycardia, or respiratory distress is present.
4. Initiate cardiac and BP monitoring.
5. Anticipate the need for arterial blood gases (ABGs).
6. Implement seizure precautions by padding side rails, keeping side rails up at all times, and having suction equipment at the bedside. Seizures may occur with conditions that result in hypoxia.
7. Administer IV fluids as ordered.
8. Inform the patient of the plan of care. Patients with environmental conditions often are anxious and fearful.
9. Support and elevate edematous extremities for comfort.
10. Determine tetanus immunization status of any patient with altered skin integrity (see Reference Guide 23).

Nursing care priorities are listed in the table on pp. 338-339.

PRIORITY DIAGNOSTIC TESTS

Arterial blood gases (ABGs): An ABG detects hypoxia and acidosis, which may occur in hypothermia, heat stroke, near drowning, and arterial gas embolus.

Coagulation profile: A coagulation profile is necessary in heat stroke and pit viper envenomation. Disseminated intravascular coagulation may occur with these conditions.

Complete blood count (CBC): A CBC is obtained to assess white blood cell (WBC) count, hemoglobin, and hematocrit levels. Hematocrit levels may elevate in heat-related emergencies. The WBC count may be elevated in reaction to an inflammatory response.

Electrolytes and glucose level: Hyperkalemia and hypoglycemia occur in heat stroke. Baseline electrolyte levels usually are obtained on patients with environmental emergencies.

Lactic acid: May be elevated in patients with exertional heat stroke.

Liver enzymes: Liver enzymes will be elevated in heat stroke.

Myoglobinuria: Myoglobin may be present if rhabdomyolysis occurs during exertional heat stroke.

NURSING CARE PRIORITIES

Potential/Actual Problem	Causes	Signs and Symptoms	Interventions
Airway compromise	• Obstruction from tongue, secretions, foreign material, or laryngeal edema • Seizure activity	• Stridor • Decreased respiratory effort	• Chin lift/jaw thrust • Insert airway adjunct if patient is unresponsive. • Suction oropharynx. • Assist with intubation. • Prepare for surgical cricothyrotomy if unable to intubate because of laryngeal edema. • Subcutaneous epinephrine 1:1000
Impaired breathing/ oxygenation	• Bronchospasms • Pulmonary edema	• Wheezing • Crackles/rhonchi • Cough • Tachypnea • Retractions • Decreased oxygen saturation	• Administer high flow oxygen by nonrebreather mask. • Ventilate with bag valve device if breathing absent or ineffective. • Tracheal suction • Bronchodilators • Monitor respiratory status, breath sounds, and oxygen saturation.

Inadequate fluid volume	• Excessive diaphoresis • Cold diuresis • Vasodilation	• Tachycardia • Tachypnea • Postural hypotension • Hypotension • Altered mental status • Pallor	• Consider oral fluids if awake and alert and no nausea or vomiting • Initiate large-bore IV • Infuse normal saline or lactated Ringer's • Monitor VS • Monitor intake and output • Monitor mental status
Altered skin/tissue integrity	• Frostbite • Sting • Bite	• Numbness • Puncture wound • Redness to site • Edema to site • Vesicles/blisters • Pain	• Oxygen • Immobilize as needed • Analgesics • Avoid further trauma to area • Antibiotics as needed • Antivenom as appropriate for snake bites
Anxiety	• Reaction to event • Fear of unknown	• Self-reports of anxiety • Difficulty answering questions • Difficulty making decisions • Difficulty concentrating • Nervousness • Denial	• Offer to contact family. • Explain all procedures. • Answer questions appropriately for age. • Comfort measures

Radiograph: A chest film may be ordered to assess lung fields for pulmonary edema. Pulmonary edema can occur in near drowning, heat stroke, and high-altitude pulmonary edema (HAPE).

CLINICAL CONDITIONS

Anaphylaxis and Anaphylactoid Reactions

Anaphylaxis is a life-threatening hypersensitivity reaction mediated by an IgE antibody response. Anaphylaxis generally involves previous exposure and sensitization to a specific substance. Anaphylactoid reactions are similar to anaphylaxis but are not mediated by an IgE antibody response. Anaphylactoid reactions result from direct stimulation of mast cells and can be triggered without prior sensitization.

An acute allergic reaction results in cutaneous symptoms. Anaphylactic and anaphylactoid reactions include the cutaneous symptoms of an acute allergic reaction **and** systemic symptoms of

---

BOX 9-1   CLASSIFICATION OF ANAPHYLACTIC AND ANAPHYLACTOID REACTIONS

Anaphylaxis (IgE Mediated)
- Food
- Drugs (penicillin, cephalosporins, insulin, sometimes aspirin and other NSAIDS)
- Insect stings and bites
- Other (exposure to antivenin or aquatic proteins)

Anaphylactoid (Non-IgE Mediated)
- Direct stimulation of mast cells
  - Drugs (opiates, vancomycin)
  - Radiocontrast material
  - Physical stimuli (exercise, cold)
  - Idiopathic
- Disturbances in arachidonic acid metabolism
  - Aspirin and other NSAIDs
- Complement activation
  - Transfusion reactions
  - Immunoglobulin

Auerbach P: Classification of anaphylactic and anaphylactoid reactions. In *Wilderness medicine,* ed 4, St. Louis, 2001, Mosby.

---

varying degrees. The symptoms are related to the release of
multiple chemical mediators that contribute to vasodilation,
increased capillary permeability, laryngeal edema, and
bronchospasm. Death is usually due to complete airway
obstruction from edema or vascular collapse.

Symptoms
- Cutaneous:
  - Diffuse hives (urticaria)
  - Pruritus
  - Flushing
- Cardiovascular:
  - Dizziness
  - Tachycardia
  - Hypotension
  - Arrhythmias
- Respiratory:
  - Rhinitis
  - Stridor
  - Hoarseness
  - Wheezing
  - Dyspnea
  - Tachypnea
  - Laryngeal and tongue edema
- Gastrointestinal:
  - Abdominal pain
  - Nausea and vomiting
  - Diarrhea

Diagnosis
- Based on physical examinations and symptoms
- May have a history of antigen exposure

Treatment
- Administer oxygen at 8 to 10 L/min via nonrebreather mask.
- Anticipate need for intubation or cricothyrotomy if laryngeal
  edema produces severe upper airway obstruction. Anticipate
  intubation if bronchospasm causes severe respiratory distress.
- Initiate two large-bore IVs.
- Administer fluid bolus of Ringer's lactate or normal saline for
  hypotension.
- Consider the use of a vasopressor such as dopamine for
  persistent hypotension.
- Administer medication as ordered:
  - Epinephrine of a 1 : 1000 solution (usually 0.3 to 0.5 mg
    for adults, 0.01 mg/kg for children) subcutaneously

or intramuscularly. It can be repeated twice at 15-minute to 20-minute intervals to control the symptoms.[4,5]

○ Epinephrine 0.1 to 0.5 ml (mg) of a 1:10,000 solution IV over 5 minutes if patient does not respond to subcutaneous or intramuscular epinephrine or if the patient is hypotensive and in severe respiratory distress.[4,5]

○ Glucagon: patients on beta-blockers may be resistant to epinephrine effects. Glucagon bolus, 1-5 mg IV over 2 minutes can be given in addition to the epinephrine to increase heart rate and contractility by pathways not related to beta-receptors.[5]

○ Antihistamines such as diphenhydramine (Benadryl); an H1 blocker and/or an H2 blocker such as cimetidine (Tagamet); famotidine (Pepcid); or ranitidine (Zantac). The combination of the H1 and H2 blockers is thought to be more effective in blocking the effects of histamine on the heart and circulatory system.[5]

○ Inhaled bronchodilators such as albuterol (beta-2 agonist)

○ Corticosteroids such as hydrocortisone (enhances beta-2 agonists, inhibits leukotriene production, stabilizes mast cell membranes). Effects are not realized for at least 6 hours, so primary function is to prevent recurrence or protracted anaphylaxis.[5]

Arachnid Envenomations and Bites
Black widow spider, brown recluse spider, scorpions: for symptoms and treatment, see Table 9-2.

Tick Bite: Lyme Disease
Lyme disease is a multisystem inflammatory disease caused by a spirochete that is transmitted by a bite from a deer tick or the related Western black-legged tick. Deer ticks are no larger than a pinhead and are difficult to see. The tick usually has to feed for 24 to 48 hours for the disease to be transmitted. The spirochete may travel by the vascular or lymph system to any organ in the body. Lyme disease affects mainly hikers or those involved in outdoor occupations such as farming and forestry. There is a higher incidence of Lyme disease in the summer and early fall and in New England and mid-Atlantic states. Lyme disease may occur in domestic animals, with a higher incidence in cats.

Symptoms
Lyme disease has three stages.

• *First stage:* Early localized infection is characterized by erythema migrans (an expanding red macular circular lesion)

TABLE 9-2 Arachnid Envenomations

Type	Location and Description	Symptoms	Treatment
Black widow spider	• Common in California and other parts of the United States • Usually found in outdoor buildings such as barns and under rocks • Black with red hourglass marking on abdomen	• Venom is neurotoxic. • Pain at bite site may be sharp and stinging or resemble light pinprick. • Limb pain, local redness and swelling • Two tiny red marks may be present. • Muscle spasms, headache, nausea, vomiting, hyperactive reflexes, ptosis, hypertension, diaphoresis, fever, seizures, shock	• 100% oxygen by mask • IV access • Diazepam and calcium gluconate for muscle spasms • Antivenin in seriously ill patient • Immobilization of the limb and cool compresses
Brown recluse spider	• Found in wood piles, attics, closets, and dark places • Found in southeastern, south central, and	• Mild or no pain with bite, local edema, erythema, bleb formation, local ischemia • Severe ulcerative necrosis appears	• Avoid further trauma to area. • Determine tetanus and diphtheria immunization status. • Antibiotics

Continued

TABLE 9-2   Arachnid Envenomations—cont'd

Type	Location and Description	Symptoms	Treatment
	southwestern states • Light brown with dark brown violin shape on back	on third to fourth day. • Fever, chills, malaise	• Debridement of necrotic areas and sterile dressings • Dapsone may be administered to inhibit neutrophil function, a major cause of skin necrosis.
Scorpion	• Found mostly in the southwestern United States • Usually brown, about 3 inches long with 8 legs, small claws, and a long tail that contains a venomous stinger	• Intense pain with little or no erythema or swelling • One species (*Centruroides sculpturatus*) injects lethal neurotoxic venom. • Symptoms may include wheezing, stridor, profuse salivation, diaphoresis, confusion, seizures, hypertension, tachypnea, tachycardia.	• Immobilize affected part. • Do not apply tourniquet. • Antihypertensives. • Ensure tetanus and diphtheria prophylaxis. • Analgesic. • Support ABCs.

usually radiating from the site of the tick bite. The rash may be solid or appear like a bull's eye with the area of the bite at the center.

- *Second stage:* The infection is disseminated. Symptoms include:
  - ○ A headache, stiff neck, enlarged lymph nodes, sore throat, joint and tendon pain
  - ○ Fatigue and malaise
  - ○ Palpitations and syncope may occur because of atrioventricular conduction blocks.
- *Third stage:* Chronic stage
  - ○ Infection may take weeks, months, or years to develop.
  - ○ Chronic arthritis may develop.
  - ○ Encephalopathy may result in mood changes and memory and sleep disturbances. Numbness may occur in the arms and hands or the legs and feet.

Diagnosis

Diagnosis is made on the basis of symptoms and evidence of a tick bite. Testing for Lyme disease is most often conducted with antigen tests (ELISA and Western blot). Serum tests will give accurate results 1 month after the initial infection.

Treatment

- Removal of the tick if it is still present
- Antibiotics, PO or IV, depending on the severity of the symptoms noted (doxycycline, amoxicillin, and Ceftin). Early antibiotic treatment prevents later stages of the disease.
- A vaccine, Lymerix, is available for those at high risk for the disease.

NURSING ALERT

Do not attempt to remove a feeding tick by using a lighted match, chemicals, or petroleum jelly. These substances may cause the tick to release more organisms (spirochetes) into the patient. One should remove ticks using tweezers placed as close to the skin as possible and, using gentle straight traction, pulling at the mouth of the tick. Squeezing the abdomen may release a greater number of spirochetes. Attach the tick to an index card using clear tape. Label the date the bite occurred, the part of the patient's body bitten, and the locale from which the tick came. The tick can be checked for the presence of spirochetes.

Cold-Related Emergencies
Frostbite
Frostbite is tissue damage from cold.
Symptoms
- Coldness of the extremity, numbness, followed by extreme pain upon rewarming
- Initially the skin is pale to waxy yellow or white.
- With rewarming, the skin becomes hyperemic, sensation returns and remains until blebs appear. Attempts at evaluating the injury severity can be made at this point.
- Edema occurs within 3 hours of rewarming and lasts for 5 days or more.
- Vesicles appear at 6 to 24 hours of rewarming.
- Black eschar may develop at 9 to 15 days.

Degrees of injury have been classified as superficial (first-degree and second-degree frostbite) and deep superficial (third-degree and fourth-degree frostbite). Initial treatment is the same regardless of the depth of injury.

Diagnosis
Diagnosis is based on history and a physical examination.

Treatment (for all degrees)
- Remove constrictive and wet clothing and jewelry.
- No vigorous rubbing of area. Handle area gently as tissue will be fragile.
- Immerse in water warmed to 104° to 108° F (40° to 42° C) for 15 to 30 minutes. Skin will become pliable and erythematous. Active motion may be helpful, but massage is not recommended.
- Pad and splint affected extremity.
- Elevate affected extremities.
- Parenteral analgesics for pain, morphine sulfate or meperidine. Extreme pain may occur during rewarming.
- Clear blisters usually are debrided. Hemorrhagic blisters are left intact; however, the fluid may be aspirated from them.
- Apply sterile dressing after area is thawed. Wrap fingers and toes separately to prevent rubbing.
- Prevent further heat loss and treat hypothermia if present. Avoid heavy blankets on injured tissues.
- Assess tetanus immunization status.
- Prepare for admission of patients with all but minor frostbite injuries.

Hypothermia
Hypothermia is defined as a core temperature below 95° F (35° C).[6]

Symptoms
See Table 9-3.

Diagnosis
- Diagnosis is based on history, core temperature, symptoms, and clinical findings.

Treatment
- Handle patients with moderate to severe hypothermia very carefully to avoid jarring the patient. Hypothermic hearts are very susceptible to ventricular fibrillation. Smooth transfers from bed to bed are necessary, and avoid actions such as kicking the stretcher and jarring side rails into place. Carefully remove clothing and cover with dry blankets.
- Evaluate for concomitant trauma.
- If intubation is necessary, it must be performed gently to prevent unnecessary stimulation and the onset of ventricular fibrillation. A good rule of thumb is to intubate the hypothermic patient as you would a patient with a possible cervical spine injury.
- Monitor core temperature continuously with an esophageal probe, rectal probe, or temperature-sensing urinary catheter. The latter may provide falsely low readings if the patient is experiencing cold diuresis.

TABLE 9-3   Hypothermia

Stage	Core Temperature[6]	Symptoms
Mild	91.4°-96.8° F (33°-36° C)	Tachypnea, tachycardia, ataxia, shivering, lethargy, confusion
Moderate	85.2°-89.6° F (29°-32° C)	No shivering; rigidity, hypoventilation, progressively decreased level of consciousness, atrial fibrillation, bradycardia, bradypnea, dilated pupils, hypovolemia, metabolic acidosis, Osborne or J-wave (positive deflection in the RT segment)
Severe	<85° F (<29° C)	Loss of reflexes, no response to pain, significant hypotension and acidosis, apnea, cyanosis, ventricular fibrillation, asystole

- Initiate IV access with two large-bore catheters. Patients can be volume depleted. Patients with temperatures of 90° F (32.2° C) or less should receive an initial fluid challenge of 250 to 500 ml of warmed D_5NS. Monitor for signs of fluid overload. Central venous catheters should not be advanced into the right atria because of the potential for cardiac muscle irritation producing arrhythmias.[6]
- Place a gastric catheter. Gastric motility is usually delayed.
- Continuous cardiac monitoring
- Institute rewarming measures (see Table 9-4).

NURSING ALERT

Apply heat to the trunk of the body and not to the extremities in patients with moderate to severe hypothermia. Warming the extremities causes vasodilation of blood vessels and could result in hypotension and movement of acidotic blood from the periphery to the core.

Diving Emergencies
Barotrauma
Barotrauma is the most common medical problem in scuba diving. Obstruction of air-containing spaces accompanied by a change in ambient pressure can result in pressure disequilibrium. Barotrauma refers to the tissue damage or changes that result from the pressure imbalance. The middle ear, sinuses, intestines, and lungs are sites often involved. (See Table 9-5 for mechanisms, symptoms, and treatment.)

Decompression Sickness
As the depth and pressure increase during scuba diving, larger and larger amounts of nitrogen and oxygen dissolve in blood and tissue. Unlike oxygen, nitrogen is not metabolized by tissue and tends to accumulate. If ascent occurs too rapidly, nitrogen quickly escapes from the tissues as gas bubbles. It is the release of the gas bubbles and the site of release that determine the symptoms. Symptoms usually present upon breaking the surface or within 4 hours of the diver surfacing.

Symptoms
- Severe joint pain
- Pruritus
- Rash
- Cough

TABLE 9-4   Patient Rewarming

Rewarming Measures	Interventions	Indications
Passive external	• Remove all wet clothing • Warm room • Blankets • Cover patient's head • Prevent drafts	• Previously healthy individuals with mild hypothermia • Patients who can still shiver are candidates for passive external rewarming.
Active external • Adding heat directly to the torso of body	• Warmed blankets • Radiant heaters • Forced-air rewarming, (e.g., Bair hugger, Arizant Healthcare) • Heat packs	• Mild to moderate hypothermia (core temperature below 89.6° F or 32°C) and in conjunction with active core rewarming in patients with moderate to severe hypothermia
Active core • Instillation of warmed fluid to internal body tissues	• Warmed, humidified oxygen • Warmed IV infusions (111° F/44°C) • Gastric lavage • Bladder irrigation • Thoracic lavage • Peritoneal lavage or dialysis • Extracorporeal blood warming (hemodialysis, arteriovenous [CAVR], venovenous, and cardiopulmonary bypass)	• Moderate to severe hypothermia

TABLE 9-5 Barotrauma

Location	Mechanism	Symptoms/Clinical Findings	Treatment
Middle ear	During descent, pressure in the middle ear may become less than the water pressure, causing the tympanic membrane to stretch and bulge inward.	• Pain • Redness of tympanic membrane (TM) • Perforation of TM in severe cases	• Decongestants • Antihistamines • Analgesics • Education on use of Valsalva maneuver immediately on submerging to equalize middle ear pressure
Sinuses	A relative vacuum may develop if there is inability to maintain the air pressure in any paranasal sinus during descent.	• Severe pain • Bleeding into the sinus	• Systemic and topical vasoconstrictors • Analgesics • Antibiotics (severe cases) • Education on importance of avoiding diving during symptoms of an upper respiratory infection or allergic rhinitis
Intestines	Expanding gas can become trapped in the GI tract during ascent.	• Abdominal fullness • Pain • Abdominal distention • Flatulence	• Comfort measures
Lungs	Pulmonary barotrauma of ascent results from expansion of gases trapped in the lungs. Intrapulmonary pressure can rise to the point where air is forced across the pulmonary capillary membrane into surrounding spaces or capillaries.	• Chest pain • Dyspnea • Respiratory distress • Pneumothorax • Subcutaneous emphysema	• Oxygen via nonrebreather mask • Chest tube if pneumothorax present • Serial chest x-rays

- Dyspnea
- Chest discomfort
- Visual disturbances
- Weakness
- Vertigo
- Headache
- Aphasia
- Coma

Diagnosis

- Diagnosis is based on a history of diving and on symptoms.

Treatment

- Place the patient in the left lateral decubitus position or supine with the head in the neutral position.
- Administer 100% oxygen by nonrebreather mask.
- Follow adult and pediatric resuscitation protocols.
- Start at least one large-bore IV with crystalloid infusion.
- Recompression is needed as soon as possible. Recompression is achieved through the use of hyperbaric (high-pressure) facilities or chambers.
- Patients with persistent symptoms may be treated with hyperbaric oxygen up to 7 days after the onset of symptoms.

Arterial Gas Embolism

Arterial gas embolism is one of the most serious injuries associated with compressed-air diving. It results from air entering the pulmonary venous circulation from ruptured alveoli. The air in the pulmonary capillary blood introduces gas bubbles into the left heart and aorta. From the aorta, the bubbles may travel through the coronary, cerebral, or systemic circulation.

Symptoms

Symptoms typically occur quickly after the diver surfaces. The symptoms will be based on the site or sites of vascular occlusion.

- Myocardial symptoms:
  - Chest pain
  - Arrhythmias
  - Cardiac arrest
- Cerebral symptoms:
  - Seizures
  - Altered level of consciousness
  - Headache
  - Visual disturbances
  - Hemiplegia

- Pulmonary symptoms:
  - Pink frothy sputum
  - Pneumothorax

Diagnosis
Diagnosis is based on history and symptoms.

Treatment
- Administer 100% oxygen by nonrebreather mask.
- Assist with intubation if there is a decreased LOC or severe respiratory compromise.
- Start at least one large-bore IV.
- Immediate recompression is a priority. Facilitate patient transfer to a facility with a hyperbaric chamber.

Heat-Related Illnesses
A variety of clinical conditions occur in heat illness. The symptoms often result from the body's attempt to dissipate heat.

Heat Cramps
Severe cramps may occur in large muscles as a result of intense activity and fatigue. This usually is seen in athletes competing in the sun for long periods of time.

Symptoms
- Painful muscle spasms in heavily exerted muscle; most often the calves, thighs, shoulders, or abdominal wall
- Nausea
- Diaphoresis
- Pallor
- Hyponatremia and hypochloremia

Diagnosis
- Diagnosis is based on history.

Treatment
- Rest in a cool environment
- Fluid replacement: water or oral electrolyte solutions such as Gatorade, PowerAde, or All Sport
- IV fluids if nausea or vomiting are present
- Replace sodium as necessary.

Heat Syncope
Heat syncope occurs when blood pooling from peripheral vasodilation results in orthostatic hypotension and a temporary reduction in cerebral blood flow. It is usually seen in people who have been standing for prolonged periods in the heat.

Symptoms
- Headache
- Lightheadedness

- Postural hypotension
- Brief loss of consciousness

Diagnosis
- Diagnosis is based on history and orthostatic vital signs.

Treatment
- Rest in a cool environment
- Fluid replacement: oral electrolyte solution such as Gatorade, PowerAde, or All Sport
- Modified Trendelenburg position (legs elevated)
- Instruct patient to avoid sudden or prolonged standing in a warm environment.

Heat Exhaustion

Heat exhaustion is caused by excessive loss of body water and electrolytes from diaphoresis and inadequate fluid intake. These losses lead to a fluid volume deficit. This usually is seen in people who have been exposed to heat over prolonged periods (hours or days), such as in strenuous activity.

Symptoms
- Muscle cramps
- Headache
- Nausea/vomiting
- Anxiety
- Elevated temperature
- Diaphoresis
- Cool, pale skin
- Mild hypotension
- Tachycardia
- Hyperventilation
- Syncope
- Hyponatremia and hypochloremia

Diagnosis
Diagnosis is based on history.

Treatment
- Rest in a cool environment
- Oral hydration if patient is alert and oriented and not experiencing nausea or vomiting
- IV fluids often are used for fluid replacement if the patient has nausea and vomiting, which can be indicative of a sodium deficit. Normal saline is preferred.

Heat Stroke

Heat stroke is a rare but life-threatening emergency. Overexposure to high environmental temperatures, especially when accompanied by high humidity and low-wind conditions, can impair the release of body heat and lead to an abnormal rise in body temperature. Temperature regulatory centers in the hypothalamus fail, which further increases body heat. Cellular breakdown begins, and all organs can be affected. Heat stroke can be categorized as classic or exertional (Table 9-6).

Symptoms
- Neurologic:
  - Confusion
  - Decreased level of consciousness
  - Visual disturbances
  - Seizures
  - Lack of muscle coordination
  - Headache
- Cardiovascular:
  - Tachycardia
  - Arrhythmias
  - Hypotension
- Pulmonary:
  - Tachypnea
  - Pulmonary edema
- Thermoregulatory:
  - Core temperature often above 104°
- Cutaneous:
  - Absence of sweating
  - Skin is dry, ashen, hot.
- Renal:
  - Decreased urinary output

Diagnosis
Diagnosis is based on history and a physical examination.

Treatment
- Support the airway, breathing, and circulation. Intubation may be necessary.
- Administer 100% oxygen.
- Cardiac monitor
- Initiate a large-bore IV.
- Administer a 1-L, normal saline, fluid bolus if the patient is hypotensive. Repeat as necessary.
- Monitor core temperature at 5-minute intervals with an esophageal or rectal probe.
- Check the glucose level and administer 50% dextrose if hypoglycemia is present.
- Begin rapid cooling: ice packs to the groin, neck, and axillae. Spray cold water over the body. Place fans close to the patient

TABLE 9-6	Two Types of Heat Stroke	
	Classic	Exertional
Age-group	Elderly and children	Usually men 15-45 yr
Medical history	Chronic medical illness(es)	Often healthy
Sweating	May be absent	Usually present
Mechanism	Poor dissipation of environmental heat. Occurs primarily during a heat wave.	Excessive heat production and overwhelming of heat-loss mechanisms. Occurs primarily in people engaging in strenuous activity (athletes) in a hot environment for a long period of time.
Onset	Usually days	Minutes or hours

to facilitate evaporative heat loss. Place hypothermia (cooling) blankets over and under the patient. Cold saline peritoneal lavage may be used in refractory cases. Consider cold saline gastric lavage.

- Monitor urine output. Monitor for myoglobinuria.

NURSING ALERT

Rapidly cool the patient to 101° F. When the temperature is 101° F, slow the cooling measures. Acetaminophen is not effective initially because its use depends on a normally functioning hypothalamus. Shivering should be avoided, because it generates heat. Diazepam or lorazepam can be used to prevent or stop shivering. Chlorpromazine (Thorazine) is not recommended to stop shivering because it is believed to lower the seizure threshold and blood pressure.

High-Altitude Illness

High-altitude illness usually occurs with rapid ascent to elevations above 8000 feet, the height at which most people's arterial oxygen saturation starts to decrease. In an unacclimated person, hyperventilation and increased erythropoietin secretion are insufficient to relieve the hypoxemia.

Acute Mountain Sickness

Acute mountain sickness (AMS) is a collection of symptoms brought on by acute exposure to high altitude.

Symptoms
- Headache
- Insomnia
- Irritability
- Anorexia
- Nausea/vomiting
- Dizziness
- Dyspnea on exertion
- Weakness
- Peripheral edema
- Symptoms peak 24 to 36 hours after onset and resolve over 1 to 5 days.

Diagnosis
- History, physical examination, and symptoms

Treatment
- Administer low-flow oxygen.
- Administer acetazolamide as ordered.
- Administer dexamethasone as ordered.
- Hyperbaric therapy

High-Altitude Pulmonary Edema (HAPE)

High-altitude pulmonary edema is a life-threatening form of high-altitude illness.

Symptoms
- Cough
- Dyspnea
- Wheezing
- Orthopnea
- Hemoptysis
- Tachycardia
- Tachypnea
- Neck veins are usually flat, and there is no hepatic engorgement.

Treatment
- Administer oxygen at 4 to 6 L/min.
- Administer nifedipine as ordered.
- Hyperbaric therapy

High-Altitude Cerebral Edema (HACE)

HACE is a life-threatening form of high-altitude illness that usually occurs at elevations above 12,000 feet. However, cases have been reported at altitudes of 8000 to 10,000 feet.

Symptoms
- Severe headache
- Ataxia
- Altered mental status ranging from confusion, to stupor, to coma
- Nausea/vomiting
- Weakness of the extremities
- Seizures

Diagnosis
Diagnosis is based on history, physical examination, and symptoms.

Treatment
- Descent remains the definitive and most successful treatment for all forms of high-altitude illness. Even a 1000-foot descent can result in the reversal of mild and moderate symptoms.
- Supplemental oxygen at 2 to 4 L/min via nasal cannula or face mask
- Administer dexamethasone as ordered.
- Hyperbaric therapy

Hymenoptera Stings (Bee, Wasp, and Fire Ant)
These insects inject venom through a stinger connected to a venom reservoir (sac). Stings are common in summer months and usually involve the head, neck, and extremities.

Symptoms
- Local reaction:
  - Immediate pain at the site of the sting
  - Erythema
  - Edema
  - Itching may be present.
- Systemic reaction:
  - Hives
  - Nausea
  - Vomiting
  - Conjunctivitis
  - Rhinitis
  - Facial swelling
  - Abdominal pain
  - Stridor
  - Wheezes
  - Anaphylactic shock

Diagnosis
Diagnosis is based on symptoms and history of an insect sting.

Treatment

- Rapid removal of the stinger by whatever method is available. The degree of envenomation increases as long as the stinger remains in place.[7]
- Cold pack for the swelling
- Home remedies such as meat tenderizer often are regarded as effective.
- Antihistamines
- For anaphylactic reactions, see treatment under Anaphylaxis.

Submersion Incident

Submersion incident refers to any submersion in water that adversely affects any person. Near drowning is defined as submersion with at least temporary survival. Secondary drowning is death occurring minutes to days after the recovery. Submersion incidents can be categorized as wet or dry. Wet drowning indicates aspiration of fluid and occurs in 80% to 90% of submersions.[1] Dry drowning accounts for 10% to 20% of cases.[1] Dry drowning victims develop laryngospasm resulting in hypoxia. Submersion incidents from either fresh water or salt water can produce intrapulmonary shunting, decreased compliance, decreased functional capacity, pulmonary edema, and hypoxia.

Symptoms

Respiratory findings include:

- Tachypnea or apnea
- Shortness of breath
- Cough
- Wheezing
- Crackles

Other Symptoms the Patient May Exhibit

- Hypotension
- Altered LOC
- Cardiac arrhythmias
- Chest pain

NURSING ALERT

Initially, the chest film may be normal. Pulmonary insufficiency related to pulmonary edema may not develop for up to 24 hours after the submersion. In dry drownings, the CXR may remain normal. Frequent pulmonary assessments for crackles, wheezing, and rhonchi along with monitoring for a decreasing P_{O_2} must be performed.

Diagnosis
Diagnosis is based on history, symptoms, and chest films.
Treatment
- Maintain a patent airway.
- Administer 100% oxygen by nonrebreather mask.

>≥ **N U R S I N G   A L E R T** ≤<

Always suspect the possibility of a cervical spine injury in a
submersion incident victim. Cervical spine injuries are a possibility
with falls, diving, or skiing events.

- Assist with intubation if respirations are absent or minimal, if
  the patient is comatose, or if the patient is unable to maintain a
  PaO_2 of 60 to 90 mm Hg with high-flow oxygen by
  nonrebreather mask.
- Positive-end expiratory pressure (PEEP) may increase the
  functional capacity of the alveoli.
- Bronchodilators to decrease bronchospasms and wheezing
- Two large-bore IV lines
- Gastric tube for stomach decompression
- Treat hypothermia (see Tables 9-3 and 9-4).
- Insert a urinary catheter to monitor the urinary output.
- Monitor and note trend of arterial blood gas results and pulse
  oximetry readings.
- Monitor for acidosis secondary to hypoxia.
- Prophylactic antibiotics (to prevent pulmonary infections) are
  not routinely used in submersion incident victims unless
  pneumonitis develops.

Venomous Snake Bites
North American envenomations result from one of two families,
pit vipers (Crotalide family) or coral snakes (Elapidae family).
Symptoms
See Box 9-2 for symptoms of pit viper and coral snake bites.
Diagnosis
Diagnosis is based on the history, symptoms, and a description of
the snake.
Treatment
- Measure the circumference of the bitten extremity. Consider
  marking the border of advancing edema every 15 to 60 minutes
  to monitor progression of the edema.
- Immobilize the extremity at the level of the heart.

BOX 9-2   VENOMOUS SNAKE BITES

Pit vipers

(Rattlesnakes, cottonmouths, copperheads)

Characteristics: Pit vipers have a heat-sensing pit midway between the eye and nostril on each side of the head; a triangular head; elliptic pupils; long, sharp, retractable fangs; and a single row of subcaudal plates.

Venom: The venom is primarily hematotoxic.

Location: Pit vipers are found in every state but Maine, Alaska, and Hawaii; they are the most common venomous snakes in the United States.

Symptoms:

Approximately 75% of pit-viper bites result in envenomation.

- Fang punctures; edema; sharp, burning pain; and erythema of the site and adjacent tissues within 1 to 30 min of the bite. Edema may spread for 12 to 24 hr.
- Minimal envenomation may cause regional lymphadenopathy and tenderness.
- Severe envenomation may be accompanied by hypotension and shock, paresthesias, anemia, and disseminated intravascular coagulation.

Coral snakes

Characteristics: Coral snakes lack facial pits. They have black snouts, round pupils, broad bands of red and black separated by yellow rings that completely circle the body, and short, fixed fangs.

Venom: The venom is primarily neurotoxic.

Location: The Arizona coral snake is found primarily in Arizona and New Mexico. The eastern coral snake is found in North Carolina, south to Florida, and west through the gulf states to Texas.

Symptoms:

- *Minimal envenomation:* There may be little or no swelling or pain immediately after the bite. There can be a delay of 1 to 5 hr before the onset of systemic symptoms.
- *Moderate envenomation:* The patient has fang punctures and minimal swelling. There is no complete respiratory paralysis.
- *Severe envenomation:* The patient experiences complete paralysis within 36 hr after the bite.

- Remove any rings or constricting items from the involved extremity.
- Apply a compression dressing over the bitten area with an elastic wrap. The wrap should be tight enough (but with fingers still able to fit and slide under the dressing) to reduce lymphatic flow.
- Administer oxygen by nasal cannula or mask.
- Insert two large-bore IVs.
- Institute cardiac monitoring and pulse oximetry.
- Administer fluid boluses of normal saline or lactated Ringer's solution if patient is hypotensive.
- Anticipate the need for antivenom for moderate to severe envenomation. Crotalidae Polyvalent Immune Fab (Crofab) received FDA approval in 2000 and is believed to have fewer adverse reactions than Antivenin (Crotalidae) Polyvalent.[8]
- Infuse albumin as ordered.

➤ NURSING ALERT ◄

Follow the antivenom package insert or appropriate drug information when preparing and administering. Any time antivenom is given, the ED nurse should anticipate possible significant adverse reactions. Airway equipment must be immediately available, and epinephrine should be available at the bedside. Skin testing for an allergic reaction can be done before antivenom is administered.

- Assess tetanus immunization status.
- Administer analgesics as ordered. Do NOT administer aspirin or nonsteroidal antiinflammatory drugs.
- Prophylactic fasciotomy is not recommended. Compartment syndrome from a venomous snakebite is rare. Subcutaneous swelling and pain on range of motion may mimic compartment syndrome.
- Do not use ice.
- Incision and suction is not recommended in the prehospital environment or ED.
- Regional poison control centers can provide information about the snakes found in a particular region.

NURSING SURVEILLANCE

Frequently assess:
- Airway patency
- Breath sounds
- Respiratory rate and pattern
- Skin perfusion
- Heart rate and rhythm
- BP
- LOC
- Amount of edema in extremities

EXPECTED PATIENT OUTCOMES

1. Patent airway
2. Bilateral equal breath sounds with absence of stridor, wheezing, and shortness of breath
3. Core body temperature between 97° and 99° F
4. Heart rate of 60 to 100 beats/min
5. Absence of life-threatening arrhythmias
6. Systolic BP of >90 mm Hg or at level needed to maintain adequate peripheral perfusion
7. Normal mentation
8. Urine output >30 ml/hr in adults, 1-2 ml/kg/hr in children
9. Decrease or no further progression of edema in extremities

DISCHARGE IMPLICATIONS

Heat-Related Illnesses
1. Teach the need to increase the intake of oral balanced salt solutions during hot, humid weather conditions.
2. Emphasize the need for frequent rest periods when participating in outdoor activities.

Cold-Related Illnesses
Frostbitten areas are very susceptible to further injury. Emphasize the importance of protecting the area from cold exposure and trauma. These patients may need to return to the ED or physician's office for dressing changes and reevaluation.

High-Altitude Illnesses
Teach the need to increase altitude gradually. This is particularly important at elevations above 8000 feet.

Diving Emergencies
Encourage divers to participate in certified diving programs and courses.

Near-Drowning Emergencies

Teach parents the importance of constant and continuous monitoring of children near pools, ponds, lakes, and other areas with water or fluid.

Venomous Snake Bites

Emphasize the need to wear boots and pants during hiking or mountain-climbing activities.

REFERENCES

1. Newman AB: Submersion incidents. In Auerbach P, ed: *Wilderness medicine*, ed 4, St Louis, 2001, Mosby.
2. American Heart Association: ACLS for experienced providers manual, Dallas, 2003, American Heart Association.
3. Erb BD: Elders in the wilderness. In Auerbach P, ed: *Wilderness medicine*, ed 4, St Louis, 2001, Mosby.
4. Patel NJ and Bush RK: Seasonal allergies. In Auerbach P, ed: *Wilderness medicine*, ed 4, St Louis, 2001, Mosby.
5. Burgess B: Anaphylaxis in the emergency department, part 1 & part 2, May, 2004, www.EMedHome.com.
6. Danzl DF: Accidental hypothermia. In Auerbach P, ed: *Wilderness medicine*, ed 4, St Louis, 2001, Mosby.
7. Minton SA, Bechtel B, and Erickson TB: North American arthropod envenomation and parasitism. In Auerbach P, ed: *Wilderness medicine*, ed 4, St Louis, 2001, Mosby.
8. Protherics. Drug insert on Crotalidae Polyvalent Immune Fab (Ovine), Melville, NY, 2000, Salvage Laboratories (a division of Atlanta, Inc.)

10 chapter

Exposures: Chemical, Radiation, and Biologic

Patty Ann Sturt

INTRODUCTION

Every emergency department (ED) should have a plan that addresses care of patients exposed to a hazardous material. A hazardous material is any substance that can cause a threat to individual safety and health. Common routes of exposure include inhalation, direct contact with skin or eyes, and ingestion.

FOCUSED NURSING ASSESSMENT

A focused assessment should be performed to address the following areas:

Oxygenation and Ventilation

- Assess for indicators of airway compromise, such as stridor and respiratory distress related to edema of the upper airways, laryngeal spasms, and oropharyngeal secretions.
- Assess for indicators of respiratory distress, such as retractions, increased or decreased depth of respirations, and pulmonary edema.
- Inhalation of hazardous chemicals may impair the airway and pulmonary system. Inhalation of high concentrations of chlorine gas can rapidly result in airway and pulmonary edema.
- Patients with cyanide inhalation will exhibit respiratory distress.
- Exposure to nerve gas vapor and sulfuric acid results in bronchoconstriction and increased respiratory secretions.

Perfusion

- Assess the patient's skin color, heart rate, rhythm, and blood pressure. Note the quality of the pulses.
- Patients with altered perfusion may exhibit pallor, tachycardia, weak peripheral pulses, and altered level of consciousness.
- Certain chemicals, such as cyanide, alter cellular function and prevent utilization of oxygen in cellular metabolism.

Cognition

- Many hazardous substances may impair cognition by impairing ventilation and perfusion.
- The patient's level of consciousness should be quickly assessed to determine whether the patient is awake, responds to verbal stimuli, responds to painful stimuli, or is unresponsive.
- After life-saving interventions have been initiated, assess the pupils for size and reactivity and evaluate the level of consciousness with the Glasgow Coma Scale (see Reference Guide 10).
- Cognition can be quickly impaired in patients exposed to cyanide and nerve gas vapors.

Sensation and Mobility

- Assess for muscle weakness and abnormal movements. Muscle weakness, spasms, and seizure activity can occur with exposure to nerve gas agents and cyanide. Muscle twitching/fasciculations are common clinical identifiers that indicate exposure to a nerve agent.

Tissue Integrity
- Assess the skin and mucous membranes for drainage, redness, blisters, open areas, and a rash.
- Patients with smallpox will have a papular rash that progresses to vesicles and pustules.
- Dermal exposure to blister agents, sulfuric acid, ammonia, and chlorine can produce skin inflammation, redness, blisters, and ulcerations.

Elimination
- Determine whether the patient has had nausea, vomiting, or diarrhea since the time of exposure. All three may occur in patients with exposure to a nerve gas agent.
- Nausea and vomiting may occur with exposure to phosgene.

Environmental Assessment/Hazard Identification
- If possible, obtain the following information from emergency medical services (EMS) personnel or first responders before arrival of the patient(s):
  ○ Number and approximate ages of victims
  ○ Name of chemicals or agents (if known)
  ○ Signs and symptoms of patients
  ○ Suspected route of exposure
  ○ Type and nature of incident (e.g., plant or industrial explosion, MVC, train derailment)
  ○ Extent of patient decontamination and treatment before arrival
  ○ Information available at the site about the chemical(s) involved. Determine availability of material safety data sheets (MSDS). MSDS sheets are provided by the manufacturer for each chemical used in a plant or industrial setting. Request information from placards or labels on vehicle or container. Placards are used when hazardous materials are stored in bulk, such as cargo tanks. Labels designate hazardous materials kept in smaller packages.
  ○ Estimated time of arrival in the emergency department.

LIFE SPAN ISSUES

Pediatric
1. Pediatric patients are more susceptible to the effects of gases/vapors of hazardous substances because of the smaller diameter of their airways and greater minute ventilation compared with adults.

2. Fluid loss from vomiting and diarrhea can lead to hypovolemia.
3. Children are more prone to hypothermia because of their large body surface area. Utilize measures such as warm blankets immediately after decontamination and in the ED to prevent hypothermia.

Geriatric
Geriatric patients are more likely to experience pain, redness, and blister formation of the skin with external exposure of chemicals because of thinning of the dermal layer and decreased collagen.

Pregnancy
Pregnant patients will require greater fluid volume replacement with vomiting and diarrhea because of their greater intravascular volume.

INITIAL INTERVENTIONS

1. Implement decontamination set-up and procedures as per written hospital or ED protocols (see Procedure 10).
2. Prevent secondary contamination of self, others, and equipment by wearing appropriate level of protection (see Procedure 10).
3. Remove all patient jewelry and clothing.
4. Decontaminate patient **before** patient enters the ED.
5. Assess patient's airway, respiratory, and circulatory status.
6. Maintain spinal immobilization if trauma is suspected.
7. In multiple-patient situations, utilize the ED or hospital mass-casualty disaster response and triage protocols.
8. Administer antidotes as appropriate for the agent. Based on the patient's condition, it may be necessary to administer the antidotes during the patient decontamination process.
9. Delay invasive procedures until the patient is decontaminated.
10. Nursing care priorities are listed in the table on pp. 368-369.

PRIORITY DIAGNOSTIC TESTS

Few diagnostic tests are readily available in EDs to identify the chemical or biologic agent involved.

Laboratory Tests
Arterial blood gas: in patients with pulmonary symptoms
Complete blood count (CBC): if infectious process or acute radiation syndrome is suspected
Electrolytes: if vomiting and diarrhea

NURSING CARE PRIORITIES

Potential/Actual Problem	Causes	Signs and Symptoms	Interventions
Skin contamination	Exposure to a chemical or biologic agent	• Burns • Urticaria • Redness • Pain • Blisters • Necrosis and deep burns • Rash	• Decontaminate the skin. • Administer antidote if available for the known substance.
Oxygenation and ventilation	Exposure to a chemical or biologic agent	• Dyspnea • Cough • Bronchospasm • Laryngospasm • Upper respiratory illness • Mild sore throat • Fever and myalgia • Respiratory failure • Pulmonary edema • Respiratory distress • Copious secretions	• Administer oxygen to maintain oxygen saturation of greater than 95%. • Continuously monitor oxygen saturation and vital signs. • Position the patient for comfort. • Prepare for intubation and ventilatory assistance/support.

Uncontrolled muscle response	Exposure to a nerve agent or cyanide	• Muscle spasms • Fasciculations • Muscle weakness	• Administer antidote if available.
Pain	Exposure to a chemical, biologic, or radiologic agent	• Complaints of pain • Crying • Meaning • Grimacing • Restlessness	• Assess pain using a pain scale, reassess after any intervention. • Position the patient for comfort. • Administer pain medication as ordered.
Altered GI function	Exposure to chemical or biologic agent	• Nausea/vomiting • Anorexia • Diarrhea • Abdominal pain	• Administer IV fluids as ordered. • Assess for hematochezia and melena. • Administer pain medication as ordered. • Administer antiemetics as ordered.
Anxiety	Potential or actual exposure to a chemical, biologic, or radiologic agent	• Behavior changes • Restlessness • Repetitive questioning about condition	• Offer reassurance and support to the patient and family. • Provide a quiet, calm environment. • Explain all procedures to the patient and family using nonmedical terms. • Administer antianxiety medication as ordered.

Liver function tests: if exposed to organic solvents

Methemoglobin level: in cyanide poisoning

Sputum and blood cultures: if inhalation anthrax, pneumonic plague, or tularemia suspected

Toxin assays of feces or gastric secretions: if botulism ingestion suspected

Radiographic Tests

Facilitate the obtaining of radiographic tests in those patients with injuries (see Chapter 21, Trauma).

Chest radiograph: In patients with pulmonary symptoms

Special Tests

Dosimeter or Geiger counter: May be used to detect radiation exposure of a patient.

CLINICAL CONDITIONS

Biologic
Anthrax

Anthrax is a bacterial spore that can be spread through inhalation, skin contamination, or gastrointestinal contamination. Inhalation exposure is the most fatal form of anthrax. Anthrax occurs naturally in animal deposits in the soil and is easily manufactured.

Signs and symptoms

- Inhalation:
  - Initial symptoms are similar to upper respiratory illness, with mild sore throat, fever, and myalgia. Respiratory failure and pulmonary edema may develop within 1 week.
- Cutaneous:
  - The presenting symptoms may be itching followed by rapid (within 2 to 3 hours) development of a papule and then a vesicle. Within a week, the tissue will become edematous and necrotic. Cutaneous anthrax is painless.
- Gastrointestinal:
  - Presents with nausea, anorexia, diarrhea (may be bloody), and severe abdominal pain.

Diagnosis

- Chest x-ray
- Blood cultures
- Oral and nasopharyngeal cultures
- Wound cultures

Treatment
- Standard precautions
- Antibiotics: May include ciprofloxacin or doxycycline
- Respiratory monitoring
- Oxygen therapy

Botulism

Botulism is a neurotoxic spore that is found naturally in soil in the form of the bacterium *Clostridium botulinum*. Botulism can be transmitted to humans through air, food, or open wounds. Mass exposure may occur by the spread of the *Clostridium botulinum* spore through aerosolization or water contamination. Symptoms may begin within a few hours to a few days after contamination and last for weeks or months.

Signs and symptoms
- Blurred vision, diplopia, ptosis, slurred speech, dysphagia, descending muscle weakness
- Botulism, when diagnosed in infants, is termed infantile botulism. The flaccid paralysis the bacteria causes in infants is known as "droopy baby syndrome."

Diagnosis
- History
- Stool cultures
- Gastrointestinal cultures
- Analysis of food

Treatment
- Ventilatory assistance including intubation and mechanical ventilation if the paralysis affects the diaphragm
- Fluid administration or resuscitation if hypovolemia is present (see Procedure 18)
- Trivalent botulinum antitoxin is available from the Centers for Disease Control (CDC)

Pneumonic Plague

Pneumonic plague is a lung infection caused by the *Yersinia pestis* bacterium. This bacterium is found in rodents and fleas and can be transmitted through a bite, but also can be manufactured in a lab. The potential for mass infection could occur with aerosolization of the spore.

Signs and symptoms
- Chest pain
- Fever
- Chills
- Headache
- Hemoptysis

- Cough
- Dyspnea
- Stridor
- Respiratory failure
- Circulatory collapse
- Bleeding diathesis

Diagnosis
- Blood and sputum cultures

Treatment
- Antibiotics: may include streptomycin, doxycycline, gentamicin, ciprofloxacin
- Respiratory monitoring
- Oxygen therapy
- Intubation and ventilatory support for respiratory failure
- IV fluids
- Strict isolation for the first 72 hours after initiation of antibiotics. (Droplet precautions)

Ricin

Ricin is a poisonous cytotoxin that is derived from the remnants of castor beans during the process of manufacturing castor oil. Infection can occur by ingestion or inhalation of ricin.

Signs and symptoms
- Inhalation:
  - Acute fever, cough, respiratory distress, nausea, myalgia approximately 3 hours after exposure
  - Pulmonary edema, respiratory failure, and circulatory collapse occur within 12 to 48 hours
- Ingestion:
  - Severe nausea and vomiting
  - Dehydration
  - GI bleeding
  - Liver and renal failure
  - Circulatory collapse

Diagnosis
- History and clinical findings
- Specific serum ELISA

Treatment
- Gastric decontamination if ingested
- Respiratory monitoring
- Oxygen therapy
- Intubation and ventilatory support for respiratory failure
- IV fluids/fluid resuscitation (see Procedure 18)
- Electrolyte replacement as needed

Smallpox

Smallpox is an extremely contagious, potentially fatal disease that has been eradicated since 1979[1] but still exists in laboratories. Many government officials are concerned that smallpox could present a bioterror threat. Direct and fairly prolonged face-to-face contact is required to spread smallpox from one person to another. Smallpox also can be spread through direct contact with infected bodily fluids or contaminated objects, such as bedding or clothing. The infected person is considered to be contagious until the last smallpox scab falls off.

If smallpox is suspected, the patient must be isolated immediately. Place the patient in a private, negative airflow room (airborne infection isolation) if available. If not available, the patient should be placed in a private room with the door closed at all times, except when patient or staff must enter or exit. Staff and visitors should wear N95 or higher quality respirators, gloves, and gowns. Patients should wear a surgical mask when outside the negative-pressure isolation room and must be gowned or wrapped in a sheet so that their rash is fully covered.

A detailed discussion of smallpox signs, symptoms, and treatment can be found in Chapter 6, Communicable Diseases.

Staphylococcal Enterotoxin B

Staphylococcal Enterotoxin B occurs after ingestion of food or water contaminated with the organism or through inhalation. It is a common source of unintentional food poisoning, but it also can be easily aerosolized, and mass contamination is possible. Hypovolemia may occur as a result of severe vomiting and diarrhea. Although rarely fatal (unless hypovolemia is not treated), it can be incapacitating for up to 2 weeks.

Signs and symptoms
- Inhalation:
  - Fever, chills, headache, myalgia, nonproductive cough, nausea, vomiting, diarrhea 1 to 6 hours after exposure
- Ingestion:
  - Vomiting, diarrhea

Diagnosis
- History and physical exam findings

Treatment
- Oxygen therapy
- IV fluids
- Cough suppressant

Tularemia

Tularemia is an infectious bacterium found naturally in the soil and carried by small animals such as rabbits and squirrels. It also can be manufactured in a laboratory setting. Tularemia can be transmitted through the bite of an infected animal, and mass contamination could occur through aerosolization.

Signs and symptoms
- Fever
- Chills
- Headache
- Malaise
- Lymphadenopathy
- Nonproductive cough

Diagnosis
- Serology testing
- Blood cultures

Treatment
- Antibiotics: may include streptomycin, gentamicin, or doxycycline
- Standard precautions

Chemical

Ammonia

Ammonia is a chemical used in the manufacture of fertilizer, pesticides, pharmaceuticals, textiles, and explosives. Exposure can occur through inhalation, ingestion, and contact with skin.

Signs and symptoms
- Respiratory:
  - ENT irritation
  - Cough
  - Bronchoconstriction
  - Pharyngeal and laryngeal edema
  - Mucosal burns
- Ingestion:
  - Vomiting
  - Epigastric tenderness
- Dermal/ocular:
  - Redness
  - Pain
  - Blisters
  - Necrosis and deep burns (concentrated solution)
  - Swelling and sloughing of surface cells of eye
  - Temporary or permanent blindness

Diagnosis
- History and physical findings

Treatment
- Decontamination
- Eye irrigation (see Procedure 17)
- ACLS measures (see Reference Guide 1)
- Aerosolized bronchodilators (for bronchospasms)
- Racemic epinephrine for pediatric patients who develop stridor

Chlorine

Chlorine is a chemical with both household and industrial uses; it also was used as a chemical weapon in World War I. Chlorine is stored as a cool liquid but when released turns into a strongly pungent gas.

Signs and symptoms
- Respiratory/cardiovascular:
  - ENT irritation
  - Cough
  - Airway constriction
  - Pulmonary edema (higher concentrations)
  - Tachycardia
  - Hypotension
- Dermal/ocular:
  - Eye irritation
  - Pain
  - Blisters
  - Ulcerations
  - Frostbite (liquefied chlorine)

Diagnosis
- History and physical findings

Treatment
- Same as ammonia
- If chlorine frostbite is present, immerse affected area in a rewarming bath at 102° to 108° F for 20 to 30 minutes (see Chapter 9, Environmental Emergencies, for further information on frostbite).

Cyanide

Cyanide is a chemical found in the form of a gas or a crystal. Cyanide is used industrially in the manufacture of plastics and paper, and in the development of photographs. The chemical was used as a weapon in World War II. Cyanide prevents the utilization of oxygen in cellular metabolism. Effects are noted in oxygen-sensitive systems such as the central nervous system and the cardiovascular system.

Signs and symptoms
- CNS:
  - Dizziness
  - H/A
  - Weakness
  - Muscle spasms
  - Convulsions
  - Loss of consciousness
- Respiratory/cardiovascular:
  - Initially hypertension and tachycardia, then bradycardia and hypotension
  - Respiratory distress that progresses to respiratory failure

Diagnosis
- History and findings
- Whole blood cyanide tests

Treatment
- Decontamination
- Oxygen therapy
- Amyl nitrite perles: broken onto a gauze and held under the nose, over the bag-valve device intake, or placed under the face mask for 30 seconds every minute until patient improves or sodium nitrite available.
- If no response to amyl nitrite and oxygen, infuse sodium nitrite, 10 ml of a 3% solution (300 mg) over at least 5 minutes. Then immediately infuse sodium thiosulfate 50 ml of a 25% solution over 10 to 20 minutes.[2]
- ACLS measures

Phosgene

Phosgene is a chemical used in the production of pesticides and plastics. In World War I, phosgene was used as a chemical warfare agent, and many deaths were linked to its use. Phosgene can cause skin and respiratory symptoms.

Signs and symptoms
- Respiratory:
  - Cough
  - Dyspnea
  - With exposure to high concentrations, progressive pulmonary edema and respiratory failure can develop within 30 minutes to 48 hours
- Eyes:
  - Diplopia
  - Watery eyes

> ⇒ **NURSING ALERT** ⇐
>
> Even though the patient may appear to be improving, the effects of phosgene may be delayed, and the patient should be closely monitored for at least 48 hours.

- Dermal:
  - Irritation and redness
  - Frostbite (liquid phosgene under pressure)

Diagnosis
- History and physical findings

Treatment
- Same as ammonia
- Serial chest radiographs
- Corticosteroids for inflammation of respiratory tract

Sulfuric Acid
Sulfuric acid is used in the manufacture of many items, including fertilizers, detergents, pharmaceuticals, and other chemicals. It can be spread through inhalation and skin contact.

Signs and symptoms
- Respiratory:
  - ENT irritation
  - Laryngeal spasm and edema
  - Bronchospasm
  - Pulmonary edema
- Dermal/ocular:
  - Pain
  - Redness
  - Blisters
  - Conjunctivitis
  - Corneal burns

Diagnosis
- History and physical findings

Treatment
- Same as ammonia

Nerve Gas Agents
Nerve gas agents manufactured as chemical weapons by the military are the most toxic of the known chemical warfare agents. The three most common agents are: Sarin, also known by the military designation GB, which is an odorless gas; VX, which is an odorless, tasteless gas; and Tabun, also known by the military

designation GA, which is a clear liquid with slightly fruity odor. These agents are chemically similar to organophosphate pesticides and exert biological effects by inhibiting acetylcholinesterase enzymes. Nerve gas agents alter synaptic transmission at certain points in the CNS.

Signs and symptoms

Exposure via contact to skin:

- Mild:
  - Sweating at exposure site
  - Localized twitching at exposure site
- Moderate:
  - May include above symptoms and generalized fasciculations (muscle spasm in a group of muscles) and muscle twitching
  - Generalized weakness
  - Nausea, vomiting, diarrhea
- Severe:
  - Extreme weakness with eventual flaccid paralysis
  - Seizures
  - Respiratory arrest
  - Loss of consciousness

Exposure via inhalation:

- Mild:
  - Miosis (pinpoint pupils)
  - Blurred vision
  - Rhinorrhea
  - Lacrimation (tearing)
  - Bronchoconstriction and tightness in chest
  - Mild to moderate respiratory distress
- Moderate: those listed above, plus:
  - Moderate to severe respiratory distress
  - Copious respiratory secretions
  - Nausea, vomiting, diarrhea, abdominal cramps
  - Fasciculations, muscle twitching
  - Muscle weakness
  - Excessive lacrimation
- Severe:
  - Extreme weakness with eventual flaccid paralysis
  - Respiratory arrest
  - Loss of consciousness

Treatment

- Decontamination (see Procedure 10)
- Airway management

> ### ➤ NURSING ALERT ◄
>
> The mnemonics SLUDGE and DUMBELS can help one remember
> the side effects of nerve agents:
>
> | | | | |
> |---|---|---|---|
> | S: | salivation | D: | diaphoresis, diarrhea |
> | L: | lacrimation | U: | urination |
> | U: | urination | M: | miosis |
> | D: | diarrhea | B: | bradycardia, bronchospasm |
> | G: | GI upset | E: | emesis |
> | E: | emesis | L: | lacrimation |
> | | | S: | salivation |

- Atropine should be administered until secretions are decreased,
  the patient is able to breathe normally, diarrhea ceases, and
  sweating ceases. When these parameters have been reached,
  the status is known as atropinization. Often large quantities of
  atropine are required to reach this point.

> ### ➤ NURSING ALERT ◄
>
> Atropine can precipitate ventricular fibrillation in the presence of
> hypoxia. Ensure a patent airway before administration.

- Pralidoxime (2-PAM chloride) also is indicated and can be
  administered intramuscularly via autoinjector or intravenously.
  2-PAM chloride helps to restore normal function and control
  of skeletal muscles.

Radiologic

Radioactive substances can be found in industry, energy
production plants, and health-care settings. The ED nurse should
obtain a history that includes the radioactive substance involved,
route (i.e., external vs. internal), and treatment before arrival. If
the exposure was internal, determine whether it involved
inhalation or ingestion of the substance. There are four types of
ionizing radiation:

- *Alpha particles:* These are slow moving and have a low energy
  field. Alpha particles can be stopped by clothing or paper.
- *Beta particles:* These particles have more penetrating ability to
  cause injury but can be stopped by plastic or aluminum.

- *Gamma rays:* These are highly penetrating but can be stopped with lead shields or concrete.
- *Neutrons:* These are the most penetrating of the radiation types and can cause significant tissue damage. Neutrons are found at nuclear reactor sites.

The effects of radiation will depend on the type, dose, time of exposure, and adequacy of shielding. A "dirty bomb," or radiologic dispersion device, is a bomb that combines a conventional explosive, such as dynamite, with radioactive materials in the form of powder or pellets. The radioactive materials used in a dirty bomb usually come from low-level radioactive sources. The greatest danger from a dirty bomb is the blast itself.

Most radiation emergencies are local or involve only a small portion of the body. Acute radiation syndrome is an acute illness caused by irradiation of the whole body or a significant portion of the body. It is characterized by signs and symptoms related to cellular deficiencies and the reaction of various organs to ionizing radiation. The higher the dose is, the greater is the severity of early symptoms.

Local Injury
Signs and symptoms
- History of possible radiation exposure such as from a radiography source, x-ray device, or accelerator
- Skin lesion without a history of chemical or thermal burn, insect bite, or skin disease
- Erythema, blistering, and/or ulceration of the skin
- Local injuries to the skin evolve slowly, and symptoms may not manifest for days to weeks after exposure.

Diagnosis
Based on history and clinical presentation.

Treatment
- Facilitate a plastic surgery or specialty consult. Conventional wound management may be ineffective.
- Administer pain and topical medications as ordered.

Acute Radiation Syndrome
Signs and symptoms
- Decreased white blood cell count
- Decreased platelet count and increased bleeding
- Nausea, vomiting, diarrhea
- Confusion, decreased level of consciousness
- Hypotension secondary to fluid loss
- Loss of dermis with "radiation burns"

Diagnosis

Based on history and clinical presentation.

Treatment

- Perform a trauma assessment if a blast or explosion is involved (see Chapter 21, Trauma).
- Patient decontamination if external contaminants are present
- If available, utilize a radiation measuring instrument before and after decontamination to ensure radioactive contaminants have been removed.
- Note areas of erythema and record on a body chart.
- Obtain and monitor CBC with differential. Repeat every 6 to 8 hours. A decrease in the initial absolute lymphocyte count may indicate recent exposure. If the initial WBC and platelet counts are significantly low, consider the possibility of exposure a few days to weeks earlier.
- Facilitate consultation with hematologist and radiation experts.
- Administer antiemetics and serotonin inhibitors.
- Institute oxygen therapy as indicated.
- Initiate and administer IV fluid therapy and blood components.
- Provide comfort measures and psychological support.

Vesicants (Blister Agents) (Sulfur Mustard, Lewisite)

Vesicants are chemical warfare agents that were originally used in World War I. These agents cause blistering of skin and mucous membranes upon contact with the agent.

Signs and symptoms

Exposure via skin contact (onset of symptoms 1 to 24 hours after exposure):

- Mild/moderate:
  - *Skin:* redness, blisters
  - *Eyes:* itching, tearing, burning, swelling of lids, photophobia, blepharospasm
- Severe:
  - *Skin:* blisters appearing shortly after contact, ulcers, necrosis, skin charring
  - *Eyes:* severe pain, severe swelling of lids, ulceration or perforation of cornea, miosis

Exposure via inhalation: (symptoms may occur 1 to 48 hours after exposure):

- Mild/moderate:
  - Burning sensation in throat, sinus pain, cough, epistaxis, hoarseness, mild dyspnea, chest tightness

- Severe:
  - Pulmonary edema, severe dyspnea, increased sputum production

Diagnosis

Based on history and clinical presentation.

Treatment

- Decontamination (see Procedure 10)
- Airway management (see Procedure 1)
- Eye irrigation (see Procedure 17)
- British Anti-Lewisite (BAL), also called dimercaprol, is a chelating agent that may reduce systemic effects from Lewisite. BAL should be administered only to those with signs of shock or significant pulmonary injury, as BAL does not affect skin or eye lesions.
- There is no antidote for sulfur mustard.

> **NURSING ALERT**
>
> Consider the possibility of a terrorist event or covert assault if one or more of the following are present:
> - ✓ Serious disease manifestations in previously healthy people
> - ✓ Higher than normal number of patients with fever and respiratory and/or GI complaints
> - ✓ Multiple people with similar complaints from a common location or function
> - ✓ Unusual number of severe or rapidly fatal cases
> - ✓ Greater number of ill or dead animals in a common location
> - ✓ Greater number of patients with severe pneumonia, sepsis, fever with rash, or cranial nerve palsies
>
> Contact the infection control department, local and/or state health department, local law enforcement, and local emergency management agency if a terrorist event is suspected.

NURSING SURVEILLANCE

1. Ongoing monitoring of airway, respiratory, and circulatory status
2. Ongoing monitoring of level of consciousness
3. Ongoing monitoring of intake and output
4. Ongoing assessment and monitoring of skin lesions, including those from dermal chemical injury or exposure to a biologic or radioactive substance
5. Be alert for and report a trend of increasing number of patients presenting to the ED with respiratory or GI symptoms

EXPECTED PATIENT OUTCOMES

1. Patient maintains a patent airway.
2. ABGs and oxygen saturation within normal limits
   (see Reference Guide 2)
3. Skin normal color, warm, and dry
4. Bilateral clear breath sounds
5. Absence of stridor, retractions, and dyspnea
6. Respiratory rate greater than 12 and less than 28 and normal
   depth
7. Palpable peripheral and central pulses
8. Vital signs within normal limits for age
9. Improved level of consciousness
10. Urine output of at least 30 ml/hr in adults, 1 to 2 ml/kg/hr
    for children
11. Pain free or at a level acceptable for patient
12. Progressive healing of skin lesions

PATIENT/FAMILY DISCHARGE IMPLICATIONS AND TEACHING

1. Provide specific instructions related to skin/wound care and
   factors to promote healing.
2. Ensure patient has contact number(s) for future questions and
   follow-up.
3. If clothes were actually or possibly contaminated, provide
   specific instructions for washing clothes. The patient should
   take the clothes home in a plastic bag and wash separately
   from other clothing.
4. Provide specific instructions related to route, dose, and side
   effects of prescriptions, such as antibiotics.
5. Encourage compliance with medication therapy and plan for
   home care.

Helpful up-to-date information about chemical and biological
exposures can be found at the following websites:

- Centers for Disease Control, www.bt.cdc.gov
- United States Army Medical Research Institute of Infectious
  Diseases, www.usamriid.army.mil/index.htm

References

1. World Health Organization, June, 2004, www.who.int.
2. Agency for Toxic Substances and Disease Registry: *Managing hazardous
   material incidents: medical management guidelines for acute exposures,*
   Washington, DC, 2001, Department of Health and Human Services.

11 chapter

Extremity Trauma

Julia Fultz
Carlos Coyle

CLINICAL CONDITIONS

Amputations
Compartment Syndrome: Acute
Dislocations
Fractures
Sprains
Strains

Hemorrhage is the most common life-threatening injury associated with musculoskeletal trauma. It may be conspicuous or concealed internally and is most often associated with pelvic, femoral, and multiple fractures. After oxygenation, ventilation, and perfusion abnormalities have been addressed, a focused nursing assessment including exposure, inspection, and palpation is performed and injuries involving the limbs and joints are evaluated.

FOCUSED NURSING ASSESSMENT

Nursing assessment of the extremities focuses on neurovascular integrity, skin integrity, mobility, and comfort. Expose the extremity. Remove anything potentially constrictive from the injured extremity, such as clothing, jewelry, or circumferential dressings. One should collect subjective information on the mechanism of injury, pain, numbness, tingling, weakness, prior efforts to treat, and normal function. Inspect the anterior, posterior, and lateral surfaces for color, bleeding, angulations, deformities, alignment, abnormal rotation or shortening of the limb, puncture wounds, avulsions, contusions, abrasions, and lacerations. Palpation includes an evaluation of pulses, capillary refill, temperature, limb movement and sensation, pitting edema, pain, bony crepitus, point tenderness, and weakness. Comparisons should be made between the injured and the uninjured extremity if possible.

Neurovascular Integrity

A neurovascular examination distal to the injury should be performed before and after any intervention involving the injured extremity and every hour otherwise. The neurovascular examination should include an evaluation of bleeding, pulses, capillary refill, color, temperature, movement, sensation, and pain.

1. Evaluate the wounds for active bleeding:
   - Evaluate dressings for success in stopping the bleeding. Note blood around the wound or soaked into clothing or temporary dressings.
   - Inspect hematomas, measure their size, and reevaluate them for expansion (circumference measurements).
   - Inspect for edema, and note any increase in amount.
2. Palpate pulses in all extremities at hourly intervals by palpation or by Doppler ultrasound.
   - Compare pulses distal to the injury with the pulses in the unaffected limb if possible. Note the amplitude of the pulse:
     - 0 = absent
     - +1 = diminished, barely palpable
     - +2 = Expected
     - +3 = Full, increased
     - +4 = Bounding

NURSING ALERT

The most important indicator of vascular injury is the quality or absence of pulses. However, the presence of pulses does not rule out vascular injury with some residual flow or compartment syndrome. Vascular injuries associated with circulatory compromise can pose a threat to limb viability.

---

3. Capillary refill in all extremities should be less than 2 seconds. In geriatric patients capillary refill may be prolonged. Environmental factors such as cold cause a delay in capillary refill, as do certain medical conditions such as arterial insufficiency.
4. Inspect each extremity for uniform color, pallor, mottling, and cyanosis. Compare the injured extremity with the contralateral extremity for each of these.

NURSING ALERT

Ischemia produces color and temperature changes.

---

5. Evaluate the extremity skin temperature. Note the temperature by touch and compare extremities. Note temperature variations within the same limb.
6. Note extremity movement and any motion limitations.
7. Evaluate sensory function distal to the injury site:
   - *Touch:* Evaluate hypoesthesia (decreased sensitivity) and hyperesthesia (increased sensitivity) by touching the skin lightly with a fine wisp of cotton, and differentiate between sharp and dull (use a sterile needle or paperclip) or two-point discrimination.
   - *Proprioception:* Receptors respond to stretch, pressure, or position. Grasp the big toe or a finger and ask the patient to determine whether you are moving it up or down. If the patient is unable to determine this, repeat with the ankle or wrist.
   - *Paresthesia (numbness and tingling):* Nerve involvement as a result of ischemia begins distally and travels proximally. Identify the area of paresthesia and perform serial examinations.
8. Pain along the distribution of affected nerve

> ### ⤳ NURSING ALERT ⤶
>
> Numbness or tingling in an extremity may be indicative of vascular or neurologic compromise.

Skin Integrity
Interruptions in skin integrity provide an entry for microorganisms. Structures under the break in skin integrity often are damaged.
1. Evaluate for continued bleeding.
2. Evaluate for potential for contamination. (What caused the injury?)
3. Determine time lapsed since injury occurred to gauge the age of wound.
4. Determine wound length and depth. A laceration over a suspected fracture site is treated as an open fracture until further assessment proves otherwise.
5. Describe break in skin integrity:
   - *Abrasion:* Area of skin that has been rubbed or worn away by friction

- *Avulsion:* Full-thickness skin loss by forcible separation or detachment
- *Puncture:* Penetration by a sharp or blunt object that produces a hole, wound, or perforation
- *Laceration:* Torn or sharply cut wound, often ragged in appearance
- *Degloving:* Full thickness of skin is peeled away from an area such as a finger, hand, or foot.

6. Evaluate for presence of foreign body.

Mobility

Loss of mobility can result from pain and/or neurovascular damage.

1. Inspect the exposed limb for the following:
   - Abnormal angulations
   - Shortening of one extremity in comparison with the other
   - External or internal rotation of an extremity
   - Discoloration (erythema, ecchymosis, paleness, or abrasions)
   - Edema
   - Exposed bone, tendons, ligaments, or muscle
2. Gently palpate the extremity, moving proximal to distal for tenderness, crepitus, and increased heat. If a fracture is known to be present, crepitus does not need to be purposefully elicited. Further movement of the bone ends can cause additional injury.
3. Evaluate for a limitation in the range of motion of the injured extremity.
4. Evaluate the extremity muscle strength. Compare it with the unaffected extremity if possible. Note any atrophy.
   - Can the patient raise the extremity without assistance?
   - Can the patient raise the extremity against gravity (dangle the leg over the bed or have the arm hang by the patient's side)?
   - Can the patient raise the extremity against resistance, such as the examiner's hand?
   - Test flexion and extension by having the patient pull and push against the examiner's hand.

Comfort
Pain

The most common complaint with musculoskeletal injuries is pain. Pain distal to the level of the injury is uncommon unless there is neurovascular damage.

⇒ NURSING ALERT ⇐

Compartment syndrome is a limb-threatening condition in which pressures in a muscle compartment rise high enough to interrupt the microvascular circulation, causing ischemia and eventual irreversible tissue damage. Symptoms include severe, progressively increasing pain that is out of proportion to what would be expected with the injury; pain on passive stretching of the muscle involved; tenseness; and a diminished sensation to touch.[1,2] It must be identified and treated swiftly (see Compartment Syndrome under Clinical Conditions).

---

1. Note the patient's pain. The most reliable indicator of pain is the patient's own interpretation of what is being experienced. Evaluation includes:
   - *Location:* Does the patient feel pain in a generalized large area, a localized small area, or a single point?
   - *Intensity:* The intensity of the pain should be evaluated on a standardized scale that can be repeated to evaluate changes in the level of pain, such as a scale of "0 = no pain" to "10 = the worst pain possible," in which the patient assigns the pain a number.
   - *Quality:* Is the pain prickling, burning, throbbing, stabbing, sharp, dull, cramping, aching, or radiating?
   - *Onset:* Did the patient feel the pain immediately after the event, or was there a delayed onset?
   - *Duration:* Is the pain continuous, steady, periodic, or momentary?
   - *Variations:* What makes the pain worse? What makes it better?
2. Point tenderness may indicate an underlying fracture.
3. Signs of discomfort include: diaphoresis, palmar sweating, dilated pupils, pallor, dry mouth, alterations in vital signs (tachycardia, tachypnea), decreased attention span, grimacing, groaning, crying, rocking, frowning, restlessness.

LIFE SPAN ISSUES

Pediatric Patients

1. Children who do not have completely developed motor skills are at an increased risk for injury.
2. A child's bones are softer and more flexible than an adult's bones. Children may sustain incomplete fractures: plastic (bend),

greenstick, physis (growth plate), and buckle (torus) fractures.[2]

3. The epiphyses are cartilaginous growth zones in children that often can be mistaken on radiographs for fractures. Because of the relative weakness of this area, it separates before other structures are torn or broken.[3] Fractures through the epiphysis with disruption of the growth plate can cause growth disturbances.

Geriatric Patients

- Geriatric patients who have decreased reaction times, a decreased range of motion, decreased muscle mass and strength, decreased endurance, and problems with balance have an increased potential for injury.
- Increased frequency of degenerative bone disease with advancing age increases the incidence of fractures.
- Fractures may occur spontaneously in osteoporotic bone.
- Geriatric patients have less subcutaneous fat padding at bony prominences and are at an increased risk for pressure sores if bed rest is needed.
- Decreased peripheral vascular circulation often is present with advancing age.
- Skin becomes thinner and more fragile.

Pregnancy

1. The hormone relaxin causes the pelvic ligaments to loosen.
2. The center of gravity changes because of the enlarged abdomen, which predisposes the woman to a loss of balance and to falls resulting in musculoskeletal injuries.

INITIAL INTERVENTIONS

The goals of extremity-injury management in the emergency department (ED) include the following:

- Hemorrhage control
- Identification of vascular injuries before irreversible ischemia develops
- Prevention of further tissue damage
- Maximizing of peripheral perfusion
- Reduction of pain
- Prevention of infection

Following are detailed discussions of each of these goals:

1. Hemorrhage control: Treat hemorrhage by placing direct pressure over the wound with a sterile dressing and finger pressure over the corresponding artery proximal to the injury. If possible, gently remove gross debris from the wound. If the

patient is hypovolemic, initiate warmed crystalloid infusion via two large-bore IV catheters attached to large-bore tubing with a maxi-drip chamber.

2. Identify vascular injuries: Perform serial neurovascular checks, remove constricting items (e.g., jewelry, clothing, dressings)

3. Prevent further tissue damage: Immobilize suspected fractures to prevent further tissue damage and blood loss resulting from movement of fractured bone ends. Include the joints above and below the suspected fracture. Assess neurovascular function before, during, and after immobilization (see Procedure 32 for specific fracture immobilization techniques). Protruding bone ends should not be disturbed. Place saline-moistened gauze over exposed bone to prevent drying. Splint as found unless neurovascular compromise is present. Stabilize an impaled object. Pressure on bony prominences from lying on a backboard can cause skin breakdown. Remove the patient from backboard as soon as possible. Skin breakdown will occur more rapidly in the geriatric patient.

4. Elevate injured extremities above the level of the heart to reduce edema unless compartment syndrome is suspected, in which case, keep the extremity at the level of the heart to maximize tissue oxygenation. Ensure adequate circulating volume.

5. Reduction of pain: Immobilization helps to reduce the amount of pain experienced by preventing the bone ends from grating together. Administer pain medication (opioids, nonsteroidal antiinflammatory agents, muscle relaxants). Apply ice packs with a barrier between the ice pack and the skin.

6. Place sterile dressings over open wounds, ensure tetanus immunization is up to date, and consider prophylactic antibiotic administration.

Nursing care priorities are listed in the table on pp. 392-393.

PRIORITY DIAGNOSTIC TESTS

Laboratory

CBC: Obtain a CBC if the break in the skin is more than 8 hours old because of the increased chance of infection.

Enzymes (serum CK, LDH, SGOT, SGPT): will be increased if skeletal muscle is damaged.

Hemoglobin and hematocrit: For patients with fractures of the pelvis, femurs, or multiple fractures, measure hemoglobin and hematocrit because of the potential blood loss (Table 11-1).

TABLE 11-1   Potential Local Blood Loss in Fractures

Injured Area	Amount
Humerus	250 ml
Forearm	150-250 ml
Pelvis	1500-3000 ml
Femur	1000 ml
Tibia/fibula	500 ml
Ankle	0.5-1.5 L
Spine or ribs	1.0-3.0 L

From Geiderman JM: General principles of orthopedic injuries. In Marx J, Hockberger RS, Wall RM, et al, eds: *Rosen's emergency medicine: concepts and clinical practice,* ed 5, St Louis, 2002, Mosby.

Type and crossmatch: obtained for potential blood transfusion if significant blood loss from the fractures has occurred or is anticipated, or for surgery to repair fractures.

Urine myoglobin: Myoglobin is a muscle protein that is released from the cell when the cell is severely damaged, such as in crush injuries or compartment syndrome. Myoglobin is excreted in the urine and will turn the urine a reddish brown color.

Radiologic Tests

Arteriogram: Confirm or rule out a suspected vascular injury in the event of diminished or absent pulses.

CT scan: often used to identify acetabulum fractures and to evaluate the integrity of articulating surfaces such as the knee, hand, wrist, and ankle. It also is used to rule out cervical spine injuries when radiographs are inconclusive and to better define the characteristics of a known fracture, such as fragment placement and bony alignment.[1]

X-rays: the mainstay in diagnosing fractures and dislocations. Anteroposterior and lateral views should be included to image the entire bone and both proximal and distal joints. Comparison with old films may be helpful.

Other Diagnostic Procedures

Magnetic resonance imaging: Magnetic resonance imaging identifies damage to bones, muscles, ligaments, cartilage, and menisci. This test is expensive and reserved for cases in which the diagnosis is in doubt and the treatment plan differs according to the test results.[1]

NURSING CARE PRIORITIES

Potential/ Actual Problem	Causes	Signs and Symptoms	Interventions
Inadequate fluid volume	Blood loss from fracture site, lacerations, or amputation	• Altered mental status • Elevated heart rate • Diaphoresis • Hypotension • Tachypnea • Cool, pale skin • Delayed capillary refill • Decreased urinary output	• Apply pressure dressings to active bleeding and use arterial pressure points if needed. • Administer oxygen. • Immobilize fractures to reduce cell/tissue damage. • Insert two large-bore IV catheters (14 to 16 gauge) connected to large-bore trauma tubing for fluid resuscitation. • Monitor intake and output, vital signs, mental status.
Inadequate peripheral tissue perfusion	Neurovascular compromise	• Decreased pulses • Cool or pale skin • Decreased motor or sensory function • Pain inconsistent with the extent of injury	• Immobilize the injured extremity. • Assess proximal and distal pulses every 30-60 minutes. • Elevate the extremity to promote venous return if not contraindicated as with compartment syndrome.
Pain	• Noxious stimuli from injury • Tissue	• Complaints of pain • Skeletal muscle tension • Restlessness/irritability	• Explain procedures and sensations to expect. • Pain medication • Ice packs

	destruction • Invasive diagnostic procedures	• Moaning • Crying • Anger/hostility • Facial grimacing • Withdrawal	• Elevate extremity (if not contraindicated). • Monitor vital signs after pain medication. • Reassess pain using a pain scale. • Prepare for sedation with analgesia.
Impaired physical mobility	• Acute extremity pain • Amputation • Fractures	• Difficulty walking • Loss of manual dexterity • Altered range of motion • Paralysis • Paresthesia • Verbalization of pain	• Immobilize fractures. • Splint joint injuries and angulated fractures as found. • Pain medication • Perform serial evaluations for neurovascular compromise. • Teach patient to use mobility aids (crutches, walker, cane).
Risk for infection	Break in skin integrity	• Exposed underlying structures • Gross debris • Lacerations	• Remove gross debris gently; if resistance is met, discontinue. • Cover opening in the skin with a sterile dressing. • Antibiotics

CLINICAL CONDITIONS

Amputations: Complete and Incomplete

A complete amputation is complete separation of some portion of the limb. An incomplete amputation is partial separation of the limb without evidence of neurovascular activity distal to the partial separation. Any tissue bridge should be left intact, no matter how small.

Symptoms

There is an obvious complete separation of the extremity or partial separation of the extremity associated with absent capillary refill, no sensation, no pulses (by palpation or by Doppler ultrasound), and no movement distal to the injury. (NOTE: If capillary refill, sensation, or movement is present to any degree, the injury does not meet the criteria of a complete or incomplete amputation. These injuries often are termed a partial amputation.)

Diagnosis

Diagnosis is based on visualization of complete separation of the extremity at any level or a partial separation of the extremity without any neurovascular activity.

Treatment (the Patient, the Stump, the Amputated Segment)

Treatment for the patient

- The only life-threatening complication of an amputation is hemorrhage.
  - *Complete amputation:* Constriction and retraction of the arteries in conjunction with a pressure dressing will usually control bleeding.
  - *Incomplete amputation:* Partial laceration of an artery prevents retraction, and the extremity may continue to bleed. Control of bleeding can be achieved through local pressure or pressure dressings and elevation of the extremity. If control of the hemorrhage cannot be obtained, a proximal tourniquet can be placed only as a temporary measure for patient resuscitation.[4,5]
- Place two large-bore IV catheters.
- Remove any constricting jewelry.
- Begin volume replacement with Ringer's lactate or normal saline (NS) as indicated.
- Implement pain management.
- Infection management includes antibiotics and tetanus toxoid. Wounds usually are tetanus prone, especially if degloving and crush injuries are involved.

- In cases of complete amputation or partial amputation with neurovascular compromise, prepare to transport the patient to a reimplantation center.

Treatment for the stump
- Apply direct pressure to control hemorrhage.
- Gently remove gross dirt or debris by rinsing the stump with Ringer's lactate or NS solution.
- Apply a sterile, moistened dressing to the stump.
- Splint fractures.
- Elevate the extremity above the level of the heart.
- Monitor dressings for hemorrhage because active bleeding can be concealed.

Treatment for the amputated part
- Collect and keep all amputated parts.
- Rinse with Ringer's lactate or NS to gently remove gross contamination.[6]
- Wrap the part in saline-moistened gauze and place it in a sealable, plastic bag.
- Place the sealed plastic bag with the amputated part in a mixture of crushed ice and water.[7] The goal is to keep the amputated part cool and not allow it to freeze. The amputated part and ice should not come into direct contact. Cooling slows chemical processes and thereby increases viability and survival. Tissue tolerance of ischemia varies. Bone, tendon, and skin tolerate 8 to 12 hours of warm ischemia and 24 hours of cold ischemia. Muscle tolerates 6 hours of warm ischemia and 12 hours of cold ischemia.[8]

NURSING ALERT

The surgeon providing definitive care will decide if any, all, or part of the amputated part can be reimplanted. All amputated pieces and parts should accompany the patient to a reimplantation center.

Compartment Syndrome: Acute

Compartment syndrome is an emergency condition that occurs when the pressure within a muscle compartment rises to a level that interferes with microvascular circulation and impairs the neurovascular integrity. Over a period of hours, the interstitial tissue pressures rise above that of the capillary bed, resulting in capillary vessel collapse, hypoxia, and ischemia of nerve and muscle tissue and eventual tissue necrosis. A histamine release in response to the reduced blood flow compounds the problem by

> ### ⤳ NURSING ALERT ⤶
>
> Determining whether a partially amputated extremity should be cooled sometimes can be difficult. An incomplete amputation should be cooled if there is no evidence of circulation in the extremity distal to the injury, as determined by palpation and Doppler. Cooling can be achieved with ice packs. Ice must not come into contact with tissue. The goal is to slow the chemical processes to increase the viability of the tissue. The extremity should not be cooled if there is any active bleeding from the cut edge of the partially amputated part[8] or if neurological or vascular activity is present. Splint the extremity after applying moistened dressings to the open wound.

increasing blood flow to the area and increasing capillary permeability. The onset of ischemia depends on the amount of pressure, the duration of increased pressure, and the hemodynamic status of the patients. Patients who have had periods of hypotension are more susceptible to compartment syndrome.[1,9] If compartment syndrome is left unrecognized and untreated, permanent disability may occur, and limb amputation may be necessary.

Causes[2,6,10]:

Compartment syndrome may result from either internal or external compression:

- Edema or bleeding into the compartment space from a crushing injury or fracture
- Prolonged compression of an extremity
- Burn (electrical or thermal)
- Bite (animal, human, snake, or spider)
- Pneumatic antishock garment (PSAG)
- Air splints
- Automatic BP cuff
- Cast or dressing that is too tight
- Malpositioned intraosseous line placement (occurs within 20 minutes of line placement)
- Thrombolytic therapy after radial artery cannulation
- Anticoagulant use

Sites

- Four compartments of the lower leg; most common site is the anterior compartment of the lower leg located lateral to the tibia[2,6,10] (Figure 11-1).

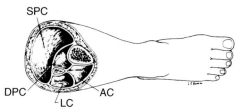

Four compartments of the leg: The anterior compartment
(AC), the lateral compartment *(LC)*, the superficial
posterior compartment *(SPC)*, and the deep posterior
compartment *(DPC)*.

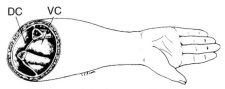

Two compartments of the forearm: The volar compartment
(VC) and the dorsal compartment *(DC)*.

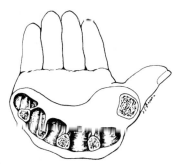

Five interosseous compartments of the hand.

Figure 11–1   Extremity compartments.

- Volar and dorsal compartments of the forearm (Figure 11-1)
- Five interosseous compartments of the hand (Figure 11-1)
- Upper arm
- Gluteal region
- Foot
- Thigh

Symptoms

- Progressive and severe pain that is out of proportion to the underlying injury; pain is aggravated by passive stretch of the involved muscles, touch, and limb elevation; pain medication does not significantly affect pain. Pain is the most sensitive symptom in awake patients.
- Diminished sensation to touch in area of affected nerves, loss of two-point discrimination
- Weakness or paralysis of the involved muscles
- Distal paresthesia
- Tenseness of the affected compartment (subjective)
- Pallor of the extremity (late sign if seen at all)
- Loss of pulses (the cause of compartment syndrome occurs at the cellular level in the capillaries, so loss of pulses is a late sign, if it is seen at all)
- Delayed capillary refill (late sign if seen at all)

Diagnosis

- Based on history and clinical symptoms **coupled** with compartment pressure measurements. There is no defining compartment pressure for which a diagnosis can be made because tolerance to the elevation of tissue pressure varies among individuals, largely related to the patient's hemodynamic status. Differential pressures (diastolic pressure to compartment pressure) of less than 30 mm Hg have been found to be indicative of compartment syndrome requiring a fasciotomy.[11] As long as the difference between the compartment pressure and the diastolic blood pressure remains greater than 30 mm Hg, there may be no need for fasciotomy.[11]
- Elevated (greater than 1000 units) serum CPK (creatine phosphokinase): Although not useful in early detection, trends may be used as an additional tool in making the difficult diagnosis or to monitor progress if a fasciotomy has been performed.
- Myoglobinuria: present with significant muscle damage

Treatment

- Remove anything that may be constricting the extremity (casts, BP cuff, PSAG, air splints, or dressings).
- Place the limb at the level of the heart. Raising the limb above the level of the heart reduces arterial flow and narrows the arterial/venous pressure gradient, thereby decreasing oxygenation of the tissue. Lowering the limb below the heart also will impede perfusion.[1,2]

- Normalize blood pressure: The lower the systemic pressure, the lower the compartment pressure, increasing the chance of compartment syndrome
- Replace blood and clotting factors as needed.
- Continue to monitor pulses, capillary refill, sensation, range of motion, skin temperature, and pain at least hourly. Monitor more often if there is a high index of suspicion that the patient is likely to develop compartment syndrome.[10]
- If appropriate equipment is available, monitor intercompartmental pressures.
- Evaluate the patient for myoglobinuria. As compartment is reperfused, damaged cells release myoblobin.[1,10]
- Monitor for hyperkalemia: Potassium released from damaged cells may cause cardiac disturbances.
- Fasciotomy: surgical opening of the affected compartment

Dislocations
- Occur when bone ends are displaced from the joints. (If the bone ends are only partially displaced, the injury is called a subluxation.)
- Considered an emergency because of the danger of damage to adjacent nerves and blood vessels.
- The most common major dislocation seen in the ED is dislocation of the anterior shoulder, followed by the elbow.[1,2]
- Dislocations also may occur in conjunction with fractures.
- An opening in the skin over a suspected dislocation, subluxation, or fracture dislocation is considered an orthopedic emergency.

Symptoms
- Severe pain to the involved joint area resulting from stretching of the joint capsule
- Deformity of the joint
- Extremity "locked" in an abnormal position
- Swelling of the joint
- Loss of range of motion
- Instability of limb if dislocation is accompanied by a fracture
- Numbness, loss of sensation, and loss of pulses distal to the injury. (A dislocation can compromise the function of arteries and nerves in proximity.)
- Delayed capillary refill if vascular involvement
- Abnormal internal or external rotation of the leg or discrepancy in the leg length if the hip is dislocated

Diagnosis
- Based on the mechanism of injury and clinical presentation
- Radiographs
- Vascular studies

Treatment
- Reassess neurovascular integrity after any limb movement.
- Immobilize the potential dislocation in the position found, use padding to fill void spots.
- Consider ice or cold packs to reduce swelling in the joint area.
- Relocation of a joint should take place as soon as possible after the diagnosis because edema and spasms make relocation more difficult with time.
- Adequate analgesia or sedation with analgesia for relocation and/or reduction.
- Straightening a dislocated joint should be done after radiographs and/or orthopedic consultation has occurred. Straightening of some joints may worsen the original injury.[1]
- Elevate the extremity.

Fractures

Any break in bony continuity is called a fracture. In addition to the bony tissue insult, injury can occur to surrounding soft tissue, blood vessels, and nerves. Shock or even death may result because of the rich blood supply found in bones. Signs and symptoms of extremity fractures are often grotesque in appearance and may lead to "tunnel vision." It is paramount to realize that, in general, fractures do not cause life-threatening situations, and that even though the injury may be "limb threatening," proper perspective, diagnosis, and treatment of life-threatening injuries must take priority. A fracture that is explained by "minimal trauma" may indicate a predisposing structural weakness (e.g., Paget's disease, tumors, osteomalacia, rickets, or scurvy) or an abusive or violent situation.

   Fractures can be classified into two broad categories: closed and open fractures:

Closed Fracture
- No associated open soft-tissue injury
- Closed fractures are classified according to their specific type: comminuted, compression impacted, greenstick, oblique, spiral, and transverse (Figure 11-2).
- Prognosis is generally better for closed fractures because of limited risk of an infection.

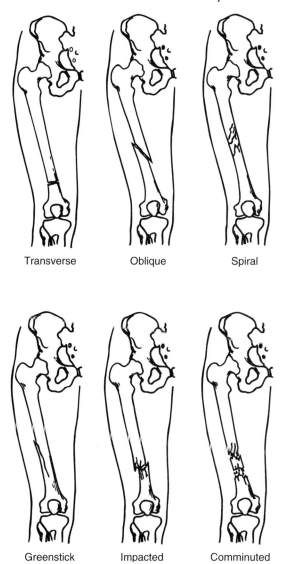

Transverse   Oblique   Spiral

Greenstick   Impacted   Comminuted

Figure 11–2   Classification of fractures.

Open Fracture
- Associated open soft-tissue injury is present.
- An orthopedic emergency because of the risk of infection; orthopedic referral should be initiated immediately.
- Injuries with a wound in close proximity to a fracture are assumed to be an open fracture until proven otherwise.
- Open fractures can defined according to severity (see Box 11-1, Open Fracture Classification).

⋙ NURSING ALERT ⋘

Patients with long-bone and pelvic fractures may develop fat embolism syndrome (FES), which manifests itself as acute respiratory distress and neurological deterioration within 24 to 48 hours after injury or after orthopedic procedure. Intravascular fat droplets can be found in most patients with bone fractures, and this is usually asymptomatic. However, a small number of patients will develop alterations in the lungs, brain, and skin functioning. These patients will develop dyspnea and/or tachypnea, pulmonary edema, hypoxemia, restlessness, altered level of consciousness, tachycardia, petechial rash (most often found on the upper torso), decreased hemoglobin, low platelet count, increased PT, and increased PTT. The pathogenesis is controversial. The diagnosis is based on clinical findings. Care is supportive; patients may require intubation and mechanical ventilation. Although uncommon, FES is life threatening. Early immobilization of fractures may help to prevent FES.[13,14]

Symptoms
The following symptoms generally are suggestive of a fracture. All need not be present to suspect a fracture:
- Pain at or around the site of injury
- Swelling at or around the site of injury
- Deformity of the extremity
- Instability of the extremity
- Crepitus (grating sound heard or felt when the ends of broken bones move together) on movement of the extremity
- Limited mobility and/or limited range of motion of the extremity
- Muscle spasms
- Numbness or tingling

BOX 11-1 OPEN FRACTURE CLASSIFICATION

Grade I: Small wound < 1 cm long that has been punctured from below

Grade II: Well-circumscribed wound up to 5 cm long with little or no contamination and no excessive soft-tissue damage or periosteal stripping

Grade III: Wound > 5 cm and associated with contamination or significant soft-tissue injury (tissue loss, avulsion, crushing injury) and often including a segmental fracture; soft-tissue stripping of bone, major vascular injury, or periosteal stripping may be present

Geiderman JM: General principles of orthopedic injuries. In Marx J, Hockberger RS, Walls RM, et al, eds: *Rosen's emergency medicine: concepts and clinical practice*, ed 5, St Louis, 2002, Mosby, p 477.

Diagnosis
- Clinical presentation
- Radiographic studies
- Determining forces involved in the mechanism of injury can help determine potential for fracture vs. sprain.

Treatment
- Establish control of the hemorrhage with sterile pressure dressings.
- Establish IV access for patients who have fractures that create the potential for fluid volume deficit.
- Cover open fracture wounds and exposed bone ends with saline-moistened sterile gauze.
- Splint the injured extremity, including the joint above and the joint below the injury. Document neurovascular status before and after splinting. If an extremity is deformed, do not force realignment. If the extremity is not easily realigned, splint in the position in which it was found.[6]
- Apply ice packs to the injured site, placing a barrier between the skin and the ice pack.
- Elevate the extremity above the level of the heart.
- Evaluate pulses frequently.
- Avoid excessive movement or manipulation of the fractured site.

In addition to the general symptoms and treatment for fractures, specific extremity fractures may have distinct symptoms and

┌───┐
│　　　　　▷ **N U R S I N G   A L E R T** ◁　　　　　│
├───┤
│ Should the neurovascular status of an angulated fracture worsen │
│ after it is realigned and splinted, the splint should be removed │
│ and the extremity returned to the position in which neurovascular │
│ status was maximized, then resplinted in this position.[6] Joint │
│ fractures often involve associated dislocations. Attempts to │
│ straighten an angulated fracture involving a joint without the │
│ benefits of radiological evaluation and orthopedic consultation │
│ may worsen the injury beyond its original presentation. │
└───┘

treatment methods (see Tables 11-2 and 11-3). Splinting techniques for specific fractures can be found in Procedure 32.

Sprains (Ligament Injury)

A sprain is a complete or partial tear of a ligament caused by sudden stretching of the joint beyond the normal range of motion. Healing is usually slow because of the limited vascularization of ligaments.

Symptoms

There are three grades of sprains. The symptoms and treatments are described in Table 11-4, p. 413.

Diagnosis

- Diagnosis is determined by history and assessment.
- Radiographs can be used to rule out fractures; avulsion fractures may occur with sprains.

Strains (Injury to a Muscle or Tendon Attachment)

A strain is an overstretching of a muscle where it attaches to a tendon. A strain is also called a pulled muscle.

Symptoms

There are three grades of strains. Symptoms and treatment are described in Table 11-5, p. 414.

Diagnosis

- Diagnosis is determined by history and assessment.
- Perform a radiographic examination to rule out a fracture. Avulsion fractures may occur with second-degree and third-degree strains.

NURSING SURVEILLANCE

1. Monitor for airway and breathing problems with patients who have fractures of long bones or the pelvis or multiple fractures.

TABLE 11-2 Lower Extremity Fractures: Symptoms and Treatment

Area of Injury	Information	Symptoms: Area Specific (Not All Symptoms May Be Present)	Treatment
Pelvis	• May be stable or unstable. Unstable fractures are a result of a great deal of force. • Potential blood loss of 1500-3000 ml • Because of the rich blood supply to the skeleton and the inability to tamponade the bleeding, pelvic fractures can result in death by exsanguination[6]	• Pain when pressure applied to the anterosuperior iliac crests and the symphysis pubis. This maneuver should be performed only once, and if a fracture is suspected, should not be repeated, to avoid additional bleeding and clot dislodgement.[6] • Hemorrhagic shock (tachycardia, delayed capillary refill, restlessness, pale skin, diaphoresis, decreased urinary output, hypotension) • Blood at the urethral meatus, vaginally and on rectal examination (rectal, urethral, and bladder injuries are complications of pelvic fractures) • Perineal ecchymosis or a scrotal hematoma	• If the pelvic fracture is an open-book type fracture, internally rotate the lower legs to reduce pelvic volume; secure the legs together.[6] • Splint the pelvis using pillows, straps, a backboard, a vacuum splint, or a pelvic girdle splint. A bed sheet also may be used for stabilizing a fractured pelvis by tightly wrapping it around the pelvis and securing it with a knot or clamps (see Splinting, Procedure 32). • Avoid unnecessary movement of the patient. • Do not insert a urinary catheter if there is blood at the urethral meatus until urethral injury has been ruled out. • Bleeding from open fracture sites must be controlled by packing of the wound. • Be prepared for rapid transport to the operating room or interventional radiology for hemodynamic instability.

Continued

TABLE 11-2 Lower Extremity Fractures: Symptoms and Treatment—cont'd

Area of Injury	Information	Symptoms: Area Specific (Not All Symptoms May Be Present)	Treatment
Femur	• Blood loss in a femur fracture may be as much as 3-4 units of blood. [6] Bilateral femur fractures may represent a life-threatening injury secondary to hypovolemia. • Fracture location is categorized as the proximal, middle,	• Abnormal rotation of the hips or legs • External bleeding if the fracture is open • Impaired distal circulation • Little external deformity may be present as a result of extensive overlying soft tissue • Pain: The patient will experience severe pain with midshaft femur fractures. • Spasms of the quadriceps muscle may cause extensive soft-tissue injury. Deformity and tightening of the thigh may be noted with the spasm. • Shortening of the affected extremity in comparison with the unaffected extremity	• Immobilize with a traction splint (Thomas, Hare traction, and Sager traction, each having its own unique application; see Procedure 32). **NURSING ALERT** Avoid the use of traction splints if joint injuries are present on the same side as the femur fracture. Immobilize with a nontraction splinting method such as a wire ladder splint.

Continued

	or distal third of the bone.[15]	• Distal femur fractures may involve the femoral or popliteal vessels, causing diminished pulses. • Internal or external rotation if the fracture is proximal
Patellar	• Commonly occur with dislocations, femur fractures, acetabular fractures, and hip dislocations as a result of high energy transmission. • May be associated with popliteal vessel injury.	• Pain: may be severe. • Decreased mobility • Numbness, tingling, cool skin temperature if neurovascular damage is present • Swelling at the site
		• Do not attempt to straighten angulation of the knee. These fractures may coexist with dislocations. • Immobilize knee fractures as found, because of the proximity of joints both proximal and distal and the potential neurovascular compromise. • When a leg that is straight is being immobilized, the knee should be flexed 10 degrees to take pressure off neurovascular structures.[6]
Tibial/ fibular	• May occur together or independently • Generally the result of a direct blow (e.g., a pedestrian struck by an automobile). • The tibia often fracture during falls because of its weight-bearing property.	• Bearing weight on the injured extremity is not possible. • Associated with the development of compartment syndrome. (See Compartment Syndrome Condition.) • Patients with a fibular fracture and a stable tibia may be able to place weight on the extremity.	• Splinting goals: provide stability and maintain neurovascular function. Any splint that immobilizes the lower leg can be employed.

TABLE 11-2   Lower Extremity Fractures: Symptoms and Treatment—cont'd

Area of Injury	Information	Symptoms: Area Specific (Not All Symptoms May Be Present)	Treatment
		Posterior examination of the lower leg may reveal symptoms consistent with a fracture.	• Dislocations may accompany fractures of the ankle, and a specialist should undertake attempts at reduction. • Immobilization of the ankle must include the foot and the distal half of the lower leg. • Pad bony prominences.
Ankle	• Often occurs with connective tissue (e.g., ligament) injuries. The most common ankle fracture is a lateral malleolar fracture.[16]	• Swelling at the injury site • Pain: may be severe. • Decreased mobility • Numbness, tingling, cool skin temperature if neurovascular damage is present	
Foot	• Usually associated with dislocations and sprains • May be virtually impossible to differentiate the fractured foot from the sprained foot without the use of radiographs • Injuries secondary to axial loading may result in calcaneal (heel) fractures.	• Pain: may be severe. • Decreased mobility • Numbness, tingling, cool skin temperature if neurovascular damage is present • Pain: The patient may experience pain and swelling at the injury site.	• Use conforming splints (e.g., pillow splint or commercial splints designed specifically for application to the foot) should be employed. • Toes should be exposed to allow for continuous reassessment.

TABLE 11-3   Upper Extremity Fractures: Symptoms and Treatment

Area of Injury	Information	Symptoms: Area Specific (Not All Symptoms May Be Present)	Treatment
Scapula	• Suspect scapular fracture with significant soft-tissue injuries to the shoulder and when the mechanism of injury suggests a high level of kinetic energy transmission. • Carefully evaluate surrounding structures. Injuries often associated with scapula fractures include shoulder dislocations, clavicle and rib fractures (potential for underlying pneumothorax, hemothorax), and pulmonary contusions.[17]	Limited range of motion in the ipsilateral extremity. **NURSING ALERT** Life-threatening and limb-threatening injuries (pneumothorax, hemothorax, pulmonary contusion) or the absence of ipsilateral extremity pulse from vascular damage may occur with scapular fractures as a result of significant blunt forces usually associated with the injury.	• Rule out or treat potentially life-threatening injuries. • Apply a sling and swathe to immobilize the arm and shoulder, thereby reducing movement of scapula. The sling cradles the arm so the elbow is bent at just less than a 90-degree angle, thus preventing extension and, to a certain extent, flexion. The swathe prevents abduction and adduction. • Frequently assess neurovascular status.

Continued

TABLE 11-3 Upper Extremity Fractures: Symptoms and Treatment—cont'd

Area of Injury	Information	Symptoms: Area Specific (Not All Symptoms May Be Present)	Treatment
Clavicle	• Often causes damage to underlying structures (i.e., lung, subclavian vein, or the airway) • Most often appears as fractures in the middle third of the bone.	• Shoulder instability as a result of a loss of support to the shoulder girdle • Signs of neurovascular compromise resulting from close proximity of subclavian vessels and brachial plexus[17]	• Rule out damage to underlying structure. • May include a figure-eight splint that takes the pressure from the rest of the shoulder girdle off the clavicle and maintains proper clavicular alignment
Humerus	• May be associated with damage to the brachial artery and damage to the radial, ulnar, and median nerves. • Direct force to the olecranon process can result in indirect fractures to the distal humerus.	• Pain • Decreased mobility • Numbness, tingling, cool skin temperature if neurovascular damage is present	• Splint with a sling and swathe. • Splint proximal shaft fractures by applying the swathe.

Radius/ulna	• Concern for fractures near the elbow and wrist related to neurovascular compromise; therefore these require meticulous neurovascular evaluation and documentation.	• Colles' fracture is one of the more common fractures of the radius and ulna. It is commonly characterized as taking on a "silver fork" type of appearance, with the wrist turned up in relation to the radius and ulna.	• Apply a rigid splint. • When splinting for a Colles' or "silver fork" fracture, use a conforming splint such as a ladder splint and pad the spaces with rolled gauze (Kling or Kerlix) to provide more stability.
Hand	• Knowing the position of the hand during the injury is essential, because this information may yield valuable insight into potential fracture sites, damage to tendons, and damage to the neurovascular system of the hand.	• Hand fractures are often associated with soft-tissue injuries. Figure 11-3 shows anatomic landmarks useful in describing injury locations.	• Remove rings promptly. • Dress the soft-tissue injury appropriately. • Place the hand in a position of function (fingers slightly flexed with the thumb abducted away from the palm), and place rolled gauze (Kling or Kerlix) in the patient's palm. • Wrap the hand, ensuring the fingertips are exposed for reassessment. • Apply a rigid splint or conforming splint, taking care to place the splint distal to the wrist to provide complete immobilization of the hand and prevent further injury.

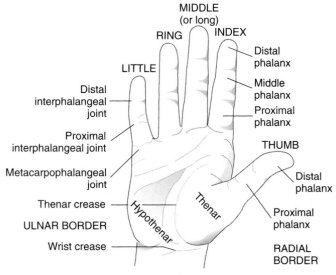

Figure 11-3 Volar view. Anatomic terminology useful in describing the hand.

2. Monitor for continued hemorrhage and hypovolemia.
3. Evaluate hematomas for expansion.
4. Evaluate pulses.
5. Monitor skin color and temperature, and capillary refill.
6. Monitor sensory function distal to the injury.
7. Evaluate the effectiveness of pain control.
8. Evaluate the effects of splint and traction splint application.
9. Monitor urine output.

EXPECTED PATIENT OUTCOMES

1. The patient's neurovascular status does not deteriorate.
2. The patient reports a decrease in pain.
3. Hemorrhage is controlled.
4. Open wounds are protected from further contamination.
5. No further tissue damage occurs.
6. The alert patient articulates an understanding of procedures to be performed in the ED.
7. Patients with open fractures that require operative intervention undergo surgery within 6 hours.

TABLE 11-4 Sprains

Grade	Cause	Symptoms	Treatment
Grade I	Mild sprains: stretching or a small tear of the ligament	• Minimal swelling and hemorrhage, local tenderness • No abnormal joint motion	• Apply ice, elevate for 12 hours, apply a compression dressing • Crutches • Analgesia
Grade II	Moderate sprains: stretching or a partial tear of the ligament	• Tenderness, edema, and moderate hemorrhage, pain associated with motion and weight bearing • Abnormal joint motion	• Apply ice for 24 hours, immobilize the joint if necessary for 48-72 hours, apply compression bandages, and direct the patient to maintain partial weight bearing with crutches. • Analgesia
Grade III	Severe sprains: complete disruption of a ligament	• Joint may be obviously deformed • Marked tenderness and swelling • Joint may be unable to bear weight • Grossly abnormal joint motion	• Apply ice for 48 hours. • Elevate the joint, and apply a compression dressing or cast for immobilization. • Surgical repair may be necessary; obtain orthopedic consultation. • Avoid weight bearing.

Data from Geiderman JM: General principles of orthopedic injuries. In Marx J, Hockberger RS, Walls RM, et al, eds: *Rosen's emergency medicine, concepts and clinical practice,* ed 5, St Louis, 2002, Mosby.

TABLE 11-5   Strains

Grade	Cause	Symptoms	Treatment
Grade I	• Mild strains: minor tearing of muscle/tendon	• Local pain, point tenderness, swelling, slight muscle spasm	• Apply an intermittent cold pack, elevate the extremity above the heart, and apply a compression bandage. • Direct the patient to maintain partial weight bearing on the extremity. • Administer analgesics.
Grade II	• Moderate strains: increased number of muscle fibers torn	• Local pain, point tenderness, swelling, discoloration, and inability to use limb for prolonged periods	• Apply cold packs for 24 hours, elevate the extremity above the heart, and apply a compression bandage. • Direct the patient to maintain only partial weight bearing on the extremity. • Administer analgesics.
Grade III	• Severe strains: complete separation of the muscle from muscle, muscle from tendon, or tendon from bone	• Localized pain, point tenderness, swelling, discoloration, and "heard a snapping noise." Sharp pain with passive stress or active contraction.	• Apply cold packs for 24 to 48 hours, elevate the extremity above the heart, and apply a compression bandage. • Direct the patient not to bear weight on the affected extremity for 48 hours. • Administer analgesics. • Obtain an orthopedic consultation.

From Geiderman JM: General principles of orthopedic injuries. In Marx J, Hockberger RS, Walls RM, et al, eds: *Rosen's emergency medicine: concepts and clinical practice*, ed 5, St Louis, 2002, Mosby.

8. Patients with fractures that benefit from operative intervention undergo surgery within 24 hours.
9. Patients discharged home must be able to:
   - Ambulate safely before discharge (Crutch Walking, Procedure 9)
   - Demonstrate an understanding of the signs and symptoms of neurovascular compromise

REFERENCES

1. American College of Surgeons: *Advanced trauma life support: student manual,* ed 6, Chicago, 1997, The College.
2. Blake R, Hoffman J: Emergency department evaluation and treatment of ankle and foot injuries, *Emerg Med Clin North Am Orthoped Emerg I* 17(4):859-876, 1999.
3. Bledsoe B, Porter RS, Cherry R: *Essentials of paramedic care,* Philadelphia, 2000, Saunders.
4. D'Heere MS, Houghton D, Ginzburg E: Fat embolism syndrome, *J Trauma Nurs* 6(3):73-76, 1999.
5. Della-Giustina K, Della-Giustina DA: Emergency department evaluation and treatment of pediatric injuries, *Emerg Med Clin North Am I* 17(4):895-922, 1999.
6. Emergency Nurses Association: *Emergency nursing core curriculum,* Philadelphia, 2000, Saunders.
7. Emergency Nurses Association: *Trauma nursing core curriculum,* ed 5, Chicago, 2000, The Association.
8. Geiderman JM: General principles of orthopedic injuries. In Marx J, Hockberger RS, Walls RM, et al. *Rosen's medicine: concepts and clinical practice,* ed 5, St. Louis, 2002, Mosby.
9. Georgopoulos G, Bouros D: Fat embolism syndrome: clinical examination is still the preferable diagnostic method, *Chest* 123(4):982-983, 2003.
10. Hoover TJ, Siefer JA: Soft tissue complications of orthopedic emergencies, *Emerg Med Clin North Am II* 18(1):115-139, 2000.
11. McQueen M, Court-Brown C: Compartment monitoring in tibial fractures: the pressure threshold for decompression, *J Bone Joint Surg* 78B(1):99-104, 1996.
12. Rudman N, McIlmail D: Emergency department evaluation and treatment of hip and thigh injuries, *Emerg Med Clin North Am Orthoped Emerg II* 18(1):29-66, 2000.
13. Schlenker JD, Koulis CP: Amputations and replantations, *Emerg Med Clin North Am* 11(3):739-753, 1993.
14. Tumbarello C: Acute extremity compartment syndrome, *J Trauma Nurs* 7(2):30-38, 2000.
15. Velmahos GC, Toutouzas KG: Vascular trauma and compartment syndrome, *Surg Clin North Am* 82(1):125-141, 2000.
16. Villarin LA, Belk KE, Fried R: Emergency department evaluation and treatment of elbow and forearm injuries, *Emerg Med Clin North Am Orthoped Emerg I* 17(4):843-858, 1999.
17. Wedmore IS, Charette D: Emergency department evaluation and treatment of ankle and foot injuries, *Emerg Med Clin North Am Orthoped Emerg II* 18(1):85-113, 2000.

12 chapter

Eye Conditions

Mark B. Parshall

INTRODUCTION

For both traumatic and nontraumatic eye conditions, a range of severity is found. True eye emergencies are those that pose an immediate threat of permanent loss of vision. In terms of triage priority, they are second only to immediate threats to life. True eye emergencies include acute angle-closure glaucoma, central retinal artery occlusion, corrosive chemical burns, and ruptured or penetrating ocular injuries. Triage categorization should be according to the degree of risk for permanent visual impairment.

Triage assessment should include the gross appearance of the eyes, particularly any obvious abnormalities of the globe, pupil, iris, lens, anterior chamber, lids, or periorbital tissues of either eye. Except in the case of a true eye emergency, visual acuity (VA), ocular motility, the severity and quality of pain, and any pattern of redness should be assessed and documented during triage. In patients with useful vision in only one eye, it is prudent to assign higher priority to any eye problem in the functional eye.

FOCUSED NURSING ASSESSMENT

A brief review of ocular anatomy and terminology is provided in Box 12-1. See Figure 12-1 for ocular anatomy.

Eye problems may present as an isolated chief complaint or may be identified in the primary or secondary survey.

Oxygenation and Ventilation

Throughout this chapter, it is assumed that airway, breathing (e.g., ventilation and systemic oxygenation), and systemic circulatory threats (e.g., major shock states) have been ruled out or stabilized, or that stabilization is under way.

Perfusion

True eye emergencies are attributable to either major trauma or ongoing or imminent threat to the circulatory supply.

Cognition

Because of the close proximity of the eyes to the brain, serious eye trauma may occur in conjunction with head injuries. Visual field defects may be among a constellation of signs and symptoms associated with stroke syndromes. Cavernous sinus thrombosis and the associated changes in cognitive or neurological function may be a sequela of orbital cellulitis.

Sensation and Mobility

Sensory deficits associated with various eye conditions may include blurred vision, diplopia, or focal neurologic deficits such as loss of light perception or visual fields (cranial nerve [CN] II). Motor deficits may include abnormal pupillary responses or loss of accommodation (CN III, parasympathetic), abnormal or absent extraocular movements (CNs III, IV, or VI), or inability to close one or both eyes (CN VII). A mixed focal neurologic defect is the loss of corneal (blink) reflex, which may involve impaired corneal sensation (CN V, ophthalmic branch) or impaired motor response of the eyelids (CN VII).

1. The patient with unequal pupil size or reactivity should be asked about any history of eye injury, surgery, or prosthesis as well as the use of any eye drops or motion-sickness patches. If there is no history that accounts for

the inequality, the patient should be assigned a higher triage priority.

2. Retinal detachment commonly is idiopathic but also may occur secondary to trauma. Patients commonly note an abnormal sensation of a curtain or veil obscuring vision in the affected eye.

BOX 12-1   OCULAR ANATOMY AND TERMINOLOGY

Globe: Three concentric roughly spherical layers make up the globe. The inner layer, the retina, is a continuation of the optic nerve. The outer fibrous shell is the sclera. It is continuous with the outer sheath of the optic nerve posteriorly and with the cornea anteriorly. Sandwiched between the retina and sclera is the uveal tract, which comprises the choroid, ciliary muscle and body, and iris.

Compartments: The interior of the globe is divided into aqueous and vitreous compartments (sometimes called, respectively, the anterior and posterior *segments*). The vitreous compartment is lined by the retina and bounded anteriorly by the back of the lens. This compartment contains a clear, colloidal gel called vitreous humor. The retina extends in all directions, lining the entire vitreous compartment, including the posterior aspects of the ciliary body and iris. The choroid is a thin, pigmented, vascular layer between the retina and sclera and is contiguous with them on each side.

Chambers: The aqueous compartment is divided into anterior and posterior *chambers*. The anterior chamber is bounded anteriorly by the posterior aspect of the cornea and posteriorly by the visible surface of the iris. The posterior chamber is bounded anteriorly by the back of the iris and ciliary body and posteriorly by the front of the lens and its suspensory ligaments. The aqueous compartment contains aqueous humor and is separated from the vitreous compartment by the lens and its suspensory ligaments.

Intraocular pressure: Aqueous humor is secreted by cells in the ciliary body in the posterior chamber. It flows through the pupil to the anterior chamber, from which it drains via the trabecular meshwork and the canals of Schlemm. These are located in the anterior chamber angle, near the corneoscleral junction (limbus). If either the anterior chamber angle or outflow from the posterior to anterior chamber is obstructed, intraocular pressure will increase.

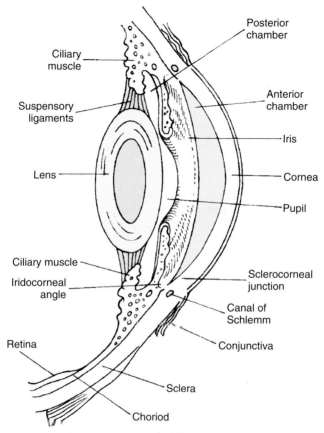

Figure 12-1 Ocular anatomy. (Modified from Thompson JM: *Mosby's clinical nursing,* ed 4, St. Louis, 1997, Mosby.

3. Pain from uveal structures (e.g., in iritis or acute glaucoma) generally is unilateral and deep and may be described as a boring or aching sensation or as a headache behind or in the affected eye.[1,2] Uveal pain often is associated with photophobia and is not relieved by topical anesthetics. In general, the patient with pain of this nature should be assigned a higher priority than the patient whose eye pain is readily relieved by a topical anesthetic.

4. Corneal pain is typically described as burning or searing.[1,3] Pain caused by a corneal abrasion is generally described as a scratching, foreign-body sensation. Pain resulting from a corneal injury is relieved promptly by topical anesthetics.

5. Pain from conjunctivitis may be described as burning or itching, or it may mimic corneal pain.

Sexuality

Some inflammatory or infectious eye conditions may result from various sexually transmitted diseases such as gonorrhea, Chlamydia, or herpes viruses.

Tissue Integrity

- Alterations of ocular or adnexal tissue integrity, such as in eyelids and tear ducts, range from major disruptions (e.g., ruptured or penetrated globe, corrosive chemical burns), to relatively minor (e.g., corneal abrasion). Between these extremes are many threats to tissue integrity that, while not true eye emergencies, nonetheless should receive prompt evaluation in the ED; some may require an ophthalmology consultation. Eye conditions commonly present with redness in addition to pain. Table 12-1 summarizes common presentations of the red eye.

- Redness associated with anterior uveitis—iritis or iridocyclitis—or acute glaucoma often is characterized by a "ciliary flush," a circular band of deeper redness at the corneoscleral limbus.[2-5] Ciliary flush generally suggests a more urgent condition than diffuse injection.

- Redness (injection) from corneal injury or conjunctival inflammation or infection is diffuse with no ciliary flush.

- Conjunctival edema (chemosis), as well as injection, may be present in conjunctivitis.

- Evidence from an increasing number of clinical trials suggests that patching the affected eye in patients with corneal abrasion or after foreign body removal is no more effective in corneal healing or pain control than not using a patch.[6-12]

- An infected eye definitely should not be patched because of the risk of a worsening infection or corneal ulceration. In addition, corneal abrasions from contact lenses should not be patched because of the increased risk of a *Pseudomonas* infection.[13-15]

- Eyelid lacerations involving the lid margin, tarsal plate, or internal canthus generally require specialty consultation for definitive repair.

TABLE 12-1 Presentation of the Painful, Red Eye

Problem	Pain Onset	Quality	Redness	Discharge	Other	Triage Category
Noncorrosive chemical	Immediate	Intense burning	Diffuse	Watery, unilateral or bilateral	• Unilateral or bilateral • Blepharospasm	Urgent
Corneal foreign body (FB)	Immediate, progressive, worsening	Scratching, FB sensation	Diffuse, but may have localized intensity	Tearing, watery, usually unilateral	• Usually unilateral • Blepharospasm	Urgent
Hyphema	Immediate, progressive, worsening	Dull pressure (boring)	Blood in anterior chamber, with or without ciliary flush	Tearing, watery may be present or absent.	• Unilateral • Often with periorbital hematoma • Lethargy	Urgent
Acute (angle-closure) glaucoma	Gradual, may progressively worsen	Dull, boring, moderate to severe; may be described as like headache around the eye	Diffuse, often with ciliary flush	Tearing, watery may be present or absent, usually unilateral	• Headache • Nausea/vomiting • Halos around lights • Pupil dilated, nonreactive to light, sluggish, may be	Emergent

Continued

TABLE 12-1 Presentation of the Painful, Red Eye—cont'd

Problem	Pain Onset	Quality	Redness	Discharge	Other	Triage Category
Anterior uveitis (iritis, iridocyclitis)	Gradual, may progressively worsen	Dull, intense, boring	Ciliary flush (limbal injection)	Minimal and watery	larger than in unaffected eye • Cornea may be hazy/steamy. • Pupil constricted, poorly reactive; smaller than in unaffected eye • Cornea may be hazy. • Photophobia	Urgent
Corneal abrasion	FB sensation that may have improved before worsening	Intense, burning	Diffuse, may have localized intensity	• Tearing, watery • Unilateral	• Unilateral • Blepharospasm • Eye rubbing	Nonurgent as long as FB no longer present
Actinic keratitis (UV exposure)	Gradual onset, 8-12 hr after	Searing, burning, very intense,	Diffuse, bilateral	• Tearing, watery • Usually bilateral	• Photophobia, eye rubbing	Nonurgent

	welding or sunlight exposure		bilateral			
Conjunctivitis	Gradual	• Burning • Itching (allergic)	Diffuse, unilateral or bilateral	• Allergic: mucoid • Viral: watery • Bacterial: purulent	• Chemosis • Blepharospasm • Possible fever • URI • Angioedema	Nonurgent
Subconjunctival hemorrhage	Usually painless	If pain present, consider other cause	Bloody: often localized	None	• Usually asymptomatic, unless associated with another problem	Nonurgent

Leibowitz HM: The red eye, *N Engl J Med* 343 (5):345-351, 2000.

Safety

Eye injuries resulting from intentional battery are among the most common seen in the ED. As with vehicular trauma, a high proportion of eye injuries associated with intentional injury are alcohol related. The risk of a serious eye injury is increased if an orbital or midfacial fracture is present.[16]

- A high proportion of serious eye injuries are related to occupational activities and could be prevented by the use of protective eyewear.[17-20] From 20% to 25% of penetrating eye injuries are work related.[21] The highest-risk occupations are construction, auto repair, and agriculture.[18-19,21] Approximately 15% of people with serious work-related eye injuries have a history of previous on-the-job eye injury.[19,21] Activities such as grinding or hammering may generate enough force to cause shrapnel to penetrate the globe.

- Sports and recreational activities are associated with hyphema, retinal detachment, and globe rupture.[18-20] The risk of injury is not reduced by the skill or experience of the individual but can be sharply reduced with proper protective eyewear and headgear.[19,22]

- Vehicular collisions are another common cause of eye injuries, both minor and serious. The use of restraint devices reduces the risk of eye injury.[18-19] A high proportion of serious eye injuries caused by vehicular collisions are alcohol related.[17,23]

- Blunt injuries to the orbital region may be associated with domestic abuse, particularly when the alleged mechanism of injury does not seem congruent with the pattern of injury.

- For any given energy level or mechanism of injury, patients with a history of eye surgery or a prior significant eye injury are at higher risk for serious ocular injury than patients without such history.[19,24,25]

LIFE SPAN ISSUES

Pediatric

1. Young children, especially toddlers, are relatively uncoordinated, lack judgment about hazards, and have a developmental need to explore their world. These factors contribute to an increased risk of eye injury.[18-19,22,26] Inadequate adult supervision is often related to pediatric eye injuries. BB gun and fireworks injuries often cause devastating eye damage in children.[1]

2. Eye injuries also are often seen in cases of child abuse and may be related to direct blows or shaking. Inconsistency of a stated mechanism of injury with a child's developmental stage and

capabilities may arouse suspicions of abuse. Intraocular or retinal hemorrhage from accidental head trauma in children is rare and should heighten the suspicion of child abuse.[4,26,27] There are some reports of retinal hemorrhage after prolonged cardiopulmonary resuscitation (CPR) in children, but there is little evidence that this is caused by CPR alone; usually there is a concomitant head injury that is most often intentional.[27]

3. On occasion, children with sickle cell disease, some leukemias, cytomegalovirus retinitis, rickettsial diseases (e.g., Rocky Mountain spotted fever), and malaria may have a retinal hemorrhage.[27] Iritis in children may be associated with juvenile arthritis, especially oligoarticular juvenile idiopathic arthritis.[28]

4. Conjunctivitis may occur in any age-group, but the viral and bacterial forms are far more prevalent in small children, probably related to droplet transmission and hand-to-face contact with inadequate hand washing.[29-31] Viral conjunctivitis generally is more contagious than bacterial conjunctivitis.[31] Nevertheless, for any infectious conjunctivitis, in addition to patient and family instructions about any medical treatment or follow-up, the importance of hand washing should be emphasized.

Geriatric

1. Adults over the age of 65 have an increased risk of eye injuries because of diminished visual and auditory acuity, changes in coordination and reflexes,[32] and greater likelihood of earlier eye surgery.[25] Falls are the most common cause of serious eye injuries for geriatric patients.

2. Especially in the elderly, for patients who wear corrective lenses, visual acuity testing should be performed with glasses on, if at all possible.

3. Central retinal artery or vein occlusion is more common in the geriatric population, especially in hypertensive patients, but occasionally may occur as a complication of certain types of eye surgery. Giant cell arteritis (which can cause blindness) is a disease affecting primarily persons who are more than 60 years of age.[33]

4. The incidence of primary acute angle-closure glaucoma and chronic open-angle glaucoma increases with age. However, it is important to distinguish between the two. Chronic open-angle glaucoma is more common in the general population but is not a true eye emergency. Chronic open-angle glaucoma usually is painless and characterized

by gradual diminution of visual acuity; therefore it rarely prompts patients to seek emergency evaluation and treatment in and of itself.

Pregnancy

- Many eye medications are of pregnancy category C, so female patients of childbearing age should be asked whether they are or might be pregnant and assessed for last menstrual period (LMP). It may be necessary to await results of pregnancy testing before administering some eye medications.

Gender

- Males have a risk for eye injury two to six times greater across all ages.[18,20] The highest incidence of eye injuries is among young adult males, which reflects an aggregated risk from occupational and recreational causes, vehicular crashes, and battery.[21]

INITIAL INTERVENTIONS

The priorities for nursing care in emergency settings are preservation of useful vision, preservation of structural integrity of the eye and its adnexa (e.g., eyelids, lacrimal system), and relief of pain. True eye emergencies are those that pose immediate threat of permanent loss of vision. They require emergent evaluation by an ophthalmologist. Most common eye problems are not true eye emergencies. Patients' eye problems that are not true emergencies often can be treated in the ED, and the patients can be discharged with follow-up by an ophthalmologist, or, in less serious problems, by a primary care provider or a planned return to the ED. The following is a summary of immediate actions that should be taken for true eye emergencies.

Chemical burns

For corrosive acid or alkaline chemical burns, high-volume irrigation, preferably with an eye fountain or eye shower, should begin immediately. It is acceptable at this stage to assess gross visual acuity (e.g., finger-counting, hand motion perception, or light perception), but no time should be lost before commencing irrigation. If there is any doubt as to the corrosiveness or pH of the chemical agent, it is safest to initiate immediate high-volume irrigation, during which time consultation with a poison center may take place. After adequate irrigation, a more detailed assessment of visual acuity may be undertaken if the patient is otherwise stable.

Open-Globe Injuries and Ocular Impalement

Treatment for an open globe should not be delayed for formal visual acuity (VA) testing (e.g., Snellen chart or near card). However, it is important initially to determine and document whether the patient can count fingers, perceive hand motion, or perceive light with each eye[7] because initial gross acuity has prognostic value (in a majority of penetrating ocular injuries, initial VA is hand motion perception or worse).[23,34] One also should document the nature of the penetrating object (e.g., organic, metal, or glass) because this information may influence diagnostic and treatment decisions.[34] The patient should be brought to an acute treatment area immediately. If possible, the head should be elevated. No attempt should be made to assess ocular motility. Topical anesthetics should not be administered if an open globe is suspected. The injured eye should be shielded at the earliest opportunity.

Sudden, Atraumatic Visual Loss

A patient with sudden, atraumatic loss of vision in one eye should be brought to an examination area for immediate examination and treatment. The patient can be screened in the treatment area for light perception and consensual pupillary response. If the visual loss is painless, it may be due to retinal artery obstruction (RAO) of either the central retinal artery (CRAO) or a branch of the retinal artery (BRAO). It may not be possible to distinguish between the two types of RAO in triage, and no time should be lost attempting to do so.

Acute Angle-Closure Glaucoma

Patients suspected of having acute angle-closure glaucoma should be triaged emergently to a treatment area in which a slit-lamp (biomicroscope) and equipment for measuring intraocular pressure are available; VA testing should be performed in triage or as soon as the patient is in the treatment area. At presentation, acute angle-closure glaucoma is less likely than CRAO to be associated with sudden loss of vision. Commonly it is associated with acute visual disturbance (notably halos around lights), acutely diminished VA in the affected eye, and pain in or around the eye that may be severe enough to provoke nausea and vomiting. Accordingly, signs and symptoms of acute angle-closure glaucoma can be mistaken for migraine in triage. The following may be helpful in differentiating these conditions in triage.

1. New-onset migraine is rare in patients over 50 years of age.[35]
2. The pain of migraine is typically pulsatile, while pain from acute angle-closure glaucoma often is characterized as fairly

continuous, boring pain. Although both conditions may be associated with photophobia, the characteristic visual disturbances of migraine (e.g., scotoma, fortification spectra)[35] and angle-closure glaucoma (halos around lights and deteriorating VA) differ.

3. The affected eye in acute angle-closure glaucoma often is injected around the limbus. Relative to the unaffected eye, the pupil of the affected eye is usually dilated to a moderate degree and is less reactive to light.[31,36-37]

Removal of Contact Lenses

Patients who are alert and oriented generally prefer to remove their own lenses. If the patient does not have a lens holder, the lenses should be covered in plain sterile saline in separate, labeled (*left* and *right*) sterile containers. If the patient is unable, or too distressed, to remove the lenses, the lenses can be removed manually or by means of a small suction cup. To remove hard lenses manually, open the lids beyond the margins of the contact lens and then close the lids with gentle, digital pressure that should pop the lens off the ocular surface. Soft lenses can be removed by gently pinching up the soft lens itself; the eye should be moist before removal. Topical anesthetics and fluorescein should not be administered until contact lenses have been removed.

Eye Irrigation

Irrigation of one or both eyes is often performed . Except in corrosive chemical injuries, the eyes should be anesthetized topically before irrigation commences and at intervals as needed (see the nursing care priorities table on p. 429). An eye fountain (eye shower) is preferred for rapid decontamination of chemical injuries. If an eye fountain or shower is not available, irrigation (a minimum of 1 to 2 L) also may be performed with IV normal saline or Ringer's lactate via irrigating lenses (Morgan lens) or manually via standard drip IV tubing (see Procedure 16). Small foreign bodies may be irrigated out with a small volume of ophthalmic irrigant.

Eye Shielding

An open-globe injury or hyphema should be protected by the securing of a metal or plastic eye shield or a disposable cup over the injured eye as soon as possible. The purpose of the shield is to prevent further injury as a result of rubbing or inadvertent contact and the reduction of stimulation from light or movement. The shield should be taped lightly to the adjacent skin in a

NURSING CARE PRIORITIES

Potential/Actual Problems	Causes	Signs and Symptoms	Interventions
Altered vision	• Eye trauma • Altered CNS function	• Decreased visual acuity	• Assess visual acuity (See Procedure 36)
Pain	• Eye trauma • Presence of foreign body • Chemical irritation	• Irritation/inflammation • Pain with eye movement	• Assess pain by using an appropriate pain scale. • Administer analgesics as ordered. • Patch as directed.
Infection	• Loss of structural integrity • Foreign bodies	• Discharge • Fever • Visual changes	• Administer antibiotics as ordered. • Administer antipyretics as ordered. • Administer tetanus prophylaxis as ordered.
Injury	• Visual impairment • Impaired depth perception • Disruption of the eye structures • Associated neurologic injury	• Visual changes	• Patch eye as directed. • Instruct patient about safety measures while eye is patched.

manner that does not exert pressure on the injured eye. The unaffected eye should be patched lightly to reduce consensual movement in the injured eye.

Comfort Measures

Patients with suspected iritis, glaucoma, hyphema, or retinal detachment or whose complaints involve photophobia should be placed, if possible, in an examination room that is quiet and can be darkened.

Patients with corneal injuries or conjunctival inflammation may have anesthetic drops administered while awaiting examination if standing protocols so direct or if the nurse obtains an order. Excessive use of topical anesthetics can aggravate corneal injuries and delay recognition of a worsening condition. Therefore patients are never discharged with topical anesthetics for self-administration; however, serial doses at appropriate intervals may be administered safely while the patient is in the ED.

Eye Patching

Patching traditionally has been a common method of treatment of corneal epithelial defects (e.g., for corneal abrasion or after corneal foreign-body removal). However, there is virtually no evidence that patching improves outcomes compared with equivalent treatment without patching in terms of pain relief or the rate of corneal healing.[6-12]

If a patch is nonetheless ordered, typically it is used in conjunction with antibiotic ointment for prophylaxis against infection. Mydriatic or cycloplegic drops may be ordered to prevent ciliary spasm and iritis.[6,13] A double-patch technique is used. The first patch should be folded in half and placed on the closed eyelid. A second patch (or more if the eye is deep-set) is placed flat on top of the folded patch. The patch is taped obliquely from the forehead to the cheek or angle of the jaw with sufficient tension that the patient cannot open the eyelid beneath the patch. A prefabricated plastic and foam patch that is secured by elastic straps (Press-Patch) is an acceptable alternative. When a patch is ordered, a follow-up examination the following day (in the ED or with an ophthalmologist) should be arranged to document evidence of healing and to determine the need for further consultation.

Reading and watching television should be discouraged while the eye is patched because scanning movements of the unaffected eye elicit consensual movements of the affected eye. Patients with corneal injuries also may need topical ophthalmic or oral antiinflammatory medication or even oral narcotic pain medication with appropriate precautions, regardless of whether the eye is patched. For medicolegal and safety reasons, the patient with an eye patch should be instructed not to drive until patching is discontinued because of the possibility of altered depth perception or peripheral vision.

Expediting Treatment, Consultation, and Transfer

Early nursing recognition (i.e., during triage or initial assessment) of presentations likely to require ophthalmologic or other specialty consultation expedites consultation and, when indicated, transfer. Any of the true eye emergencies will require immediate ophthalmologic consultation (or emergent transfer if no such capability is available locally). Presentations that generally require urgent specialty consultation or transfer include hyphema, retinal detachment, corneal or scleral lacerations, complex lid lacerations (e.g., disrupting a lid margin, tarsal plate, or canthal region), orbital cellulitis, ophthalmic shingles, and blowout fractures. Adherence to legal and institutional requirements for interfacility transfers is both an ethical and a medicolegal duty.

PRIORITY DIAGNOSTIC TESTS

Cultures: Conjunctival cultures are helpful in cases of rapidly progressing conjunctivitis or chronic conjunctivitis that has been refractory to treatment.[30]

Direct ophthalmoscopy: A direct ophthalmoscopic examination is used to diagnose conditions of the vitreous compartment and retina, as well as intraocular manifestations of other conditions (e.g., papilledema).

Fluorescein staining for cobalt blue, Wood's lamp, or slit lamp examination: Fluorescein dye has increased uptake in an area of corneal epithelial defect (e.g., abrasion and keratitis). Fluorescein strips are preferred to drops for infection-control reasons. A drop of topical anesthetic is placed on the end of the strip, the lower lid is retracted, and the strip is touched to the palpebral conjunctiva.

Slit-lamp examination: A slit lamp (biomicroscope) is a binocular microscope that is used to diagnose an anterior chamber inflammation and injury or the depth of a corneal injury. The patient must be cooperative and able to sit up for a slit-lamp examination. Children and toddlers usually must be held in a parent's lap for this examination to be performed. For bedside examination, a Wood's lamp and magnifying loupe may be used.

Tonometry (Schiötz or applanation): Normal intraocular pressure (IOP) is 12 to 21 mm Hg. IOP can be measured by any of several applanation tonometry devices or by a Schiötz tonometer. Before tonometry is performed, a topical anesthetic should be administered and the patient should be instructed not to rub the eye.

Applanation tonometers measure pressure either by transduction of a pressure signal sufficient to flatten a known area of direct contact with the cornea (e.g., slit lamp cone or Tono-Pen), or by delivering calibrated puffs of air and measuring corneal reflectance, which is maximal at an air pressure sufficient to flatten a small area of the cornea (e.g., Perkins-type). Applanation tonometers are more accurate, albeit more expensive, than Schiötz tonometers. An Internet search using "applanation tonometer" is useful in locating various types and brands of applanation tonometers.

A Schiötz tonometer measures pressure indirectly by the displacement of a weighted plunger that moves an indicator needle along a calibrated scale. A conversion table, based on the plunger weight and scale reading, is necessary to determine the IOP in mm Hg.

One can decontaminate an applanation tonometer cone by soaking for 10 minutes in a 1:10 bleach solution, after which it should be rinsed, blotted dry, and replaced. A Tono-Pen uses sterile, disposable, single-use covers. A Schiötz tonometer can be swabbed off and decontaminated in its own sterilization unit. Department policies should specify whether tonometer decontamination is a physician or a nursing responsibility.

Diagnostic Imaging

Plain radiographs are helpful in the diagnosis of some orbital and midfacial injuries, but a computed tomography (CT) scan is more definitive. A CT scan is preferred for complex facial injuries, orbital cellulitis, and suspected optic nerve trauma.

CLINICAL CONDITIONS

True Eye Emergencies
Acute Angle-Closure Glaucoma

The incidence of primary acute angle-closure glaucoma is higher in patients of African or Asian ancestry and in Alaska natives than in white or Native American patients. In white patients, the incidence is substantially higher in women than men (approximately 3:1), a gender difference that is not seen in other racial groups.[36] An acute episode may be precipitated by anticholinergic or sympathomimetic (beta-agonist) medications (e.g., in patients with asthma or chronic obstructive pulmonary disease) or by the administration of topical mydriatic agents.[38]

Signs and symptoms

- Acute glaucoma often is accompanied by conjunctival injection and a ciliary flush. In contrast to iritis, however, the pupil of the affected eye tends to be moderately dilated, or midposition, and poorly reactive.
- The cornea may be edematous, giving rise to a clouded, hazy, or "steamy" appearance.[38]
- The patient may report visual alterations such as diminished acuity, blurred vision, or halos around light sources.
- Often the pain is described as an intense, periorbital headache and may be associated with nausea and vomiting. As such, the pain must be discriminated from migraine headache, which also may have symptoms of nausea, vomiting, and visual disturbance, but is not associated with altered appearance of the eye or increased IOP.[29,36,38]

Diagnosis

- An acute elevation of IOP above 20 mm Hg is diagnostic for acute glaucoma.
- Determination of the acuity of the elevation is based on the history and progression of symptoms. The outcome of an episode is less dependent on the degree of pressure elevation than on its duration.[38]
- Several different underlying mechanisms have been described for primary acute angle closure glaucoma. The most common is pupillary block, which can be caused by the lens coming in contact with the iris or by formation of synechiae between the iris and posterior aspect of the cornea. Other patients may be predisposed by a narrow anterior chamber angle in which there is a more anterior insertion of the iris to the ciliary body (plateau iris), or as a consequence of hyperopia, which tends to be associated with a shallow anterior chamber. Secondary causes of acute angle-closure glaucoma include ocular trauma (or past history thereof), tumors, iritis, and other inflammatory diseases affecting the eye.[36]

Treatment

- ED therapy is directed toward reducing IOP by decreasing the production and improving the outflow of aqueous humor, as well as by osmotically reducing the volume of vitreous humor.[38] Definitive treatment is surgical (laser iridotomy or gonioplasty or peripheral iridectomy).[36]

- Ophthalmologic consultation is necessary and may require the transfer of the patient, but ultimately the patient may be discharged.
- A topical beta-blocker, such as timolol or betaxolol, or beta 2-agonist (brimonidine or apraclonidine) may be ordered to reduce the production of aqueous humor, thus reducing IOP.[36-38] The onset of the pressure decrease takes approximately 30 minutes, with maximal decrease in 1 to 2 hours. Caution is advised for patients with chronic obstructive pulmonary disease or reactive airway disease and for patients with a heart block.[37,38]
- Pilocarpine ophthalmic solution (1% to 4%) is a topical miotic (muscarinic parasympathomimetic) that also may be ordered acutely (1 drop every 15 minutes for 1 to 2 hours[37,39]) to constrict the pupil, thus improving the outflow of aqueous humor.[3,40] Higher concentrations may be advantageous in patients with darkly pigmented irises.[36,37] IOP may begin to decrease before miosis is evident.[38] Maintenance dosage is 1 to 2 drops, three to four times each day.[36,37]
- Several topical prostaglandin analogs are available (latanoprost, travoprost, unoprostone) that enhance outflow of aqueous humor via the trabecular meshwork and uveoscleral drainage.[36]
- A combination of topical agents may be used. If so, it is recommended that instillations be staggered approximately 10 minutes apart.[36,37]
- Cycloplegic or mydriatic medications are contraindicated.
- The carbonic anhydrase inhibitor acetazolamide (Diamox), up to 500 mg PO, IM, or IV, also may be ordered to reduce the rate of production of aqueous humor, often in conjunction with a topical beta-blocker.[36-38,40] Several topical carbonic anhydrase inhibitors also are available (brinzolamide, dorzolamide).
- If IOP has been found to be elevated and the patient is not vomiting, oral glycerol (1 to 1.5 g/kg) may be ordered for its osmotic effect.[36-38] Because glycerol is metabolized to glucose, it should be used cautiously in diabetics.[38]
- If the patient is vomiting, IV mannitol (20%; 1.5 to 2 g/kg) may be administered.[36-38,40] Both glycerol and mannitol draw water from vitreous humor, thus reducing its volume. Because both are nonspecific in their osmotic effects, they increase the circulating blood volume. Therefore they should be used

cautiously in patients with congestive heart failure (CHF) or chronic renal failure.[37]

- Specific guidelines regarding medications, activity restrictions, and follow-up should be clarified with the consultant before discharge.

Corrosive Chemical Burns

Chemical burns can be caused by a variety of chemicals. Common acids include sulfuric acid (car batteries), hydrochloric acid (drain openers), and muriatic acid (swimming pool chemicals). Common alkalis include lye (drain openers and oven cleaners), lime (plaster and concrete), and ammonia.[41] Some detergents used for restaurant or institutional dishwashing contain bleach or alkaline corrosives; if constituents are not immediately known, they should be presumed corrosive.

Signs and symptoms
- Severe, burning pain, rapid onset of visual impairment, inflammation and swelling of the lids, and severe chemosis of the eye(s).
- Corneal haziness or opacification may be evident.[41]

Diagnosis
- Initial diagnosis of a chemical burn is presumptive, based on symptoms and known or suspected exposure.

Treatment
- If the chemical is in powder or crystalline form, it should be rapidly, but gently, brushed from the ocular region and face before irrigating.
- Initial decontamination should employ whatever method of irrigation achieves the highest delivered volume in light of concomitant injuries (e.g., an eye shower would not be feasible if the patient is unconscious or if a cervical spine fracture has not been ruled out).
- Strong acids cause the coagulation of proteins with which they come into contact, which limits the depth of injury.[41] An exception is hydrofluoric acid, which burns more deeply than other acids.[3,4,41]
- Strong alkaline chemicals cause liquefaction of proteins with which they come into contact and so have a tendency to penetrate through to the anterior chamber, where they can damage the iris, ciliary body, and lens.[41] Therefore alkaline ocular exposures often need a longer period of irrigation than acids.
- One should continuously attend to the patient with a chemical burn during irrigation to provide emotional support and ensure the adequacy of irrigation.

- Irrigation should be continued for as long as required to get the conjunctival pH to normal range (7.4 to 7.6).[4]
- To test the pH, retract the lower lid gently and touch a test strip to the conjunctiva (much in the manner of a fluorescein strip). The pH should be retested several times after irrigation to make sure the pH is not changing.
- After initial decontamination, anesthetic drops may be instilled as needed until the irrigation and initial examination are complete.
- Some particulates (e.g., plaster and concrete powders) may embed in the lids or conjunctival fornices and cause ongoing release. Fine-forceps debridement of such particles by the physician may be necessary.[41]
- Cycloplegic agents generally are ordered to reduce pain from a ciliary spasm. Topical steroids are helpful in this setting but should be administered only on the recommendation of the ophthalmologist.[3,41]
- Acetazolamide (PO or IV) or topical beta-blockers may be ordered after irrigation to decrease IOP.[41]
- Topical antibiotics and patching are commonly ordered.
- Systemic narcotic analgesics often are necessary.[4]
- Tetanus prophylaxis should be administered if indicated.

Globe Injuries (Open: Rupture and Penetration)

Globe injuries may result from blunt or penetrating injuries, or through acceleration or deceleration forces.

Signs and symptoms

- Symptoms include severe pain and sudden, severe visual impairment or loss in the affected eye.[20,23] Small, intraocular foreign bodies may be attended by a more subtle visual impairment.
- Signs of an open globe may include:
  - Enophthalmos
  - Proptosis (a globe protrusion caused by retrobulbar hemorrhage)
  - Obvious asymmetry of the globe
  - Iridodialysis or pupil herniation (disruption of the iris at, respectively, the ciliary or pupillary margin)
  - Complete ("eight ball") hyphema
  - Severe chemosis
  - Extrusion of aqueous or vitreous humor

Diagnosis

- The diagnosis of an open globe is based primarily on gross appearance, history, and the mechanism of injury.

- The IOP may be decreased below 10 mm Hg.
- Intraocular metal or glass foreign bodies can be diagnosed radiographically.
- CT scanning is helpful in determining whether the optic nerve has been severed or avulsed.

Treatment

- Open-globe injuries should be covered with a metal or plastic eye shield or a paper cup.[4]
- The unaffected eye should be patched or shielded to reduce consensual movement.[4]
- Tetanus and preoperative antibiotic prophylaxis are indicated.
- If the patient has an impalement of the globe or orbit, manual stabilization of the impaling object should be immediate.
- As soon as concomitant threats to ABCs have been ruled out, or as they are being treated, dressings may be applied to stabilize the object in a manner that does not put pressure on the object or the globe.
- Removal should be undertaken only by the appropriate surgical specialist in the operating room.

Retinal Artery Occlusion, Central and Branch

Central retinal artery occlusion (CRAO) is a sudden, painless, unilateral visual loss caused by an embolus lodging in the central retinal artery. Patients are most often elderly, and the prevalence is slightly higher among men.[39] Episodes are more common at night and in the early morning.[39,42] Smaller emboli may lodge in a branch of the retinal artery rather than centrally. CRAO accounts for a majority of RAO events; branch retinal artery occlusion BRAO accounts for less than 40%.[39]

In BRAO, loss of vision in the affected eye may occur only in a visual field corresponding to the retinal region supplied by the arterial branch.[39] Approximately one quarter to one third of patients with CRAO can have some degree of useful vision restored with prompt recognition and treatment, but salvage is rare after 2 hours from onset. Therefore CRAO is a true ophthalmic emergency that requires immediate triage and ophthalmological examination.[39] Although BRAO is less devastating to subsequent useful vision, differentiation from CRAO depends on complete ophthalmological examination; therefore it is reasonable and prudent to triage suspected BRAO as though it were CRAO. Approximately two thirds of patients with RAO have a history of hypertension, and approximately one quarter have diabetes mellitus. Other conditions that may predispose include arteriosclerosis or conditions associated with embolization from the left side of the heart (e.g., atrial tachyarrhythmias, mitral or aortic valve disease), coagulopathy, endocarditis, carotid insufficiency, or glaucoma.[39]

Signs and symptoms

- Sudden onset of painless complete or partial unilateral visual loss that does not resolve within a few minutes of onset. Absence of direct, but normal, consensual light reflex in the affected eye[11] or paradoxical pupil dilation of the affected eye when an examination light is swung from the unaffected to the affected eye (afferent pupillary defect).[39]

Diagnosis

- Diagnosis is based on the patient's description of the vision loss. In addition to lack of spontaneous resolution, signs and symptoms are confined to the affected eye (e.g., in distinction to a transient ischemic attack).
- Afferent pupillary defect is an early sign that may occur almost immediately after the occlusion.[39] The characteristic funduscopic findings (e.g., an edematous, pale-milky, or ground-glass retina with a "cherry red" fovea) take longer to become evident.[39,42]
- RAO is painless. If the visual loss is associated with head pain, then migraine or temporal (giant cell) arteritis should be considered; an elevated erythrocyte sedimentation rate (ESR) may suggest the latter, a history of migraine in younger patients suggests the former.[39,42]
- Cerebrovascular disease, methanol ingestion, or hysterical blindness should be considered if the visual loss is bilateral.[29]
- Diagnosis of RAO per se is based primarily on the history and nature of visual loss and associated physical findings. However, because of the variety of predisposing risk factors and because patients with RAO have substantially diminished life expectancy compared with age-matched controls, ancillary studies that may be ordered in the ED include an electrocardiogram, complete blood count with differential, ESR, coagulation studies, and blood cultures.[39]

Treatment

- Ophthalmological specialty consultation should be initiated as soon as RAO is suspected.
- Intraocular pressure (IOP) should be measured early and treated rapidly with some combination of medication, ocular massage, and anterior chamber paracentesis.
- Firm ocular massage through closed lids may be performed by the physician for 3 to 4 seconds with abrupt release of pressure in an attempt to dislodge a thrombus.[3,39,42]

- Anterior chamber paracentesis is performed under slit-lamp visualization. A pinhole puncture of the cornea at the limbal margin with a 27-gauge needle and tuberculin syringe is made.[3,39,42] The purpose is to extrude a small amount of aqueous humor, thereby suddenly lowering IOP. This should be performed only by a specialist or emergency physician experienced in the procedure.[42]

- If carbogen gas (95% O_2 + 5% CO_2) is available, it can be administered as a vasodilator for three 10-minute intervals with 5 minutes off between administrations. Otherwise, rebreathing into a paper bag for 10 to 15 minutes each hour may raise the patient's $Paco_2$.[39,42]

- There is no evidence from randomized clinical trials that any of the above approaches is any more or less effective than the others.[43] As noted above, salvage of useful vision in CRAO occurs in only about one quarter to one third of cases, even when recognition, diagnosis, and emergent and definitive specialist care are immediate.

- In tertiary centers other possible treatments include hyperbaric oxygen and angiographic injection of a thrombolytic agent into the proximal ophthalmic artery. However, time to treatment is critical, so the utility of these approaches and decisions about transfer are best made by the consulting ophthalmologist.[39]

Other Eye Conditions
Amaurosis Fugax (Fleeting Blindness)
Amaurosis fugax is a symptom, not a disease, that presents as a transient, painless, unilateral loss of vision. In essence, it is a visual transient ischemic attack (TIA) that indicates a need for evaluation of the underlying cause, most often ipsilateral carotid disease (e.g., an ulcerated plaque). For patients with carotid stenosis, there is an increased risk of stroke, although this risk is not as great as with hemispheric TIA. Amaurosis fugax also may be a prodromal symptom of BRAO.[39]

Signs and symptoms
- Transient, painless, unilateral loss of vision often described as the sensation of a curtain descending and then being raised[33] or constriction and expansion of the visual field
- Unlike CRAO, there is spontaneous improvement, generally within minutes of onset.
- Unlike migraine, amaurosis fugax generally is painless and not associated with fortification spectra (the scintillating, zigzag

scotoma of classic migraine).[33] Episodes of amaurosis fugax generally are briefer than migraine episodes.

Diagnosis
- The diagnosis is based on the rapid onset and resolution of the episode and on funduscopic examination.

Treatment
- Noninvasive carotid flow studies may be ordered or scheduled, and the patient may be started on one 325-mg ASA per day.[33]
- Vascular and ophthalmologic consultations or referral is indicated.
- Other less common causes of transient, monocular blindness (e.g., giant cell arteritis) may call for different work-ups (e.g., an erythrocyte sedimentation rate for screening purposes) and referral.[29,33]

Anterior Uveitis (Iritis and Iridocyclitis)

Iritis suggests that inflammation largely is confined to the anterior chamber. Iridocyclitis implies that the ciliary body and iris both are involved (i.e., both anterior and posterior chambers of the aqueous compartment). Anterior uveitis may be idiopathic (approximately 40% of cases)[44] or secondary to recent or old eye trauma; autoimmune, inflammatory, or granulomatous conditions; infection; or malignancies. It is a common feature of autoimmune processes associated with human leukocyte antigen B27 (HLA-B27) seropositivity, especially ankylosing spondylitis and reactive arthritis, but also including psoriatic arthritis, inflammatory bowel and Crohn's diseases, and Reiter's syndrome.[28,50-52]

Other inflammatory or granulomatous conditions of which anterior uveitis may be a feature include juvenile idiopathic arthritis[28] Rosenberg, 2002 or juvenile rheumatoid arthritis,[44] sarcoidosis,[28] and Sjögren's syndrome. Infectious causes account for only approximately 10% of anterior uveitis.[44] A wide variety of organisms have been implicated, including herpes simplex or zoster, chlamydia, cytomegalovirus, syphilis, and tuberculosis.[44] Anterior uveitis also may be a feature of some leukemias, lymphomas, or malignant melanomas.[2] Recreational nasal cocaine use also has been reported as a cause.[48] Patients with Behçet's syndrome are predisposed to developing panuveitis (i.e., iridocyclitis plus involvement of the choroid).[28]

Signs and symptoms
- Anterior uveitis (iritis and iridocyclitis) is generally unilateral and associated with an acute decrease in pupillary responsiveness.
- The pupil of the affected eye is constricted and may be irregular.

- The affected iris may have a muddy, grayish cast relative to the unaffected eye.[5]
- The pain is of gradual onset, aching in nature, and associated with intense photophobia and watery discharge. The pain also may be increased in the affected eye when it responds consensually to elicitation of the light reflex in the unaffected eye.[2,5,38]
- In severe cases, aqueous humor may be cloudy and associated with a complaint of blurred vision.[37]

Diagnosis

- Although iridocyclitis is more serious, there is little difference in terms of initial evaluation and treatment in the ED.[2,5]
- Patients with anterior uveitis will have inflammatory vasodilation and increased vascular permeability of the iris (or iris and ciliary body), causing protein and fibrin exudation into the anterior chamber. This causes a characteristic flare on slit lamp examination that is diagnostic for the condition.[2,3,5,38] In severe cases, a hypopyon may be evident even without a slit lamp; this a collection of leukocytic/inflammatory debris that settles inferiorly in the anterior chamber (as opposed to a hyphema, a hypopyon is atraumatic and light in color).[31]
- In contrast to angle-closure glaucoma, in which the pupil is moderately dilated, the pupil of the affected eye with anterior uveitis typically is constricted and smaller than the pupil of the unaffected eye.[31]
- Fibrin deposits may cause the formation of synechiae (adhesions) of the iris and ciliary body that can interfere with the flow or drainage of aqueous humor and may lead to pupillary block and acute angle-closure glaucoma[2,3,5,38] or chronic glaucoma.[38]

Treatment

- ED treatment involves the administration of topical corticosteroids (e.g., prednisolone acetate or phosphate 1%) to reduce inflammation.[39,44] Initial dosage may be as frequent as 1 to 2 drops every 30 to 60 min or 5 drops every hour administered 1 minute apart.[44,45] If prednisolone acetate (a suspension) is used, it is essential to shake the container vigorously for about half a minute immediately before administration.[44]
- Fluorometholone ointment may be ordered for use at bedtime for a longer duration of action.[45] Although corticosteroid dosage will be tapered eventually, that decision is best left to the ophthalmologist to whom the patient is referred for follow-up.

- Dexamethasone ophthalmic preparations can increase anterior chamber pressure to a greater extent than prednisolone; therefore dexamethasone is less desirable as a first-line agent.[44]
- A topical cycloplegic/mydriatic agent (e.g., homatropine 2% to 5% or scopolamine 0.25% drops for more severe inflammation, or cyclopentolate HCl 1% or tropicamide 1% for less severe cases) often is ordered in conjunction with topical corticosteroids. As referral to an ophthalmologist for follow-up care is important, the choice of agent potentially can be discussed with the consultant. The purposes of these agents in the setting of anterior uveitis include relief of pain and photophobia (cycloplegia) and prevention of posterior synechiae (mydriasis).[44,45]
- Pilocarpine and latanoprost exacerbate anterior chamber inflammation and, for that reason, should not be used.[44] Ophthalmic nonsteroidal antiinflammatory drugs (NSAIDS) theoretically reduce pain and inflammation, but efficacy in anterior uveitis has not been demonstrated.[44]
- The eye should not be patched but may be shielded; the patient may instead use dark glasses to reduce discomfort from light.[3]
- Warm compresses may afford some symptomatic relief.[3]
- The patient may need oral narcotics and should be counseled not to drive while the eye is shielded or while the pupil is dilated by cycloplegic/mydriatic medication.

Cellulitis: Periorbital and Orbital

Periorbital (preseptal) cellulitis is an infection of the eyelids and surrounding tissues anterior to the orbital septum. Preseptal cellulitis is most often caused by trauma to the lids and surrounding tissues or as a sequela to an upper respiratory infection. It is common in children. If the infection affects structures posterior to the orbital septum, it is called orbital cellulitis. This is a potentially life-threatening infection that can lead to blindness, cavernous sinus thrombosis, or an intracranial abscess. Orbital cellulitis may result from dentoalveolar infection, sinusitis, periorbital trauma, or an infection of the eyelids or lacrimal system.

Signs and symptoms

- In general, VA, pupil reflexes, and extraocular movements (EOM) are unaffected in preseptal cellulitis. Proptosis and chemosis are absent.[49]
- Because structures anterior to the orbital septum also may be involved, look for signs that may distinguish orbital cellulitis from preseptal infection. These include a more toxic appearance, fever,

pain on eye movement, limitation of EOM, abnormal pupil reflexes, diminished VA, chemosis, and proptosis.[49]

Diagnosis
- A CT scan of the orbit is often necessary to evaluate the depth of the infection.

Treatment
- Infants and young children with periorbital cellulitis should be hospitalized because the condition may be associated with sepsis or meningitis.
- For adult patients with periorbital cellulitis, the condition can be managed on an outpatient basis if they are capable of complying with antibiotic therapy and follow-up. If it is managed on an outpatient basis, the patient should be reevaluated within 24 hours. If there is no evidence of improvement, patients may require a CT scan to ascertain the depth of the infection; they also may require admission.[49]
- Patients of any age with orbital cellulitis require admission for administration of IV antibiotics.[3,29,49]

Chemical Injuries, Noncorrosive
Noncorrosive chemicals are painful and irritating to the eyes but are less likely to cause permanent visual impairment than corrosive chemicals (e.g., acids and alkalis).

Signs and symptoms
- Symptoms generally include burning pain, blepharospasm, and tearing.
- Visual acuity may be unaffected or mildly diminished.
- Hyperemia (injection) is usually present, but chemosis usually is not.

Diagnosis
- Common noncorrosive exposures involve petroleum distillates, alcohol-based products, and detergents. The triage classification of noncorrosive chemical exposures is theoretically at a less emergent level; however, as a practical matter the pain and emotional distress caused by the contamination may necessitate relatively rapid initiation of treatment.

Treatment
- Again, if an eye fountain or shower is available, it is the best method of initial decontamination, followed by Morgan lens irrigation.
- The physician may order a topical antibiotic and patching; however, there is no evidence from controlled clinical trials of patching for mechanical superficial corneal injuries

(e.g., abrasion, foreign body) that patching is any more effective than not patching, and it is reasonable to suppose that cautions about patching deeper-than-superficial corneal defects merit consideration (see p. 430, Eye Patching).

- A patient may have gotten "super glue" in the eye, which can cause the lids to adhere together. This usually can be manually debrided by the physician.
- The importance of protective eyewear when using potentially injurious chemical agents at home, school, or work should be emphasized in discharge instructions.
- Depending on the nature of the agent and the extent of corneal injury, follow-up consultation with an ophthalmologist may be advisable.

Conjunctivitis

The principal types of conjunctivitis are bacterial, viral, and allergic. They are differentiated by the presence and type of discharge and whether symptoms are present unilaterally or bilaterally.

Signs and symptoms

- Bacterial conjunctivitis is usually bilateral, with a purulent, matting discharge that is usually worse upon awakening.[31]
- Viral conjunctivitis usually begins in one eye but often spreads to the other. It has a more mucoid discharge and often is associated with fever and sore throat.[3,29-31]
- Pain from infectious conjunctivitis is burning or itching but is generally less intense than corneal pain.
- The patient may complain of blurry vision resulting from a blepharospasm or discharge, but visual acuity is generally unaffected.[29]
- Allergic conjunctivitis is generally associated with itching, puffy eyelids, and a watery to mucoid discharge.[29-31] Allergic conjunctivitis may be unilateral or bilateral.

Diagnosis

- Diagnosis is made by clinical presentation and progression.
- Cultures may be indicated for infants, for conjunctivitis of rapid onset or progression, and for chronic cases.[23] For bacterial conjunctivitis, infection with gram-positive organisms is more common than with gram-negative organisms.[31]
- Hyperacute bacterial conjunctivitis (i.e., of abrupt onset with rapid progression, copious purulent discharge, and severe chemosis) generally is gonococcal. An ophthalmologist best manages this form of conjunctivitis, and a consultation should be requested while the patient is being evaluated in the ED.

If not treated aggressively, the infection can rapidly progress to corneal ulceration and perforation.[31]

- Inclusion conjunctivitis is a sexually transmitted infection (STI) caused by exposure to genital secretions (by direct contact or via the hands) infected with *Chlamydia trachomatis*.[50] In this form, follicular swelling may be evident in the inferior conjunctival fornix.[31,50] The organism is the same as that which causes trachoma (which is not an STI, but which is an infectious cause of blindness endemic in many parts of the underdeveloped world). Unlike trachoma, inclusion conjunctivitis does not cause blindness.

Treatment

- Viral conjunctivitis is self-limiting but highly contagious. Treatment focuses on alleviation of discomfort with warm compresses and topical decongestants. Some practitioners prescribe topical antibiotic prophylaxis. Steroids and patching are contraindicated. Patients or parents should be advised of the importance of careful hand washing and of not sharing towels.[30] Medical and nursing staff also need to be scrupulous about hand washing and disinfection.
- Uncomplicated bacterial conjunctivitis is treated with antibiotic drops or ointments and warm compresses. Steroids and patching are contraindicated.[30]
- Hyperacute (gonococcal) conjunctivitis requires both topical (bacitracin, macrolide, or quinolone) and systemic antibiotics appropriate for gonorrhea, as well as a full STI work-up and tracing and treatment of recent sexual contacts.[31]
- Inclusion (chlamydial) conjunctivitis requires systemic antibiotic therapy (tetracycline, doxycycline, or erythromycin), which may be supplemented, but not replaced, by topical antibiotic therapy. Although signs and symptoms are less dramatic than those of gonococcal conjunctivitis, a full STIs work-up, contact tracing, and treatment are still important.[31,50]
- Allergic conjunctivitis is treated with antihistamines and topical decongestants. Steroids are controversial, and their use is discouraged in episodic care.[30]

Eyelid Lacerations

The priority given to eyelid lacerations depends on their complexity and on whether a facility has appropriate consultants (e.g., ophthalmology or plastic surgery). Lid lacerations that disrupt the tarsal plate or lid margin, as well as those that involve the lacrimal drainage system or lateral or medial canthus of the eye, usually require specialty consultation.[4]

Herpes (Varicella Zoster Virus [VZV; Shingles] or Herpes Simplex Virus [HSV])

Ophthalmic shingles are caused by varicella zoster virus (VZV), a late, latent sequela of herpes varicella infection (chickenpox). Herpes simplex virus (HSV) also may infect the eye from direct contact with infected oral or genital secretions.

Signs and symptoms

- VZV is characterized by unilateral, intense pain and herpetic lesions disposed linearly along the distribution of one of the facial nerves.
- Pain and lesions from HSV do not necessarily follow a facial nerve distribution. Patients with HSV should be screened for STIs.
- Both VZV and HSV also can cause anterior uveitis and jointly constitute the most common form of infectious anterior uveitis in developed countries.[47]

Diagnosis

- The distribution of the pain and lesions and the characteristic appearance of the lesions are diagnostic.
- A history of chickenpox supports, but does not make, a diagnosis of ophthalmic shingles, nor does absence of a known history of chickenpox rule it out.

Treatment

- Although herpetic infections may be confined to extraocular tissues, there is a risk of corneal involvement that can lead to blindness.
- Ophthalmologic consultation is essential; hospitalization may be necessary.
- Treatment with oral acyclovir is common.[40]
- While awaiting consultation, the patient will be more comfortable in a darkened room.

Hyphema

Hyphema is a collection of blood in the anterior chamber, usually caused by a direct blow to the globe, such as by a ball or a fist, that causes bleeding from the vessels of the ciliary body. Because the blood is denser than the aqueous humor, it tends to settle in the lower half of the anterior chamber and is generally visible as a distinct blood fluid level.

Signs and symptoms

- Hyphema is graded according to how much of the anterior chamber is filled with blood (Table 12-2).

TABLE 12-2   Grades of Hyphema

Grade	Blood Level in Anterior Chamber
Microscopic	Blood-tinged aqueous humor; no layering
Grade I	$<\frac{1}{3}$ anterior chamber height
Grade II	$>\frac{1}{3}$, but $<\frac{1}{2}$ of anterior chamber height
Grade III	$\geq\frac{1}{2}$ of anterior chamber but not complete
Grade IV	Complete ("eight ball") hyphema

From Sankar PS, Chen TC, Grosskreutz CL, et al: *Int Ophthalmol Clin* 42:57, 2002.

- Pain resulting from hyphema is a deep aching, but concomitant injury to the cornea or orbit may cause mixed pain presentations.[1,51] The degree of visual impairment is proportional to the grade of hyphema.
- Hyphema often is accompanied by somnolence, especially with children. The etiology of this association is not certain.[51]

Diagnosis

- Although hyphema usually is easy to identify, a few confounding circumstances may occur. Hyphema is, at times, difficult to discern if a patient has dark brown eyes because there is less contrast. Because it is a unilateral injury, comparison with the uninjured eye is always helpful.
- A second difficulty occurs if a patient is under spinal precautions or has been lying supine. In this instance, the blood may settle more diffusely in the anterior chamber, with a less distinct layering.
- Patients with sickle-cell anemia or trait are at increased risk for serious complications from a hyphema. Patients of African ancestry should be screened if their sickle-cell status is unknown.[52]

Treatment

- Clinical management of hyphema is directed toward preventing complications and reducing the risk of rebleeding.
- The injured eye should be shielded (not patched) to prevent further injury (e.g., from rubbing). Patients being discharged should be advised to wear the shield continuously until the hyphema resolves and an ophthalmologist recommends discontinuation.[52]
- If possible, the patient should be positioned sitting upright or with the head of the bed elevated.

- There is a risk of renewed bleeding. This risk is greatest 2 to 5 days after the injury. Although the blood is usually reabsorbed spontaneously, it can cause staining of the cornea.
- Cycloplegic or mydriatic drops may be ordered to reduce or prevent ciliary spasm[41] and inflammation of the ciliary body.[52] Clinical experience suggests this may improve patient comfort, but solid evidence is lacking with respect to the effectiveness of cycloplegia in improving outcomes or reducing complications such as rebleeding.[52]
- A topical ophthalmic corticosteroid may be ordered, depending on consultant preferences. The use of oral corticosteroids is controversial.[52] There are some reports of experimental use of antifibrinolytic and thrombolytic agents in the literature, but evidence of effectiveness to date is insufficient.[52]
- A patient with hyphema requires prompt, but not emergent, ophthalmologic consultation. If not properly treated and given follow-up care, hyphema may cause permanent corneal staining.
- A patient with higher-grade hyphema may be hospitalized on bed rest.
- Ophthalmologists increasingly are treating lesser grades of hyphema at home if the patient will comply with activity restriction and daily follow-up visits and is not taking anticoagulants.[4,51,52] Treatment and disposition decisions for children and for patients with a known history of sickle-cell anemia or a positive screen for sickle-cell trait should be determined by the ophthalmological consultant.[52]
- A patient being discharged home should be advised not to take aspirin or nonsteroidal antiinflammatory medications.[4] Although there is no experimental evidence that these agents actually increase the risk of rebleeding in hyphema, there is, at least, a theoretical justification for this concern.[52]
- Anyone who has suffered hyphema has an increased lifetime risk of glaucoma in the injured eye.[51]

Orbital Blowout Fracture

Orbital blowout fractures occur as a result of injury; generally a blunt retrograde displacement of the globe, which is relatively noncompressible because it is fluid filled. This can cause the orbital floor (ethmoid bone) or the lateral or medial orbital walls to fracture.

Signs and symptoms

- The classic symptoms of a blowout fracture are binocular diplopia and infraorbital anesthesia after trauma to the orbital region.

- Signs may include a gaze limitation as a result of the entrapment of ocular muscles or enophthalmos resulting from herniation of periorbital fat.
- Gaze limitation and enophthalmos may occur as late signs that may not be evident acutely, and they may occur independently or in combination.

Diagnosis
- A blowout fracture is suspected on the basis of the mechanism of injury and on signs and symptoms and is confirmed radiographically by plain films or a CT scan.

Treatment
- A cold pack applied to the orbital area is helpful.
- After the cervical spine has been cleared, the head should be elevated to reduce swelling.
- The patient should be instructed not to blow his or her nose.
- Specialty consultation by a plastic or maxillofacial surgeon is indicated, but surgical repair is not always necessary. Surgical repair often is performed on a delayed elective basis after swelling has gone down.

Retinal Detachment

Retinal detachment may be idiopathic or caused by trauma or degenerative changes associated with aging.

Signs and symptoms
- The detachment is painless and gradual in onset unless it is associated with an acute injury.
- The classic symptom description is clouded vision or the sensation of a veil or curtain interfering with vision; visual alterations can range from total loss of vision to relatively minor decreases in visual field and VA.[42] Patients also may indicate that they are perceiving "floaters" or flashing lights.[42]

Diagnosis
- Diagnosis is based primarily on history, progression, and a funduscopic examination.
- Specific funduscopic findings are beyond the scope of this chapter.

Treatment
- The treatment for retinal detachment is ultimately surgical; nowadays surgical treatment often can be performed as an outpatient or office procedure (e.g., pneumatic or laser retinopexy).
- Guidelines for treatment will depend, to some degree, on the preferences of the consultant, but emergency care may involve the patching or shielding of both eyes to reduce eye movements

pending examination by the consultant. If the eyes are not covered, patients may be less distressed by their visual symptoms if ambient lighting can be reduced or by wearing sunglasses.

- If the patient is to be discharged, a careful assessment must be made of the resources that are available to the patient at home for assistance with self-care.

Superficial Injuries (Corneal Foreign Bodies, Abrasions, and Actinic Keratitis)

Superficial injuries may occur secondary to the presence of foreign bodies in the eye.

Signs and symptoms

See Table 12-1.

Diagnosis

- Diagnosis is based on fluorescein staining and Wood's lamp, cobalt blue light, or slit-lamp examination.

Treatment

- Superficial corneal foreign bodies may be removed by irrigation or with a cotton swab.
- The physician can remove embedded foreign bodies with a spud or the bevel of a 25-gauge hypodermic needle. Often this is performed under slit-lamp visualization. This can be disquieting to the patient even though the cornea is anesthetized. It is often helpful for the nurse to remain with the patient during the removal to assist the patient to sit still.
- If the foreign body was metallic, it can leave a rust ring behind; rust rings often are removed in the ED with a rotary burr.
- If the patient is deemed reliable and understands the necessity of follow-up, the eye can treated with antibiotic ointment for 24 to 36 hours and the ring can be removed by an ophthalmologist the next day.[4]
- Treatment for a corneal abrasion or actinic injury involves antibiotic drops or ointment, oral analgesics, or topical ophthalmic NSAID such as indomethacin,[12] ketorolac,[53] or diclofenac.[55] Patching of the eye has not been shown to improve outcomes in adults[10] or children[11] (see above under Interventions, Eye Patching) but may on occasion still be ordered.
- Patients with contact lenses should be advised not to reinsert them until cleared by an ophthalmologist or optometrist. Treatment is with antibiotic ointment or drops. Corneal abrasion or ulceration from contact lenses definitely should **not** be patched.[15]

NURSING SURVEILLANCE

1. Monitor pain relief and administer analgesics or topical aesthetics as ordered.

2. Expedite examination and treatment. As indicated above, true eye emergencies require immediate care and direct involvement of an ophthalmologist at the earliest opportunity. In smaller communities, transfer to a higher level of care may be necessary for true eye emergencies. As with other transfers, protocols should be in place to guarantee prior acceptance of the patient by the receiving physician and facility, adequate documentation of stabilizing care, and adequate report to nursing personnel at the receiving facility.

3. For conditions such as anterior uveitis and hyphema, follow-up care with an ophthalmologist is essential, and the patient must understand its importance before being discharged. If there are doubts about the capacity or willingness of the patient to obtain follow-up care as directed, the matter should be discussed with the ophthalmologist before discharge, and those concerns and the results of the consultation should be documented.

4. Coaching, guiding, and teaching of the patient and family throughout the emergency visit are essential. Concrete information about the eye examination and what sensations the patient is likely to experience improves coping by giving the patient objective expectations against which the experience and any uncomfortable sensations can be gauged. Offering clear information about the nature of the eye problem and usual functional outcomes helps to reduce uncertainty about what is in store in the short and long term.

5. For patients being discharged with any topical ophthalmic medications, proper instillation technique should be taught to, and understood by, the patient or a household member.

EXPECTED PATIENT OUTCOMES

1. Pain and emotional distress (e.g., fear and anxiety) are reduced.
2. Ocular pH is normal (7.4 to 7.6) in chemical injury.
3. There is no evidence of rebleeding in hyphema.
4. IOP is stabilized.
5. The patient should feel secure in the ability to cope with the problem and in treatment expectations.
6. The patient, family, or household member understands the importance of hand washing before and after instillation of

topical ophthalmic medications and understands proper
instillation technique.
7. The patient understands functional limitations imposed by
treatment (e.g., cycloplegia or patching), as well as the plan of
treatment and follow-up.

DISCHARGE IMPLICATIONS

1. The patient and family should understand expected time
frames for improvement and the significance of any signs or
symptoms that may represent a developing complication or
other departure from the predicted course. It is important to
establish with whom the patient should obtain follow-up care
(e.g., ED, family physician, or ophthalmologist) and whether
follow-up care is essential (e.g., hyphema, anterior uveitis) or
discretionary (e.g., non-STI conjunctivitis).
2. The relation of the problem to risk-taking behaviors (such as
the failure to use protective eyewear) and measures the patient
can take to prevent recurrent injury should be explored in a
nonjudgmental fashion.
3. Patients with RAO or amaurosis fugax will likely require a
more thorough evaluation for cardiovascular disease and
stroke risk than may have been feasible in the ED, but
appropriate referrals may be initiated in the ED.
4. Patients, especially children, with anterior uveitis may benefit
from referral to a primary care physician in addition to an
ophthalmologist as they may require HLA testing or
rheumatological evaluation.
5. Patients with infectious or inflammatory eye conditions caused
by STIs should have the same kind of work-up, referral, and
follow-up as other STI patients.
6. Patients with corneal injuries who wear contact lenses should
be instructed not to reinsert their contacts until they are
cleared to do so in a follow-up examination.

REFERENCES

1. Hitchings R: Eye pain. In Wall PD and Melzack R, eds: *Textbook of pain,*
ed 2, Edinburgh, Scotland, 1989, Churchill Livingstone.
2. O'Brien JM, Albert DM, and Foster CS: Anterior uveitis. In Albert DM and
Jakobiec FA, eds: *Principles and practice of ophthalmology: clinical practice,*
Philadelphia, 1994, WB Saunders.
3. Goodenberger D and Greer D: Ophthalmic emergencies, *Top Emerg Med*
6 (3):1, 1984.
4. Janda AM: Ocular trauma: triage and treatment, *Postgrad Med* 90 (7):51, 1991.

5. Miller SJH, ed: *Parson's diseases of the eye,* ed 18, Edinburgh, Scotland, 1990, Churchill Livingstone.

6. Campanile TM, St Clair DA, and Benaim M: The evaluation of eye patching in the treatment of traumatic corneal epithelial defects, *J Emerg Med* 15:769, 1997.

7. Patterson J, Fetzer D, Krall S, et al: Eye patch treatment for the pain of corneal abrasion, *South Med J* 89:227, 1996.

8. Kirkpatrick JN, Hoh HB, and Cook SD: No eye pad for corneal abrasions, *Eye* 7:468, 1993.

9. Hulbert MF: Efficacy of eye pad in corneal healing after corneal foreign body removal, *Lancet* 337:643, 1991.

10. Le Sage N, Verreault R, and Rochette L: Efficacy of eye patching for traumatic corneal abrasions: a controlled clinical trial, *Ann Emerg Med* 38 (2):129-134, 2001.

11. Michael JG, Hug D, and Dowd MD: Management of corneal abrasion in children: a randomized clinical trial, *Ann Emerg Med* 40 (1):67-72, 2002.

12. Solomon A, Halpert M, and Frucht-Pery J: Comparison of topical indomethacin and eyepatching for minor corneal trauma, *Ann Ophthalmol* 32 (4):316-319, 2000.

13. Bertolini J and Pelucio M: The red eye, *Emerg Med Clin North Am* 13:561, 1995.

14. Schein OD: Contact lens abrasions and the nonophthalmologist, *Am J Emerg Med* 11:606, 1993.

15. Pfaff JA and Moore GP: Eye, ear, nose, and throat, *Emerg Med Clin North Am* 15 (2):327-340, 1997.

16. Joseph E, Zak R, Smith S, et al: Predictors of blinding or serious eye injury in blunt trauma, *J Trauma* 33;19, 1992.

17. Feist RM and Farber MD: Ocular trauma epidemiology, *Arch Ophthalmol* 107:503, 1989.

18. Schein OD, Hibberd PL, Shingleton BJ, et al: The spectrum and burden of ocular injury, *Ophthalmology* 95:300, 1989.

19. Schein OD and Vinger PF: Epidemiology and prevention. In Shingleton BJ, Hersh PS, and Kenyon KR, eds: *Eye trauma,* St Louis, 1991, Mosby.

20. Sternberg P: Prognosis and outcomes for penetrating ocular trauma. In Shingleton BJ, Hersh PS, and Kenyon KR, eds: *Eye trauma,* St Louis, 1991, Mosby.

21. Dannenberg AL, Parver LM, Brechner RJ, et al: Penetrating eye injuries in the workplace: the national eye trauma system registry, *Arch Ophthalmol* 110:843, 1992.

22. Semonin-Holleran R: Trauma in childhood. In Neff JA and Kidd PS, eds: *Trauma nursing: the art and science,* St Louis, 1993, Mosby.

23. Parver LM, Dannenberg AL, Blacklaw B, et al: Characteristics and causes of penetrating eye injuries reported to the national eye trauma system registry, 1985-1991, *Public Health Rep* 108:625, 1993.

24. Joseph E, Zak R, Smith S, et al: Predictors of blinding or serious eye injury in blunt trauma, *J Trauma* 33:19, 1992.

25. Klopfer J, Tielsch JM, Vitale S, et al: Ocular trauma in the United States: eye injuries resulting in hospitalization: 1984 through 1987, *Arch Ophthalmol* 110:838, 1992.

26. Hoover DL and Smith LEH: Evaluation and management strategies for the pediatric eye trauma patient. In Shingleton BJ, Hersh PS, and Kenyon KR, eds: *Eye trauma,* St Louis, 1991, Mosby.

27. Gayle MO, Kissoon N, Hered RW, et al: Retinal hemorrhage in the young child: a review of etiology, predisposed conditions, and clinical implications, *J Emerg Med* 13:233, 1995.

28. Rosenberg AM: Uveitis associated with childhood rheumatic diseases, *Curr Opin Rheumatol* 14 (5):542-547, 2002.

29. Lawlor MC: Common ocular injuries and disorders, *J Emerg Nurs* 15:32, 1989.

30. Wagoner MD, Sadun AA, and Bienfang DC: Acute disorders of the eye. In May HL, Agnababian R, Fleisher GR, et al, eds: *Emergency medicine,* ed 2, Boston, 1992, Little, Brown.

31. Leibowitz HM: The red eye, *N Engl J Med* 343 (5):345-351, 2000.

32. Newman R: Trauma in the elderly. In Neff JA and Kidd PS, eds: *Trauma nursing: the art and science,* St Louis, 1993, Mosby.

33. Amaurosis Fugax Study Group: Current management of amaurosis fugax, *Stroke* 21:201, 1990.

34. Linden JA and Renner GS: Trauma to the globe, *Emerg Med Clin North Am* 13:581, 1995.

35. Blanda M and Wright J: *Headache, migraine,* June, 2003, www.emedicine.com/emerg/topic230.htm.

36. Noecker R and Patterson E: *Glaucoma, angle-closure, acute,* June, 2003, www.emedicine.com/oph/topic255.htm.

37. Bertolini J: *Glaucoma, acute angle-closure,* June, 2003, www.emedicine.com/emerg/topic752.htm.

38. Bertolini J and Pelucio M: The red eye, *Emerg Med Clin North Am* 13:561, 1995.

39. Huang E and Gordon K III: *Retinal artery occlusion,* June, 2003, www.emedicine.com/emerg/topic777.htm.

40. Ellis PP: Commonly used eye medications. In Vaughan DV, Asbury T, and Riordan-Eva P, eds: *General ophthalmology,* ed 13, Norwalk, Conn, 1992, Appleton & Lange.

41. Wagoner MD and Kenyon KR: Chemical injuries. In Shingleton BJ, Hersh PS, and Kenyon KR, eds: *Eye trauma,* St Louis, 1991, Mosby.

42. LaVene D, Halpern J, and Jagoda A: Loss of vision, *Emerg Med Clin North Am* 13:539, 1995.

43. Fraser S and Siriwardena D: Interventions for acute non-arteritic central retinal artery occlusion (Cochrane Review), *The Cochrane Library,* issue 2, Oxford, 2003, Update Software.

44. Dodds EM: Treatment strategies in patients with anterior uveitis, *Int Ophthalmol Clin* 40 (2):55-68, 2000.

45. DiLorenzo AL: *HLA-B27 syndromes,* June, 2003, www.emedicine.com/oph/topic721.htm.

46. Martin TM, Smith JR, and Rosenbaum JT: Anterior uveitis: current concepts of pathogenesis and interactions with the spondyloarthropathies, *Curr Opin Rheumatol* 14 (4):337-341, 2002.

47. Siverio CD Jr, Imai Y, and Cunningham ET Jr: Diagnosis and management of herpetic anterior uveitis, *Int Ophthalmol Clin* 42 (1): 43-48, 2002.

48. Wang ESJ: Cocaine induced iritis, *Ann Emerg Med* 20:192, 1991.

49. Rubin S and Hallagan L: Lids, lacrimals, and lashes, *Emerg Med Clin North Am* 13:631, 1995.

50. Bashour M: *Chlamydia*, June, 2003, www.emedicine.com/oph/topic494.htm.

51. Shingleton BJ and Hersh PS: Traumatic hyphema. In Singleton BJ, Hersh PS, and Kenyon KR, eds: *Eye trauma*, St Louis, 1991, Mosby.

52. Sankar PS, Chen TC, Grosskreutz CL, et al: Traumatic hyphema, *Int Ophthalmol Clin* 42 (3):57-68, 2002.

53. Goyal R, Shankar J, Fone DL, et al: Randomised controlled trial of ketorolac in the management of corneal abrasions, *Acta Ophthalmol Scand* 79 (2):177-179, 2001.

54. Szucs PA, Nashed AH, Allegra JR, et al: Safety and efficacy of diclofenac ophthalmic solution in the treatment of corneal abrasions, *Ann Emerg Med* 35 (2):131-137, 2000.

13 chapter

Genitourinary and Renal Conditions

Cyndi Baxter

INTRODUCTION

Genitourinary (GU) conditions are encountered often in the emergency department (ED). GU complaints may result from a primary disease process or from a secondary injury and often are associated with trauma and hypotension. The most common conditions presenting to the ED include genitourinary trauma, urinary tract infections (UTIs), renal calculi, renal failure, and epididymitis.

> **NURSING ALERT**
>
> Although few GU conditions are medical emergencies, patients with severe pain, tachypnea, or hypertension should be triaged immediately to the treatment area.

FOCUSED ASSESSMENT

Oxygenation and Ventilation

- Tachypnea may be present related to increased fluid volume, acidosis (to remove CO_2), or pain and anxiety.

- Deep and rapid respirations may indicate metabolic acidosis secondary to renal failure.
- The presence of rales or crackles that do not clear with cough may indicate pulmonary edema related to heart failure secondary to fluid overload.

Perfusion
- Tachycardia may occur related to pain or increased fluid volume.
- Hypertension may be related to pain, anxiety, increased fluid volume, or a history of hypertension.
- Fever related to inflammation or infection
- Presence of jugular venous distention may indicate renal failure.
- Diaphoresis or pale, clammy skin may result secondary to sympathetic nervous system action, which can result from renal calculi, testicular torsion, epididymitis, and GU trauma.
- The presence of S_3 or S_4 may indicate acute heart failure related to fluid overload.
- Weak peripheral pulses and moderate peripheral edema may be present as a result of fluid overload.

Cognition
- Disorientation may occur related to decreased cerebral circulation secondary to heart failure and fluid overload or as a result of accumulated toxins.

Sensation and Mobility
- If pain is suprapubic in location, it may indicate bladder or urethral trauma or a lower UTI.
- If pain is located in the flank, it may indicate renal or ureter trauma, an upper UTI, or renal calculi.
- Pain radiating to the shoulder may indicate intraperitoneal leakage of urine.
- Pain from urinary colic occurs most often at night or in the early morning.

Sexuality
- Pain during or after intercourse may be present with sexually transmitted infections (STIs) (see Chapter 18) and in epididymitis.
- Unilateral testicular pain is associated with testicular torsion.
- Scrotal pain is present in epididymitis.
- Penile discharge may occur with STIs and epididymitis.
- Swelling may be present in testicular torsion. Table 13-1 contrasts symptoms of torsion and epididymitis.

TABLE 13-1   Differentiating Testicular Torsion and Epididymitis

Factor	Torsion	Epididymitis
History	Previous episode common	Recent sexual activity
Age	Most common from 12-18 years	Age at onset of sexual activity and older
Pain	Sharp, sudden onset	Gradual onset
Fever	Absent (usually)	Present
Edema	Elevated testis (to assess this, stand at foot of patient's bed and have patient fold his arms over his chest)	Swollen scrotum
Urethral discharge	Absent	Possible
CBC	Normal	Elevated WBC count
Urinalysis	Normal	Bacteriuria
Testicular scan	Hypoperfused	Hyperperfused
Prehn's sign (amount of pain elicited on testis elevation)	Negative (pain increases)	Positive (pain decreases)

- Inspect the genitalia for the presence of vaginal bleeding, penile discharge, or evidence of incontinence.

Tissue Integrity
- Inspect the flanks for ecchymotic areas and abrasions, which may suggest renal trauma. If evidence of trauma is present, auscultate the flank for the presence of a bruit. Mark the size of any hematoma.
- Inspect for bruising around the umbilicus (Cullen's sign) and bruising over the flank (Grey Turner's sign) that results from a retroperitoneal hemorrhage.

Safety
- The presence of dialysis access devices (arteriovenous [AV] shunt, fistula, or graft) may indicate current or previous renal deficiency (Figure 13-1).
- One should assess the shunt, fistula, or graft for patency by palpating the length of the graft for a strong thrill (constant

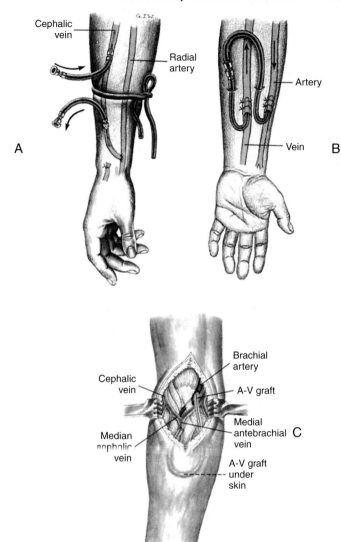

Figure 13–1 Circulatory access for hemodialysis. **A,** External (temporary) arteriovenous cannula (shunt). **B,** Internal (permanent) arteriovenouss fistula. **C,** Internal (permanent) arteriovenous graft. (From Thompson JM, McFarland GK, Hirsch JE et al: *Mosby's clinical nursing,* ed 5, St. Louis, 2001, Mosby.)

vibration), which is indicative of adequate blood flow. Auscultate for a bruit, which is produced by blood flow through the graft.
- A patient presenting with a clotted access device requires declotting through instillation of fibrinolytics or surgical intervention.

NURSING ALERT

Frequent assessment of the clotted graft site is necessary because of the risk of graft rupture. Monitor for redness of extremity, warmth, or tenderness. Extreme hypertension may exacerbate the condition.

- Peritoneal dialysis patients may present with an infection of the insertion site of the peritoneal dialysis catheter or peritonitis.

NURSING ALERT

Signs and symptoms of peritonitis include abdominal pain, fever, nausea and vomiting, and the presence of cloudy dialysate fluid.

- Maintain the integrity of peripheral devices by avoiding use of the extremity for obtaining blood pressure (BP) measurement, blood specimens, or venous access.

Elimination
- A decrease in or cessation of the urinary stream may indicate obstruction. Increased frequency may indicate infection.
- Increased or decreased urinary output may indicate acute renal failure (ARF).
- Hematuria may be present in cases of infection, calculi, or trauma. Medications such as analgesics, anticoagulants, busulfan, cyclophosphamide, extended-spectrum penicillins, oral contraceptives, quinine, and vincristine also can cause hematuria.[1]
- Nonhematuric causes of red or dark red urine include medications such as Dilantin, phenothiazines, or rifampin. Foods such as beets and blackberries also may cause the urine to change to a dark red color.

- Palpate the bladder to determine whether distention is present. Urgency, pain on voiding, and bladder distention suggest a bladder or urethral injury.

LIFE SPAN ISSUES

1. *Pediatric:* Testicular torsion is most common in adolescence. Ureter rupture is most common in pediatric patients with blunt injuries (e.g., pedestrian run over by motor vehicle). UTIs are more common among young females.
2. *Geriatric:* UTIs are common among postmenopausal women. Older men may experience problems with starting, with the force of the urinary stream, or with dribbling and/or inadequate emptying of the bladder because of prostrate enlargement. A UTI may be the first manifestation of sepsis in the elderly.
3. *Pregnancy:* UTI and renal calculi are more prone to occur during pregnancy.

INITIAL INTERVENTIONS

Regardless of the source of the GU condition, the following interventions will not harm the patient and may be beneficial:
1. Raise the head of the patient's bed 30 degrees if cervical spine injuries have been ruled out. The patient should assume the semi-Fowler's position to facilitate urine drainage in urinary tract trauma if cervical spine injury has been ruled out.
2. If the patient can void, obtain a midstream clean-catch specimen. Split the specimen with sterile technique to provide samples for a urinalysis (UA) and a culture and sensitivity if the UA result is positive for infection. Examine the specimen for hematuria, protein, glucose, and pH with a clinical reagent strip. If possible, examine the specimen for the presence of leukocytes with a clinical reagent strip. Females during heavy menses should have a catheterized specimen obtained if no sign of urethral injury is present.
3. A urinary catheter may be ordered to monitor urine output. If blood is present at the urinary meatus, do not pass the catheter until a retrograde urethrogram has been performed. In selecting a urinary catheter, examine the urethral opening and select an appropriate size for the opening (usually a size 12 to 18 Fr in adults).
4. Initiate intake and output recording.
5. In cases of testicular swelling, elevate the scrotum on a pillow or towel and apply ice. Place a protective barrier between the ice and the skin.

6. If renal failure is suspected, record the patient's weight. Measure the circumference of edematous extremities and initiate neurovascular checks. Maintain NPO status until the patient is examined by a physician. The patient may require rapid fluid removal through hemodialysis or peritoneal dialysis. Pulmonary edema, hyperkalemia, uncontrolled hypertension, and pericarditis are indicators for rapid fluid removal.

7. Monitor vital signs every 30 minutes (or by policy) if renal failure is suspected.

8. Continuous cardiac monitoring should be initiated if the patient has a history of chronic renal failure and requires dialysis. An ECG usually is obtained in acute or chronic renal failure to check for life-threatening arrhythmias secondary to hyperkalemia.

9. Nursing care priorities are listed in the table on pp. 463-464.

PRIORITY DIAGNOSTIC TESTS

Laboratory Tests

If renal failure or fluid volume excess is suspected, obtain enough blood for a complete blood count and electrolytes. If possible, fill an additional tube for potential type and crossmatch (transfusion may be necessary if anemia is severe). Clotting profiles may be needed. If an infection or obstruction is suspected, a complete blood count should be adequate. A differential should be performed if infection is suspected.

Arterial blood gases: Metabolic acidosis (pH less than 7.35, HCO_3^- less than 22, and $Paco_2$ less than or equal to 35) may be present in renal failure.

Blood urea nitrogen (BUN) and creatinine: BUN can increase with diuretics, dehydration, or renal failure. Creatinine is specific for renal function, as it is not influenced by diet or fluid intake. Changes in the glomerular filtration rate produce an increase in creatinine.

Complete blood count: A decreased hematocrit may be present in chronic renal failure. An increased white blood cell count is associated with infection. If the infection is acute and bacterial in origin, an increased level of neutrophils and a decreased level of lymphocytes will be present.

Electrolytes and basic metabolic profile: Hyperkalemia may be present in renal failure. If so, assess for hyperactive reflexes and electrocardiogram changes such as peaked T waves, a prolonged PR interval, and prolonged QRS duration (Figure 13-2).

NURSING CARE PRIORITIES

Potential/Actual Problem	Causes	Signs and Symptoms	Interventions
Fluid volume overload	• Primary renal damage • Decreased cardiac output	• Pulmonary edema • Peripheral edema • Hypertension • Tachypnea • Hyperphosphatemia • Hyperkalemia • Metabolic acidosis • Jugular venous distension • Oliguria	• Monitor breath sounds. • Monitor oxygen saturation. • Monitor intake and output. • IV at keep open rate, preferably saline lock • Anticipate diuretic order. • Anticipate need for Foley catheter.
Pain	• Inflammation • Tissue trauma • Spasms	• Tachycardia • Facial expressions • Frequent changes of position • Verbal reports of pain	• Place patient in position of comfort. • Initiate imagery, relaxation exercises, or other coping mechanisms. • Administer NSAIDs or narcotics per order.

Continued

NURSING CARE PRIORITIES—cont'd

Potential/Actual Problem	Causes	Signs and Symptoms	Interventions
Urinary elimination alterations	• Infection • Trauma	• Involuntary urine loss associated with urge to void	• Monitor voiding patterns (factors, amount, time). • Document mishaps. • Assess symptoms associated with voiding.
Risk for urinary retention	• Chronic obstruction	• Bladder distension • Decreased urine output	• Assess breath sounds for crackles. • Assess edema. • Percuss/palpate bladder for degree of distension. • Monitor intake and output • Insert urinary catheter per physician's order.
Infection	• Invasive procedures • Urine retention • Insertion of urinary catheter • Decreased immunocompetence	• Fever • Site swelling, edema, and warmth • Foul-smelling urine	• Maintain sterile technique. • Document baseline temperature. • Monitor temperature. • Assess for evidence of infection.

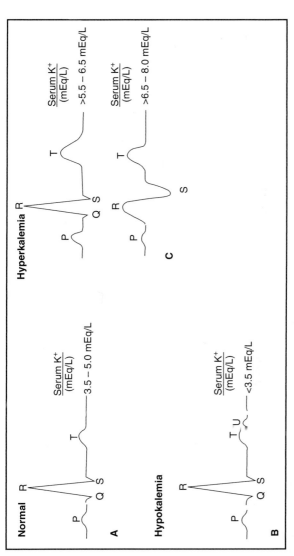

Figure 13-2 Electrocardiogram abnormalities associated with potassium changes. **A,** Electrocardiogram with potassium range. **B,** In hypokalemia, the T wave becomes flatter, and the U wave is seen. **C,** In hyperkalemia below 6.5 mEq/L, the QRS becomes widened and the T wave large and rounded. The P wave flattens and the PR interval increases. When the potassium level is >8.0 mEq/L, cardiac arrest is imminent. (From Bullock BL: Pathophysiology: adaptations and alterations in functions, Philadelphia, 1996, JB Lippincott, p. 201.)

TABLE 13-2 Categories of Acute Renal Failure and Related Laboratory Values

	Prerenal	Intrarenal (ATN)	Postrenal
Urine			
Volume	Low	Low or high	Low or high
Sodium	<20 mEq/L	>20 mEq/L	>40 mEq/L
Osmolality	>350 mOsm	<300 mOsm (fixed)	<350 mOsm (varies)
Specific gravity	>1.020	<1.010	1.008-1.012
Creatinine	~Normal	Low	Low
FE na	≤1%	>1%	>1%
Sediment	Normal	Normal	Cells, casts, protein
Plasma			
Urea (BUN)	High	High	High
Creatinine	~Normal	High	High
BUN:creatinine	20:1 or more	10:1 to 15:1	10:1

ATN, acute tubular necrosis; *BUN,* blood urea nitrogen; *FE na,* fractional excretion of sodium.
From Stillwell SB: *Mosby's critical care nursing reference,* St Louis, 2002, ed, 3 Mosby.

Urinalysis and urine culture and sensitivity: The presence of casts indicates pyelonephritis (upper UTI). The presence of white blood cells and RBCs is nonspecific for infection and calculi. Urine specific gravity and osmolality vary depending on the origin of renal failure. Table 13-2 contrasts these differences. Urine cultures usually are reserved for patients with chronic disease and pregnant, geriatric, pediatric, and immunosuppressed patients.

Radiographic Tests

Intravenous pyelogram: This test is used to assess upper urinary tract function. A contrast medium is injected intravenously, and serial x-ray films are obtained. Expect a 30-minute to 45-minute procedure. If the patient's BP is unstable and he or she is to be taken out of the department for the test, the nurse or physician should accompany the patient. A "one-shot" intravenous pyelogram (IVP) just before laparotomy is useful for patients too unstable to await CT scanning. This film checks for two functioning kidneys and gross renal trauma.

NURSING ALERT

Assess any allergies. Iodine and seafood allergies may require cancellation of IVP or premedication (steroids, antihistamines, and acetaminophen) to minimize reaction.

Cystography: Cystography is used to assess bladder function. Radiopaque dye is injected through a urinary catheter. X-ray films are obtained to determine whether the bladder is distended with dye or the dye is extravasated. Extravasation may occur intraperitoneally or extraperitoneally. A cystogram is typically a 15-minute to 20-minute procedure.

NURSING ALERT

The patient may complain of severe burning and discomfort if a bladder laceration or rupture is present. Prepare the patient for this pain, and use distraction, imagery, and medication as appropriate to facilitate patient coping.

Retrograde pyelogram: This test is used to assess ureter function. Dye is injected through catheters placed in ureters. Note the same concerns as with IVP.

Retrograde urethrography: This test usually is performed in conjunction with cystography. Radiopaque dye is injected through a urinary catheter as the catheter is inserted to detect urethral lacerations. Note the same concerns as for an IVP.

CT/renal scan: This test is rapidly replacing the IVP and arteriography because it is noninvasive. A spiral, or helical, CT without contrast is now the gold standard for diagnosis of renal colic or calculi. Depending on the type of scanner, this procedure may take 15 to 30 minutes. It is difficult to use with an agitated patient because clear films cannot be obtained with patient movement. The test is used when gross hematuria is present on UA and is the most accurate modality available for staging renal injuries.

Renal angiography: This test is used when a renal vascular injury is suspected and when the patient has a mechanism of injury severe enough to cause renal damage (e.g., fracture of lower ribs) and unstable vital signs. If the IVP shows absent or poor visualization of contrast medium, an angiogram may be performed.

Renal ultrasonography: This test may be used to assess for obstruction, stones, and abscesses. The test is a noninvasive procedure performed at the bedside, using reflection of high-frequency sound waves to produce an organ image.

Radionuclide imaging: Radionuclide is administered via IV, and a radioactivity-detecting device records the radionuclide uptake to evaluate alterations in blood flow. This test is used for both renal and testicular problems.

NURSING ALERT

Use gloves when handling the patient's urine after this procedure because the excretion of the radionuclide may take 24 hours.

CLINICAL CONDITIONS

Genitourinary Conditions

Acute Cystitis (Lower Urinary Tract Infection)

Lower urinary tract infections are caused most often by bacteria and occur in the urethra or bladder. Females are more susceptible to UTIs because of their anatomically shorter urethra, which allows bacteria to enter more readily.

Symptoms
- Irritability in children and the elderly with dementia
- Dysuria
- Urinary frequency
- Suprapubic tenderness
- Foul odor to urine

Diagnosis
- The UA shows an increased level of neutrophils. A positive UA result has greater than 2 to 5 leukocytes, greater than 2 to 5 RBCs, and greater than 1+ bacteria.

Treatment
- Administer antibiotics as ordered. Amoxicillin often is used to treat cystitis as it concentrates well in the bladder.

NURSING ALERT

Assess for potential sensitivity before administration of an antibiotic or before discharge with prescription.

- Increased fluid intake and frequent resting periods may be ordered.

Acute Pyelonephritis (Upper Urinary Tract Infection)

Acute pyelonephritis is a bacterial infection that occurs in the pelvis or parenchyma of the kidney. It occurs more often in females.

Symptoms
- The symptoms are the same as those for cystitis, plus:
- Fever
- Nausea and vomiting
- Flank pain

Diagnosis
- Casts will be present in the urine. A complete blood count with differential will show an increased number of white blood cells. Electrolytes, blood urea nitrogen, and creatinine also should be measured.

Treatment
- Administer oral antibiotics if the case is mild.
- IV antibiotics are administered if the case is severe or if the patient cannot tolerate PO medications secondary to nausea and vomiting.
- Cephalosporins, ampicillin, quinolone drugs (ciprofloxacin, ofloxacin, enoxacin, and norfloxacin), aminoglycosides, and IV trimethoprim may be ordered.
- Increased fluid intake and analgesics may be ordered.
- Pregnant females will usually be hospitalized because of an increased chance of premature labor. Children also may be hospitalized.

Epididymitis

Epididymitis results from inflammation of the epididymis caused by an infection such as an STI. The most common causative organisms are *Escherichia coli, Chlamydia trachomatis,* and

Neisseria gonorrhea. Extreme exertion and trauma also may cause epididymitis.

Symptoms

See Table 13-1.

The symptoms have a gradual onset and include:

- Edema of the scrotum
- Fever
- Urethral discharge
- Dysuria
- Recent history of sexual activity

Diagnosis

- Diagnosis is made with an enhanced image on a testicular ultrasound.
- A Doppler stethoscope will show increased blood flow to the testicular area.
- A radionuclide testicular scan may reveal normal or increased perfusion of the testis.

Treatment

- Administer oral antibiotics as ordered.
- Implement scrotal elevation and support.
- Apply ice packs to the scrotum.
- Administer pain medication as ordered.

Testicular Torsion

Testicular torsion occurs when the testicles twist, causing compression of blood and lymphatic vessels, nerves, and the spermatic cord. This results in cessation of blood flow and ultimately tissue necrosis if not diagnosed and treated rapidly. This condition often results from failure of one or both testicles to descend into the scrotum. Other causes may include injuries to the groin or scrotum. Testicular torsion may occur during sleep.

Symptoms

See Table 13-1.

- Acute onset of pain and a positive Prehn's sign (increased pain that occurs with testicular elevation). Pain occurs most often after physical activity or during sleep.
- Nausea and vomiting
- Scrotal swelling

Diagnosis

- Torsion is a surgical emergency and must be repaired within 6 hours to maintain testis viability.
- Diagnosis is based on a decreased image on testicular ultrasonography. A Doppler blood flow study shows

diminished blood flow. A radionuclide testicular scan shows a hypoperfused testis.

Treatment
- Administer IV pain medication.
- Prepare the patient for transfer to the operating suite.

Urinary Calculi

Urinary calculi result from the formation of a stone from substances such as uric acid or calcium. The stones can occur at any point along the genitourinary tract; however, the most common area for calculi formation is the renal pelvis. Risk factors associated with calculi formation include a history of gout, previous episodes of calculi, a large amount of calcium or protein in the diet, pregnancy, or dehydration.

Symptoms
- Sudden, severe pain and extreme restlessness with costovertebral angle tenderness. Pain may radiate to the groin, thigh, abdomen, and genital area.
- Nausea and vomiting
- Hematuria may be present.
- Fever is not present unless an infection accompanies the calculi.

Diagnosis
- CT/renal scan
- Diagnosis is based on a history of calculi.
- Perform an IVP to identify site and renal function.
- A renal ultrasound may be used.

Treatment
- Administer IV analgesics and antiemetics as ordered.
- IV fluids may be required if there is an associated dehydration.
- Strain all urine.
- Send passed stone for analysis.
- A prostaglandin inhibitor such as Ketorolac may be ordered to reduce ureteral peristalsis.
- Stones up to 5 mm may pass spontaneously.
- Extracorporeal shock-wave lithotripsy may be used if calculi are in the renal collecting system or upper ureter and are less than 2 cm.
- Stones greater than 2 cm in the upper renal poles or those greater than 1 cm in the lower renal poles may be removed by percutaneous nephrolithotomy.

Genitourinary Trauma

Genitourinary trauma is associated with a pelvic fracture. Acceleration and deceleration forces (e.g., falls or a one-car motor vehicle crash where the car hits a stationary object such as a tree) and blunt force trauma are associated with renal and bladder injury.

Renal vascular injuries may present without hematuria (e.g., renal thrombosis).

Symptoms
- Pain
- Swelling
- Ecchymosis in the scrotum, perineum, or flank
- Bladder distention
- Pain on voiding
- Hematuria and blood at the urinary meatus
- Gross hematuria does not indicate the severity of the injury

Diagnosis
- Diagnosis is based on an IVP, retrograde pyelogram, cystography, retrograde urethrogram, and CT scan.

Treatment
- Conservative management of the patient with urinary tract trauma includes placement of a urinary catheter and admission until the hematuria is cleared.[2]
- Surgery is indicated when vital signs cannot be maintained with fluid or blood replacement, and when expanding flank mass, decreased urine output, decreased central venous pressure, and continuing gross hematuria are noted. Renal vascular emergencies require immediate surgical intervention, so the patient should be prepared for transfer to the operating suite.
- Penetrating trauma of the urinary tract usually is surgically explored. Blunt bladder trauma with intraperitoneal extravasation usually is surgically explored.

Genitalia Injuries

Genitalia injuries usually result from blunt trauma, although penetrating injuries also may occur. Risks from genitalia injuries include infection and potential for sexual dysfunction.

Symptoms
- Severe pain
- Nausea and vomiting

Diagnosis
- Most genitalia injuries are diagnosed by history and observation.
- A urethral injury may be present and is evaluated by retrograde urethrogram.
- Transillumination of the scrotum should be performed to determine whether testicular rupture is present.

Treatment
- Bleeding from lacerations is treated with application of direct pressure.
- Crush injuries are treated with elevation and ice.
- Most scrotal and vaginal lacerations are cleansed and repaired under anesthesia in the operating suite.

RENAL CONDITIONS
Renal Failure
There are two types of renal failure: chronic renal failure (CRF) and acute renal failure (ARF). CRF results from progressive, irreversible damage to the kidneys that occurs over a long period of time. The most common etiologies are diabetes, hypertension, and autoimmune disease.

Acute renal failure (ARF) is defined as a sudden, rapid decline in renal function. The renal dysfunction causes a buildup of waste products, specifically creatinine and urea nitrogen. ARF also causes metabolic and electrolyte disturbances. Renal failure may occur secondary to a prerenal, intrarenal, or postrenal cause (Table 13-3).

- *Prerenal:* caused by hypoperfusion of the kidneys resulting from hypovolemic shock or renal artery damage. Other causes of prerenal ARF include congestive heart failure, liver failure, and sepsis.
- *Intrarenal:* results from damage to the renal parenchyma. This type of ARF can occur secondary to agents such as nephrotoxic drugs, contrast media, myoglobin, nonsteroidal antiinflammatory drugs (NSAIDs), pesticides, trauma, or inflammation. Acute tubular necrosis is the most common type of ARF and may occur secondary to trauma, acute infection, or a prolonged prerenal state.
- *Postrenal:* results from a urinary flow obstruction. In the ED patient, this usually is related to a tumor or renal calculi

Symptoms
- Symptoms are diverse with multisystem involvement. Refer to Table 13-4.
- Initially oliguria (<400 ml in 24 hours) may be exhibited. This is followed by a diuretic phase in which urine output may increase to 3 to 5 liters in 24 hours.
- Patients in the diuretic phase may exhibit fluid volume deficit and hypotension.

Diagnosis
- Diagnosis is confirmed by BUN and creatinine levels.

TABLE 13-3   Common Causess of Acute Renal Failure

Prerenal	Intrarenal	Postrenal
Hypovolemia caused by:	Nephrotoxic injury	Calculi formation
Hemorrhage	from the following:	Benign prostatic
Burns	Drugs (aminoglycosides	hyperplasia
Dehydration	[gentamicin,	Prostate cancer
Prolonged diarrhea	lobramycin amikacin],	Bladder cancer
or vomiting	amphotericin B, cisplatin)	Trauma (to back,
Decreased cardiac	Radiographic contrast	pelvis, or perineum
output caused by:	agents	Strictures
Myocardial infarction	Hemolytic blood trans-	Spinal cord disease
Cardiac dysrhythmias	fusion reaction	
Congestive heart failure	(hemoglobin	
Cardiogenic shock	blocks tubules)	
Pericardial tamponade	Severe crushing injury	
Surgery (e.g., open	(myoglobin released from	
heart)	muscles blocks tubules)	
Decreased peripheral	Chemicals (ethylene	
vascular resistance	glycol, mercuric chloride,	
caused by:	carbon tetrachloride,	
Septic shock	lead, arsenic)	
Anaphylaxis	Acute glomerulonephritis	
Neurologic injury	Acute pyelonephritis	
Renal vascular	Toxemia of pregnancy	
obstruction caused by:	Malignant hypertension	
Thrombosis of renal	Systemic lupus	
arteries	erythematosus	
Bilateral renal vein	Interstitial nephritis	
thrombosis	Allergic (antibiotics	
Embolism	[sulfonamides,	
	rifampin], nonsteroidal	
	antiinflammatory drugs,	
	ACE inhibitors)	
	Infection (bacterial [e.g.,	
	acute pyelonephritis],	
	viral [e.g., CMV], fungal	
	[e.g., candidiasis])	

From Lewis SM, Heitkemper MM, Dirksen SR: *Medical-surgical nursing: assessment and management of clinical problems*, ed 5, St. Louis, 2000, Mosby.
ACE, Angiotensin-converting enzymes; *CMV*, cytomegalovirus.

TABLE 13-4 Clinical Manifestations of Acute Renal Failure

Symptom	Pathophysiology
Cardiovascular • Arrhythmia • Heart failure • Metabolic acidosis • Hypertension	• Hyperkalemia, hypocalcemia • Hypertension, fluid retention, decreased H^+ secretion • Decreased Na^+ reabsorbtion/HCO_3^- reabsorption/generation • Increased Na^+ retention • Activation of renin
Pulmonary • Pulmonary edema • Kussmaul's respirations	• Left ventricular dysfunction • Increased capillary permeability • Fluid retention • Metabolic acidosis
Hematopoietic • Anemia • Altered coagulation • Immunosuppression	• Decreased erythropoietin • Platelet dysfunction secondary to toxins • Decreased neutrophils
Gastrointestinal • Anorexia/nausea and vomiting • Gastritis/GI bleed	• Breakdown of urea, release of ammonia • Ammonia produces ulcerations.
Neuromuscular • Decreased LOC • Tremors/hyperreflexia	• Metabolic acidosis • Uremic toxin accumulation • Hyperkalemia
Integumentary • Pallor • Yellow skin • Pruritis • Purpura • Uremic frost	• Anemia • Urochrome excretion • Calcium and phosphate deposits, platelet dysfunction • Terminal sign • Urea skin crystals
Skeletal • Hypocalcemia	• Hyperphosphatemia resulting from decreased excretion • Decreased Ca^+ absorption from decreased conservation of vitamin D

- Table 13-2 compares the laboratory values in the three categories of ARF.

Treatment

- If the origin of the renal failure can be determined, therapy should be directed toward correction of the cause of ARF. The goal is to improve cardiac output and renal perfusion.
- Infusion of IV fluids or blood products should be initiated to correct hypovolemia.
- Fluid restriction, diuretics, IV nitroglycerin, and dialysis may be used in intrarenal and postrenal etiologies.
- Electrolyte abnormalities and metabolic acidosis must be treated. Bicarbonate is given when the bicarbonate level is less than 10 mEq/L.
- Hyperkalemia ($\geq$6.5 mEq/L) is the most serious electrolyte abnormality among ARF patients in the ED. IV administration of calcium, insulin, and glucose will cause the potassium to shift into the intracellular space. Potassium-binding ion exchange resins (Kayexalate) may be given either orally or rectally. Inhaled beta agonists such as albuterol also may be administered to help shift potassium intracellularly.
- Hyperphosphatemia and hypocalcemia also may be present. Oral calcium-based antacids will bind phosphorus in the gut. IV calcium may be administered to correct hypocalcemia.
- Hemodialysis may be initiated in the ARF or CRF patient. Hemodialysis removes waste products through an external filtration device utilizing either a temporary or permanent dialysis access device (see Figure 13-1).
- Peritoneal dialysis may be initiated in the patient with CRF. Peritoneal dialysis is accomplished by gravity instillation and draining of dialysate fluid through a port in the peritoneal space, while toxins are removed from the bloodstream through osmosis (Figures 13-3 and 13-4). Strict sterile technique must be maintained during peritoneal dialysis, and the procedure should be performed according to institutional policy and procedure.
- If the patient presents in the diuretic phase of ARF, hypokalemia may occur. Patients in this condition require volume and potassium replacement.

Renal Transplant Rejection

Renal transplant rejection can occur weeks to years after transplant and is related to an antigen–antibody reaction after the body recognizes the organ as being foreign. Renal transplant

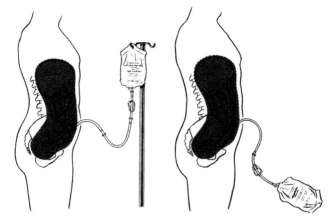

Figure 13–3 Peritoneal dialysis **A,** Inflow. **B,** Outflow (drains to gravity). (From Thompson JM, McFarland GK, Hirsch JE et al: *Mosby's clinical nursing,* ed 5, St. Louis, 2001, Mosby.)

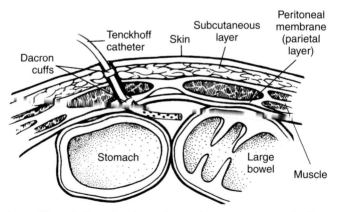

Figure 13–4 Peritoneal catheter. (From Thompson JM, McFarland GK, Hirsch JE et al: *Mosby's clinical nursing,* ed 5, St. Louis, 2001, Mosby.)

patients are maintained on immunosuppressant drugs to reduce the risk of rejection. Two types of rejection are most likely to be seen in the ED, acute and chronic.

- Acute rejection occurs within 12 weeks after transplant and is manifested by elevated serum BUN and creatinine, oliguria, fever, and pain at the graft site.
- Chronic rejection can occur months or years after transplant. Symptoms of chronic rejection include hypotension, proteinuria, and a gradual loss of renal function.

Symptoms

- In addition to the symptoms seen in ARF, a fever will be present.
- Urine output may drop suddenly.
- A 2-lb to 3-lb weight gain may be noted in a 24-hour period.
- Unexplained increase in serum creatinine

Diagnosis

- Diagnosis is confirmed by a renal biopsy, but a renal scan may be performed to assess blood flow while the patient is in the ED.

Treatment

- Drug therapy may include steroids, azathioprine (Imuran), cyclosporine (Sandimmune), and monoclonal antibodies such as OKT3. These drugs require careful patient monitoring because of the potential for serious side effects. See the company's drug insert for information.

NURSING SURVIELLANCE

1. Monitor hematuria.
2. Monitor vital signs.
3. Monitor intake and output to assess fluid balance.
4. Observe and mark ecchymotic areas and expanding masses.
5. Monitor BUN, creatinine, and electrolytes.

EXPECTED OUTCOMES

1. Urinary output is maintained at 30 ml/hr in adults and 1 ml/kg/hr in children.
2. Mean arterial pressure is maintained at 70 to 105 mm Hg.
3. Fever decreases.
4. Pain decreases in severity as documented by a pain scale.
5. Resolution of nausea and vomiting occurs.
6. The patient has diminished crackles and rales upon auscultation.
7. Electrolyte values are within normal limits.

PATIENT/FAMILY DISCHARGE IMPLICATIONS AND EDUCATION

Urinary Tract Infections

1. Teach good hygiene. Instruct the patient to void after intercourse.
2. Stress follow-up care after treatment in 7 to 14 days to examine for reinfection.
3. Cranberry juice may reduce bacterial adherence to the bladder wall and increase urine acidity, thereby reducing the incidence of UTIs. The recommended amount is 3 oz per day for prevention of UTI and 8 to 16 oz per day for treatment of an active UTI.[3]
4. Increase fluids to 2 qt/day.
5. Instruct the patient to return if fever or chills persist or nausea and/or vomiting precludes the taking of antibiotics.

Discharged with Indwelling Catheter

Patients with indwelling urinary catheters do not benefit from routine catheter changes.[4] Irrigate a catheter only if a decreased flow is noted. Catheters should be changed only if a blockage is present. To reduce the incidence of blockage, patients should consume 2 qt of fluids daily to dilute urine. Vitamin C tablets (1 g/day) or three 8-oz glasses of cranberry juice daily decrease encrustation on catheter surfaces, thus reducing the incidence of blockage.

Renal Calculi

1. Stress increasing hydration to 2 qt/day.
2. Provide a strainer and teach the patient how to strain urine.
3. Dietary modifications may need to be made (e.g., decreased calcium intake, decreased oxalate intake, and a low purine diet) if the source of the stone formation has been identified.

Genitourinary Trauma

1. Instruct the patient to increase fluid intake.
2. The patient should return to the ED if urine output decreases.
3. If hematuria is present, bed rest is suggested until the hematuria clears.
4. Emphasize the need for follow-up care to assess renal function and potential complications such as hypertension.

REFERENCES

1. Mazhari R and Kimmel PL: Hematuria: an algorithmic approach to finding the cause, *Cleveland Clin J Med* 69 (11):870-884, 2002.
2. Ruja E: Renal and genitourinary trauma. In Newberry L, ed: *Sheehy's emergency nursing principles and practice,* ed 5, St Louis, 2003, Mosby, pp 304-313.
3. Newton M, Combest W, and Kosier JH: Select herbal remedies used to treat common urologic conditions, *Urol Nurs* 21 (3):232-233, 2001.
4. Bates P: Renal and urologic problems. In Lewis SM, Heitkemper MM, and Dirksen SR, eds: *Medical/surgical nursing,* St Louis, 2000, Mosby, pp 1261-1298.

chapter *14*

Hematologic and Oncologic Conditions

Lisa Collins-Brown
Patty Ann Sturt

INTRODUCTION

Most patients who present to the emergency department with a hematologic or oncologic emergency need urgent or emergent treatment (see Table 14-1).

FOCUSED NURSING ASSESSMENT (HEMATOLOGIC AND ONCOLOGIC CONDITIONS)

Oxygenation and Ventilation

- Pleural effusions may develop in neoplastic cardiac tamponade and SVCS, diminishing breath sounds in the affected area.

- SVCS is more likely to develop in a patient with right-side rather than left-side lung or bronchogenic cancer.
- The patient's respiratory rate and pattern may be altered if airway compromise is occurring secondary to retropharyngeal bleeding.
- Tachypnea may indicate an acute chest crisis in patients with sickle cell anemia (SCA).

Perfusion

- A systolic murmur may be present in patients with SCA as a result of chronic anemia.
- The apical pulse may be shifted in patients with SCA because of congestive heart failure (CHF) that develops from pulmonary hypertension secondary to repeated pulmonary infarcts.
- With SCA patients, neck veins may be distended because of cor pulmonale.
- Muffled heart sounds may be present in neoplastic cardiac tamponade. Tamponade may result from primary or secondary tumors and mediastinal radiation treatments.
- Assess for facial, neck, and periorbital edema. In superior vena cava syndrome (SVCS), edema in these areas may be present and may worsen with bending over or lying down.
- With cancer patients, distended neck veins may suggest neoplastic cardiac tamponade or SVCS.
- Hypotension may be present in acute sequestration syndrome in patients with SCA. In this syndrome, blood pools in an organ, depleting circulating blood volume. Disseminated intravascular coagulation (DIC) may produce hypotension as a result of excessive bleeding. Hypotension also may occur in cases of hypercalcemia because of the polyuria it produces.
- Assess for signs of hemorrhage (petechiae, ecchymoses, hematomas, or swelling). If detected, pressure and cold should be applied and the site elevated if possible.
- The degree of swelling present is not a good indicator of the degree of bleeding.

Cognition

- Perform a neurologic assessment and assign the patient a Glasgow Coma Scale score (see Reference Guides 10 and 16). A patient with a score of less than 15 may need CT brain scanning.
- Assess level of consiousness because meningitis is common in pediatric patients with SCA. If the condition is present, anticipate a lumbar puncture (see Procedure 22) and cerebrospinal fluid cultures.

- If the patient is disoriented, suspect an intracranial bleed, metastatic tumor, or electrolyte abnormality.
- Patients with SCA are at risk for cerebrovascular attacks. Altered mental status or coma may occur as a result of cerebral hypoxia.

Sensation and Mobility

- Stiffness of the joints, a limited range of motion, and joint edema are common in hemarthroses (joint bleeding).
- Weakness on ambulation may be a sign of spinal cord compression (SCC) and may be present for several weeks before the patient seeks treatment. Patients with SCC who are ambulatory at the time they seek treatment have a better chance of remaining mobile.
- Numbness and tingling in the extremities may be another sign of SCC. Extension of the extremities may elicit an electrical sensation down the back. Examine the patient's extremities for deformity and angulation.
- Pathologic fractures may be present in malignancy. Pain is present on weight bearing.
- Patients with hemophilia and SCA have symptoms inconsistent with a minor trauma history.
- With hemophilic patients, any injury to the head and spinal column, no matter how trivial, should be viewed as significant.

Sexuality

- Priapism (a painful sustained erection) may be present in SCA. Because erectile dysfunction and impotence may occur if the condition is left untreated, hydration and analgesia are initiated quickly.

Tissue Integrity

- Some hemophiliacs are at increased risk of human immunodeficiency virus (HIV) secondary to blood products received from multiple donors (blood products were not tested for HIV before 1986). Immunosuppression and active infections may be present in addition to their presenting complaint.
- A low-grade fever may be present in sickle cell crisis and indicate infection. For the cancer patient, infection is defined as one temperature measurement greater than 101° F (38.5° C) or three readings greater than 100.4° F (38° C) in a 24-hour period.
- Assess for blood in the anterior chamber of the eyes (hyphema). For patients with SCA, hyphema can have

devastating complications because of the increased intraocular pressure (IOP) caused by the blockage of outflow tracts by sickled cells.

Pain

- For a patient with cancer, back pain is a critical symptom. Back pain is the first symptom in neoplastic spinal cord compression (SCC). Rest does not relieve the pain.
- In hemophilia, pain is present on rest and movement of the affected extremity or muscle group. Immobilization and the application of ice and a pressure dressing (elastic bandage) may relieve the pain.
- In patients with SCA, pain may be precipitated by alcohol use, physical activity, changes in temperature or altitude, and emotional stress. Pain results from obstruction of the blood flow and its resulting hypoxia and ischemia. Pain from SCA may be relieved by IV hydration. Ask the patient what usually relieves the pain based on the severity of the episode. Distraction, imagery, and relaxation techniques can be initiated immediately. Seek an order for administration of acetaminophen, antiinflammatory agents, and narcotics.

LIFE SPAN ISSUES

Children

1. Hemophilia, when not diagnosed at birth, is usually detected when the child begins to walk and joint swelling occurs.
2. Cutting teeth and losing deciduous teeth may precipitate bleeding in hemophilia.
3. The death of patients under 6 years of age with SCA may be related to pneumococcal sepsis and can be prevented with prophylactic penicillin.[1] If the patient is receiving penicillin, this should be noted, because clinical presentation and bacterial studies may be altered in the presence of an infection.
4. Acute chest crisis is more common among pediatric patients with SCA.
5. Bladder control regression may be the first symptom for children who have SCC because of cancer.

Women

Postpartum bleeding may occur on a delayed basis after hospital discharge with women who have von Willebrand's disease.

TABLE 14-1 Oncologic Emergencies

Emergency	Symptoms	Consideration
Tumor Lysis Syndrome		
Hyperuricemia	• Dysuria • Anuria • Anorexia • Vomiting • Lethargy • Pain and swelling of joints	• Recent initiation of chemotherapy for treatment of leukemia or lymphoma
Hyperkalemia	• Bradycardia • Hypotension • ECG changes: • Tall peaked T waves • Depressed ST segment • Widening of QRS • Diarrhea • Muscle weakness	
Hyperphosphatemia/hypocalcemia	• Carpopedal spasms • Hyperactive deep tendon reflexes • Seizures • Irritability	

Continued

TABLE 14-1 Oncologic Emergencies—cont'd

Emergency	Symptoms	Consideration
Hypercalcemia	• Photophobia • Diarrhea • Nausea\Vomiting • Constipation • Abdominal pain • Polyuria • Bradycardia • Mental changes • ECG changes: • Prolonged PR interval	• History of breast cancer with bony metastatic disease
Spinal Cord Compression Syndrome Cervical region: symptoms listed in order of appearance	• Motor impairment of arm • Motor impairment of ipsilateral leg • Motor impairment of contralateral leg • Motor impairment of opposite arm • Pain is worse on lying down	• Results from compression from metastasis of a tumor • Most often occurs in the thoracic spine
Thoracic region	• Stiff and weak legs • Altered pain and temperature sensation on side opposite from maximum motor weakness	

Radicular or nerve root

- Pain over affected spinal process that is aggravated with coughing, sneezing, straight-leg raising, spasms, loss of deep tendon reflexes

Superior Vena Cava Syndrome

Increased venous pressure

- Edema
- Erythema of face and neck
- Visual changes
- Headache
- Conjunctival hemorrhage
- Engorged neck veins
- Dyspnea

- Symptoms are worse on awakening.
- May be compressed externally by a mass or internally by a thrombus (e.g., forming on a central venous catheter).

Pericardial Tamponade

Hypotension

- Dyspnea
- Chest pain
- Cough
- Tachycardia
- Distant heart sounds (possible)
- Jugular venous distension

- Other symptoms typical of tamponade seen in traumatic injury (e.g., pulsus paradoxus or pericardial rub) may be absent.

Anemia

Decreased oxygen transport

- Dyspnea
- Fatigue

- History of radiation to pelvic area or chemotherapy

Continued

TABLE 14-1 Oncologic Emergencies—cont'd

Emergency	Symptoms	Consideration
Thrombocytopenia		
Bleeding	• Dizziness • Pallor • Tachycardia	
	• Petechiae • GI/GU bleeding • Epistaxis	• History of radiation or chemotherapy
Disseminated Intravascular Coagulation		
Coagulopathy	• Fever • Petechiae • Conjunctival hemorrhage • Melena • Hematemesis • Headache • Change in mentation • Hematuria	• Bleeding from three unrelated sites

ECG, Electrocardiogram; *GI/GU,* gastrointestinal/genitourinary.

Adults

1. With adult hemophiliac patients, intracranial bleeding may occur spontaneously (without an injury history).
2. Adult patients with SCA often die from bone marrow and fat embolization.

INITIAL INTERVENTIONS (HEMATOLOGIC AND ONCOLOGIC CONDITIONS)

1. Initiate oxygen administration as needed to relieve dyspnea and impaired gas exchange. If dyspnea is present (as in suspected SVCS), elevate the head of the bed and administer low-flow oxygen. Initiate pulse oximetry. For SCA patients only, administer oxygen if they have signs and symptoms related to respiratory distress or decreased oxygen saturation.
2. Initiate IV access. Oncologic and hematologic emergencies require fluid resuscitation, factor replacement, pain control, electrolyte replacement or removal, or diuretics. Patients with SCA and hemophilia have had multiple IV catheters, and their veins may be sclerosed. Ask the patient for the "best vein site." Place the largest IV catheter that vein integrity will allow. Hydration in the SCA patient is initiated with D_5W or D_5 $\frac{1}{2}$NS because these allow free water to enter the cells and thus reduce the hemoglobin concentration, improving tissue oxygenation. For unsuccessful IV attempts, apply pressure to the puncture or injection site for at least 10 minutes in hemophilic patients. While starting the IV in hemophilic patients, obtain blood for a complete blood count (CBC) and coagulation studies. This allows for the prediction of the amount of factor replacement necessary based on the severity and location of the bleed and the degree of factor activity present.
3. Administer antibiotics as ordered.
4. Administer diuretics and vasoactive drugs as ordered.
5. Use imagery, distraction, or relaxation techniques for patients with pain.
6. Administer narcotics, acetaminophen, or antiinflammatory drugs. Schedule pain medications on a regular basis and document pain assessment, including a pain scale, before each administration of medication.
7. Immobilize and elevate joints if appropriate.
8. Apply cold compresses to affected areas.
9. Implement spinal immobilization when necessary until radiographic tests are completed.

10. Initiate blood product replacement. Hemophilic patients may need factor replacement in cases in which they come to the ED with a primary problem (e.g., laceration) and will require an invasive procedure (e.g., suturing). When in doubt, initiate factor replacement while awaiting laboratory results. Hemophilic patients may have administered several units of factor replacement at home, thus alerting ED personnel that additional medication or blood products may be necessary.

11. Simple or partial exchange transfusions may be administered in SCA to improve local blood flow to infarcted areas. A hemoglobin S level of less than 30% is desired.[1] In DIC, clotting factors may be replenished using platelets, fresh frozen plasma, or packed cells.

12. Use standard precautions. Hemophilic patients have a high rate of HIV and hepatitis B infection. Cancer patients' white blood cell (WBC) count may be below 2000 cells/mm^3, increasing their susceptibility to opportunistic and nosocomial infections. Patients with a low WBC count should be placed in a private room. Wash your hands well before and after each patient contact.

13. If the patient is complaining of chest pain, obtain an electrocardiogram (ECG). Several oncologic emergencies produce the symptom of chest pain (e.g., neoplastic cardiac tamponade and hypercalcemia).

14. Nursing care priorities can be found in the table on p. 491.

PRIORITY DIAGNOSTIC TESTS

Laboratory Tests

Complete blood count: A CBC may be ordered to detect dehydration (high hematocrit) and infection in patients with SCA. A WBC count greater than 20,000 mm^3 has been associated with a higher infection and death rate with SCA. Hemoglobin levels will be extremely low in acute sequestration syndrome in SCA.[1]

Electrolytes: The potassium and phosphorus levels may be elevated in tumor lysis syndrome (TLS). The calcium level may be increased in malignancy and decreased in TLS.

Fibrin split products: Increased in DIC

Hemoglobin S level: Elevated in cases of acute crisis in patients with SCA

Platelets: Decreased in DIC

Prothrombin time: Increased in DIC

Partial thromboplastin time: Increased in DIC

NURSING CARE PRIORITIES

Potential/Actual Problem	Causes	Signs and Symptoms	Interventions
1. Impaired gas exchange	• Pulmonary infiltrates • Pleural effusion • Cor pulmonale • Compression by tumor	• Shortness of breath • Decreased level of consciousness	• Administer oxygen to maintain oxygen saturation of greater than 94%. • Continuously monitor oxygen saturation. • Position the patient for comfort. • Prepare for intubation. • Administer diuretics as ordered to relieve fluid overload.
2. Pain	• Poor tissue perfusion or ischemia • Obstruction of blood flow	• Complaints of pain • Crying • Moaning • Grimacing • Restlessness	• Assess pain using a pain scale; reassess after any intervention. • Position the patient for comfort. • Administer pain medication as ordered. • Give pain medication on a schedule to prevent acute pain crisis. • Provide teaching of nonpharmacologic pain-control measures, such as guided imagery, relaxation, and distraction. • Immobilize and elevate joints if appropriate and apply cold compresses to affected area.

Reticulocyte count: A reticulocyte count may be ordered for patients with SCA to detect an aplastic crisis.

Uric acid: Increased in TLS

Urinalysis: A urinalysis may be ordered to detect dehydration or infection in the patient with SCA.

Radiographic Tests

Lateral soft-tissue neck films: To rule out retropharyngeal bleeding in hemophilia

Chest film: To rule out infection and infiltrates in patients with SCA. A widened mediastinum may be present in patients with SVCS.

CT scan: Head: may be used to detect intracranial bleeding in hemophilia and SCA. A scan of the chest may show collateral circulation in SVCS.

Long-bone films: May be obtained in hemophilia and SCA to detect acute joint effusions

Spinal films: Most cases of vertebral body involvement by tumor can be identified through spinal films.

Special Diagnostic Studies

Abdominal ultrasound: To evaluate abdominal pain in patients with SCA

ECG: The direction or size of the QRS complex and T wave may change with every other beat in cardiac tamponade. In hypercalcemia, first-degree or second-degree heart block may be present. In hyperkalemia associated with TLS, tall, peaked T waves may be present.

Echocardiogram: This test may be useful in diagnosing the degree of pericardial effusions.

Venography: Venography may be used to identify the degree of obstruction in patients with SVCS.

CLINICAL CONDITIONS

Hematologic Conditions

Acute Sickle Cell Pain Crises

In the United States, SCA occurs predominantly among the African-American population. It is characterized by the presence of an abnormal type of hemoglobin, termed hemoglobin S, in the red blood cell. When the cell becomes hypoxic, these red blood cells assume an irregular, crescent shape, causing an increase in blood viscosity that results in stasis of blood flow and in sludging. This leads to microvascular obstruction and tissue ischemia. The sickling process can also occur with local tissue hypoxia, dehydration, and acidosis and with exposure to cold, infection, or emotional stress.

Sickle-cell crisis encompasses a variety of acute symptomatic events that result from the sickling process associated with SCA. The most common emergency is the pain associated with vascular occlusion. Aplastic crises normally follow a viral infection, causing bone-marrow suppression with worsening anemia. Splenic sequestration crises result from sudden trapping of blood in the spleen. Splenic function may be altered, which increases the patient's susceptibility to infection.

Symptoms

ABDOMINAL CRISES CAUSED BY ISCHEMIA OR INFARCTS OF THE MESENTERIC AND ABDOMINAL VISCERA

- Abdominal pain
- Nausea, vomiting, and diarrhea

APLASTIC CRISIS

- Fatigue and dyspnea
- Decreased number of RBCs and hemoglobin
- Decreased number of or absence of reticulocytes

BONE CRISES CAUSED BY SLUDGING OF BLOOD

- Acute long-bone pain
- Back pain (common in pediatric patients)
- Nonpitting edema

CENTRAL NERVOUS SYSTEM CRISES RELATED TO THROMBOTIC STROKE

- Headache
- Visual changes
- Change in LOC

PULMONARY CRISIS

- Chest pain
- Dyspnea and tachypnea
- Pleural effusions
- Nonproductive cough
- Hemoptysis (suggests a pulmonary infarction)

SPLENIC SEQUESTRATION CRISES

- Left upper quadrant tenderness and enlarged spleen
- Infections

Other Symptoms

- Priapism

Diagnosis

- Diagnosis is based on the patient's history of SCA, clinical presentation, and laboratory values (CBC and reticulocyte count).

Treatment
- Initiate hydration. If the crisis episode is mild and the patient is able to tolerate oral fluids, hydration can be given orally. If intravenous administration is required, D_5W or $D_5\frac{1}{2}NS$ are recommended as the fluids of choice. Begin at a rate of 150 to 200 ml/hr for adults.[2]
- Provide oxygen therapy at 2 to 4 L/min per nasal cannula for those patients who have respiratory distress symptoms or low oxygen saturation.
- Administer pain medications as ordered. Narcotic analgesics, such as morphine and fentanyl, are the preferred medications for pain management. These should be administered on a scheduled basis until pain control is achieved. A patient-controlled analgesia (PCA) pump can be used either in demand or controlled infusion modes. Document a pain assessment before pain medication administration, including the use of a pain scale.
- Administer antiemetics for nausea as ordered.
- Administer antibiotics as ordered if an underlying infection is present.
- Patients with aplastic or splenic sequestration crises may require blood transfusions.
- Administer folate for anemia per physician order.
- Consider using or creating a plan of care for your frequent patients with SCA (Figure 14-1).

≥ NURSING ALERT ≤

Aspirin products should not be administered to hemophilic patients because of their interference with platelet function. Meperidine (Demerol) is not used in SCA patients because repeated doses usually are necessary, resulting in accumulation of narcotic metabolites and subsequent seizures. Toradol (ketorolac) has had mixed success in treating SCA pain.

Disseminated Intravascular Coagulation (DIC)

In DIC the pace of the clotting cascade is accelerated and fibrinolysis is unable to keep pace with thrombus formation. Injury results from thrombi in the microcirculation and from bleeding as a result of the consumption of clotting factors in the microcirculation. DIC may be associated with sepsis, traumatic injury, or a complication of malignancy.

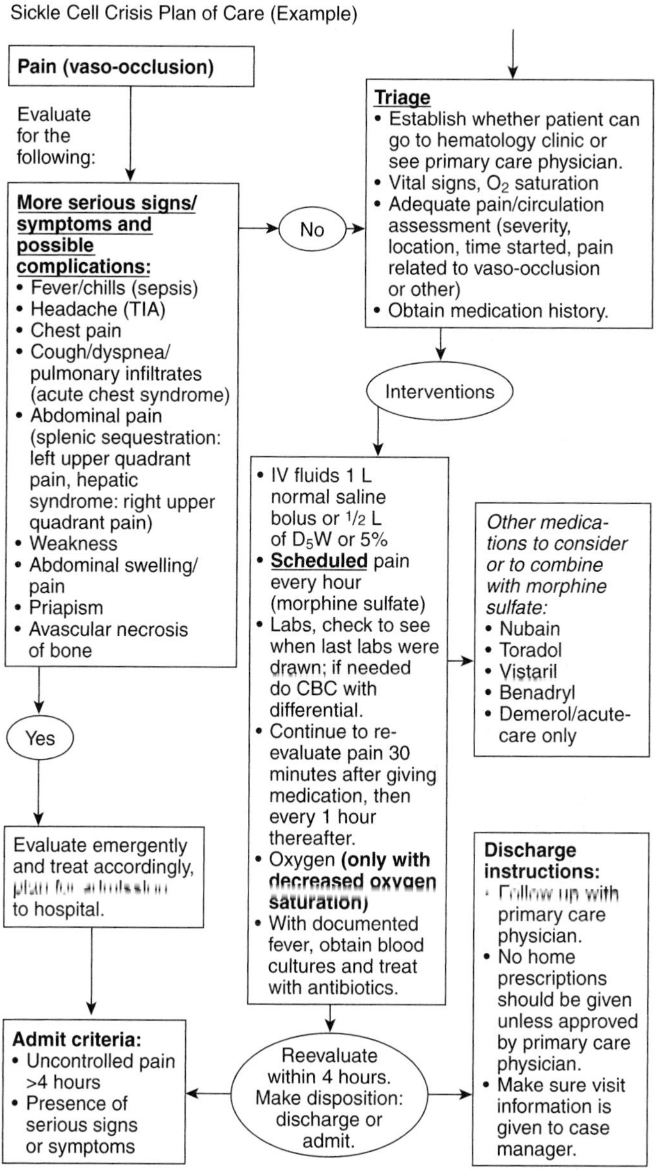

Sickle Cell Crisis Plan of Care (Example)

Figure 14–1 Sickle cell crisis plan of care.

Symptoms
- Bleeding generally occurs from three or more sites.
- Petechiae, epistaxis, abdominal pain and distension, melena, hematuria, hemoptysis, and level-of-consciousness (LOC) changes may be present.
- The bleeding site(s) determine the symptoms.

Diagnosis
- Laboratory data show increased prothrombin and partial thromboplastin times.
- Levels of fibrin split products are elevated.
- The level of platelets and fibrinogen is decreased.
- Elevated D-dimer assay.

Treatment
- Heparin therapy is used to block microthrombus formation.
- In malignancy, patients may be resistant to heparin therapy. Oncology patients with solid tumors usually suffer greater problems from hypercoagulability.[3] Aspirin and dipyridamole may be used.
- Platelets (when the platelet count is less than 50,000/mm³), packed red blood cells, fresh frozen plasma, or factor VIII may be given.

Hemophilia

Hemophilia is a genetic disorder characterized by a clotting factor deficiency. Hemophilia affects primarily males, but females carry the trait. It results in prolonged or excessive bleeding in response to varying degrees of physical injury. Hemophilia A is the most common type and results from a factor VIII deficiency. Hemophilia B (Christmas disease) results from a factor IX deficiency. In von Willebrand's disease, there is a deficiency of factor VIII and von Willebrand's factor. These two factors usually circulate together as a complex. Clinical manifestations of all types of hemophilia are similar.

Symptoms
- The bleeding sites and respective symptoms of the various types are listed in Table 14-2.

Diagnosis
- Table 14-3 lists the laboratory values in most types of hemophilia.
- Factor levels should be determined to calculate the factor replacement that is adequate for the type and severity of factor deficiency and the type, severity, and location of the bleeding (see Box 14-1).

Treatment
- Bleeding of the mucous membranes of the mouth and nose is treated with both factor replacement and antifibrinolytic agents

TABLE 14-2	Common Manifestations of Bleeding in Hemophilia Disorders	
Bleeding Site	Symptoms	Special Considerations
Muscle	• Pain at site on movement or rest • Numbness, tingling if nerve compression occurs • Decreased or absent deep tendon reflexes (DTRs)	• Potential for compartment syndrome
Hemarthrosis	• Edema at site • Pain—usually in knee, elbow, shoulder, ankle, or wrist • Limited range of motion	• More factor replacement is required for weight-bearing joints. • Hypovolemia may occur if bleeding into shoulder or hips.
Central nervous system	• Altered level of consciousness, headache, vomiting, seizures	• May have 24-hr symptom-free interval after injury
Gastrointestinal	• Melena, hematemesis	
Retropharyngeal	• Sore throat, dysphagia, dyspnea, change in voice quality	• Usually occurs after dental procedures
Retroperitoneal	• Abdominal tenderness • Absent bowel sounds • Rigid abdomen • Flank pain with hematoma • Hypovolemic signs	

TABLE 14-3   Laboratory Values in Bleeding Disorders

Condition	Activated Partial Thromboplastin Time (aPTT)	Bleeding Time	Factor VIII	Factor IX	Von Willebrand's Factor
Hemophilia A	Increased	Normal	Decreased	Normal	Normal
Hemophilia B	Increased	Normal	Normal	Decreased	Normal
von Willebrand's disease	Normal or increased	Increased	Decreased	Normal	Decreased

(e.g., Amicar) because saliva contains high levels of fibrinolytic enzymes, making clots unstable.

- Ice, elastic bandages (pressure dressings), packing, and immobilization and elevation may be used in addition to medication and factor administration to control bleeding in joints and muscles.
- Acute bleeding episodes should be treated with intravenous administration of recombinant factor VIII or IX. Hemophilia A can be treated with either plasma or recombinant factor VIII. The treatment of choice for hemophilia B is recombinant factor IX, such as Autoplex T.
- Mild episodes of acute bleeding in patients with hemophilia A and von Willebrand's disease may be treated with desmopressin (DDAVP), which can be given parenterally or via nasal spray. DDAVP is a synthetic analog of vasopressin that may be used to stimulate an increase in factor VIII and von Willebrand's factor.[4]

BOX 14-1   HOW TO CALCULATE FACTOR REPLACEMENT

Amount of factor VIII required = (wt in kg) × (0.5) × (% change desired in factor activity).

Amount of factor IX required = (wt in kg) × (1.0) × (% change desired in factor activity).

- Cryoprecipitate is no longer recommended for acute bleeding episodes because of the potential for infection with the HIV virus or hepatitis C and should be given only in the event of a life-threatening hemorrhage.

Thrombocytopenia

Thrombocytopenia occurs when the platelet count is below 150,000 mm^3. Thrombocytopenia can result from diseases such as DIC, leukemia, or severe infections, may result from a congenital disorder, or may be idiopathic. A variety of medications also can cause a reduced platelet count, including: heparin, low-molecular-weight heparins, glycoprotein IIb/IIIa inhibitors, typical antipsychotics, chemotherapy drugs, estrogen, digoxin, and Lasix.

Symptoms
- Bruises easily
- Ecchymosis
- Petechiae
- Hematuria
- Melena
- Hematemesis

Diagnosis
- History and physical exam
- Presence of a decreased platelet count

Treatment
- If drug induced, discontinue the medication
- Platelet transfusion for severe bleeding

Oncologic Conditions

An oncologic emergency is a clinical situation in which the condition is secondary to a malignancy or its treatment (see Tables 14-4 and 14-5). Rapid assessment and interventions are often necessary to prevent continuing patient deterioration. Aggressive treatment may be appropriate when there is potential for a cure or prolonged survival.

Hypercalcemia

Hypercalcemia is one of the most common oncologic emergencies, occurring in 10% to 20% of oncology patients. Solid tumors, lung cancer, and breast cancer account for 80% of malignancies related to hypercalcemia. These tumors may produce a parathyroid-hormone–like substance, resulting in elevated calcium levels. The remaining 20% include causes from multiple myeloma, leukemia, and lymphoma. Patients being treated with estrogens or antiestrogens may experience

TABLE 14-4 Complications of Cancer	
Primary Cancer Site and Type	**Associated Oncologic Emergency**
Breast cancer	• Hypercalcemia • Neoplastic cardiac tamponade • SCC • SVCS • Pleural effusion • Brain tumor
Lung cancer	• Pleural effusion • SCC • Brain tumor • SVCS
Adenocarcinoma	• Pleural effusion • SCC • Brain tumor
Oat cell	• SVCS • Pleural effusion
Multiple myeloma	• Hypercalcemia
Lymphoma	• Hyperkalemia • Hypercalcemia • Neoplastic cardiac tamponade • TLS • SCC • SVCS • Pleural effusion
Leukemia	• Hypercalcemia • TLS • Hyperkalemia • Thrombocytopenia • Hemorrhage
Prostate	• SCC • Brain tumor • DIC
Pancreatic	• DIC • Thrombocytosis
Bone	• Hypercalcemia

DIC, Disseminated intravascular coagulation; *SCC*, spinal cord compression; *SVCS*, superior vena cava syndrome; *TLS*, tumor lysis syndrome.

TABLE 14-5	**Complications of Chemotherapeutic Agent**	
Agent	**Side Effects**	**Use**
Doxorubicin	• Chemical pericarditis • Arrhythmia	• Leukemia • Breast cancer
Daunorubicin	• Chemical pericarditis • Arrhythmia	• Leukemia
Cisplatin	• Nephrotoxicity • Neurotoxicity • Ototoxicity	• Oat cell lung cancer • Ovarian and testicular cancer
Cyclophosphamide	• Hemorrhagic cystitis • Myelosuppression	• Breast cancer • Lymphoma
Methotrexate	• Nephrotoxicity • Hepatic toxicity • Pulmonary fibrosis	• Breast cancer • Bladder cancer • Lymphoma • Leukemia
Bleomycin	• Pulmonary fibrosis • Pneumonitis	• Gynecologic cancers • Lung cancer
Carboplatin	• Neurotoxicity • Nephrotoxicity	• Ovarian cancer • Leukemia
Etoposide	• Myelosuppression • Neuropathy • Hepatic damage	• Lung cancer • Testicular cancer • Leukemia

progressive hypercalcemia. Hypercalcemia also may result from direct bony destruction by tumor cells, resulting in the release of calcium from bone into the serum.

Lack of recognition and interventions can lead to renal failure, coma, cardiac arrhythmias, and cardiac arrest.

Symptoms
• Nausea, vomiting, and polyuria. These contribute to the hypovolemia associated with hypercalcemia.
• Abdominal pain and distension
• Muscle weakness
• Diminished or absent deep tendon reflexes (DTRs)
• Restlessness, confusion, or a decreased LOC

Diagnosis
- Elevated serum calcium levels (greater than 11 mg/dl)
- ECG changes of short ST segments, first-degree or second-degree heart block, and wide T waves may be present.

Treatment
- Medications such as, plicamycin, etidronate disodium (Didronel), and calcitonin are used to treat hypercalcemia.
- IV hydration with isotonic (0.9%) saline
- After volume is restored, loop diuretics such as furosemide may be ordered to increase urinary excretion of calcium.
- Medications aimed at preventing bone breakdown (e.g., pamidronate, calcitonin, plicamycin, and gallium nitrate)
- Radiation and chemotherapy aimed at the primary tumor may be instituted.
- Dialysis with hypercalcemia and renal failure.

> **⇒ NURSING ALERT ⇐**
>
> Hypokalemia may occur with saline hydration and diuretic use in treatment of hypercalcemia. Monitor the patient for muscle weakness, paralytic ileus, and flattening of the T wave (T-wave inversion) on an ECG.

Neoplastic Cardiac Tamponade

Neoplastic cardiac tamponade occurs when a tumor or postirradiation pericarditis causes fluid to accumulate within the pericardial sac. The fluid accumulation causes a marked rise in intrapericardial pressure. This pressure around the heart prevents adequate cardiac filling during diastole, which results in decreased cardiac output.

Symptoms
- Pallor
- Tachycardia
- Pulsus paradoxus
- Decreased LOC
- Hypotension
- Elevated central venous pressure
- Muffled heart tones
- Oliguria

Diagnosis
- Diagnosis is based on clinical presentation and echocardiogram.

Treatment
- Pericardiocentesis is an emergency treatment option in the patient with clinical deterioration evidenced by indicators of shock (see Procedure 26).
- Continuous drainage by an indwelling catheter may be initiated and used until surgery can be performed.
- IV fluid administration and vasoactive medications (e.g., dopamine)
- Pericardial sclerosis may be instituted via chemotherapeutic agents.

Spinal Cord Compression (SCC)
SCC usually results from metastatic tumors that compress the spinal cord or cauda equina. Cancers of the lung, breast, and prostate carry the highest risk. Early recognition and treatment may prevent permanent neurologic deficits such as paralysis.

Symptoms
- Localized back pain is the most common symptom. The pain often is unrelieved by rest and exacerbated by lying flat, straining, or coughing.
- Vertebral tenderness at or near the level of compression
- Decreased motor function
- Decreased sensation to pain and touch
- Bowel and bladder dysfunction
- DTRs initially may be hyperreflexic but eventually diminish.

Diagnosis
- Diagnosis is based on clinical history and findings and one or more diagnostic studies, including spine films, bone scan, myelography, and MRI.

Treatment
- High-dose steroids (dexamethasone 100 mg/day IV) may be given.
- Radiation and surgery may be used.

Superior Vena Cava Syndrome
The superior vena cava is a large venous vessel that returns blood to the right side of the heart. It may be compressed externally by a mass, internally by a thrombus (as in cases of indwelling central venous catheters), or by direct invasion by the disease process.

Symptoms
- Dyspnea, cough, dysphagia, hoarseness, and chest pain
- Edema of the face and neck
- Engorgement of veins across the upper torso
- In severe obstruction, syncope and a decreased LOC

- Symptoms are worse upon rising in the morning or when bending forward.

Diagnosis
- Diagnosis is based on clinical history and findings, and is confirmed by chest film and venography.

Treatment
- Oxygen therapy if dyspnea or indicators of respiratory distress are present
- Chemotherapy and radiation are used if SVCS is caused by external compression.
- Fibrinolytic therapy with agents such as TPA to resolve thrombus obstruction secondary to a central venous catheter
- Specific surgical procedures such as stent placement or SVC bypass
- Diuretics to reduce edema of head and neck

Tumor Lysis Syndrome

TLS is caused most often by treatment or therapy that results in tumor cell death. As tumor cells are killed, levels of potassium, phosphate, and uric acid rise. Calcium levels will fall in response to the elevated phosphate levels.

Symptoms

Symptoms are listed in Table 14-1.
- Joint pain secondary to accumulation of uric acid
- Decreased renal function resulting from uric acid crystal formation
- Cardiac symptoms of tachycardia, hypotension, tall T waves, prolonged ST segment, and delayed conduction secondary to hypocalcemia and hyperkalemia.
- Hyperactive DTRs and muscle cramps

Diagnosis
- Diagnosis is based on serum electrolyte levels and the uric acid level.

Treatment
- IV hydration
- Diuretics, such as furosemide, to promote excretion of potassium in urine
- Potassium restriction in both IV fluids and diet
- Cation-exchange resins, such as Kayexalate, to reduce serum potassium level
- Calcium gluconate to correct hypocalcemia
- Regular insulin and glucose IV to facilitate the movement of potassium into the cells

- Sodium bicarbonate to reduce the likelihood of uric acid precipitation
- Phosphate-binding gels, such as aluminum hydroxide

NURSING SURVEILLANCE

1. Monitor the patient for complications of factor or blood replacement. Allergic reactions may range from wheezing, fever, chills, and hives, to dyspnea. Flushing, tachycardia, nausea, and headaches may occur if the drugs are infused too rapidly.
2. Monitor the patient for response to fluid administration. Fluid overload can occur quickly, especially in malignancy where radiation treatment has been administered to the mediastinum and chest. Hydration is a common treatment for oncologic emergencies (e.g., hypercalcemia, TLS, and cardiac tamponade). Fluid overload also can occur in SCA in cases of multiple pulmonary infarcts and pulmonary hypertension.
3. Monitor the patient for changes in the LOC.

EXPECTED PATIENT OUTCOMES
Hematologic Conditions
1. Factor activity levels are at least 50% (in cases of hemophilia).
2. The hemoglobin S level is 30% or less.
3. The LOC returns to baseline.
4. Seizure activity is diminished.
5. Pain diminishes.

Oncologic Conditions
1. Serum electrolyte levels normalize.
2. Pain diminishes.

DISCHARGE IMPLICATIONS
Hematologic Conditions
1. Teach prevention of acute episodes.
2. In SCA, avoid changes in temperature, hydration, and stressful situations.
3. In hemophilia, avoid injury (e.g., wear protective devices such as helmets and kneepads, as appropriate for activity) and use of products that contain aspirin. Home environments (e.g., playground areas) may need alteration to promote safety. Only electric razors should be used. Good dental hygiene may prevent the need for tooth extractions and subsequent bleeding.

4. Teach recognition of acute episodes. Hemophiliacs should be taught how to examine their urine for microscopic hematuria (using urine reagent strips). A tingling sensation may precede any objective signs of bleeding. A change in the LOC, vomiting, severe headache, mood changes, and gait changes may signal intracranial bleeding. Pallor, weakness, and restlessness may indicate internal bleeding.

5. Encourage health-care evaluation after what is perceived to be a "minor" injury. Major bleeding may occur hours after minor trauma.

6. Help the patient obtain a "Medic Alert" tag.

Oncologic Conditions

1. Teach prevention of acute episodes.
2. Encourage patient mobility and fluid intake of 3 to 4 L of fluid/day to prevent hypercalcemia.

REFERENCES

1. Platt A, Eckman JR, Beasley J, et al: Treating sickle cell pain: an update from the Georgia Comprehensive Sickle Cell Center, Atlanta GA, *J Emerg Nurs* August, 2002.
2. Otto K: *Oncology nursing,* ed 4, St Louis, 2001, Mosby.
3. Nevidojan B and Sowers K: *Cancer care,* 2000, Lippincott Williams and Wilkins.
4. Mara AM, Whedon MB: Hematologic problems. In Lewis SM, Heitkemper MM, Dirksen SR, eds: *Medical-surgical nursing,* St. Louis, 2002, Mosby.

chapter *15*

Neurologic Conditions

Steve Talbert

INTRODUCTION

Neurologic emergencies can result from trauma or a disease process that impairs brain or spinal cord function. Many neurologic emergencies result from risk-taking behaviors or noncompliance with medications such as antihypertensives or anticonvulsants.

FOCUSED NURSING ASSESSMENT

In the focused assessment, one should briefly reassess the ABCs for changes and necessary interventions. Nursing assessment should focus on ventilation, perfusion, cognition, and associated signs and symptoms.

Oxygenation and Ventilation

- Assess respiratory rate, depth, and rhythm. Abnormal respiratory patterns often are seen with lesions involving the pons and midbrain (respiratory centers of the brain). Refer to Table 15-1.
- Respiratory irregularities are a late sign of increased intracranial pressure (ICP). An abnormal respiratory rate and pattern indicates impending herniation of the respiratory centers located in the brainstem.
- Assess breath sounds for crackles and wheezes. Decreased breath sounds may indicate hypoventilation.
- Assess chest and abdominal movement.

Perfusion
Pulses

- Note the rate and quality of the pulses. Bradycardia can be seen in cases of neurogenic shock and is a late finding of increased ICP.

TABLE 15-1	**Abnormal Respiratory Patterns**
Patterns	**Characteristics**
Cheyne-Stokes	• Rhythmic waxing and waning in the depth and rate of the respirations followed by apnea • Lesions often are bilateral and involve the basal ganglia, thalamus, or hypothalamus.
Central neurogenic hyperventilation	• Respirations are increased in depth and rate. • Usually related to lesions in the midbrain or upper pons
Apneustic breathing	• The patient pauses 2 to 3 seconds after a full or prolonged inspiration. • The lesion is located in the lower pons.
Cluster breathing	• Clusters of irregular breaths with periods of apnea at irregular intervals • The lesion is located in the lower pons or upper medulla.
Biot's (ataxic) breathing	• The pattern is completely irregular and unpredictable with deep and shallow random breaths and pauses. • The lesion is located in the medulla.

Bradycardia related to unopposed parasympathetic nervous system stimulation occurs in cases of neurogenic shock.

Cardiac Rhythm
- Atrial and ventricular arrhythmias can occur with patients who have a subarachnoid hemorrhage.[1]

Blood Pressure
- Obtain a blood pressure (BP) reading. Hypotension is seen in cases of neurogenic shock.
- Hypertension is a late finding of increased ICP. As ICP rises, the blood pressure rises reflexively to maintain cerebral blood flow.
- Hypotension is a symptom of neurogenic shock secondary to loss of vasomotor tone below the level of the injury, which causes vasodilation.

Neurological Functioning
Level of Consciousness
- The level of consciousness (LOC) is the most important factor in the neurologic assessment.
- Assess the LOC with the Glasgow Coma Scale (see Reference Guides 10 and 16). The range of possible scores is 3 to 15. A score of 15 indicates a fully alert and oriented person. A score of 3 indicates a deep coma.
- Behavior changes, sleepiness, memory loss, or confusion may indicate decreased cerebral perfusion.

NURSING ALERT

Inform the physician immediately if there is a decrease in the score on the Glasgow Coma Scale. This may indicate an increase in ICP.

Pupils/Eye Movements
- Assess pupil size and reactivity to light. The millimeter scale often is used to record pupil size (Figure 15-1).
- When light is shined into the eye, the pupil should constrict immediately. Pupillary reaction is described as brisk, sluggish, nonreactive, or fixed.
- Pupils normally are of equal size; however, a few people have unequal pupils without any associated pathology. See Box 15-1

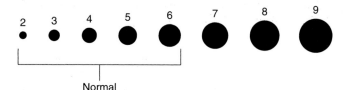

Normal

Figure 15–1 Pupil gauge in millimeters. (From Stillwell SB: *Mosby's critical care nursing reference,* ed 3, St Louis, 2002, Mosby.)

BOX 15-1 COMMON ABNORMAL PUPILLARY RESPONSES

Oculomotor Nerve Compression
Observation
One pupil (R) is larger than the other (L), which is of normal size. The dilated pupil (R) does not react to light, although the other pupil (L) reacts normally.

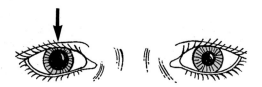

Meaning
A dilated, nonreactive (fixed) pupil indicates that the controls for pupillary constriction are not functioning. The parasympathetic fibers of the oculomotor nerve control pupillary constriction. The most common cause of interruption of this function is compression of the oculomotor nerve, usually against the tentorium or posterior cerebral artery. The compression of the oculomotor nerve against these structures is caused by a lesion, such as a hematoma, tumor, or cerebral edema, on the same side of the brain as the dilated pupil. This causes downward pressure so that the uncus of the temporal lobe herniates, trapping the oculomotor nerve between it and the tentorium.

Action
The nurse must check previous assessments to determine the past pupil size and reaction to light. If the dilated pupil is a new finding, it should immediately be reported to the physician because the process of rostral-caudal downward pressure must be treated without delay.

BOX 15-1 COMMON ABNORMAL PUPILLARY RESPONSES—cont'd

Changes also can be expected in the level of consciousness, motor function, and other parameters of the neurologic assessment.

Bilateral Diencephalic Damage

Observation

Upon examination, the pupils appear small but equal in size, and both react briskly to direct light, contracting when light is introduced and dilating when light is withdrawn.

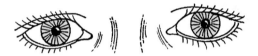

Meaning

The sympathetic pathway that begins in the hypothalamus is affected. Because both pupils are equal in size and respond equally to light, the damage is bilateral. Therefore it can be assumed that there is bilateral injury in the diencephalon (thalamus and hypothalamus). Because metabolic coma also can cause bilaterally small pupils that react to light, this diagnostic possibility must be explored and ruled out.

Action

The findings should be compared with previous assessments to determine whether this is a new development. One should consider the possibility of metabolic coma by reviewing blood electrolyte and blood glucose levels. For example, diabetic acidosis may cause a metabolic coma because of an excessive amount of glucose in the blood. The abnormal glucose level would be evident upon checking. A review of blood chemistry values is particularly important if the patient was a recent emergency admission, for whom an adequate history may not have been collected. If the small, reactive pupils are a new finding, this information should be reported.

Horner's Syndrome

Observation

One pupil (L) is smaller than the other (R), although both pupils react to light. The eyelid on the same side as the small pupil droops (ptosis). There may be a sweating deficiency (anhidrosis) on the

Continued

BOX 15-1   COMMON ABNORMAL PUPILLARY RESPONSES—cont'd

same side of the face as the ptosis. The collective symptoms of a small reactive pupil, ptosis, and anhidrosis are called Horner's syndrome.

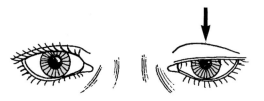

Meaning
An interruption of the ipsilateral sympathetic innervation to the pupil can be caused by hypothalamic damage (posterior or ventrolateral portion), a lesion involving the lateral medulla or the ventrolateral cervical spinal cord, and sometimes occlusion of the internal carotid artery. Downward displacement of the hypothalamus along with a unilateral Horner's syndrome may be an early sign of transtentorial herniation.

Action
● If this is a new finding, it should be reported.

Midbrain damage
Observation
● Both pupils are at midposition and are nonreactive to light.

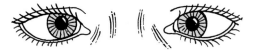

Meaning
When the pupils are midposition in size and nonreactive, neither the sympathetic nor parasympathetic innervation is operational. This finding often is associated with midbrain infarction or transtentorial herniation.

Action
The pupils should be evaluated in conjunction with other neurologic assessments. The change in pupil size and reaction should be reported if this represents a new finding.

BOX 15-1   COMMON ABNORMAL PUPILLARY RESPONSES—cont'd

Pontine Damage
Observation
Very small (pinpoint), nonreactive pupils are noted.

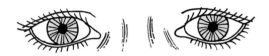

Meaning
This finding most often indicates hemorrhage into the pons, a grave
   occurrence because the pons controls many motor pathways and
   vital functions. Bilateral pinpoint pupils also may occur with
   opiate drug overdose, so this possibility should be considered
   and ruled out.

Action
Report this finding if it is new. The prognosis for patients with
   pontine damage is grave. Other changes in neurologic status,
   such as a decreased LOC and respiratory abnormalities, also
   would be expected.

Dilated Nonreactive Pupils
Observation
Both pupils are dilated and nonreactive (fixed).

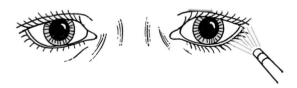

Meaning
This finding is characteristic of the terminal stages of severe anoxia,
   ischemia, and death. Because atropine-like drugs cause dilated

Continued

BOX 15-1   COMMON ABNORMAL PUPILLARY RESPONSES—cont'd

pupils, this possibility must be considered. An intact ciliospinal reflex can produce momentary bilateral dilation.

Action

Emergency action is necessary to reverse the anoxic state and prevent death. Oxygen therapy at high concentrations and a patent airway must be ensured to provide oxygen to the ischemic cerebral cells.

From Hickey JV: *The clinical practice of neurological and neurosurgical nursing*, ed 5, Philadelphia, 2003, Lippincott Williams & Wilkins, pp 174-175.

for a description of various pupil findings and their significance.

- Abnormal eye movements often occur with seizure activity.

Headache

- Headache is a symptom often associated with increased ICP caused by intracranial hemorrhage, cerebral edema, or an intracranial mass.

Gait

- A staggered gait, uncoordinated movements, and ataxia often are indicative of cerebellar dysfunction secondary to a stroke, TIA, or trauma.

Speech

- Slurred speech or difficulty expressing thoughts may indicate an impairment of the Broca's area in the frontal lobe.
- Suspect a stroke, a transient ischemic attack (TIA), or an intracranial mass if the patient has slurred speech or difficulty speaking.

Drainage

- Basal skull fractures can enter the paranasal air sinuses of the frontal bone or the middle ear within the temporal bone, resulting in a dural tear. Cerebrospinal fluid (CSF) then is able to leak through the dural tear and drain from an ear or the nose.

Motor

- Assess motor ability and strength, focusing on the arms and legs. Noting changes is important to identifying deterioration, improvement, or stabilization in the patient's condition.

- Motor strength on both sides should be compared.
- To assess the upper extremities, extend the middle and index fingers of your hands and ask the patient to squeeze with his or her hands. Crossing the index and middle fingers may help to reduce pain if the patient is expected to have a strong grasp. Hand grasps should be strong and equal. Next, have the patient attempt to move his or her shoulders, forearms, and wrists against resistance. To assess strength in the patient's lower extremities, have the patient flex and extend the upper leg, knee, and ankle on each side against gravity and against resistance. Instruct the patient to press his or her feet against your hands. The following scale can be used to measure motor strength and movement:
  0 = None
  1 = Trace
  2 = Not against gravity
  3 = Against gravity
  4 = Against some resistance
  5 = Against strong resistance
- For spinal cord injury (SCI) patients, the motor assessment helps identify the level of injury and assess the function of the corticospinal tract within the cord. Table 15-2 lists the levels of the spinal cord and their associated muscle functions.
- Abnormal flexion or extension may occur in cases of severe brain injury. Abnormal flexion (also known as decorticate posturing) presents as a rigid flexion of the upper extremities

TABLE 15-2   Motor Assessment of the Corticospinal Tract

Spinal Level	Motor Assessment
C5	Shoulder abduction
C5-C6	Elbow flexion
C7	Finger and elbow extension
C6-C7	Wrist dorsiflexion
C8	Thumb-finger pinch
L2-L4	Hip flexion
L5-S1	Knee flexion
L2-L4	Knee extension
L5	Foot dorsiflexion
S1	Foot plantar flexion

toward the center of the chest and extension of the lower extremities. Abnormal extension (also known as decerebrate posturing) presents with rigid extension of both the upper and lower extremities.

Sensation
- Assessing sensory function helps in identifying the level of spinal involvement for SCI patients.
- Start at the feet and systematically work upward, comparing both sides. Determine the patient's ability to detect light touch and pain (pinprick). Ask the patient to tell you when he or she feels the sensation.
- Record the highest level of function on each side of the body. Figure 15-2 matches the areas of sensation with their levels of the cord.
- Unilateral or bilateral abnormalities in sensation (e.g., numbness, tingling, or decreased sensation) or movement (e.g., weakness, paralysis, or posturing) may be associated with stroke, TIA, trauma, or decreased cerebral perfusion.

Skin
- Fever can be associated with lesions of the hypothalamus, increased ICP affecting the hypothalamus, central nervous system infections (meningitis or encephalitis), or status epilepticus.
- Hypothermia may occur in cases of neurogenic shock as a result of vasodilation and a loss of the ability to shiver below the level of the injury.

GI
- Vomiting can result from increased ICP caused by a mass, intracranial hemorrhage, or brain trauma.

LIFE SPAN ISSUES

1. Brain injury occurs most often among those 15 to 30 years old. Males are affected more often than females.
2. Home falls contribute significantly to the incidence of head trauma, particularly among the geriatric population.
3. Persons 16 to 30 years of age account for 60% of SCIs. Most of those affected are males.

INITIAL INTERVENTIONS

1. Maintenance of a patent airway is the highest priority. Assume that the head-injured patient has a cervical spine injury. Open the airway with techniques that require no movement of

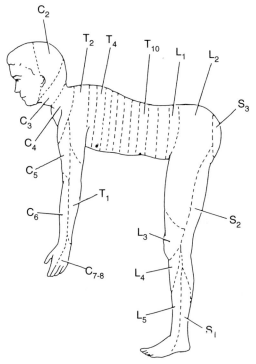

Figure 15–2 Arrangement of dermatomes is more easily understood when an individual is considered in quadruped (crouched) position. It is important to correlate the level of injury with the area of the body surface that is affected (dermatome). (Adapted from Zejdlik CP: *Management of spinal cord injury*, Boston, 1992, Jones & Bartlett.)

the head (e.g., jaw thrust). If endotracheal intubation is required, care should be taken to maintain neutral spinal alignment, which may require manual stabilization during the intubation procedure.

2. Head injuries should be treated based on the GCS score. Head injuries are rated as mild, moderate, or severe, and treatment centers on maintaining ABCs, performing neurologic evaluation, and providing intervention as follows:
   Treatment of mild head injury (GCS score 14 to 15)[2]:
   - Perform an ongoing neurologic evaluation.
   - The patient may be discharged or admitted.

Treatment of moderate head injury (GCS score 9 to 13)[3]:
- Perform a neurosurgical evaluation.
- Perform an ongoing neurologic evaluation.
- Obtain a CT examination of the head.
- Be prepared to intubate should neurologic status deteriorate.
- Prepare the patient for admission or transfer.

Treatment of severe head injury (GCS score ≤8)[1,4-22]:
- Prepare for endotracheal intubation (consider rapid sequence induction protocol; see Procedure 1).
- Obtain a neurosurgical consult.
- Obtain a CT examination of the head.
- Maintain adequate oxygen saturation (≥95%).
- Maintain an adequate mean arterial pressure (MAP) (>90 mm Hg).
- Maintain adequate cerebral perfusion pressure (CPP) as prescribed (usually 70 mm Hg in adults and 50 mm Hg in children).
- Control ventilation to maintain adequate oxygenation and a $PaCO_2$ of 30 to 35 mm Hg.

➤ NURSING ALERT ◄

Prophylactic use of hyperventilation should be avoided. Hyperventilation may be used acutely if signs of impending herniation are present. Other measures to improve cerebral perfusion (adequate oxygenation and adequate MAP) should accompany hyperventilation efforts. If hyperventilation is used, it should be used on a short-term basis only.

- Administer osmotic diuretic (mannitol) as an IV bolus (0.25 to 1 g/kg).
- Perform gastric decompression (oral or nasal gastric tube).
- Place an indwelling urinary catheter.
- Perform an ongoing neurologic evaluation.
- Prepare the patient for admission or transfer.
- Prepare for placement of an intraventricular catheter (IVC) to monitor ICP and CPP and to drain CSF.
- Sedate the patient as prescribed by the physician. Monitor BP closely because many sedatives may cause hypotension.
- The use of steroids has not proved beneficial in clinical studies, and their administration is not recommended.
- Ensure adequate ventilation by providing the appropriate amount of oxygen to meet the patient's needs. If cerebral

> **NURSING   ALERT**
>
> Any patient with an altered level of consciousness must be
> monitored carefully for airway compromise.

perfusion is compromised, the patient should receive 100%
oxygen until a lower oxygen concentration is determined to be
adequate. If ventilation is inadequate, assist the patient with a
bag-valve-mask device and 100% oxygen.

> **NURSING   ALERT**
>
> The two-person technique is the preferred method for use of a
> bag-valve-mask device. Airway adjuncts (preferably an oral
> airway and 2 nasal airways) are strongly recommended to
> facilitate ventilation with a bag-valve-mask device.

- Establish intravenous access for patients experiencing
  neurologic emergencies. Intravascular volume resuscitation
  and/or medication administration often are indicated.
- When appropriate, maintain spinal immobilization until a
  physician has ruled out a spinal cord injury. Patients should
  not be left on backboards for long periods of time, because
  this promotes decubitus formation.

> **NURSING   ALERT**
>
> Complete spinal immobilization requires a rigid cervical collar
> of appropriate size, head immobilization devices, tape or straps
> across the forehead, straps across the shoulders and hips and
> above the knees if the patient is on a backboard, and in-line
> spinal alignment.

- Have suction available at all times.
- Anticipate the need for the insertion of a ventricular drainage
  catheter for patients with signs and symptoms of increased
  ICP. The signs and symptoms of increased ICP include a
  decreased LOC, pupil changes, weakness, nausea, vomiting,
  headache, seizures, and an abnormal respiratory pattern.

- Anticipate the need for a computed tomography (CT) scan. Notify the CT scan technician.
- Nursing care priorities are listed in the table on p. 521.

PRIORITY DIAGNOSTIC TESTS

Laboratory Tests

ABG: A Pco_2 of 30 to 35 mm Hg should be maintained if the patient's GCS score is less than or equal to 8. Reduction of the Pco_2 results in vasoconstriction of the cerebral vessels, thereby reducing cerebral blood volume and ICP. Reducing the Pco_2 below 25 mm Hg is associated with cerebral ischemia, so Pco_2 should be monitored closely (e.g., via continuous capnography). Measures to reduce Pco_2 should be combined with other interventions directed at optimizing cerebral perfusion.[1,4]

Blood alcohol level: A high serum alcohol level may alter the LOC and reduce the patient's ability to cooperate during the examination and treatment.

Cerebrospinal fluid (CSF): CSF may be obtained via a lumbar puncture or intraventricular catheter (IVC) to assess color, white blood cell count, protein content, glucose content, and culture and sensitivity. The presence of more than 5 to 10 white blood cells/mm³ indicates an inflammatory process such as meningitis. Cloudy fluid indicates infection. CSF glucose normally is approximately 80% of the blood glucose level. A reduced CSF glucose level is suggestive of bacterial meningitis.

The normal protein count is 15 to 45 mg/100 ml. The protein count may be elevated with tumors, viral meningitis, and hemorrhage. A culture can be obtained to identify the invading organism. Sensitivity also can be determined to identify the most effective drug therapy. Activities to drain CSF should not be attempted before obtaining a head CT scan.

Complete blood count: Expect an increase in the white blood cell count with central nervous system (CNS) infections such as meningitis.

Electrolyte levels: Mannitol can cause electrolyte imbalances (especially hypokalemia). Vomiting can cause hypokalemia and other electrolyte imbalances.

Type and crossmatch: This is necessary if the patient has other system involvement such as chest or pelvic injuries. Patients do not become hypovolemic from a closed-head injury.

Urine and serum drug screen: Many drugs can alter the LOC and pupil size.

NURSING CARE PRIORITIES

Potential/Actual Problem	Causes	Signs and Symptoms	Interventions
1. Airway compromise	• Decreased LOC • Seizure activity	• Sonorous, irregular or shallow respirations • Inability to handle secretions	• Maintain a patent airway (jaw thrust, oral airway, nasopharyngeal airway, or intubation). • Provide suction for the patient as needed.
2. Impaired breathing	• Increased ICP affecting the respiratory centers of the brain • SCI with impairment of the diaphragm or intercostal muscles	• Irregular or shallow respirations • Use of accessory muscles	• Administer 100% oxygen. • Assist breathing with a bag-valve-mask device as needed. • Prepare to assist with intubation if the patient is hypoventilating or in respiratory distress.
3. Altered cerebral perfusion	• Increased ICP	• Altered LOC • Altered pupillary reaction	• Maintain PaCO$_2$ at 30 to 35 mm Hg if GCS score is less than 8. • Anticipate the need to insert a ventricular drainage catheter. • Closely monitor the patient's score on the Glasgow Coma Scale.
4. Safety	• Cerebral edema • Seizure activity • Noncompliance with anticonvulsants	• Signs of increasing ICP • Seizure activity	• Keep side rails up at all times. • Pad the side rails of the bed. • Have suction and oxygen available at all times. • Administer anticonvulsants as ordered by the physician.
5. Altered tissue peripheral perfusion	• Hypotension associated with neurogenic shock	• Hypotension • Bradycardia	• Insert two large-bore IVs. • Administer fluid bolus and vasopressors as ordered by the physician.

Radiographic Tests

CT scan: The CT scan is extremely useful in locating and diagnosing various cranial lesions such as abscesses, cysts, infarctions, hematomas, and tumors. IV radiopaque material (contrast) may be given to improve the clarity of images.

MRI: The MRI is efficient in identifying cerebral and spinal cord edema, CNS ischemia or areas of infarction, hemorrhage, and tumors in the brainstem, basal skull, and spinal cord.

Skull x-rays: Skull films may be used to rule out skull fractures. The films include anteroposterior and lateral views. Skull films generally are not recommended, as most patients with suspected skull fractures will undergo a head CT.

Spine x-rays: Cervical, thoracic, lumbar, and sacral views may be ordered to determine the presence of fractures and dislocations. C7 to T1 often is difficult to visualize in obese or heavily muscled patients. It may be necessary to pull the shoulders downward toward the feet while the x-ray examination is being conducted. The swimmer's view (one arm above the head) also can help in visualizing the cervical spine. An open-mouth view can be used to visualize the odontoid process, the upward extension of the body of C2.

CLINICAL CONDITIONS

Central Nervous System Infections

Suspect meningitis or a brain abscess with patients who have a recent history of infection involving the ears, sinuses, or respiratory tract.

Encephalitis[23]

Encephalitis is an inflammation of the brain caused by viruses, bacteria, or parasites. The etiology is most often viral.

Symptoms

- Fever
- Headache
- Stiff neck
- Changes in the LOC
- Hemiparesis
- Facial weakness
- Ataxia
- Nystagmus
- Generalized seizures

Diagnosis

- Diagnosis is based on symptoms and CSF analysis.

Treatment

- Reduce stimuli such as noise and lights.

- Administer analgesics and antipyretics.
- Initiate seizure precautions.
- Treat any increased ICP.
- There is no definitive drug treatment for viral encephalitis. Steroids may reduce cerebral edema. Prophylactic anticonvulsants often are used to prevent seizures.

Meningitis[23]

Meningitis is an inflammation of the meninges (coverings of the brain and spinal cord) as a result of viral or bacterial invasion.

Symptoms

- Fever
- Severe headache
- Changes in LOC
- Stiff neck
- Photophobia
- Seizure activity
- Increased ICP (because of cerebral exudate, cerebral edema, and hydrocephalus)
- Petechiae may be seen in meningococcal meningitis.
- Infants may have bulging fontanels, irritability, temperature instability, and poor feeding.
- Geriatric patients may experience only low-grade fever and confusion.

Diagnosis

- Diagnosis is based on history (a recent history of head trauma, ear infections, sinus infection, or respiratory illness), symptoms, and CSF analysis.

Treatment

- Maintain the ABCs.
- Initiate IV antibiotic therapy as soon as possible. Antibiotics used for bacterial meningitis may include penicillin, cefotaxime, or ceftriaxone. Ampicillin may be used for infants and children.
- Reduce stimuli such as noise and lights.
- Initiate seizure precautions.
- Administer antipyretics and analgesics.
- Use droplet precautions until bacterial meningitis has been ruled out.

Head Injuries
Basal Skull Fractures[24]

Basal skull fractures involve the base of the skull. The frontal and temporal bones often are affected. The fracture can be linear, comminuted, or depressed. Fractures involving the sinus areas often result in CSF leaks.

Symptoms
- Drainage from the ears or nose
- Periorbital ecchymosis (raccoon's eyes)
- Ecchymosis over the mastoid bone (Battle's sign; usually does not develop for 24 hours)
- Subconjunctival hemorrhage
- Hearing loss
- Agitation
- Headache
- Nausea and vomiting

Diagnosis
- Diagnosis is based on history, symptoms, results of a skull x-ray examination, and CT scan findings.
- The halo sign (blood encircled by a yellow stain on bed linens) is highly suggestive of a CSF leak. Most leaks resolve in 2 to 10 days.

Treatment
- Anticipate the need for prophylactic antibiotics if there is a CSF leak (prevent meningitis).
- Do not pack the ears or nose.
- Instruct the patient not to blow his or her nose.
- Ensure tetanus and diphtheria prophylaxis.
- Prepare for admission for observation.
- Monitor for symptoms of an epidural hematoma if the fracture involves the temporal bone.
- Monitor for increased ICP from a possible underlying tissue injury.

NURSING ALERT

Never insert a nasogastric tube in a patient with head or facial injuries with nasal drainage. The tube may enter the brain, resulting in damage and/or infection.

Concussion

Concussion is a transient, temporary loss of consciousness caused by an impact to the skull that injures the brain. Consciousness returns within minutes of the impact.

Symptoms

These symptoms may last several minutes to days.

- Temporary loss of consciousness
- Amnesia
- Headache
- Dizziness
- Drowsiness
- Irritability
- Visual disturbances

Diagnosis

- Diagnosis is based on history and symptoms.
- The result of a CT scan will be normal.

Treatment

- Monitor the patient for changes in neurologic status.
- Administer non-narcotic analgesics as ordered for headache.
- Give head-injury instructions if the patient is discharged from the ED.

Contusion

A contusion is a bruising of the brain. Edema of brain tissue is a concern.

Symptoms

- Symptoms are related to the amount of bruising and swelling and to the area involved.
- Symptoms may include an altered LOC, headache, nausea, vomiting, visual disturbances, seizures, and hemiparesis.

Diagnosis

- Diagnosis is based on a history of head trauma, symptoms, and CT scan findings.

Treatment

- Treat increased ICP and maintain a CPP of at least 70 mm Hg.
- Anticipate the need for anticonvulsants.
- Initiate seizure precautions.

Diffuse axonal injury

A diffuse axonal injury is a severe injury that results in widespread brain damage. Shearing forces disrupt axons in the cerebral white matter.

Symptoms

- A GCS score of 3 to 5
- Hypertension
- Hyperthermia
- Abnormal flexion or extension

Diagnosis

- Diagnosis is based on CT scan findings and symptoms.

Treatment
- Maintain adequate oxygenation and ventilation and prepare for intubation.
- Provide measures to control ICP and maintain CPP above 70 mm Hg.

Epidural Hematoma

An epidural hematoma results from bleeding between the skull and dura mater (outer meningeal layer). Many patients have an associated skull fracture. Often there is a fracture in the temporal bone with a tear in the meningeal artery or vein under the bone. Medications such as anticoagulants and oral contraceptives place the patient at increased risk for epidural hematoma.

Symptoms
- Initial loss of consciousness followed by a lucid interval that lasts a few hours. A rapid deterioration in the LOC then occurs. At least 15% of patients do not have a lucid interval.
- Headache
- Dilated pupil
- Hemiparesis
- Other symptoms of increased ICP may be present.

Diagnosis
- Diagnosis is based on history, symptoms, and CT scan findings.

Treatment
- Treat increased ICP and maintain CPP of at least 70 mm Hg.
- Prepare the patient for surgical evacuation of the clot.

⋙ NURSING ALERT ⋘

The ICP can increase quickly to a dangerous level with arterial epidural bleeds. Herniation is a concern. Death may result if surgery is delayed.

Increased Intracranial Pressure[25]/Herniation Syndrome
- Three main components (volumes) create ICP: brain tissue, blood volume, and CSF. Brain tissue constitutes 80% of the volume, while blood and CSF each account for 10%.
- An increase in one volume (e.g., edema or hyperemia) may increase ICP unless it is accompanied by an equal decrease in one or more of the other components.
- The body is able to compensate for mild to moderate ICP elevations (increased intracranial volume) by increasing absorption of CSF and shunting of cerebral blood volume.

- Rapid or significant elevations in ICP are not tolerated well and may result in herniation, the protrusion of brain tissue outside its normal compartment.[25] Herniation is a terminal event (Table 15-3).
- Cerebral edema, intracranial blood, tumors, and abscesses can increase brain tissue volume.
- Blood volume can be increased by hypercapnia and hyperthermia. Overproduction or decreased absorption of CSF can result in hydrocephalus.
- Conditions associated with hydrocephalus are tumors, subarachnoid hemorrhage, meningitis, and Guillain-Barré syndrome.
- Normal ICP is 0 to 14 mm Hg.
- Patients with an existing ventricular peritoneal shunt may present with signs and symptoms of increased ICP (e.g., mental status changes and vomiting) if the shunt becomes dislodged, infected, or blocked.

NURSING ALERT

Early recognition of elevated ICP and measures to maintain cerebral perfusion are important to maintaining brain function.

Symptoms[25]

- Symptoms vary with the magnitude of the insult, the time over which the insult occurs, and the effectiveness of compensatory mechanisms.
- Early symptoms of increased ICP may include the following:
  - Headache
  - Nausea and vomiting
  - Muscle weakness
  - Hemiplegia
  - Hemiparesis
- As cerebral perfusion is further compromised, symptoms will include the following:
  - A decrease in the LOC
  - Seizures
  - Pupillary changes (see Box 15-1, Common Abnormal Pupillary Responses)
- Severe increases in ICP may include the following:
  - Profoundly abnormal motor response (flexing, extending, or absent)
  - Changes in respiratory rate and depth (see Table 15-1)

TABLE 15-3 Herniation Syndrome

Type of Herniation	Description	Symptoms
Supratentorial cingulate herniation	An expanding lesion in one cerebral hemisphere causes pressure medially, placing pressure on the cingulate gyrus under the falx cerebri; displacement of the falx compresses the internal cerebral vein; if untreated, can lead to central or uncal herniation.	• Changes in mental status and level of consciousness • A midline shift may be present on the CT scan
Central (transtentorial) herniation	Downward displacement of the cerebral hemispheres, basal ganglia, diencephalon, and midbrain through the tentorial notch.	• *Early signs:* Decreased level of consciousness, small but reactive pupils, Cheyne-Stokes respirations, increased motor spasticity, hemiparesis • *Late signs:* Abnormal flexion or extension, pupils progress from unequal and nonreactive to dilated and fixed

Uncal (lateral transtentorial) herniation	A large lateral lesion at the middle fossa causes lateral displacement of the medial portion of the temporal lobe through the tentorial notch.	• *Early signs:* Ipsilateral dilated pupil resulting from pressure on the oculomotor nerve, contralateral hemiplegia or hemiparesis, decreased level of consciousness, respiratory changes • *Late signs:* Unconsciousness, bilateral fixed dilated pupils, abnormal flexion or extension, absence of oculocephalic and oculovestibular reflexes
Subtentorial herniation	Can occur by either upward displacement of the cerebellum through the tentorial notch or downward movement of brain tissue (brainstem or cerebellar tonsils) through the foramen magnum	• Abnormal respiratory patterns and pupillary changes depending on area involved, coma, hemiparesis, hemiplegia, and abnormal flexion or extension

- ○ Hypertension
- ○ Hyperthermia
- ○ Bradycardia
- ○ Loss of brainstem reflexes occurs, including the corneal, oculocephalic, and oculovestibular reflexes.
- ○ Test of the oculocephalic reflex (doll's-eye reflex) may be performed only by the physician after the cervical spine has been cleared by x-ray or CT scan. The physician performs the exam by rotating the head while holding the eyelids open. The reflex is intact if the eyes move in the opposite direction of the head.
- ○ Injecting cold water into the external auditory canal of the ear assesses the oculovestibular reflex. If the reflex is intact, the eyes will move toward the side being irrigated.

Diagnosis
- The preferred method for monitoring ICP is through an IVC (see Procedure 20).[5-7] The catheter affords the opportunity to drain CSF if necessary to maintain an appropriate ICP and facilitate CPP management.
- The CPP also may be calculated and monitored if an IVC has been inserted. The CPP is an indirect measurement of cerebral blood flow and is determined by subtracting the ICP from the mean arterial pressure (MAP) (CPP = MAP − ICP). Normal CPP is 60 to 100 mm Hg. A CPP of 70 mm Hg is generally the therapeutic goal.[4]
- Treatment for herniation is the same as for increased ICP. Specific treatment is based on the location and cause of the increased ICP.

Treatment[8]
- Maintain the head in a neutral position to facilitate venous outflow.
- Avoid extreme hip and knee flexion, which can increase intraabdominal and intrathoracic pressures.
- Use the logroll technique to position the patient.
- Suction the endotracheal tube for no longer than 10 to 15 seconds at a time. The number of suction passes should be limited to a maximum of two during any one suction episode.
- The position of the head of the bed is controversial. The head of the bed should be positioned based on the individual's ICP and CPP. If a spinal injury has been ruled out, elevating the head of the bed 30 to 45 degrees may facilitate venous outflow.

- Reduce loud stimuli and bright lights.
- Administer mannitol, sedatives, and paralytics, as ordered.

Subdural Hematoma

A subdural hematoma is a condition in which blood collects between the dura and arachnoid meningeal layers. The hematoma can result from the rupture of vessels or from bleeding from contused or lacerated areas. Anticoagulants and oral contraceptives place the patient at increased risk for subdural hematomas. Subdural hematomas are common in the geriatric population. There are three categories: acute, subacute, and chronic.

- Acute: associated with major cerebral trauma. Symptoms occur within 48 hours.
- Subacute: associated with less severe contusions. Symptoms appear within 2 days to 2 weeks.
- Chronic: symptoms appear within 2 weeks to several months. Chronic hematomas are seen in patients who fall frequently because of alcohol abuse.

Symptoms
- Headache (which gradually worsens)
- Drowsiness
- Confusion
- Slow thought processes
- Hemiparesis (late sign)
- Seizures

Diagnosis
- Diagnosis is based on history, symptoms, and CT scan findings.

Treatment
- Treat increased ICP.
- Administer nonnarcotic and nonaspirin analgesics.
- Small hematomas rarely require surgery because they often are absorbed.
- Larger hematomas require surgical evacuation.

Seizures

Seizures are produced by intermittent, sudden, massive neuronal discharge (electrical activity) in various parts of the brain.[25] The clinical manifestations depend on the type.

Focal (Jacksonian) Seizure[25]

Symptoms
Focal (Jacksonian) seizures begin with slow, repetitive jerking of a body part that increases in strength and rate over a period of 5 to 15 seconds.

Diagnosis
- Diagnosis is based on history and symptoms.

Treatment
- Protect the patient from injury.
- Anticipate the need for anticonvulsants.

Generalized Tonic-Clonic (Grand Mal)

Symptoms
- Tonic phase: sudden loss of consciousness with rigidity of the trunk and extremities
- Clonic phase: violent rhythmic muscular contractions
- Apnea and cyanosis often occur.
- The seizure lasts approximately 2 to 5 minutes.
- Afterward, the patient may experience a headache, confusion, weakness, and motor or sensory deficits, which may persist for minutes to hours. These symptoms are commonly known as the postictal phase of a seizure.

Diagnosis
- Diagnosis is based on history (tonic-clonic seizures may occur with tumors, head injuries, overdoses, infections, electrolyte imbalances, ventriculoperitoneal shunt malfunction, febrile illness with children, subtherapeutic anticonvulsant levels, or hypoxic events) and symptoms.

Treatment
- Turn the patient to the side to facilitate drainage of secretions.
- If the cause of the seizure is unknown, administer Narcan as ordered. Dextrose 50% (dextrose 25% for children) may be administered *if* a finger-stick blood glucose test reveals hypoglycemia.
- Pad side rails to prevent injury. Keep the bed in a low position.
- Establish IV access for medication administration.
- Administer anticonvulsants such as diazepam, lorazepam, and phenytoin as ordered. Phenobarbital is used frequently for children.
- Administer acetaminophen 10 to 15 mg/kg for the febrile child.
- Carefully observe and record the activity associated with the seizure.

Petit Mal Seizures[25]

Petit mal seizures generally occur with children who are 4 to 12 years of age.

Symptoms
There is an abrupt cessation of activity and a glassy stare (the child may stare straight ahead for 5 to 30 seconds). The child resumes activity after the seizure.

Diagnosis
Diagnosis is based on history and symptoms.

Treatment
Administer anticonvulsant medication as prescribed by
a physician.

Status Epilepticus

Symptoms
- Status epilepticus is defined as continuous seizures or seizures
  that occur at a frequency that prevents the patient from fully
  recovering from one seizure before having another.[26]

Diagnosis
- Based on history and examination
- Common causes include the sudden withdrawal of
  anticonvulsants, subtherapeutic levels of anticonvulsants,
  meningitis, encephalitis, hypoxia, or withdrawal from
  alcohol.

Treatment
- The treatment is the same as for generalized tonic-clonic
  seizures.

Spinal Injuries[27-29]

Motor vehicle crashes are the most common cause of SCIs.
Respiratory assessment is extremely important for patients with
cervical spine injuries. An injury at C4 or above will impair
phrenic nerve innervation and will result in paralysis of the
diaphragm. In these cases, air movement will be inadequate and
mechanical ventilation will be necessary. Injuries involving T1 to
T6 spare the diaphragm but impair the intercostal muscles,
placing the patient at increased risk for respiratory problems.
Injuries involving T6 to T12 may impair the abdominal muscles
and reduce the ability to generate a cough.

Autonomic Hyperreflexia[30]

Autonomic hyperreflexia (also known as autonomic dysreflexia)
is a serious hypertensive emergency that arises in the postacute
phase of SCI. This condition occurs after reflex activity has
returned in patients who have injuries at or above T6. Autonomic
hyperreflexia is caused by noxious stimuli that result in mass
reflex stimulation of the sympathetic nerves below the level of the
injury. Causes of noxious stimuli include: bladder distention,
constipation, fecal impaction, cystitis, urinary calculi, pressure
ulcers, and stimulation from skin lesions. If left untreated, this
condition can lead to a cerebrovascular accident (CVA), seizure
activity, or myocardial infarction.

Symptoms
- Sudden hypertension is a primary symptom (i.e., systolic BP as high as 240 to 300 mm Hg); there may be a significant rise in the patient's BP when compared with usual baseline.
- Anxious appearance
- Pounding headache
- Blurred vision
- Flushed face and neck
- Profuse sweating above level of injury
- Nasal congestion
- Nausea

Diagnosis
- Diagnosis is based on a history of previous SCI and on symptoms.

Treatment
- Treatment is directed toward removing the noxious stimuli and lowering the BP.
- If a urinary catheter is in place, attempt to irrigate if a plug or obstruction is suspected.
- Replace the catheter if irrigation does not remove the obstruction.
- Other treatment measures that should be considered include digital removal of any fecal impaction and removal of pressure from areas of irritated or broken skin.
- Elevate the head of the bed and administer an antihypertensive as ordered by the physician.

Cord Syndromes[27-29]

See Figures 15-3 to 15-5.

Diagnosis
- Diagnosis is based on a history of spinal trauma and on symptoms.

Treatment
- Maintain spinal immobilization.
- Administer 100% oxygen.
- Initiate two large-bore IVs.
- Insert a nasogastric tube and urinary catheter.
- Administer IV methylprednisolone.
- Assist with the application of cervical skeletal traction or the halo immobilization device.

Cord Transection

Complete transection of the spinal cord results in spinal and neurogenic shock with a complete loss of motor, sensory, reflex, and autonomic function below the level of the injury. The level of the injury influences the severity of spinal shock. Injuries above

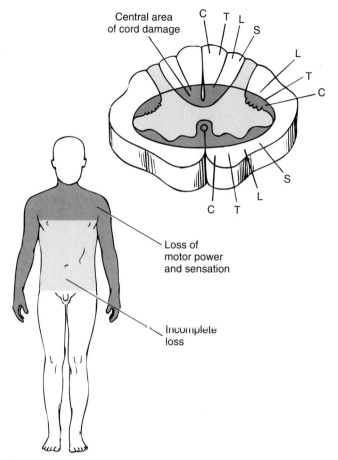

Central area
of cord damage

Loss of
motor power
and sensation

Incomplete
loss

Figure 15–3 Central cord syndrome. A cross section of the cord shows central damage and the associated motor and sensory loss. C, Cervical; T, thoracic; L, lumbar; S, sacral. (Modified from Hickey JV: *The clinical practice of neurological and neurosurgical nursing,* Philadelphia, 1992, JB Lippincott.)

T6 disrupt sympathetic nervous system activity below the level of the injury. Thus there is unopposed parasympathetic nervous system activity. The extent of the loss of function is less with partial cord transections. Varying degrees of spinal shock may be seen with cord injuries resulting from contusions, compression, lacerations, and hemorrhage.

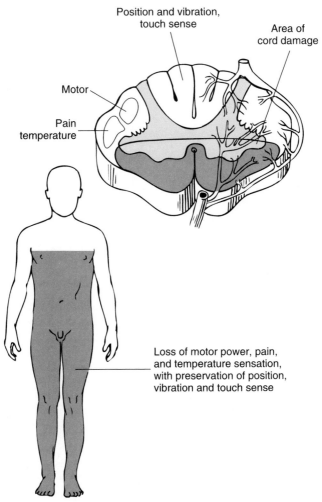

Position and vibration, touch sense

Area of cord damage

Motor

Pain temperature

Loss of motor power, pain, and temperature sensation, with preservation of position, vibration and touch sense

Figure 15–4   Anterior cord syndrome. Cord damage and associated motor and sensory loss. (Modified from Hickey JV: *The clinical practice of neurological and neurosurgical nursing,* Philadelphia, 1992, JB Lippincott.)

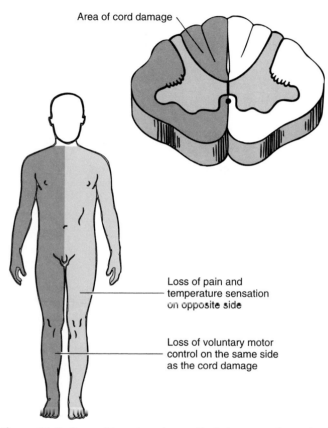

Figure 15-5 Brown-Séquard syndrome. Cord damage and associated motor and sensory loss. (Modified from Hickey JV: *The clinical practice of neurological and neurosurgical nursing,* Philadelphia, 1992, JB Lippincott.)

Symptoms
- Loss of sensation below the level of the injury
- Flaccid paralysis below the level of the injury
- Hypotension
- Vasodilation below level of injury
- Bradycardia
- Lack of sweating below the level of injury

- Loss of all spinal reflexes below the level of injury
- Atonic bladder and bowel

Diagnosis
- Physical assessment
- Evidence of injury on MRI and spine films

Treatment[28,29]
- Maintain spinal immobilization.
- Maintain a patent airway.
- Prepare to intubate patients who have cervical cord injuries above C4.
- Administer 100% oxygen.
- Apply two large-bore IVs with Ringer's lactate or normal saline.
- Maintain systolic BP of at least 80 to 90 mm Hg. Mental status and urine output are useful parameters in evaluating perfusion.
- Administer an IV fluid bolus if BP is less than 90 mm Hg or is inadequate to maintain perfusion.
- Titrate vasopressor agents such as dopamine if IV fluids are not successful in maintaining BP.
- Initiate cardiac monitoring.
- Treat bradycardia with atropine.
- Insert a nasogastric tube to reduce the risk of vomiting and aspiration.
- Insert a urinary catheter to monitor urine output.
- Implement measures to keep the patient warm (vasodilation and a lack of the ability to shiver can reduce body temperature).
- Assist with the application of cervical skeletal traction.
  A general rule is to use 5 lb of weight for each level of injury beginning with C1 (e.g., a fracture of C3 would require 15 lb of weight). Weights should be free hanging.

Vascular Injuries
Hemorrhagic Stroke and Injury[27]
- Subarachnoid hemorrhage is the most common hemorrhagic stroke. This condition, a sudden bleeding into the subarachnoid space, most often results from the rupture of an aneurysm.[7] An aneurysm is an outpouching of the wall of a blood vessel. Other causes include severe brain injury and the rupture of an arteriovenous malformation.

Symptoms
- Sudden and severe headache
- Sudden transient loss of consciousness (occurs in 45% of all subarachnoid hemorrhage patients)
- Nausea

- Vomiting
- Stiff neck
- Photophobia
- Signs of increased ICP
- Elevated temperature
- Elevated blood pressure (BP)

Diagnosis
- Diagnosis is based on symptoms and CT scan findings.

Treatment[31,32]
- To prevent further bleeding, treatment is geared toward controlling the BP until the patient goes to surgery (1 to 3 days after hemorrhage).
- The patient must have bed rest.
- The patient should remain in a quiet environment.
- Maintain systolic BP at no more than 150 mm Hg. Systolic pressures above this level can be treated with hydralazine or nitroprusside.
- Use anticonvulsants as prophylaxis against seizures if prescribed by the physician.
- Use analgesics to control any headaches.
- Monitor the patient for complications such as diabetes insipidus.
- Treat increased ICP.

Ischemic Stroke[33]

Ischemic stroke is a condition in which a blood vessel supplying the brain is occluded. The majority of ischemic strokes are caused by blood clots that develop within the brain artery itself (cerebral thrombosis). Ischemic strokes also occur when clots arise elsewhere in the body and migrate to the brain (embolic stroke). The result is ischemia to the cerebral tissue. TIAs, hypertension, hypercholesterolemia, hyperlipidemia, diabetes mellitus, cigarette smoking, and alcoholism all are considered risk factors for strokes. Other risk factors for the development of cerebral emboli include a history of atrial fibrillation and medications such as anticoagulants and oral contraceptives.

Symptoms
- Box 15-2, Correlation of Cerebral Artery Involvement and Common Manifestations, describes symptoms based on the cerebral artery occluded.

Diagnosis
- Diagnosis is based on history or risk factors for stroke, on symptoms, and on the results of diagnostic procedures, including a CT scan, angiography, and carotid studies.
- The CT scan may be normal initially.

BOX 15-2 CORRELATION OF CEREBRAL ARTERY INVOLVEMENT AND COMMON MANIFESTATIONS

Internal Carotid Artery

- Contralateral paresthesia (abnormal sensations) and hemiparesis (weakness) of arm, face, and leg
- Eventual complete contralateral hemiplegia (paralysis) and hemianesthesia (loss of sensation)
- Visual blurring or changes, hemianopsia (loss of half of visual field), repeated attacks of blindness in the ipsilateral eye
- Dysphasia with dominant hemisphere involvement

Anterior Cerebral Artery

- Mental impairment such as perseveration, confusion, amnesia, and personality changes
- Contralateral hemiparesis or hemiplegia with leg loss greater than arm loss
- Sensory loss over toes, foot, and leg
- Ataxia (motor uncoordination), impaired gait, incontinence, and akinetic mutism

Middle Cerebral Artery

- Level of consciousness varies from confusion to coma.
- Contralateral hemiparesis or hemiplegia with face and arm loss greater than leg loss
- Sensory impairment over same areas of hemiplegia
- Aphasia (inability to express or interpret speech) or dysphasia (impaired speech) with dominant hemisphere involvement
- Homonymous hemianopsia (loss of vision on the same side of both visual fields) and inability to turn eyes toward the paralyzed side

Posterior Cerebral Artery

- Contralateral hemiplegia with sensory loss
- Confusion, memory involvement, and receptive speech deficits with dominant hemisphere involvement
- Homonymous hemianopsia

Vertebrobasilar Artery

- Dizziness, vertigo, nausea, ataxia, and syncope
- Visual disturbances, nystagmus, diplopia, field deficits, and blindness
- Numbness and paresis (face, tongue, mouth, one or more limbs), dysphagia (inability to swallow), and dysarthria (difficulty in articulation)

From Stillwell SB: *Mosby's critical care nursing reference,* St Louis, 2002, Mosby.

Treatment[33]

The goals are to restore cerebral perfusion and minimize loss of cerebral function. Priorities of care include:

- Support of airway and ventilation with supplemental oxygen administration
- Maintain adequate circulating volume and perfusion pressure. Antihypertensives should be avoided unless the systolic BP is greater than 220 mm Hg or the diastolic BP is greater than 120 mm Hg. Avoid medications that cause a precipitous reduction in BP.
- Reduction of fever if present
- Rule out hypoglycemia as a cause of neurologic dysfunction. Diabetes mellitus is a risk factor for stroke.
- Other interventions may include:
  - Anticoagulant therapy to reduce further development of thrombi
  - Treat increased ICP as necessary.
  - Supportive therapy, such as support for flaccid limbs and proper body alignment, should be implemented.
  - Elevate the head of the bed to facilitate the drainage of oropharyngeal secretions.
  - Thrombolytics[33-35] should be considered for patients who present to the ED within 3 hours of the onset of symptoms. A CT scan of the head should be obtained within 25 minutes of arrival at the ED to rule out hemorrhagic stroke. Hypertension (systolic BP >185 or diastolic BP >110) should be controlled *before* administration of fibrinolytics. One to two inches of nitropaste or one to two doses of 10 to 20 mg of labetalol may reduce the BP. Heparin *should not* be given before or 24 hours after thrombolytic administration.

NURSING SURVEILLANCE

Monitor the trend of the following:

- Vital signs
- GCS score
- Pupil size and reactivity to light
- ICP and CPP
- Motor and sensory function
- Urine output

EXPECTED PATIENT OUTCOMES

1. Patent airway will be maintained
2. Bilateral equal breath sounds

3. Systolic BP between 80 and 150 mm Hg or as needed to maintain perfusion
4. Heart rate between 60 and 100 beats/min
5. Equal and reactive pupils
6. No deterioration in the LOC
7. ICP of 0 to 15 mm Hg
8. CPP of 70 to 100 mm Hg
9. Urine output of at least 30 ml/hr in adults, 1 to 2 mg/kg in children
10. Patient will remain normothermic
11. Absence of seizure activity

DISCHARGE IMPLICATIONS

- Instruct on the importance of medication (anticonvulsant) compliance.
- Teach geriatric patients to be aware of fall hazards: rugs, slick floors, similarly colored floors and walls (contrasting colors are better), and stairways.
- Emphasize the hazards of drinking alcohol before or during driving or swimming.
- Encourage helmet use when participating in recreational and sports activities.
- Give discharge head-injury instructions: Patient should return to the ED for the following signs and symptoms:
  - Drowsiness or lethargy (Wake patient every 2 hours for the first 24 hours. The patient should be capable of being aroused to a normal state of alertness.)
  - Forceful vomiting or vomiting more than three times
  - Pupil changes
  - Confusion
  - Vision changes
  - Difficulty with coordination
  - Severe headache
  - Slurred speech

  Patient should avoid alcohol or sedative medications for 24 hours.

REFERENCES

1. The Brain Trauma Foundation, the American Association of Neurological Surgeons, the Joint Section on Neurotrauma and Critical Care. Hyperventilation, *J Neurotrauma* 17 (6-7):513-520, 2000.
2. Cushman JG, Agarwal N, Fabian TC, et al: Practice management guidelines for the management of mild traumatic brain injury: the EAST practice management guidelines work group, *J Trauma* 51 (5):1016-1026, 2001.

3. Fearnside M and McDougall P: Moderate head injury: a system of neurotrauma care, *Aust N Z J Surg* 68 (1):58-64, 1998.

4. The Brain Trauma Foundation, the American Association of Neurological Surgeons, the Joint Section on Neurotrauma and Critical Care: Guidelines for cerebral perfusion pressure, *J Neurotrauma* 17 (6-7):507-511, 2000.

5. The Brain Trauma Foundation, the American Association of Neurological Surgeons, the Joint Section on Neurotrauma and Critical Care: Indications for intracranial pressure monitoring, *J Neurotrauma* 17 (6-7):479-491, 2000.

6. The Brain Trauma Foundation, the American Association of Neurological Surgeons, the Joint Section on Neurotrauma and Critical Care: Recommendations for intracranial pressure monitoring technology, *J Neurotrauma* 17 (6-7):497-506, 2000.

7. The Brain Trauma Foundation, the American Association of Neurological Surgeons, the Joint Section on Neurotrauma and Critical Care: Intracranial pressure treatment threshold, *J Neurotrauma* 17 (6-7):493-495, 2000.

8. The Brain Trauma Foundation, the American Association of Neurological Surgeons, the Joint Section on Neurotrauma and Critical Care: Critical pathway for the treatment of established intracranial hypertension, *J Neurotrauma* 17 (6-7):537-538, 2000.

9. The Brain Trauma Foundation, the American Association of Neurological Surgeons, the Joint Section on Neurotrauma and Critical Care: Age, *J Neurotrauma* 17 (6-7):573-581, 2000.

10. The Brain Trauma Foundation, the American Association of Neurological Surgeons, the Joint Section on Neurotrauma and Critical Care: Computed tomography scan features, *J Neurotrauma* 17 (6-7):597-627, 2000.

11. The Brain Trauma Foundation, the American Association of Neurological Surgeons, the Joint Section on Neurotrauma and Critical Care: Glasgow coma scale score, *J Neurotrauma* 17 (6-7):563-571, 2000.

12. The Brain Trauma Foundation, the American Association of Neurological Surgeons, the Joint Section on Neurotrauma and Critical Care: Hypotension, *J Neurotrauma* 17 (6-7):591-595, 2000.

13. The Brain Trauma Foundation, the American Association of Neurological Surgeons, the Joint Section on Neurotrauma and Critical Care: Initial management, *J Neurotrauma* 17 (6-7):463-469, 2000.

14. The Brain Trauma Foundation, the American Association of Neurological Surgeons, the Joint Section on Neurotrauma and Critical Care: Methodology, *J Neurotrauma* 17 (6-7):561-562, 2000.

15. The Brain Trauma Foundation, the American Association of Neurological Surgeons, the Joint Section on Neurotrauma and Critical Care: Nutrition, *J Neurotrauma* 17 (6-7):539-547, 2000.

16. The Brain Trauma Foundation, the American Association of Neurological Surgeons, the Joint Section on Neurotrauma and Critical Care: Pupillary diameter and light reflex, *J Neurotrauma* 17 (6-7):583-590, 2000.

17. The Brain Trauma Foundation, the American Association of Neurological Surgeons, the Joint Section on Neurotrauma and Critical Care: Resuscitation of blood pressure and oxygenation, *J Neurotrauma* 17 (6-7):471-478, 2000.

18. The Brain Trauma Foundation, the American Association of Neurological Surgeons, the Joint Section on Neurotrauma and Critical Care: Role of

antiseizure prophylaxis following head injury, *J Neurotrauma* 17 (6-7):549-553, 2000.

19. The Brain Trauma Foundation, the American Association of Neurological Surgeons, the Joint Section on Neurotrauma and Critical Care: Role of steroids, *J Neurotrauma* 17 (6-7):531-535, 2000.

20. The Brain Trauma Foundation, the American Association of Neurological Surgeons, the Joint Section on Neurotrauma and Critical Care: Trauma systems, *J Neurotrauma* 17 (6-7):457-462, 2000.

21. The Brain Trauma Foundation, the American Association of Neurological Surgeons, the Joint Section on Neurotrauma and Critical Care: Use of barbiturates in the control of intracranial hypertension, *J Neurotrauma* 17 (6-7):527-530, 2000.

22. The Brain Trauma Foundation, the American Association of Neurological Surgeons, the Joint Section on Neurotrauma and Critical Care: Use of mannitol, *J Neurotrauma* 17 (6-7):521-525, 2000.

23. Padgett K: Alterations of neurologic function in children. In McCance KL and Huether SE, eds: *Pathophysiology: the biologic basis for disease in adults and children*, ed 4, St Louis, 2002, Mosby, pp 566-596.

24. Samii M and Tatagiba M: Skull base trauma: diagnosis and management, *Neurol Res* 24 (2):147-156, 2002.

25. Boss BJ: Concepts of neurologic dysfunction. In McCance KL and Huether SE, eds: *Pathophysiology: the biologic basis for disease in adults and children*, ed 4, St Louis, 2002, Mosby, pp 438-486.

26. Lowenstein DH and Alldredge BK: Status epilepticus, *N Engl J Med* 338 (14):970-976, 1998.

27. Boss BJ: Alterations of neurologic function. In McCance KL and Huether SE, eds: *Pathophysiology: the biologic basis for disease in adults and children*, ed 4, St Louis, 2002, Mosby, pp 487-549.

28. Buckley DA and Guanci MM: Spinal cord trauma, *Nurs Clin North Am* 34 (3):661-687, 1999.

29. Belanger E and Levi AD: The acute and chronic management of spinal cord injury, *J Am Coll Surg* 190 (5):603-618, 2000.

30. Acute management of autonomic dysreflexia: individuals with spinal cord injury presenting to health-care facilities, *J Spinal Cord Med* 25 suppl 1:S67-S88, 2002.

31. Tuhrim S: Management of hemorrhagic stroke, *Curr Cardiol Rep* 4 (2):158-163, 2002.

32. Butcher K and Laidlaw J: Current intracerebral haemorrhage management, *J Clin Neurosci* 10 (2):158-167, 2003.

33. Adams HP Jr, Adams RJ, Brott T, et al: Guidelines for the early management of patients with ischemic stroke: a scientific statement from the Stroke Council of the American Stroke Association, *Stroke* 34 (4):1056-1083, 2003.

34. Hickenbottom SL and Barsan WG: Acute ischemic stroke therapy, *Neurol Clin* 18 (2):379-397, 2000.

35. Lang ES: Evidence-based emergency medicine. Use of thrombolytic therapy in patients with acute ischemic stroke, *Ann Emerg Med* 39 (3):296-298, 2002.

chapter 16

Obstetric and Gynecologic Conditions

Kelly Gandee

INTRODUCTION

When a patient presents to the emergency department (ED) with a chief complaint of vaginal bleeding, the nurse should assess the patient to determine the cause of the bleeding. Potential etiologies of vaginal bleeding include: pregnancy, menstrual cycle disturbances related to endocrine changes, systemic problems such as a hematologic disorder, use of anticoagulants, and traumatic injury.

A pertinent history and primary assessment should be obtained. The history should include questions about the nature of vaginal bleeding, which may help determine the etiology of the gynecologic and/or obstetric problem. The primary assessment should encompass the initial vital signs and general observations.

FOCUSED NURSING ASSESSMENT (OBSTETRIC CONDITIONS)

To effectively assess abnormal clinical signs in pregnancy, the nurse must be aware of normal physiologic changes in pregnancy.

Cardiovascular
- Increased heart rate caused by a state of hypervolemia. Heart rate can increase by 10 to 20 beats per minute.
- Decreased blood pressure caused by hormonal changes and adaptive changes that occur in the cardiovascular system.
- Anemia resulting from an increase in plasma volume

Respiratory
- Increased respiratory rate
- Hyperventilation and mild respiratory alkalosis
- Vascularity of the upper respiratory passages increases, which can cause epistaxis.

Abdominal
- Decrease in gastric motility, delayed gastric emptying time, and relaxation of the gastroesophageal sphincter predisposes the pregnant patient to aspiration in the second and third trimesters.

Urinary
- Increased urination resulting from an increase in glomerular filtration rate and compression of the bladder by the uterus.
- The bladder is more susceptible to injury because of anatomic changes.

NURSING ALERT

Because of the normal physiologic changes that occur during pregnancy, the patient will not demonstrate the classic signs and symptoms of hypovolemic shock until the shock state is advanced. "Normal vital signs" may indicate a shunting of blood from the uterus to maintain core maternal body functions, causing fetal deterioration. Changes in fetal activity and fetal heart rate may be the first signs of maternal hypovolemia.

Ventilation
Breath Sounds
- Pulmonary edema can occur rapidly in a patient who has preeclampsia or who receives fluid resuscitation.
- Coarse or fine crackles may be auscultated.

Perfusion
Blood Pressure and Pulse
- Tachycardia is a normal finding in pregnancy and therefore may mask the signs and symptoms of hypovolemia. Maternal hypervolemia allows the pregnant woman to tolerate acute blood loss of up to 15% without a major change in blood pressure and heart rate.
- Hypotension may be present related to hypovolemia; hypertension may be related to pregnancy-induced vascular changes.
- A single systolic blood pressure (BP) reading of 140 mm Hg or greater before 20 weeks' gestation indicates a higher-than-normal risk of pregnancy-induced hypertension, preeclampsia, and premature delivery.[1]
- A systolic BP of at least 140 mm Hg and/or a diastolic BP of 90 mm Hg or higher on two occasions, 6 hours apart after the 20th week of pregnancy is the criteria for a diagnosis of hypertension in pregnancy.[2,3]
- A systolic BP greater than 160 mm Hg or a diastolic BP greater than 109 mm Hg for at least 6 hours is considered an emergency, and hydralazine, labetalol, or nifedipine should be administered.[2,3]

Fetal Heart Rate (FHR)
- The FHR may increase or decrease in situations in which fetal hypoxia is occurring, such as placenta previa, abruptio placentae, uterine rupture, sepsis, and preeclampsia.

NURSING ALERT

Fetal heart tones must be assessed, although they may not be audible in the first trimester.

Assessment of Fetal Heart Tones (FHTs)[4]
Supplies and equipment
- Fetoscope with tubing <10 inches long or Doppler ultrasound
- Water-soluble ultrasound gel

Recommended technique
1. Ensure a quiet, private environment.
2. The patient should void before auscultation of FHTs.
3. The patient may be supine, or if past 28 weeks' gestation, a small rolled towel may be placed under the right hip to tilt her slightly to her left side.
5. If using Doppler ultrasound, apply a small amount of gel to the end of the instrument.

6. If using a fetoscope, place the padded cone on the woman's abdomen just above the pubic bone and the headpiece solidly against the forehead.
7. Exert a little pressure as the instrument is placed immediately above the pubic bone.
8. Slowly rotate it 360 degrees until the fetal heart rate is heard.
9. If nothing is heard, move the instrument 1 cm at a time up toward the umbilicus until the position is halfway between the pubic bone and the umbilicus. If the heart beat is not yet heard, move 1 cm to one side of the midline, and proceed back down toward the pubic bone. If the FHTs still are not heard, do the same on the opposite side.
10. Rotate the instrument at each new position because it must be directed at the fetal heart.
11. Count the FHTs for 15 seconds and multiply by four to obtain the rate per minute.
12. Document the fetal heart rate (FHR) rate on the record.
13. In late pregnancy, also chart the location on the woman's abdomen at which FHTs were heard.
14. If no FHTs are heard with Doppler ultrasound by 13 weeks or with a fetoscope by 20 weeks, a sonogram should be obtained to confirm fetal viability.

Sexuality

- Obtain a brief reproductive history and investigate chief complaint.
- Determine the type of contraceptives used and the patient's sexual history. Vaginal bleeding has been associated with the use of intrauterine devices and also may occur with some sexually transmitted infections (STIs).
- Ascertain the type and amount of vaginal discharge. Some STIs may be associated with vaginal discharge.
- Determine the date of last menstrual period. Irregular menstrual cycles often are a sign of dysfunctional uterine bleeding. Assess reproductive history by obtaining the number of pregnancies (gravidity), live births (parity), and abortions (spontaneous and elective). If the patient is pregnant, the estimated date of confinement (EDC) or due date should be ascertained.
- Assess the amount of vaginal bleeding. Severe bleeding is defined as soaking more than 8 pads or super tampons in an 8-hour period.[5] Bleeding may be associated with self-induced abortion attempts. Document the number of pads/tampons used per hour.

- Question the patient about use of anticoagulants, hormones, or oral contraceptives, as these may induce vaginal bleeding.
- Passing of blood clots or tissue (hamburger-looking substance) is associated with miscarriage.
- Assess the fetal heart rate.
- By pelvic exam, assess the percentage of effacement, centimeters of dilation, and station of the fetus.
- Assess the status of the amniotic fluid membrane (intact or ruptured) in the pregnant patient. If membranes have ruptured, document color of fluid.
- Mucoid, watery, or blood-tinged discharge is associated with preterm labor.
- Test the vaginal discharge for amniotic fluid (turns blue on contact with nitrazine paper). The presence of amniotic fluid indicates the rupture of membranes and an increased risk for maternal infection and fetal deterioration.
- Meconium staining, a green coloration of the amniotic fluid, may be associated with fetal airway compromise.

Skin
- Pregnancy-induced hypertension (PIH) may produce facial flushing.
- The pregnant patient in shock may present with warm or dry extremities.
- Fever related to infection (STI, ruptured ectopic, premature rupture of membranes in pregnancy).

LIFE SPAN ISSUES (GYNECOLOGIC CONDITIONS)

1. Vaginal bleeding may occur in early adolescence because of irregular menstrual patterns rather than because of a pathologic condition.
2. Vaginal bleeding may occur in middle age as a result of the beginning of menopause rather than because of a pathologic condition.

INITIAL INTERVENTIONS

1. Ascertain pregnancy status through a urine or blood human chorionic gonadotropin (HCG) test if the patient is of childbearing age.
2. Initiate IV access (large bore for compromised patients), and send a blood specimen to the laboratory for a type and crossmatch and complete blood count (CBC) for all patients

with vaginal bleeding and abnormal vital signs. If the patient
is pregnant, the Rh factor and clotting studies also should be
checked.

3. Initiate cardiac, BP, and pulse oximetry monitoring for
   patients with significant vaginal bleeding.
4. For compromised patients complaining of vaginal bleeding,
   administer high-flow oxygen using a nonrebreather mask at
   10 to 15 L/min.
5. Prepare the patient for a bimanual and/or speculum
   examination. Obtain culture media, swabs, and specimen
   containers for conception products examination.

➤ N U R S I N G   A L E R T ➤

Internal vaginal exam is contraindicated if placenta previa is
suspected

---

6. Initiate IV access and send a complete blood count
   (CBC) for all patients with vaginal bleeding and abnormal
   vital signs.
7. Pregnant patients in the second trimester or beyond should
   be placed on the left side to facilitate venous return and
   reduce pressure on the inferior vena cava. If the patient is on
   a backboard because of traumatic injury, elevate the right
   side of the backboard with a wedge.
8. In the hypertensive pregnant patient, anticipate the
   possibility of seizure activity. Pad the side rails and keep
   the bed in a low position. Have suction and airway materials
   available.
9. If available, initiate external fetal monitoring for pregnant
   patients with vaginal bleeding.
10. Treat the pregnant patient's fear and anxiety by explaining all
    procedures and offering support from clergy, family, and/or
    significant others.
11. Nursing care priorities are listed in the table on pp. 552-553.

PRIORITY DIAGNOSTIC TESTS
(GYNECOLOGIC AND OBSTETRIC
CONDITIONS)

Many of the tests in this section are initiated in the ED, but
results may take several days. The information is provided to
support patient teaching.

Laboratory Tests

Complete blood count (CBC): A CBC may indicate infection if the white blood cell count is elevated or may indicate bleeding if hemoglobin and hematocrit are low.

Human chorionic gonadotropin (HCG) test: Detection of HCG in the blood indicates pregnancy; the higher the level, the longer the gestation period. The level of HCG for a woman with an ectopic pregnancy is lower than for a woman with an intrauterine pregnancy of the same gestation.

Iron level: The iron level is low when vaginal bleeding has been excessive or chronic.

Kleihauer-Betke test: A positive test result suggests fetomaternal hemorrhage, usually resulting from abdominal trauma. This is indicative of fetal blood entering the maternal circulation.

Platelet level: The platelet level may be low if the cause of vaginal bleeding is leukemia, preeclampsia, idiopathic thrombocytopenic purpura, or disseminated intravascular coagulation (DIC).

Prothrombin time: This level may be high if vaginal bleeding is associated with von Willebrand's disease and other clotting disorders such as disseminated intravascular coagulation (DIC), which is associated with abruptio placentae and uterine rupture.

Serum gonadotropins: A follicle-stimulating hormone level greater than 40 IU/L suggests impending ovarian failure (menopause), while a luteinizing hormone/follicle-stimulating hormone ratio that is greater than 2 suggests chronic anovulation.

Type and crossmatch: A type and crossmatch may be ordered if a blood transfusion is needed as a result of bleeding.

Special Diagnostic Studies

Endometrial biopsy: An endometrial biopsy is used to determine the presence of ovulation by measuring progesterone and estrogen levels in the endometrial lining.

Ultrasound: An ultrasound examination is used for identification of ovarian cysts, for early diagnosis of ovarian tumors, for evaluation of abnormal uterine bleeding, for ectopic pregnancy, and for guidance during aspiration procedures (e.g., pelvic and ovarian abscesses). A transabdominal scan may be performed with a full urinary bladder. The patient then voids, and a transvaginal scan is conducted if indicated.

NURSING CARE PRIORITIES

Potential/Actual Problem	Causes	Signs and Symptoms	Interventions
1. Fluid volume deficit	• Hemorrhage	• Vaginal bleeding • Delayed capillary refill • Decreased skin turgor • Pale or flushed color	• Initiate IV access. • Administer IV crystalloids and blood components as ordered. • Anticipate surgical intervention.
2. Pain	• Uterine contractions • Peritoneal irritation	• Complaints of pain • Crying • Moaning • Facial grimacing • Restlessness	• Administer analgesics as ordered. • Use imagery techniques and distraction if they are helpful to the patient.
3. Fear	• Unknown pregnancy outcome	• Increased heart rate • Increased respiratory rate	• Allow the mother to hear the FHTs. • Encourage participation in

			maternal tests and treatments by explaining the benefits to the fetus.
4. Grieving	• Loss of pregnancy • Loss of reproductive abilities	• Elevated blood pressure • Nervousness • Feelings of helplessness • Crying	• Explain treatment options and probable consequences. • Maintain a support base as identified by the patient.
5. Injury	• Infection from peritoneal contamination • Infection from retained placental fragments	• Fever • Elevated WBC count • Skin warm to touch	• Administer antibiotics as ordered. • Anticipate dilation and curettage (D & C) or surgery. • Monitor fever and leukocytosis.

> **NURSING ALERT**
>
> The patient must have a full bladder for a transabdominal ultrasound examination and an empty bladder for a transvaginal ultrasound examination.

CLINICAL CONDITIONS (GYNECOLOGIC)

Dysfunctional Uterine Bleeding

Dysfunctional uterine bleeding is defined as abnormal bleeding from the lining of the uterus that occurs without an underlying disease or problem with the size or shape of the uterus.[6]

Symptoms

- The most common symptom is abnormal uterine bleeding associated with anovulation, either acute (menarche and menopause) or chronic.

Diagnosis

- Diagnosis is based on clinical findings and presentation.
- An endometrial biopsy may be performed.

Treatment

- If the bleeding is significant or the patient is hemodynamically unstable, a dilation and curettage (D & C) should be performed in the operating suite. Estrogen and progesterone medications may be administered.

Ovarian Cysts

Ovarian cysts are difficult to identify on the physical examination. The clinical presentation is similar to that of ectopic pregnancy and appendicitis. Hormonal changes, endometriosis, and neoplasms may produce ovarian cysts.

Symptoms

- A wide range of pain severity may be experienced with ovarian cysts. The pain generally is worse during the latter half of the menstrual cycle and is worse with movement. The pain may be localized to the right or left lower abdominal quadrant.
- If the cyst has ruptured, the patient may experience severe pain.
- Patients may report discomfort with intercourse, particularly deep penetration.

Diagnosis

- A pelvic ultrasound examination is the diagnostic tool of choice; however, a CT scan or MRI is sometimes helpful in defining ovarian cysts.
- A CBC and HCG test may be performed.

- If rupture is suspected, a type and crossmatch and prothrombin time may be ordered.
- Nausea and vomiting (N/V), fever, leukocytosis, and a firm to rigid abdomen without bowel sounds may be present.

Treatment

- Hormone supplements/oral contraceptives may be ordered.
- Pain medication usually is prescribed to accompany OTC antiinflammatory medications.
- A follow-up ultrasound examination is essential to detect enlargement of the cyst.
- Depending on the size of the ruptured cyst, surgery may be required to remove products and irrigate the peritoneal cavity.
- One or two large-bore IV catheters should be inserted, and Ringer's lactate or normal saline solution should be infused.
- IV antibiotics may be initiated in the ED.
- Monitor for shock via BP, central venous pressure (if available), base deficit (ABG), and urine output.

CLINICAL CONDITIONS (OBSTETRIC)

Abruptio placentae

Abruptio placentae is more common after 20 weeks' gestation. Tearing and bleeding into the inner layer of the endometrium compresses and impairs the functioning of the placenta. Abruptio placentae may be concealed (rarely) because of internal uterine bleeding or revealed (in 80% of cases) where bleeding dissects the membrane from the uterine wall[7] (Figure 16-1).

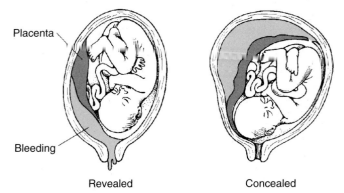

Figure 16-1   Abruptio placentae. (From Murphy P: *J Emerg Med Serv* 17[9]:48-49, 1992.)

Smoking, uterine trauma, substance abuse with alcohol or cocaine, and hypertension are risk factors for abruptio placentae.

Symptoms
- Sharp, sudden generalized pain over the abdomen
- Rapid, continuous, or intermittent uterine contractions may occur.
- Vaginal bleeding may be present. If present, it is usually dark in color.
- Fetal activity is decreased and the FHR will decrease as fetal hypoxia occurs. Fetal death may occur rapidly.
- Signs of hypovolemic shock may be present.
- DIC is common in cases of abruption.

Diagnosis
- Diagnosis is usually based on clinical presentation and ultrasound examination.
- A prolonged PT and the presence of fibrin degradation products may indicate DIC.

Treatment
- The goal of treatment is to maintain maternal blood volume through fluid resuscitation with crystalloids and blood components. Two large-bore IV lines infusing Ringer's lactate solution may be necessary if significant bleeding is present.
- High-flow oxygen (10 to 15 L/min) is administered.
- Initiate fetal monitoring.
- Delivery of the fetus may be necessary if fetal distress is noted. Anticipate the need for resuscitation if delivery is required.

Ectopic Pregnancy

An ectopic pregnancy occurs when a fertilized ovum implants on tissue other than the uterine endometrium, usually because of impaired passage through the fallopian tubes. A history of infertility or previous abdominal surgery increases the risk of an ectopic pregnancy.

Symptoms
- Amenorrhea, pelvic or abdominal pain, and abnormal vaginal bleeding are the most common symptoms.
- A pelvic mass can be palpated in some cases.
- Symptoms occur most often at 4 to 6 weeks' gestation.
- An ectopic rupture with intraperitoneal bleeding occurs at 6 to 10 weeks' gestation. Thus symptoms may include hypotension, tachycardia, nausea/vomiting, a rigid abdomen without bowel sounds, fever, and leukocytosis.

Diagnosis

- An ultrasound examination may detect an ectopic pregnancy before clinical symptoms appear.
- Ultrasound examination findings are compared with HCG levels.

Treatment

- Surgery usually is performed for a ruptured ectopic to remove the products of conception and to repair the damaged fallopian tube.
- Stable patients with an unruptured ectopic may be candidates for treatment with methotrexate.
- Rh testing of the mother should be performed and Rh immunoglobulin given if the patient is Rh negative.

Emergency delivery

The multiparous pregnant patient is at the greatest risk for precipitous delivery.

NURSING ALERT

If the cord presents (prolapses) before the baby appears, place the mother in the knee-chest position or Trendelenburg position. Administer high-flow oxygen (10 to 15 L/min) to the mother.

Symptoms

- Question the patient about amniotic fluid rupture. If the water has broken, ascertain the length of time since rupture and color of the fluid. Fluid that is green or has a greenish tint may indicate meconium, which when aspirated can cause respiratory distress in the newborn.
- The patient will have bloody show secondary to rapid dilation of the cervix.
- A bulging perineum and anus are indicative of fetal descent and the fetus will display crowning of the head.
- If the baby's head remains visible between contractions, birth is imminent.

Diagnosis

- Diagnosis is based on clinical presentation.

Treatment

- See Box 16-1, Steps in Emergency Delivery.
- After delivery, document the time the fetus and placenta were delivered. The placenta should be sent to the laboratory for examination, and the time sent to lab also should be documented.

BOX 16-1   STEPS IN EMERGENCY DELIVERY

1. Place the mother on her left side to slow fetal descent.
2. Have the mother open her mouth and pant to slow progress.
3. Have a neonatal resuscitation bag and oxygen supply available. Suction equipment also is needed.
4. Wash your hands and put on gloves.
5. Wash the patient's perineum, then reglove.
6. Ease the perineum back until the head emerges.
7. As the baby's head emerges, check for the umbilical cord. If it is around the baby's neck, slip it over the head or back over the shoulders.
8. Suction the baby's mouth first, then the nose. Suctioning the nose first may elicit a reflex gasp and force fluids in the lungs.
9. Place your hand under the cord as the baby emerges.
10. If the cord is extremely tight, clamp the cord with two clamps and cut between the clamps.
11. Keep the baby's head lower than its trunk during birthing to promote drainage.
12. Do not pull the baby out; allow the baby to advance on its own.
13. Cut the cord after clamping $1\frac{1}{2}$ inches from the infant's umbilicus after the cord stops pulsating. Use two clamps to prevent cord bleeding.
14. Document the time of delivery and the baby's Apgar score (see Table 16-1 on p. 569).
15. Delivery of the placenta will occur within a few minutes of fetal delivery and will be preceded by a sudden discharge of blood. Gently depress the uterus by applying pressure over the suprapubic area. When the placenta appears in the vaginal area, maintain gentle traction on the cord until the placenta is delivered. The cord should never be pulled, as this can cause inversion of the uterus and subsequent bleeding.

- The fundus (top of the uterus) should be assessed for position in relation to the umbilicus and is measured in fingerbreadths above or below the umbilicus. Massage the fundus every 15 minutes to help reduce the amount of bleeding. Bleeding can cause the fundus to feel soft or boggy. If the fundus feels boggy, fundal massage should continue until the uterus contracts and becomes firm to stop the bleeding. The uterus should remain firm and in the midline position, centered at the umbilicus. If deviated to the right, assess the patient for

the need to void, as bladder fullness can shift the uterus and cause increased bleeding.
- The color and amount of vaginal discharge or lochia as well as the appearance of the perineum should be assessed every 15 minutes for the first hour postpartum, then hourly.

Miscarriage (Abortion)

Vaginal bleeding is very common in early pregnancy, with approximately one of every four women experiencing bleeding during the first trimester. Bleeding in early pregnancy may be classified as a threatened abortion if the vaginal bleeding is mild and not associated with cervical dilation. Approximately half of these women stop bleeding and complete a normal pregnancy.

A miscarriage or spontaneous abortion is defined as the passing of fetal tissue through the dilated cervical opening. Miscarriage occurs before the twentieth week of pregnancy and may be classified as one of the following:

- *Incomplete miscarriage (abortion):* Heavy vaginal bleeding and cramping with cervical dilation and expulsion of a small amount of the products of conception.
- *Complete miscarriage (abortion):* Mild vaginal bleeding and cramping with an open cervix and expulsion of the products of conception.
- *Septic miscarriage (abortion):* Severe abdominal pain associated with intrauterine infection and a malodorous vaginal discharge.

Symptoms
- Crampy lower abdominal pain may be present.
- Vaginal bleeding with or without the passage of tissue may occur. Bleeding can range from slight spotting to severe hemorrhage.

Diagnosis
- An HCG test is performed to confirm pregnancy.
- A CBC may be performed to assess for anemia.
- An ultrasound examination is performed to determine whether a gestational sac is present and to determine the location of the sac.
- A speculum examination is performed to determine whether the cervix is dilated and to determine the source of the bleeding.

Treatment
- Oxytocin or Methergine may be administered to promote expulsion of all products of conception.

- Antibiotics and analgesics may be ordered.
- A dilation and curettage (D & C) may be needed. If a D & C procedure is performed in the emergency department, all products of conception should be sent to the lab for pathology evaluation.
- The patient should be tested for Rh status, and Rh immunoglobulin should be administered if the mother is Rh negative.

Newborn Resuscitation

Approximately 90% of newborns transition from intrauterine to extrauterine life without difficulty. However, 10% will require some assistance, and 1% will require extensive resuscitation measures.[8] Many fetal and maternal factors place the newborn at risk for requiring resuscitation (Box 16-2). Initial care of the newborn is described in Box 16-3. Newborn resuscitation should be initiated in the event of ineffective respirations or bradycardia that persists after the initial assessment and resuscitation efforts.

Symptoms

- Ineffective or absent respiratory effort
- Irregular, decreased, or absent pulse

BOX 16-2 RISK FACTORS THAT MAY PRECIPITATE THE NEED FOR NEONATAL RESUSCITATION IN THE ED

- Abruptio placentae
- Gestational diabetes
- Maternal substance abuse
- Meconium staining
- Multiple gestation
- Precipitous labor
- Pregnancy-related hypertensive disorder
- Premature rupture of membranes
- Preterm labor
- Prolapsed cord
- Third-trimester bleeding
- Underlying maternal cardiac, renal, pulmonary, neurologic, or thyroid disease

---

BOX 16-3   INITIAL RESUSCITATION OF THE NEWBORN

1. Rapid assessment of airway/breathing. Position the neonate on the back or side with the head slightly extended in the "sniffing position" and clear the airway by suctioning first the mouth and then the nose.
2. Dry the neonate to minimize heat loss. If possible use warm blankets to dry the neonate.
3. To prevent hypothermia, provide warming measures such as radiant heat.
4. Record neonatal assessment and treatment. Calculate an Apgar score at 1 and 5 minutes after delivery. The Apgar score is based on the scoring of the following parameters: heart rate, respirations, muscle tone, reflex irritability, and color (see Table 16-2).
5. Be aware that the neonate is at risk for hypothermia, hypoglycemia, and ineffective airway clearance.

Diagnosis
- Based on history and physical exam findings

Treatment
Ineffective or absent respiratory effort:
- After the airway is suctioned, administer 100% oxygen as necessary using a blow-by device or bag-valve mask.
- Intubation should follow if spontaneous effective respirations are not established.

Irregular, decreased, or absent pulse:
- If the heart rate is less than 60 beats/min, chest compressions should be initiated.
- An IV line must be initiated. The umbilical cord may be used.
- Epinephrine 0.01 mg/kg of a 1:10,000 solution may be given endotracheally, or may be given through the umbilical catheter in cases of cardiac arrest.

Placenta Previa
Placenta previa generally is defined as the implantation of the placenta over or near the internal os of the cervix. This obstetric complication occurs in the second and third trimesters of pregnancy. Almost half of all placenta previa patients have their first episode of bleeding before 30 weeks' gestation. Initial bleeding usually is self-limiting.

The earlier this episode occurs in the pregnancy, the less likely the pregnancy is to reach term. The placenta may cover the os partially or completely (Figure 16-2). The danger in placenta previa is a separation of the placenta from the uterine wall and subsequent hemorrhage. Perinatal mortality is greater because of reduced fetal perfusion, both from the implanted placenta and from decreased circulating blood volume of the mother. The risk factors for placenta previa include: smoking, age greater than 35, previous cesarean section, uterine trauma, diabetes, and substance abuse.

Symptoms
- Bright red, painless bleeding, which may or may not occur simultaneously with contractions
- Hypotension, tachycardia, a soft and non-tender uterus, and normal fetal heart tones (usually) are all characteristics of placenta previa.

Diagnosis
- A speculum examination may be performed, but a bimanual examination is not advisable because of the potential for exacerbating hemorrhage.
- An ultrasound examination is used to determine placental location.
- A Kleihauer-Betke test is performed if there is concern for fetal-maternal transfusion.

Treatment
- The goal is to postpone labor to promote fetal maturation.
- The ED goal should be directed at the hemodynamic stability of the patient. The primary therapeutic agents should be IV crystalloids and/or transfusions.
- Bed rest may be initiated.
- If the patient continues to bleed, the baby may be delivered by cesarean section.
- Vaginal delivery is possible if previa is marginal.

Postpartum Hemorrhage

Postpartum hemorrhage (PPH) is defined as any bleeding that results in signs and symptoms of hemodynamic instability, or bleeding that could result in hemodynamic instability if untreated.[9] PPH can be categorized as early or late onset. Early PPH occurs during the first 24 hours after delivery, and late PPH occurs more than 24 hours and less than 6 weeks after delivery.

Symptoms
- Vaginal bleeding with the presence of clots

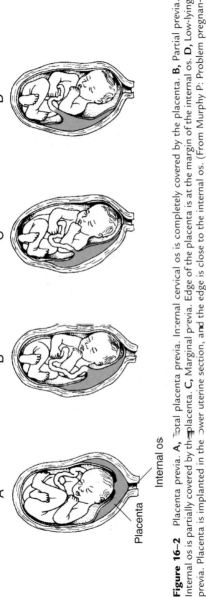

Figure 16–2 Placenta previa. Internal cervical os is completely covered by the placenta. **B,** Partial previa. Internal os is partially covered by the placenta. **C,** Marginal previa. Edge of the placenta is at the margin of the internal os. **D,** Low-lying previa. Placenta is implanted in the lower uterine section, and the edge is close to the internal os. (From Murphy P: Problem pregnancies, *J Emerg Med Serv* 17[9]:48-49, 1992.)

- A soft, boggy uterus indicates atony.
- Tissue may be passed vaginally.

Diagnosis

- Diagnosis usually is based on clinical presentation.
- A speculum examination is made to determine the presence of cervical and vaginal lacerations.
- Laboratory studies including a CBC may be performed. PT/PTT and D-dimer may be assessed to determine whether a coagulation disorder is present.

Treatment

- If bleeding occurs early in the postpartum period, the physician may perform uterine massage, with one hand externally massaging and the other gloved hand supporting the lower uterine segment through a vaginal approach (Figure 16-3).
- Oxytocic drugs are administered (e.g., Methergine, Ergotrate, and Pitocin).
- Breastfeeding (if appropriate) helps the uterus to contract.
- Fluid resuscitation with two large-bore IV lines infusing crystalloids or blood components may be indicated.

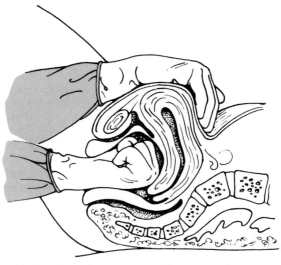

Figure 16–3   Bimanual compression of the uterus and massage with the abdominal hand usually will control hemorrhage resulting from uterine atony. (From Cunningham FG, Grant NF, Levero KF, et al: *Williams obstetrics,* ed 20, Norwalk, Conn, 1998, Appleton & Lange.)

- High-flow oxygen (10 to 15 L/min) may be necessary.
- Initiate cardiac, blood pressure, heart rate, and pulse oximetry monitoring.

Pregnancy-Induced Hypertension (PIH)

Pregnancy-related hypertension is divided into 4 categories.

- Preeclampsia and eclampsia (see Box 16-4)
- Chronic hypertension, which begins before pregnancy. A BP greater than 140/90 occurs before the twentieth week of gestation, is not associated with significant proteinuria or end-organ damage, and continues well after delivery.[10]
- Chronic hypertension with superimposed preeclampsia.
- Gestational hypertension results in a BP greater than 140/90 without proteinuria or end-organ damage. Initially normotensive women may become hypertensive late in pregnancy, during labor, or within 24 hours postpartum, and their BPs return to normal within 10 days postpartum.[2]

Symptoms

- The patient may exhibit a variety of clinical signs.
- Visual changes, edema, persistent vomiting, or reduced urine output
- A classic sign is seen in the second trimester—the mean arterial pressure (MAP) does not drop lower than the first-trimester MAP.
- Papilledema and seizures may occur.
- Epigastric pain (resulting from liver edema) and severe headache can be associated with impending seizure.
- Fetal movement may decrease.
- Reflexes are hyperactive.

BOX 16-4   PREECLAMPSIA VS. ECLAMPSIA

- Preeclampsia is defined as BP greater than 140/90 mm Hg at two readings taken 6 or more hours apart. Proteinuria is present.[2]
- Eclampsia is the development of seizures in a preeclamptic patient.[11] The arterial wall responds differently to angiotensin II and renin, resulting in arterial spasms.

Diagnosis
- BP changes occur as described earlier in the section.
- Urine protein levels increase (1+ in mild cases, up to 3+ or greater in severe cases). A urine protein level of more than 0.3 g/day is the criterion for diagnosis of proteinuria.[2]
- Platelet levels may be low, fibrin degradation products may be present, and liver enzyme levels may be elevated if the preeclampsia has progressed into HELLP (hemolysis, elevated liver enzymes, low platelets) syndrome.

Treatment
- Seizures are treated as outlined in Chapter 15.
- Severe cases are treated with magnesium sulfate to prevent seizures.

➤ NURSING ALERT ◄

Valium should never be administered to treat seizures in the pregnant patient because it causes depression of the fetus and increases the risk of maternal aspiration.

- Hydralazine, labetalol, or nifedipine may be given to reduce the BP.[2,3]
- Terbutaline may be given to prevent contractions.
- Milder cases are treated with bed rest, a no-added-salt diet, and home monitoring of BP and urine protein levels.
- Delivery may be necessary to decrease the blood pressure.

Preterm Labor
Many women ignore the signs of preterm labor and come to the ED after the membranes have ruptured or cervical dilation has occurred. The gestational age of the fetus may be reflected in the baseline FHR, a pattern of reactivity, and changes in the behavioral state of the fetus.

Symptoms
- The symptoms associated with preterm labor may include an elevated FHR (150-160 beats/min).[11]
- If fetal monitoring is available in the ED, preterm fetuses will be seen to have fewer accelerations and less amplitude with acceleration.
- Painless contractions and a change in vaginal discharge (mucoid, watery, or blood-tinged appearance) are the best predictors of preterm labor.

Diagnosis
- Preterm labor is diagnosed by labor pattern and not by FHR alone.
- A speculum examination is conducted to rule out premature rupture of the membranes as the cause of the change in vaginal discharge, followed by a digital examination of the cervix to evaluate cervical dilation and effacement.

Treatment
- Tocolytic agents (e.g., nifedipine or magnesium sulfate) can be administered.
- The patient is placed on bed rest in the left lateral recumbent position.
- Fetal monitoring is used to detect activity and heart rate variability.

Ruptured Uterus

A ruptured uterus may be considered complete when a tear occurs through the uterus and peritoneal covering, allowing intrauterine contents to be "spilled" into the peritoneal cavity. An incomplete (occult) tear also may occur. Rupture of the healthy uterus occurs most often during labor with oxytocin administration. Rupture of a previously scarred uterus (e.g., by a cesarean section) may occur as pregnancy advances.

Symptoms
- Bleeding may be great if the tear is complete but not visible; thus the patient will have signs of hypovolemia (an increased heart rate with decreased BP and oxygen saturation).
- Parts of the fetus may be palpable in the abdomen.
- If the tear is partial, minor bleeding may occur and seal itself off by hematoma formation.
- Sharp shooting abdominal pain or a tearing sensation may be present.
- Contractions may suddenly stop.
- Fetal mortality is high, ranging from 50% to 75%.

Diagnosis
- Diagnosis is based on clinical presentation.

Treatment
- Emergency surgical delivery by cesarean section is indicated for delivery of the fetus and repair of the peritoneum and uterus.
- Rapid fluid resuscitation is indicated.
- Two large-bore IV lines are inserted, and crystalloids and blood components are administered.
- Administer high-flow oxygen (10 to 15 L/min).

Trauma in Pregnancy

Trauma caused by accidents and violence is a common and important complication of pregnancy, involving 5% to 20% of pregnancies. Recent studies demonstrate that trauma is more likely to cause maternal death than any other medical complication in pregnancy.[12]

Symptoms

- Any event with the release of energy resulting in physical trauma may injure the mother and fetus.
- Warning symptoms include vaginal bleeding, uterine contractions, and abdominal tenderness.
- Domestic and sexual abuse must be considered as possible causes of trauma.
- Complications of traumatic injury in pregnancy are uterine rupture, abruptio placentae, emergency delivery, and neonatal compromise. Common traumatic injuries in pregnant women include liver and splenic lacerations and pelvic fractures (see Chapter 21).

Diagnosis

- The degree of diagnostic testing used depends on the severity of the precipitating event.
- External fetal monitoring should be performed for a minimum of 6 hours if fewer than 6 contractions occur in an hour. In pregnancies of less than 25 weeks' gestation, continuous fetal monitoring should be performed for 24 hours after major trauma because signs of fetal compromise can occur as long as 24 hours after injury.[12]
- Pregnant women with trauma should receive a Kleihauer-Betke test to estimate the volume of fetal-to-maternal transfusion.
- An ultrasound examination may be used to assess fetal status.

Treatment

- Monitor the fetus and uterine contractions.
- Provide hemodynamic stabilization. Two large-bore IV lines are inserted, and crystalloids and blood components may be administered.
- Administer high-flow oxygen (10 to 15 L/min).
- Anticipate an emergency cesarean section and surgery.
- The patient usually can be discharged after 6 hours of monitoring if there are no signs of fetal or maternal distress.[12]

NURSING SURVEILLANCE

1. Monitor the trend of vital signs and oxygen saturation.
2. Monitor contractions for timing and duration.

3. Monitor the FHR during contractions.
4. Monitor the level of consciousness.
5. Monitor the trend of pain.
6. Diligent pulmonary assessment is crucial in a pregnant patient who has been receiving IV fluids to avoid the risks of pulmonary edema.
7. Monitor arterial blood gases and beware of an increased CO_2 level because respiratory alkalosis is normal for pregnancy.

EXPECTED PATIENT OUTCOMES

1. The patient's level of consciousness improves or remains stable.
2. Vaginal bleeding decreases.
3. Pain decreases or stops.
4. Urine output is greater than 30 ml/hr.
5. Fever decreases or is absent.
6. Vital signs improve, and the systolic BP remains greater than 90 mm Hg but less than 140 mm Hg.
7. Seizure activity is absent.
8. The FHR is normal for gestational age.
9. The newborn infant's Apgar score is greater than 5 at 1 minute and improves at 5 minutes (Table 16-1).

DISCHARGE IMPLICATIONS

1. When discharging a patient with vaginal bleeding, instruct to the patient to monitor temperature and to seek follow-up care with a fever greater than 100.4° F.
2. Instruct the pregnant patient to avoid tampon use.

TABLE 16-1	Apgar Score		
Sign	**0**	**1**	**2**
Heart rate	Absent	Slow: below 100 beats/min	Above 100 beats/min
Respirations	Absent	Slow, irregular	Good crying
Muscle tone	Flaccid	Some flexion of extremities	Active motion
Reflex irritability	None	Grimace	Vigorous cry
Color	Pale blue	Body pink with blue extremities	Completely pink

3. Patients with a threatened abortion should be instructed to abstain from sexual intercourse until the bleeding stops.

4. Pregnant patients with PIH should receive education about a low-salt or no-added-salt diet. They should be taught how to take their BP and to perform urine reagent testing for protein content.

5. Patients who are found to be Rh negative should be told to wear a medical alert bracelet with this information.

REFERENCES

1. Broughton-Pipkin F, Sharif J, and Lal S: Predicting high blood pressure in pregnancy: a multivariate approach, *J Hypertens* 16:221-229, 1998.

2. Sibai BM: Diagnosis and management of gestational hypertension and preeclampsia, *Obstet Gynecol* 102(1):181-192, 2003.

3. Yankowitz J: Pharmacologic treatment of hypertensive disorders during pregnancy, *J Perinat Neonat Nurs* 18(3):230-240, 2004.

4. Roark M: *Listening to fetal heart tones, procedure checklists to accompany Rosdahl & Kowalski's textbook of basic nursing,* ed 8, Philadelphia, 2003, Lippincott Williams & Wilkins.

5. Youngerman-Cole S: Dysfunctional uterine bleeding, *WebMD Journal* 2002, www.my.webmd.com/content/healthwise/43/10669.

6. Bravender T and Emans SJ: Menstrual disorders: dysfunctional uterine bleeding, *Pediatr Clin North Am* 46:3, 1999.

7. Murphy P: Problem pregnancies, *J Emerg Med Serv* 17(9):44-60, 1992.

8. American Academy of Pediatrics: *Neonatal resuscitation textbook,* Elk Grove Village, Ill, 2000, American Academy of Pediatrics.

9. Wainscott M: Pregnancy, postpartum hemorrhage, *eMedicine Journal* 2002, www.emedicine.com/EMERG/topic481.htm.

10. Brooks M: Pregnancy, preeclampsia, *eMedicine Journal* 2001, www.emedicine.com/EMERG/topic480.htm.

11. Eganhouse D and Burnside JS: Nursing assessment and responsibility in monitoring the preterm pregnancy, *J Obstet Gynecol Neonatal Nurs* 21:355-363, 1992.

12. Newton E: Trauma and pregnancy, *eMedicine Journal* 2003, www.emedicine.com/med/topic3268.htm.

chapter *17*

Respiratory Conditions

Steve Talbert

CLINICAL CONDITIONS

Acute Respiratory Distress Syndrome (ARDS)
Asthma
Bronchitis
Chronic Obstructive Pulmonary Disease (COPD)
Pneumonia
Pulmonary Edema
Pulmonary Embolism
Spontaneous Pneumothorax

INTRODUCTION

A patient who presents to the emergency department
(ED) with respiratory symptoms or distress should be
considered a high-acuity patient, because many such patients
may require airway management or ventilatory support.
Patients with respiratory distress should be taken immediately
to the treatment area for further evaluation and intervention.
Obtain a history of any activity or exposure that may have
precipitated respiratory distress. Acute exacerbations of
chronic conditions often are triggered by infection, antigen
exposure, stress, or exertion. Other factors that can precipitate
respiratory distress include trauma, electrical injury, overdose,
paralysis secondary to cerebrovascular attack or spinal cord
injury, carbon monoxide poisoning, and smoke inhalation.

FOCUSED NURSING ASSESSMENT

Oxygenation and Ventilation
Respirations
- Determine the depth, rate, and character of respirations.
- A change in respiratory rate or pattern may be an early
  sign of respiratory insufficiency.
- Tachypnea occurs secondary to hypoxemia and impaired
  ventilation.

- Bradypnea is a sign of respiratory failure and impending cardiopulmonary arrest.
- Suprasternal, supraclavicular, and sternocleidomastoid muscle retractions may be noted. Intercostal retractions are indicative of increased work of breathing. Patients with chronic obstructive pulmonary disease (COPD) often use accessory muscles to assist with breathing.
- Inward chest movement noted on inspiration and/or outward abdominal movement noted on inspiration indicates increased work of breathing.
- Nasal flaring indicates increased work of breathing.
- Tripod positioning (torso upright with elbows placed on a supporting object) is common for patients with respiratory distress.
- Determine SpO_2 levels with continuous pulse oximetry. An SpO_2 level of 91% or less is highly predictive of hospital admission.
- Note any history of productive cough, wheezing, dyspnea, smoking, or exposure to environmental pollution (suspect COPD).
- Assess for a history of any form of dyspnea. Dyspnea can be assessed by use of a standardized scale (Figure 17-1).
  - Paroxysmal nocturnal dyspnea (PND): a sudden episode of dyspnea or orthopnea that awakens the patient from sleep, usually 1 to 2 hours after going to bed. Subsides spontaneously, but may recur at about the same time on subsequent nights.
  - Orthopnea: shortness of breath occurring when the patient is lying down, improves with sitting up.
  - Dyspnea on exertion (DOE): dyspnea occurring with mild activity. Can be related to a pulmonary disease, anemia, or deconditioning.

Breath Sounds

- Assess breath sounds.
- Abnormal inspiratory sounds are consistent with an upper airway obstruction and often are heard if the underlying problem is an upper airway infection or a foreign-body aspiration. Figure 17-2 shows the relationship between anatomy and type of stridor.
- Lower airway sounds are consistent with lower airway obstruction and often are heard if the underlying problem is asthma or COPD. Table 17-1 summarizes common respiratory conditions and their associated breath sounds.

Circle the Number That Best Matches Your Shortness of Breath	
0	None at all
0.5	Very, very slight (just noticeable)
1	Very slight
2	Slight
3	Moderate
4	Somewhat severe
5	Severe
6	
7	Very severe
8	
9	Very, very severe (almost maximal)
10	Maximal

Figure 17-1 Borg dyspnea scale.

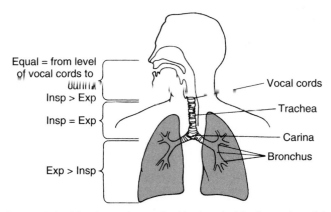

Figure 17-2 The airway. Types of stridor heard with obstruction of the airway. *Insp*, Inspiratory; *Exp*, expiratory. (Redrawn from Josephson GD, Josephson JS, Krespi YP, et al: Airway obstruction: new modalities in treatment, *Med Clin North Am* 77 (3):542, 1993.)

TABLE 17-1   Determining Source of Airway Obstruction

Origin	Etiology	Symptoms
Nasal • URI • Allergy • Foreign bodies/tumors	• Related to inflammation of nares • Incidence may be increased during certain seasons if related to allergens or infection.	• Absence of stridor • Rarely life threatening • Patient demonstrates mouth breathing.
Pharyngeal • Infection • Foreign bodies	• Regurgitation of gastric contents • Dislodged or broken teeth • Nasal, oral, and pharyngeal bleeding • Occlusion of tongue in unconscious patient	• Snoring • Inspiratory stridor
Laryngeal • Infection • Foreign bodies and tumors • Trauma	• Spasm may result from foreign body or may be related to suctioning. • Edema may result from intubation attempts or inhalation of caustic substances.	• Crowing • Inspiratory stridor is equal to expiratory stridor.
Tracheal • External pressure on trachea	• Hematoma from repeated attempts at internal jugular cannulation • Compression of neck by hanging or strangling	• Inspiratory stridor is equal to expiratory stridor.
Bronchial • Inflammation	• Exposure to allergens • Exposure to caustic substances • Foreign-body inhalation	• Expiratory stridor and wheezing

- Crackles (rales) or wheezing can be heard with many respiratory conditions and often are heard in the presence of alveolar edema. Crackles that do not clear with coughing may indicate heart failure.
- Unilateral absent or diminished breath sounds are consistent with a spontaneous pneumothorax.
- Absent or diminished breath sounds also are significant findings and may indicate a pneumothorax or some form of alveolar consolidation.
- Breath sounds may be absent or diminished as a result of bronchoconstriction caused by foreign-body aspiration. The right mainstem bronchus is a common site for foreign-body lodgment or passage because of the lesser angle at which it comes off the trachea compared with the left mainstem bronchus. Wheezing is not a reliable indicator of the severity of obstruction.

NURSING ALERT

If wheezing decreases, check to see whether the patient's condition is worsening because of decreased airflow. Stridor indicates a life-threatening problem.

Sputum
- Describe sputum production, including amount and color.
- A change in sputum production or appearance in those with COPD indicates an acute pulmonary infection.
- Pink, frothy sputum is a sign of cardiogenic pulmonary alveolar edema (PAE).
- Patients who have pneumonia may produce green, yellow, or rust-colored sputum.

Perfusion
Pulse
- Assess peripheral pulses, edema, skin temperature and color, and capillary refill.
- A paradoxical pulse (a fall in systolic BP of at least 12 mm Hg during inspiration) indicates severe asthma related to the negative intrapleural pressure created as an asthmatic patient inspires.
- Tachycardia may result from hypoxemia, fever, pain, or a change in cardiac output.
- Bradycardia may be a sign of severe hypoxemia.
- Suspect atrial fibrillation if there is a discrepancy between the radial and apical pulses.

Heart Sounds
- A third heart sound often is noted in cases of heart failure.

Jugular Venous Distension (JVD)
- Determine the presence of JVD. Place the patient in the semi-Fowler's position with the head turned to the right or the left. Observe the jugular vein at the posterior border of the sternocleidomastoid muscle. Right atrial congestion is suspected when jugular veins distend 2 inches or more above the sternal notch (Figure 17-3). Jugular veins may be distended and the trachea shifted away from midline if a spontaneous pneumothorax has resulted in a tension pneumothorax.

Cardiac Rhythm
- Identify the cardiac rhythm.
- Individuals who have cardiogenic pulmonary edema may experience tachycardic or bradycardic arrhythmias.

Blood Pressure
- Hypotension may be caused by heart failure.

Skin Color
- Cyanosis is a very late sign and signals impending respiratory failure.

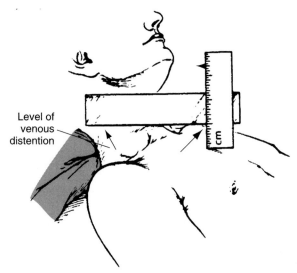

Level of venous distention

Figure 17-3   Jugular venous distension. (From Barkauskas VH, Baumann LC, Darling-Fischer CS: *Health and physical assessment,* ed 2, St Louis, 1998, Mosby.)

- Signs of venous insufficiency include pedal edema and brown, leathery extremity skin. Venous insufficiency is a risk factor for pulmonary embolism.
- Observe for peripheral and central cyanosis.

Cognition

- A decreased LOC should be considered a sign of respiratory failure, and the patient should be taken immediately to the treatment area.
- Anxiety may be a sign of hypoxemia.
- Perform a neurologic assessment and document a Glasgow Coma Scale (GCS) score (see Reference Guides 10 and 16).
- Medications used to treat pulmonary disorders can produce central nervous system effects such as nervousness, tachycardia, and agitation.
- Hypoxemia and hypercapnia can cause restlessness and a decreased LOC.

Sensation and Mobility

- Chest pain that increases on inspiration with respiratory movement that is limited to one side is suggestive of spontaneous pneumothorax.
- Chest tightness often is associated with airway inflammation and bronchoconstriction.

> ### NURSING ALERT
>
> Patients with respiratory conditions can quickly decompensate. Those with severe dyspnea, tachypnea, chest pain, or other signs of acute respiratory distress should be taken to the ED treatment area immediately.

Safety

- Patients with severe dyspnea often are extremely anxious and frightened.

Elimination

- Monitor the patient's urinary output. Patients who have cardiogenic pulmonary edema can experience hypervolemia and a decreased urine output. Hypovolemia or hypervolemia also may occur in cases of noncardiogenic pulmonary edema. Document renal response to diuresis.

LIFE SPAN ISSUES

Pediatric Patients

1. Newborns are at risk for a spontaneous pneumothorax related to hyaline membrane disease and meconium aspiration.

2. Infants younger than 4 months are obligate nose breathers.
3. Pediatric patients will deteriorate rapidly with desaturation.
4. Young children and adolescents may experience acute respiratory distress syndrome (ARDS) secondary to trauma.
5. The incidence of staphylococcal pneumonia is greatest in children younger than 2 years of age. Respiratory syncytial virus (RSV) is the most common cause of viral pneumonia in children.
6. Children with a history of cystic fibrosis have a higher incidence of spontaneous pneumothorax.
7. Infants and children exposed to passive smoking experience a higher incidence of asthma.
8. A respiratory rate of greater than 50 breaths/min in infants or greater than 40 breaths/min in children over 3 years of age is sensitive and specific for infections of the lower respiratory tract.

Pregnancy
One third of pregnant women with asthma have increased symptom severity, particularly during the gestation period of 19 to 36 weeks.

Geriatric Patients
1. COPD occurs mainly among middle-aged and older adults. It is often associated with asthma.
2. Geriatric patients are at risk for pneumonia.
3. For patients older than 40 years, a spontaneous pneumothorax is associated with a history of COPD or pulmonary tuberculosis.
4. A blunted perception of breathlessness has been found in geriatric patients. Patients may not be dyspneic with respiratory conditions. If a patient complains of dyspnea, the condition may be severe.

INITIAL INTERVENTIONS
Airway Management
1. Administer supplemental oxygen as prescribed. The delivery system and amount of oxygen used for improving oxygenation outcomes depend on the severity of the disease process (see Reference Guide 14). Be prepared for intubation because respiratory conditions can rapidly deteriorate.
2. Place the patient in high Fowler's position for maximal lung expansion. If heart failure is suspected, the lower extremities may be dangled to help reduce venous return.
3. Perform the Heimlich maneuver if appropriate.

> ### NURSING ALERT
> Do not place the obtunded patient supine with a pillow under the head because this position can precipitate airway obstruction.

4. Obstruction below the larynx requires emergency bronchoscopy or surgery for foreign-body removal.
5. Perform the head-tilt/chin-lift or jaw-thrust maneuver to open the airway. Maintain cervical spine stabilization if spinal injury is suspected.
6. If the patient is not breathing, administer two breaths by bag-valve-mask device. If resistance is met, perform the head-tilt/chin-lift or jaw-thrust maneuver a second time to ensure an open airway.
7. Insert an artificial airway to help maintain airway patency and to reduce gastric inflation.
8. One can estimate the proper size of an oral airway by measuring from the corner of the patient's mouth up to the tragus of the ear. An oral airway can be inserted more easily if it is wet. Do not tape the oral airway. The patient should be able to cough out the airway if the gag reflex returns.

> ### NURSING ALERT
> Oral airways are used only with an unconscious patient. Have suction equipment available because placement may stimulate the gag reflex, producing vomitus.

9. Nasopharyngeal airways may be used if the patient is awake but not alert. The use of a nasopharyngeal airway is contraindicated when the patient is receiving anticoagulants because of the potential for bleeding. Apply lubricant to the device before insertion. Figure 17-4 shows proper insertion technique.
10. The nasopharyngeal airway can be connected to a bag-valve-mask device via an endotracheal tube adaptor inserted into the nares' end of the airway (Figure 17-5). The mouth and opposite naris must be occluded while one squeezes the bag. If the patient's heart rate decreases during passage, suspect that the airway is too long and is compressing the epiglottis against the laryngeal entrance, producing vagal stimulation.

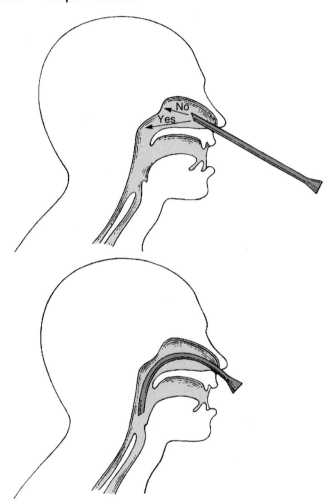

Figure 17–4   To insert a nasal airway: Insert the airway into the nostril and advance it along the floor of the nose *(top)*; not upward toward the frontal sinus, which will increase the risk of epistaxis. Slide it forward to place it in the posterior pharynx *(bottom)*. (Redrawn from Whitten: *Emerg Med* March 15, p 115, 1990.)

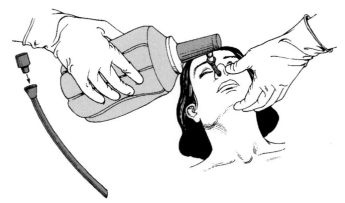

Figure 17–5 Nasal ventilation. When bag-and-mask ventilation is difficult, insert an endotracheal tube connector into a nasal airway *(left)*, place the airway, close the opposite nostril and mouth, attach the bag, and ventilate *(right)*. (Redrawn from Whitten CE: Management of the airway, *Emerg Med* 22:5, 1990.)

11. Ventilate the patient by applying a mask over the mouth and nose with the airway in place (pocket mask with one-way valve for mouth-to-mask ventilation). The most effective way of ventilating the patient is by connecting the mask to a manual resuscitation bag with an oxygen reservoir attached The bag should be connected to oxygen at a 10-L to 15-L rate. Ventilate the adult patient 12 times a minute.

12. Anticipate endotracheal intubation. Rapid sequence induction (RSI) may be considered. RSI is a method of inducing anesthesia and neuromuscular blockade just before performing endotracheal intubation. RSI facilitates success of the procedure by producing a fully relaxed state (see Procedure 1).

NURSING ALERT

If resistance is encountered during bag mask ventilation, suspect that obstruction or the patient's preexisting illness (e.g., CHF, bronchospasm, or pneumothorax) has produced increased pulmonary resistance. The underlying cause must be treated. If no resistance is encountered, suspect a leak in the ventilation system. Check all tubing and connections, the integrity of the bag-valve device, and, if appropriate, the fit of the mask.

13. When the endotracheal tube is in place, correct placement must be confirmed by auscultation of equal and bilateral breath sounds, fogging of the endotracheal tube, equal rise and fall of the chest, no epigastric gurgling with ventilations, and improved oxygenation of the patient.

14. End tidal CO_2 (ET_{CO_2}) detectors may be used for secondary confirmation of tube placement in both adult and pediatric patients. These devices detect the presence of exhaled CO_2 to confirm tracheal tube placement in the lungs. The detectors contain litmus paper, and when the patient is ventilated, the color will change in the presence of CO_2 (see Procedure 1, Figure 2). The detector has two connector ports, and when intubation has been accomplished, the detector should be connected between the tracheal tube and bag-valve device. The patient then is ventilated with six breaths. If the tube is in the correct position, the color will change. If there is no color change, the tube should be removed, as no CO_2 is being detected. If the color changes marginally, only a small amount of CO_2 has been detected and the patient should be ventilated with six more breaths. If the color still does not change, patient may need to be reintubated. If fluid enters the detector, it will no longer be accurate and should be discarded. The detectors can stay in place for up to 2 hours. End tidal CO_2 monitoring, or capnography, can also be performed via an external sensor attached to the ventilator circuit. The CO_2 level then can be translated into a graphic waveform, which represents the level of carbon dioxide present.

15. One should document the depth of the endotracheal tube by noting the centimeter mark on the endotracheal tube at the level of the teeth. The tube should be firmly secured (see Procedure 1).

Cricothyroidotomy

1. In the presence of massive emesis or bleeding associated with facial injuries, upper airway edema, or a known cervical spine fracture, the physician may elect to perform a surgical cricothyroidotomy.

2. This procedure is performed at the level of the larynx through the cricothyroid membrane. A 1-cm to 2-cm transverse incision is made through the skin and cricothyroid membrane. A #4 Shiley tracheostomy tube or a #7 or smaller endotracheal tube is inserted and connected to a bag-valve device. A needle cricothyroidotomy may be done as a temporizing measure to oxygenate the patient, especially in the prehospital setting (Figure 17-6).

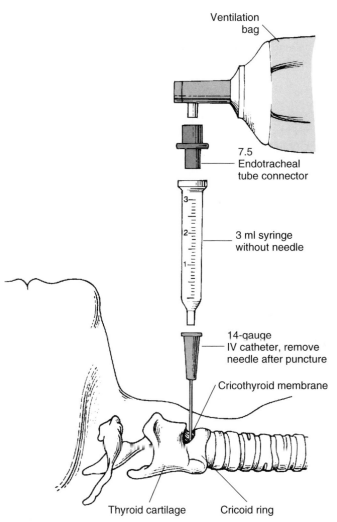

Figure 17–6 Emergency needle cricothyrotomy. Identify the cricothyroid membrane, and puncture it with a large intravenous catheter-over-needle. To attach the ventilation bag, place the connector from a #7.5 endotracheal tube into the barrel of a 3-ml syringe and attach that to the catheter hub. (Redrawn from Whitten CE: Management of the airway, *Emerg Med* 22:5, 1990.)

GENERAL INTERVENTIONS

1. Initiate cardiac monitoring.
2. Monitor oxygen saturation with continuous pulse oximetry.
3. Monitor end tidal CO_2 values.
4. Assess vital signs as dictated by acuity.
5. Keep the patient NPO until stabilized. In some instances, surgery or invasive tests may be required.
6. Monitor urine output. Place a urinary catheter according to the physician's prescription. Patients with cardiogenic pulmonary edema require diuretics and accurate urinary output measurement.
7. Obtain a sputum sample in a sterile container. Sputum cultures may be ordered.
8. Suction the patient's airway as needed. Hyperoxygenate and ventilate before suctioning.
9. Reassure the patient. Severe dyspnea often produces anxiety.
10. If the patient has a history of COPD or asthma, obtain the peak expiratory flow rate via a peak flow meter.
11. Initiate IV access. Two IV lines are preferable in cases of severe respiratory distress. An intermittent infusion device may be substituted for continuous IV fluids if fluid volume overload is suspected.
12. Nursing care priorities are listed in the table on pp. 586-587.

PRIORITY DIAGNOSTIC TESTS

Laboratory Tests

Activated partial thromboplastin time (aPTT): An aPTT test is used to evaluate the effectiveness of heparin therapy in cases of pulmonary embolism. The goal is to maintain aPTT at 1.5 to 2 times the control time.

Antibody titers and blood serology: These tests are used to determine the cause of pulmonary infection.

Arterial blood gases: An ABG test is used to evaluate oxygenation and the acid–base balance. It is useful in most respiratory conditions. The test is not definitive for pulmonary embolism. Supplemental oxygen may be adjusted according to ABG test results and clinical symptoms. Respiratory alkalosis is common in mild to moderate cases of asthma. If the PCO_2 starts to return to normal, it may indicate respiratory muscle fatigue.

Brain natriuretic peptide (BNP): BNP is a hormone that is secreted primarily by the ventricles. The level is elevated in congestive heart failure (CHF) and is a useful tool along with clinical correlation to confirm the diagnosis of CHF.

Blood cultures: Blood cultures are used to diagnose bacteremia and the causative agent for those with pneumonia.

Complete blood count: White blood cell counts are elevated or decreased in cases of pulmonary inflammation or infection. An elevated hemoglobin level may indicate polycythemia, a clinical indicator of prolonged hypoxemia.

D-dimer: The presence of D-dimer in the blood is indicative of thrombus formation in the body. The test is not specific for DVT or pulmonary embolism, as the D-dimer may be elevated as a result of infection, trauma, recent surgery, or pregnancy. D-dimer is considered to be a test of exclusion for DVT and pulmonary embolism because a normal level indicates that there is no abnormal clot formation.

Plasma DNA assay: This test is used to diagnose a pulmonary embolism in the event of inconclusive lung scans.

Prealbumin, transferrin levels: These levels are used to evaluate nutritional status.

Prothrombin time (PT)/international normalized ratio (INR): PT and INR typically are reported simultaneously. The PT test is used to evaluate the effectiveness of oral anticoagulation for patients receiving Coumadin. The goal is to maintain PT at approximately 2.5 times the control time. The INR is a standardized, international test that corrects for the various reagents that are used for testing prothrombin. The target INR is 2.0 to 3.0.

Serum electrolyte levels: Potassium, chloride, and sodium levels fluctuate with diuresis and impaired renal function. Diuretics are used to treat fluid volume excess in cases of pulmonary edema.

Sputum culture and sensitivity: These are used to determine the causative agent of pneumonia and other respiratory infections. If pneumonia is suspected, broad spectrum antibiotics are started before culture results return in most instances. More organism-specific antibiotics are ordered when culture results become available.

Radiographic Tests

Chest x-ray: A chest x-ray examination is used to evaluate heart and lung structures. It is nonspecific for a pulmonary embolus. Infiltrates may be present with cases of pneumonia. Hyperinflation, a flattened diaphragm, and cardiomegaly are present with cases of COPD. Negative lung expansion is present in cases of spontaneous pneumothorax. Some foreign bodies

NURSING CARE PRIORITIES

Potential/Actual Problem	Causes	Signs and Symptoms	Interventions
1. Impaired gas exchange	• Decreased pulmonary ventilation and/or perfusion	• Decreased pO_2 • Decreased/increased pCO_2 • Dyspnea • Cyanosis • Decreased O_2 saturation	• Administer oxygen. • Monitor $ETCO_2$ levels. • Report changes in ABGs. • Administer bronchodilators as ordered.
2. Ineffective airway clearance	• Airway obstruction • Mucociliary dysfunction • Muscle weakness • Fatigue	• Nonproductive cough • Decreased breath sounds • Adventitious breath sounds • Tachypnea • Airway noises	• Relieve airway obstruction. • Prepare to assist with intubation. • Suction as needed. • Administer mucolytics as ordered. • Instruct in technique for cough and deep breathing.
3. Ineffective breathing	• Muscle weakness • Alveolar hypoventilation	• Tachypnea • Hyperventilation • Dyspnea	• Position in high Fowler's. • Administer O_2. • Reduce anxiety. • Encourage fluids.
4. Altered tissue perfusion	• Hypoxemia	• Central or peripheral pallor • Cool extremities	• Administer O_2. • Reduce activity.

		• Chest pain	• Administer analgesics as needed.
		• Mental status changes	
5. Pain	Pleural irritation	• Pleuritic pain	• Administer analgesics as needed.
		• Chest wall tenderness	• Teach splinting.
		• Restlessness	
6. Infection	Bacterial, viral, or fungal organisms	• Fever	• Administer antibiotics.
		• Tachypnea	• Administer antipyretics.
		• Positive sputum cultures	
		• Productive cough	
		• Dyspnea	
7. Activity intolerance	Decreased pulmonary function	• Shortness of breath	• Gradually increase activity.
		• Fatigue	• Monitor vital signs.
		• Chest pain	• Assist with movement.
		• Vital sign changes	• Anticipate home health referral if help is needed with ADLs.
8. Knowledge deficit	Lack of understanding about disease process and treatment	• Unable to describe home care	• Determine level of understanding of disease process and treatment.
			• Instruct patient and/or family on disease process and treatment.

may be radiopaque. Atelectasis of the involved lung may be present in cases of foreign-body aspiration.

Pulmonary angiogram: Dye is injected into the pulmonary vasculature. This is the most definitive test for a pulmonary embolism. Emergency medications may be administered if complications occur during the procedure; therefore IV access is required.

Venography: A venography is the injection of dye into the veins to detect deep venous thrombosis (DVT), a risk factor for pulmonary embolism. IV access is necessary for this procedure.

⇒ NURSING ALERT ⇐

Determine that the patient is not allergic to radiographic dye, iodine, or seafood before dye tests. If the patient has an allergy to contrast dye, the patient may be premedicated with Benadryl, Tylenol, and/or corticosteroids, or a less allergenic substance may be required.

OTHER DIAGNOSTIC TESTS

Bronchoscopy: In this test, a fiberoptic or rigid scope is inserted for examination of the internal structures of the airway and lungs. The patient is maintained NPO after the procedure until the gag reflex returns. Rigid bronchoscopy is performed in the operating room. Bronchoscopy may be used to remove foreign bodies.

Doppler ultrasonography: When Doppler ultrasonography is used, a handheld transducer that produces high-frequency sound waves is moved across the skin of the extremity being examined. Audible tones proportional to blood velocity help in the detection of thrombi.

Echocardiogram: The echocardiogram is used to assess right ventricular function.

Electrocardiogram (ECG): An ECG is used to detect heart failure, arrhythmias, and strain on the right side of the heart.

Peak expiratory flow rate (PEFR): This is the greatest flow that can be obtained during forced exhalation starting from full-lung inflation. A peak flow meter is used to measure this value. The patient can monitor the PEFR at home. A normal peak flow ranges from 400 to 600 L/min. A peak flow of less than 200 L/min indicates obstruction or respiratory fatigue. PEFR correlates well with forced expiratory volume (FEV_1) obtained by spirometry. The PEFR may not be reliably obtained from children. Oxygen saturation values may be more useful in determining the severity of the situation.

Spirometry (pulmonary function test): Use a spirometer to determine lung capacities, lung volumes, and flow rates. This is useful for determining the severity of airway obstruction in cases of COPD and other respiratory problems. Airway obstruction is confirmed by a reduction in the ratio of FEV_1 to forced vital capacity (FEV_1/FVC).

Ventilation and perfusion scan: A lung scan is performed after the inhalation of xenon-127. The perfusion scan is completed after the IV injection of technetium-97 macroaggregated albumin. Areas of poor ventilation and inadequate perfusion are identified.

CLINICAL CONDITIONS

Acute Respiratory Distress Syndrome (ARDS)

Acute respiratory distress syndrome (ARDS) is caused by either direct or indirect lung injury and may result from recent trauma, a major burn, toxicant inhalation, hemorrhage, drug overdose, altitude changes, massive infection, or near drowning. There is an inflammatory response in the lungs, which leads to a decrease in oxygenation or complete collapse of the alveoli. This results in severe, refractory hypoxemia. ARDS is characterized by respiratory failure and noncardiogenic pulmonary edema and also is called noncardiogenic pulmonary edema.

Symptoms
- Respiratory distress
- Tachypnea
- Orthopnea
- Crackles
- Hypovolemia or hypervolemia
- Hypotension
- Faint heart sounds

Diagnosis
- Chest x-ray examination demonstrates bilateral fluffy infiltrates, which have a "ground glass" appearance.
- Severe hypoxemia as documented by ABGs.
- Pulmonary artery catheterization reveals low or high pulmonary artery pressures.

- The patient has a history of risk factors for noncardiogenic pulmonary edema (e.g., recent trauma, hemorrhage, drug overdose, or infection).
- Clinical symptoms are demonstrated.

Treatment[1]
- Initiate supplemental oxygen.
- Continuous positive airway pressure (CPAP or bilevel positive airway pressure [BiPAP]) by mask or positive end-expiratory pressure (PEEP), or pressure support for the intubated patient may be necessary to improve alveolar inflation.
- Steroids may be administered.
- Inhaled surfactant can be administered.
- Careful diuresis or fluid replacement may be used, depending on preload measurements.

Asthma[2]

Asthma is a chronic respiratory condition characterized by airway inflammation (mucus hypersecretion), increased airway responsiveness to stimuli (airway edema), and reversible airway obstruction. The goal of treatment is to reduce inflammation, thereby reducing obstruction. Any history of exercise limitations, current steroid use, and prior hospitalization for acute asthma should be obtained. A history of intubation for respiratory failure is highly significant for fatal asthma. Patients with asthma tend to have other allergic signs, such as dark circles around the eyes, watery eyes, clear nasal discharge, eczema, and dermatitis. The use of beta-blocking agents (e.g., propranolol, timolol, and pindolol) may precipitate bronchoconstriction in patients with asthma.

Symptoms
- Wheezing
- Paradoxical pulse
- PEFR less than 400 L/min
- Nocturnal dyspnea is associated with severe asthma.

Diagnosis[3,4]
- Diagnosis is based on clinical presentation. See Box 17-1 for asthma classification according to severity.

Treatment[3-7]
- Inhaled beta-agonist (e.g., albuterol) agents in either inhaler or nebulizer form are used initially. Continuous nebulization is more effective than intermittent nebulization for patients with PEFR of less than 200 L/min[3,4,6,8]
- Systemic beta-adrenergic agonist agents (e.g., subcutaneous epinephrine) should be used cautiously for asthmatic patients

---

BOX 17-1   ASTHMA CLASSIFICATION BY SEVERITY

Mild asthma
- More than two exacerbations weekly
- Good exercise tolerance
- Awakened from sleep with symptoms less than twice monthly

Moderate asthma
- More than two exacerbations weekly
- Fewer than three severe episodes requiring urgent care annually

Severe asthma
- Daily symptoms
- More than three episodes requiring urgent care annually
- More than two hospitalizations per year

---

less than 35 years old whose airways are so narrowed by bronchoconstriction that inhaled medication may not penetrate far enough into the lungs. These agents should not be used to treat older patients or patients with a positive cardiac history because of their cardiovascular side effects, such as increased heart rate and contractility. The response to beta-agonists decreases with age.

- Patients who are taking steroids on a long-term basis need close monitoring for signs of adrenal suppression.
- Hospitalization may be indicated for patients with the following
  - A respiratory rate greater than 30 breaths/min
  - A heart rate greater than 120 beats/min (bradycardia may be present if severely hypoxic)
  - PEFR less than 120 L/min
  - FEV_1 less than 1000 ml
  - O_2 saturation less than 91%
- The best indicator of a good response to treatment is improvement in the PEFR or FEV_1 within 2 hours of treatment.[3]

Bronchitis[2]
Bronchitis results from an inflammation of the bronchi and may be caused by a virus, bacteria, smoking, or the inhalation

---

> ### ⇥ NURSING ALERT ⇤
>
> If an asthmatic patient requires intubation and mechanical
> ventilation, monitor the patient closely for barotrauma and
> pneumothorax, as high airway pressure may be required to
> ventilate the patient. Significant sedation and medical paralysis
> may be necessary for effective mechanical ventilation of the
> asthma patient.

---

of chemical pollutants or dust. When the cells of the bronchial-
lining tissue are irritated beyond a certain point, the cilia stop
functioning, allowing the air passages to become clogged by
debris. As the irritation increases, mucus development increases,
resulting in the characteristic cough of bronchitis.

Symptoms
- Substernal chest discomfort
- Dyspnea
- Wheezing
- Fatigue
- Fever
- Chills
- Scattered wheezes and rhonchi

Diagnosis
- Diagnostic tests usually are not necessary unless the
  symptoms have lasted for 2 weeks or longer or CHF is
  possible. In these cases a chest x-ray is obtained.
- A CBC and chest x-ray may be obtained in cases in which
  pneumonia could be more serious (e.g., child, elderly, or
  immunosuppressed patient).

Treatment[8]
- Rest, fluids, and humidification of heat
- Cough suppressant should be used only at night.
- Acetaminophen
- Administer albuterol via nebulizer, inhaler, or syrup
  (children).
- Antibiotics should be initiated in the presence of purulent
  sputum in a smoker or if sputum has changed from clear to
  purulent in a nonsmoker.

Chronic Obstructive Pulmonary Disease[2,9]
COPD is a disease of obstructive airflow that is associated with
chronic bronchitis, emphysema, or asthma. Diagnostic criteria for

COPD include the presence of a productive cough that is
3 months in duration for 2 to 3 consecutive years. Smoking,
air pollution, and occupational dust exposure also may lead to
the development of COPD. Patients with emphysema often are
thin and may exhibit muscle wasting.

Symptoms
- Dyspnea
- Productive cough
- Wheezing
- Pursed-lip exhalation (see Discharge Implications)
- Tripod positioning
- Use of accessory respiratory muscles
- Increased chest anteroposterior diameter
- Diminished breath sounds
- Jugular vein distension (JVD) suggests right-side heart failure, a common problem in those with severe COPD.

Diagnosis
- Pulmonary function tests show a reduced FEV_1/FVC ratio.
- ABG test results indicate hypoxemia and/or hypercapnia.
- A chest x-ray examination reveals hyperinflation.
- Presence of clinical symptoms

Treatment
- Initiate supplemental oxygen based on ABG results.

➤ NURSING ALERT ◄

If the patient has a history of pulmonary disease, administer
a low concentration of oxygen, preferably 2 L or less, although
oxygen never should be withheld if the patient's condition
warrants a higher concentration. Reference Guide 14 lists
oxygen devices and their possible oxygen-delivery ranges.

- Administer inhaled anticholinergics (e.g., ipratropium bromide [Atrovent]) to aid in bronchodilation.
- Provide antibiotics for infection.
- Steroids may be administered, but their use is controversial.
- Provide mucolytics to mobilize secretions.
- Administer beta-adrenergic agonists (e.g., albuterol) to bronchodilate.

- Subcutaneous epinephrine or terbutaline is administered in cases of severe airway obstruction for those who are unable to receive aerosol bronchodilating agents.
- If the patient is using home oxygen, the same dosage is used in the ED. Home oxygen is indicated when PaO_2 is less than 55 mm Hg or O_2 saturation is less than 85%.

Pneumonia[2,8]

Pneumonia may result from bacterial, viral, or fungal organisms as well as chemicals. Pneumonia may affect the entire lung or a portion of the lung. The risk for pneumonia is greater in people who are institutionalized or have a depressed gag or cough reflex, which can result in aspiration pneumonia. Multiple sexual partners and IV drug abuse increase the risk of AIDS and *Pneumocystis carinii* pneumonia (PCP) (Chapter 6).

Symptoms
- Fever
- Shaking
- Chills
- Pleuritic chest pain
- Tachypnea
- Diaphoresis
- Crackles
- Productive cough with purulent or rust-colored sputum

Diagnosis
- Diagnosis is based on infiltrates on a chest x-ray examination, positive results from sputum cultures, a CBC showing leukocytosis, and the presence of clinical symptoms.

Treatment[8]
- Initiate the administration of supplemental oxygen.
- Administer broad-spectrum antibiotics.
- Use bronchodilators (e.g., theophylline) and mucolytics such as acetylcysteine (Mucomyst) to mobilize secretions.
- Administer analgesics for pleuritic chest pain.
- Provide chest physiotherapy.
- Provide nutritional support.
- Initiate oral or IV hydration.
- Implement bed rest to reduce oxygen demands.

Pulmonary edema[10]

Pulmonary edema results from a sudden increase in left ventricular filling pressures, which produce a rapid movement of fluid into pulmonary capillaries and subsequently into the interstitial spaces and alveoli. People with cardiovascular diseases such as CHF or atrial fibrillation are prone to develop cardiogenic pulmonary edema.

Symptoms

- Tachypnea
- Dyspnea (orthopnea, DOE, PND)
- Lower extremity edema
- Crackles
- Wheezes
- Unexplained fatigue
- Pink and frothy sputum
- High pulmonary artery pressures
- Hypervolemia, signs of heart failure (e.g., JVD, peripheral edema, and organomegaly)
- Hypertension

Diagnosis[10]

- Diagnosis is based on the presence of clinical symptoms.
- Arterial blood analysis reveals hypoxemia and, eventually, hypercarbia secondary to fatigue.
- Infiltrates can be seen on a chest x-ray film.
- Pulmonary artery catheterization reveals high pulmonary artery pressures.
- History of cardiovascular disease

Treatment[10]

- Initiate supplemental oxygen, intubation, and mechanical ventilation in cases of severe respiratory distress. A trial of CPAP or BiPAP may be used before intubation and mechanical ventilation.
- Preload and afterload may be reduced by administration of the following medications:
  - Diuretics (e.g., furosemide)
  - Vasodilators (e.g., nitroprusside or hydralazine [direct acting])
  - Calcium channel blockers (e.g., verapamil or diltiazem)
  - Angiotensin-converting enzyme inhibitor (e.g., captopril)
  - Nitroglycerin sublingually, by paste, or by IV
- Bronchodilators (e.g., albuterol by inhaler) may be used to increase alveolar ventilation.
- Administer cardiac glycosides (e.g., digoxin) and inotropes to improve cardiac contractility.
- IV morphine sulfate is administered to reduce venous return and alleviate anxiety. Beware of respiratory depression if the patient is not intubated.

Pulmonary Embolism[2,11]

Pulmonary embolism occurs when a thrombus enters the microcirculation of the lungs and lodges in the pulmonary circulation. Patients with prolonged immobility, obesity, or recent orthopedic surgery are at risk for pulmonary embolism, as are those who are pregnant, who are receiving estrogen therapy, or who have cardiovascular disease such as CHF or atrial fibrillation. The most common precursor of pulmonary embolism is DVT. Warfarin (Coumadin) is used to prevent clot formation with patients who are at risk for pulmonary embolism.

Symptoms[11]

- Dyspnea
- Sudden pleuritic chest pain
- Cough
- Hemoptysis
- Diaphoresis
- Apprehension
- Tachypnea
- Tachycardia
- Crackles
- The triad of petechiae (chest, axilla), dyspnea, and mental confusion is suggestive of fat emboli.

Diagnosis[11]

- Elevated D-dimer indicates an abnormal clotting process.
- Ventilation/perfusion scan reveals a ventilation/perfusion mismatch.
- Chest x-ray examination
- Pulmonary angiography is the gold standard for diagnosis.
- ABG analysis will reveal hypoxemia.
- Presence of clinical symptoms
- Diagnostic tests include those such as Doppler ultrasound (color duplex ultrasonography) of the lower extremities to assess for DVT.

Treatment[12,13]

- Initiate supplemental oxygen.
- Initiate intubation and mechanical ventilation in cases of severe respiratory distress.
- Fluid and vasopressor support should be administered in cases of severe hypotension.
- Initiate anticoagulation (e.g., heparin IV or low-molecular-weight heparin, then PO warfarin).
- Fibrinolytics such as streptokinase, urokinase, and tPA may be administered IV or via intrapulmonary route in cases of severe pulmonary embolism, via intrapulmonary route.

- Surgical embolectomy may be necessary if other treatment is unsuccessful.
- Apply antiembolic devices (e.g., elastic, gradient, or intermittent compression stockings) on lower extremities in the absence of DVT.

Spontaneous Pneumothorax

Spontaneous pneumothorax may occur as a primary disorder not associated with pulmonary disease, or as a secondary condition, usually related to pulmonary fibrosis or pulmonary bullae and blebs. Symptoms for both types of spontaneous pneumothorax are similar, but severity is greater when the pneumothorax is caused by a preexisting pulmonary condition. Recurrence of a spontaneous pneumothorax is common. Regardless of the size of the spontaneous pneumothorax, it can progress into a tension pneumothorax, which is a life-threatening emergency (see Chapter 20).

Symptoms

- Pain on inspiration on the same side as the pneumothorax.
- Dyspnea may be present, but severity will depend on the size of the pneumothorax and the remaining pulmonary reserve. Continuous dyspnea unrelieved with rest may indicate a spontaneous pneumothorax.
- In cases of secondary spontaneous pneumothorax, the PaO_2 may be less than 55 mm Hg and the $PaCO_2$ may be greater than 50 mm Hg.
- FEV_1 may be less than 1000 ml.
- Subcutaneous emphysema may be present.
- Percussion over the affected area produces tympany.

Diagnosis

- The size and location of the pneumothorax are confirmed by chest radiography.

Treatment

Observation

If the patient is not dyspneic and the respiratory rate is within normal limits, observation may be preferred. The pneumothorax usually is less than 15% of the hemithorax, as confirmed by chest radiography.[3] This type of treatment is used for first occurrences without the presence of preexisting pulmonary disease.

Aspiration (using unidirectional valve device)

Aspiration of air from the pleural space is more successful in patients who have a primary spontaneous pneumothorax.

A guide wire is inserted over a 16-gauge needle. An 8-Fr aspiration catheter then is inserted over the guide wire, and the guide wire is removed. A 60-ml syringe is attached to the catheter with a three-way stopcock. Before removal, the stopcock is closed to the patient and a repeat chest radiographic film is obtained. If no lung expansion occurs, a Heimlich valve is attached to the catheter. If no lung reexpansion is seen on the second radiograph, the Heimlich device is connected to a chest catheter draining system (e.g., Pleurovac) at a negative pressure of 20 cm H_2O.[3,13]

>■ **N U R S I N G   A L E R T** ◄

Aspiration is rarely successful in cases of iatrogenic pneumothorax from central venous line placement. Anticipate the need for chest tube insertion.

Chest tube insertion
A 16-Fr to 24-Fr thoracostomy tube may be placed in the fourth to sixth intercostal space, midaxillary line, for air expulsion. The patient should be placed in the supine position with the head of the bed elevated 30 degrees. The patient's arm nearest the procedure should be placed behind the patient's head. The tube is connected to a closed draining system (see Procedure 8).

>■ **N U R S I N G   A L E R T** ◄

If reexpansion is not occurring after placement of the chest tube, check to see whether the connecting tubing is kinked or clogged. Confirm that the tubing is connected to the suction apparatus correctly, if appropriate.

Chest tube insertion with instillation of sclerosing agent
A sclerosing agent such as minocycline or doxycycline is injected through the chest tube to reduce the chance of recurrence of a spontaneous pneumothorax. This procedure, also known as chemical pleurodesis, is painful, and the patient should be sedated before the instillation. Lidocaine may be injected into the pleural space before the instillation of the sclerosing agent to reduce pain.
Thoracotomy
Surgical intervention may be required with severe unilateral pneumothorax or simultaneous bilateral pneumothoraces that have been unresponsive to reexpansion by other modalities.

NURSING SURVEILLANCE

1. Monitor respiratory function, including breath sounds.
2. Monitor dyspnea.
3. Note the trend of vital signs and oxygenation status (SaO_2, PaO_2, $PaCO_2$).
4. Monitor intake and output.
5. Monitor the patient for cardiac arrhythmias.
6. Analyze laboratory tests, and report significant changes to the physician.
7. Assess the patient for therapeutic response and adverse reactions to medications.
8. Evaluate and support effective coping strategies.
9. Monitor PEFR (if appropriate).

EXPECTED PATIENT OUTCOMES

1. Shortness of breath improves compared with initial assessment.
2. The ABG levels trend toward normal.
3. The heart rate ranges from 60 to 100 beats/min.
4. The mean arterial pressure remains at 70 to 100 mm Hg.
5. Urinary output is greater than 30 ml/hr or 0.5 ml/kg/hr.
6. Life-threatening arrhythmias are absent.
7. Wheezing and stridor are absent, and spontaneous ventilation is present.

DISCHARGE INSTRUCTIONS

General

1. If the patient is receiving home oxygen, instruct on oxygen safety. There must be no open flame within 6 feet of the oxygen.
2. Offer appropriate resources for smoking cessation. These may include medications, support groups, and relaxation training. Instruct the patient to avoid secondhand smoke.
3. Encourage adequate nutrition and hydration to support respiratory function.
4. The geriatric population and those with COPD may benefit from annual influenza vaccines and from the one-time pneumococcal pneumonia vaccine (Pneumovax). The pneumococcal pneumonia vaccine is contraindicated for those with an active pulmonary infection.
5. Environmental pollutants should be avoided by all patients with or without respiratory disease.

6. Infection control can be supported by frequent hand washing, the appropriate use of tissues, and the use of masks for those who are immunosuppressed.
7. Instruct patients in the home administration of medications.

Asthma

1. Involve children in the management of their asthma.
2. Teach the use of metered dose inhalers (MDIs). MDIs may be difficult to use for persons with impaired mental function, poor motor coordination, or weakened, arthritic hands. The use of spacers attached to the MDI allows the drug to be expelled into a large plastic chamber. The patient can inhale the medication from the chamber so activation of the MDI does not have to be coordinated with inhalation. Spacers also reduce the incidence of thrush and hoarseness associated with steroid MDI. Box 17-2, Properly Metered Dose Inhaler Technique, explains proper technique.
3. Emphasize to pregnant, asthmatic patients that hypoxia is a greater risk to the fetus than are inhaled medications.
4. Teach parents about the effect of passive cigarette smoke on children with asthma.
5. Teach home monitoring of PEFR. PEFR is best measured with the patient in the standing position. The patient breathes deeply and blows out fast and hard through the peak flow meter. This maneuver is performed three times, and the highest value is recorded. Portable peak expiratory flow

---

BOX 17-2   PROPERLY METERED DOSE INHALER TECHNIQUE

- Shake the canister.
- Hold the canister approximately 2 inches (4 to 5 cm) in front of the mouth.
- Exhale completely.
- Begin to inhale.
- Activate the canister.
- Continue to breathe deeply and hold your breath for 5 sec. Exhale.
- Wait for response (1 to 10 min), depending on your symptoms.
- Repeat as prescribed.

meters should be calibrated regularly because accurate readings depend on a spring mechanism that can stretch with time. PEFR should be measured at the same time each day for patients with severe asthma (twice daily to four times daily during acute exacerbations). Values obtained in the morning usually are lower than those obtained in the evening.

6. Many patients believe that asthma medication is harmful and addictive. Emphasize that the continuous use of medication is the key to prevention and is required for this chronic illness. Instruct the patient on the correct use of control inhalers (e.g., steroids) and rescue inhalers (e.g., albuterol).

7. Teach patients when to seek urgent care. Classic symptoms are the need for frequent use (greater than four times/day) of a rescue inhaler (e.g., albuterol) without sustained improvement, frequent nocturnal awakening with symptoms, and a drop in PEFR to 50% or less of the predicted value at any time.

8. Teach patients to reduce the amount of allergens in their environment by removing all carpeting, washing animals weekly, and covering mattresses and pillows with impermeable covers.

9. Advise the patient to use the prescribed inhaler before exposure to known allergens or exercise.

10. Warn patients that there is an increased risk of bronchospasm associated with use of aspirin and nonsteroidal antiinflammatory medication. Acetaminophen should be used for pain and fever relief. Sulfite sensitivity also may be present. Sulfating agents are found in processed potatoes, shrimp, dried fruits, beer, and wine.

Pulmonary Alveolar Edema
1. Teach the patient about home administration of respiratory and cardiac medications.
2. Patients with severe PAE are hospitalized.

Pulmonary Embolism
1. Advise the patient to avoid long periods of immobility.
2. Instruct the patient in home administration of warfarin when applicable, as follows:
   - Wear a medical alert bracelet indicating anticoagulation therapy.
   - Use an electric razor and a soft toothbrush.
   - Watch for bleeding and report black or maroon stools to a physician.

- Avoid foods high in vitamin K (e.g., green leafy vegetables, tomatoes, cauliflower, and fish) to maintain anticoagulation.
3. Encourage the patient to wear loose-fitting clothes.
4. Instruct the patient in the use of elastic or gradient stockings.

Pneumonia
1. Pneumonia often is slow to resolve, especially in geriatric patients. Instruct the patient to schedule frequent rest periods to minimize oxygenation needs.
2. Instruct the patient to avoid exposure to people known to have URIs.
3. Ensure that the patient understands home administration of antibiotics. Reinforce the importance of finishing antibiotic prescriptions.

Chronic Obstructive Pulmonary Disease
1. Ask the patient to demonstrate use of the inhaler to determine the proper technique.
2. Teach breathing techniques to enhance oxygenation as follows:
   - *Pursed-lip breathing.* Breathe in slowly through nose, purse the lips (as if to whistle), and then breathe out slowly through pursed lips.
   - *Diaphragmatic breathing.* In an upright position, place one hand on the abdomen just above the waist, place the other hand on the upper chest, and breathe in through the nose. The lower hand should push out and the hand on the chest should not move. Then breathe out through pursed lips and feel the lower hand move in.[6]
3. Avoid alcohol, spicy foods, and dairy products that increase bronchospasm and sputum production.
4. Avoid extremes in temperature. Wear a mask when going from warmth indoors to coldness outdoors.
5. Increase fluids to 3 L each day to aid in sputum liquefaction.
6. Instruct the patient to avoid exposure to people known to have URIs.

Spontaneous Pneumothorax
1. Symptoms may take up to 10 days to resolve.
2. Instruct the patient to avoid air travel and scuba diving until total lung reexpansion has been confirmed by chest radiography. Follow-up care is recommended 7 to 10 days after the event.
3. Alert the patient that recurrences are likely and that treatment should be sought if symptoms return.

REFERENCES

1. Colucci WS: *Noncardiogenic pulmonary edema*, June, 2002, www.utdol. com/application/topic.asp?file=hrt_fail/12162&type=A&selectedTitle= 3~54.

2. Brashers VL: Alterations of pulmonary function. In: McCance KL and Huether SE, eds: *Pathophysiology: the biologic basis for disease in adults & children*, ed 4, St Louis, 2002, Mosby; pp 1105-1144.

3. Boushey HA and Venkayya R: *Pathogenesis and management of status asthmaticus*, September, 2002, www.utdol.com/application/topic/ print.asp?file=asthma/7775.

4. Fanta CH: *Treatment of acute exacerbations of asthma*, June, 2002, www.utdol.com/application/topic/print.asp?file=asthma/12318.

5. Phanareth K, Hansen LS, Christensen LK, et al: A proposal for a practical treatment guideline designed for the initial two hours of the management of patients with acute severe asthma and COPD using the principles of evidence-based medicine, *Respir Med* 96 (9):659-671, 2002.

6. Marik PE, Varon J, and Fromm R Jr: The management of acute severe asthma, *J Emerg Med* 23 (3):257-268, 2002.

7. Adams BK and Cydulka RK: Asthma evaluation and management, *Emerg Med Clin North Am* 21 (2):315-330, 2003.

8. Ward MA: Emergency department management of acute respiratory infections, *Semin Respir Infect* 17 (1):65-71, 2002.

9. Stoller JK: *Overview of management of acute exacerbations of chronic obstructive pulmonary disease*, June, 2002, www.utdol.com/application/ topic/print.asp?file=copd/8006.

10. Colucci WS: *Cardiogenic pulmonary edema*, December, 2002, www.utdol. com/application/topic/print.asp?file=hrt_fail/11440& type= A&selectedTitle=1~54.

11. Thompson BT and Hales CA: *Clinical manifestations of and diagnostic strategies for acute pulmonary embolism*, May, 2003, www.utdol.com/ application/topic.asp?file=vascular/6608&type=A&selectedTitle=1~98.

12. Valentine KA and Hull RD: *Treatment of acute pulmonary embolism*, May, 2001, www.utdol.com/application/topic.asp?file=vascular/ 7738&type=A&selectedTitle=5~98.

13. Tapson VF: *Massive pulmonary embolism*, January, 2003, www.utdol.com/ application/topic.asp?file=misclung/18989&type=A&selectedTitle=2~98

18 chapter

Sexually Transmitted Infections

Deborah M. Anderson

CLINICAL CONDITIONS

Candida Infection
Chancroid (Genital Ulcer Disease)
Chlamydia Infection
Gonorrhea
Hepatitis B Virus Infection
Herpes Simplex Virus Infection
Human Papillomavirus Infection
Pelvic Inflammatory Disease
Syphilis
Trichomonas Infection
Vaginal Bacteriosis (VB)

INTRODUCTION

Sexually transmitted infections (STIs) are those that are contracted by intimate sexual contact. Patients may be infected with more than one STI. Some STIs can be spread by other means, such as through contaminated blood products or unintended inoculation. Risk factors for STIs are listed in Box 18-1. In the United States, gonorrhea, syphilis, chlamydia, HIV, and chancroid are among the infections reportable to state or local health officials. The local or national health authority determines what is reportable in a specific geographic location.

FOCUSED NURSING ASSESSMENT

Nursing assessment should center on pain, elimination, metabolic changes, sexuality, and tissue integrity.

Pain
1. Where is the pain located?
2. What are the characteristics of the pain?

BOX 18-1 RISK FACTORS ASSOCIATED WITH STIs

1. Vaginal douching has been associated with PID, *Candida* infection, and bacterial vaginosis.[1]
2. Smoking has been associated with PID and other STIs.[2]
3. Having multiple sexual partners (defined as more than three in a lifetime[3]) increases the risk for PID.
4. Diabetes is associated with a higher incidence of *Candida* infection.
5. The use of tight undergarments or feminine hygiene sprays is associated with vaginitis and *Candida,* as are hyperglycemia and increased sugar intake.
6. The early onset of sexual activity is associated with human papillomavirus (HPV).
7. Pregnancy may activate HPV and herpes.

---

3. Auscultate bowel sounds, and then palpate the abdomen for rigidity and tenderness. A rigid abdomen and absent bowel sounds may indicate pelvic inflammatory disease (PID), a ruptured ectopic pregnancy, or a ruptured ovarian cyst (see Chapter 16). Alert the physician to the urgency of evaluating this patient.

Elimination

- When was the last time the patient voided? A urinalysis can detect nonspecific urethritis in men if they have not voided for 1 hour. If the patient needs to void while waiting for evaluation and treatment, provide a sterile container and instructions on clean catch urine collection. Menstruating women may need to be catheterized to obtain a specimen.
- Does the patient have constipation or rectal drainage? Give the patient a stool specimen container if necessary.

Metabolic and Vital Signs

Blood pressure (BP) may be decreased, and the patient's pulse may be elevated in cases of hemorrhage (rigid abdomen). Fever is common if a disease has progressed to salpingitis, particularly if the causative agent is gonorrhea. When genital infection has progressed to systemic sepsis, fever may be present, depending on the causative organism and the patient's immune status.

TABLE 18-1 Differential Diagnosis of STIs

Diagnosis	Nodes	Lesion
Syphilis	Firm, painless, usually not enlarged	Single, painless lesion
Herpes	Tender, bilateral inguinal node enlargement	Multiple, tender vesicles that ulcerate
Chancroid	Tender, unilateral or bilateral nodes that may not be enlarged	Multiple painful, leaking lesions with ragged edges
HPV (genital warts)	Possible enlarged inguinal lymph nodes	Pinhead papules to cauliflower-like masses that are flesh colored, pink, or red and that may cluster

Sexuality

Depending on the privacy of the triage area, several of these questions may have been explored at triage. If the information has not been collected, ask the following:

- The date of onset of sexual activity and of the last sexual activity
- The number of partners and number of the significant other's partners
- The type of sexual activity (e.g., oral or anal)
- The type of protection used to prevent STIs and pregnancy
- The date of the last menstrual period
- Any symptoms associated with the sexual activity

Tissue Integrity

- Examine skin for color, rashes, lesions, and texture.
- Note lymph node enlargement (see Table 18-1) (see Reference Guide 21 for descriptions of non-STI rashes).
- Note the characteristics of any abnormalities found.

LIFE SPAN ISSUES

Pediatric Patients

1. It is not typical for children to experience genital problems or vaginal discharge. Ask whether there has been a change in the child's behavior. Maintain a high index of suspicion for sexual abuse (see Chapter 2).

2. Females between the ages of 15 and 19 have the highest incidence of gonorrhea and *Chlamydia*.[3] Gonorrhea preferentially infects columnar epithelial cells. In adolescence, these cells are everted over part of the ectocervix, increasing the amount of susceptible tissue exposed during intercourse. For this same reason, HPV incidence is greatest among women 15 to 24 years old.[2]

Women

1. Pregnancy increases the incidence of STIs because of metaplasia and relative immunosuppression.
2. STIs in women may be associated with cervical cancer.

INITIAL INTERVENTIONS

1. Monitor vital signs closely. If the patient has a fever and a rigid, painful abdomen, anticipate the need for a large-bore IV catheter. Normal saline or Ringer's lactate solution may be administered for fluid resuscitation, for hydration, or at a rate to keep a vein open (e.g., 30 ml/hr). While starting the IV, obtain blood specimens for possible type and crossmatch, complete blood count, hemoglobin, hematocrit, rapid plasma reagin/Venereal Disease Research Laboratory (VDRL) testing, and a serum pregnancy test.
2. Anticipate a pelvic examination.
   - Determine whether the patient prefers to have certain individuals remain in the room during the examination. Prepare the patient by having the patient undress and put on a gown. Note any discharge on the undergarments.
   - Prepare the equipment (e.g., speculum; slide; slide cover; fixative; KOH; culture media and DNA probe for *Chlamydia* and gonorrhea; viral culturette; bacterial culturette; gauze sponges; swabs; wooden spatula or brush, if a Pap smear is to be performed; lubrication for bimanual examination; Hemoccult testing for stool).
   - Follow the procedure described in Box 18-2, Pap Smear Procedure. Make sure the bed allows for performance of a pelvic examination (i.e., breaks down with stirrups). Have a high-powered light source available.
   - When obtaining a wet smear, use the technique described in the Box 18-3, Wet Smear Procedure. Refer to the section Priority Diagnostic Tests for more information.
3. Obtain a clean-catch urine specimen. If the patient is menstruating, obtain a catheter specimen. Test the specimen

---

BOX 18-2   PAP SMEAR PROCEDURE

Nursing Action
1. Warm the speculum or wet it with warm tap water.
   Do not use lubricants.

Physician Actions
2. Use a cotton swab to remove excess discharge.
3. With a cytobrush or a wooden spatula, scrape the cervix.
4. Use the cytobrush to brush the endocervical canal.
5. Smear the brush or spatula on a slide.

Nursing Action
6. Spray the slide with a fixative (95% alcohol may be used).

BOX 18-3   WET SMEAR PROCEDURE

1. Place one drop of vaginal discharge on each end of a plain, unfrosted microscope slide or use two slides.
2. Add one drop of 10% KOH. Note the odor when KOH is applied. (A fishy smell is present in cases of vaginitis.)
3. Cover the KOH drop with a coverslip.
4. Add enough saline to the remaining drop of vaginal secretion to dilute the specimen.
5. Place a coverslip over the saline specimen.

---

with a urinary reagent strip for blood, protein, pH, and glucose. Using sterile technique, split the specimen into two containers in anticipation of microscopic analysis, culture, and urine pregnancy test.
4. Provide pain and anxiety relief:
   - Use nonpharmacologic strategies to reduce pain and anxiety.
   - Administer pain medication as ordered.
   - Provide reassurance; treat the patient in a nonjudgmental manner.
   - Explain all procedures.
5. Nursing care priorities are listed in the table on pp. 610-611.

PRIORITY DIAGNOSTIC TESTS

Laboratory Tests

Blood cultures: Cultures may be conducted in cases of suspected PID and disseminated gonorrhea.

Complete blood count (CBC): In cases of systemic symptoms (e.g., fever), a CBC is obtained to detect leukocytosis. The WBC count is elevated in cases of PID.

Direct fluorescent antibody test (DFA): Monoclonal antibodies are used to detect *Chlamydia* and herpes.

DNA probe: A DNA probe may be used to identify *Chlamydia* and gonorrhea. DNA probes tend to have false-positive results with children. Nonculture tests (Gram stain smear and DNA probe) should not be used alone in diagnosing gonorrhea in children.[2]

Erythrocyte sedimentation rate (ESR): The erythrocyte sedimentation rate is obtained in cases of suspected PID. The value is elevated with any inflammatory condition.

Genital cultures: Vaginal, cervical, rectal, and urethral drainage may be cultured.

1. *Gonorrhea:* Thayer-Martin or Martin-Lewis culture media usually are used and contain antibiotics against other organisms that often invade genital sites. Discharge is obtained on a swab and applied directly to the culture medium with a back-and-forth motion. The inoculated culture should be sent to the laboratory as soon as possible to be placed in a CO_2-rich environment or incubator. With children, specimens from the vagina, urethra, pharynx, and rectum should be obtained.

2. *Chlamydia:* A special culture medium is used for this organism. A cytologic swab is used to obtain the specimen. The swab is placed in the test tube of medium. This specimen should be obtained last during the pelvic examination because epithelial cells are needed and all discharge must be swabbed away. The specimen must be refrigerated quickly. Place the specimen in a cup of ice until it is taken to the lab.

Glucose level, serum: The blood glucose level may be obtained if the woman complains of several episodes of *Candida* infection.

Gram stain: Gram staining of cervical and urethral specimens (with men) is conducted to determine the presence of gonorrhea. This test has a low sensitivity and is followed by a culture. It also is used to determine the source of the organism in cases of vaginitis.

Joint aspiration: Joint aspiration is indicated in cases of suspected disseminated gonorrhea with symptoms of joint pain and swelling, fever, and rash (gonorrheal arthritis).

Lumbar puncture: A lumbar puncture may be performed to obtain a cerebrospinal fluid specimen to test for syphilis if neurologic symptoms are present.

NURSING CARE PRIORITIES

Potential/Actual Problem	Causes	Signs and Symptoms	Interventions
Altered fluid volume	• Anorexia • Nausea resulting in a decreased intake • Diarrhea • Intraperitoneal hemorrhage	• Delayed capillary refill • Elevated heart rate • Altered mental status • Decreased urine output • Dry mucous membranes • Furrowed tongue • Decreased skin turgor • Depressed fontanel in infants • Pale or flushed color	• Monitor vital signs, including orthostatic vital signs. • Monitor intake and output. • Check specific gravity and color of urine. • Perform occult blood test on all vomitus and stool. • Assess for signs and symptoms of dehydration. • Assess neck veins (collapsed when lying flat). • Administer IV fluid. • Prepare patient for surgical intervention if necessary.
Pain	• Infection • Inflammation • Burning • Vomiting • Diarrhea	• Complaints of pain, self-reporting pain scale • Crying, moaning • Irritability • Facial grimacing	• Pain medications as ordered IV or PO • Monitor vital signs after pain medication. • Reassess pain using a pain scale. • Apply warm compresses to genital lesions after diagnostic procedures.

		Listen to patient concerns.
	• Restlessness	• Explain all procedures and answer questions.
	• Hostility	• Provide reassurance and comfort.
	• Inability to relax	• Provide a calm, quiet environment.
Changes in body image and self-concept	• Nervousness	• Suggest alternative sexual activities during exacerbations.
	• Increased heart rate	• Refer to infertility specialists as necessary.
	• Increased respiratory rate	
	• Elevated blood pressure	
	• Potential for surgery	
	• Invasive procedures	
	• Alteration in sexual function or reproductive abilities	
Lack of knowledge	• Lack of integration of treatment plan into activities	• Initiate patient and family teaching.
	• Requests for information	• Use family to enforce teaching whenever possible.
	• Diet	• Dietary consultation: nutritionist visit
	• Fluid intake	
	• Medication use	

Pregnancy test, serum (human chorionic gonadotropin; HCG): A pregnancy test should be completed for all females with suspected STIs because some treatments differ during pregnancy.

Rapid plasma reagin (RPR): This test is used to detect syphilis. Results yield a nonreactive or reactive state. A nonreactive reading does not rule out an incubating disease. If the disease is suspected, the RPR should be repeated at 1-week, 1-month, and 3-month intervals. A reactive test may indicate a past infection inadequately treated or a new infection. Treated individuals should be retested at 3-month intervals for 1 year or until a nonreactive test occurs. If the RPR test result is positive, a VDRL test is performed because of its increased specificity for syphilis.

Throat culture: A throat culture is indicated with symptoms of pharyngitis in sexually active patients who engage in oral sex.

Urinalysis and urine culture: Several STIs may infect the urethra as well as other genital areas. Urethral leukocytosis with pyuria may be present in male patients who have *Chlamydia* infection or gonorrhea.

Venereal Disease Research Laboratory test: A VDRL test is used to detect syphilis.

Wet Prep: This test is a microscopic examination with normal saline and KOH. This test will show the presence of clue cells, yeast, and trichomoniasis.

CLINICAL CONDITIONS

Candida Infection
Also known as a yeast infection, this is considered a sexually associated, but not sexually transmitted, disease.

Symptoms
- Itching
- Burning
- Vulvovaginal pain
- Irritation
- Inflammation
- Thick, white, cottage-cheesy substance may coat the vaginal walls; there is no foul odor.
- Urination and intercourse may be painful.

Diagnosis
- Culture of vaginal secretions: Microscopic examination is performed to confirm the diagnosis and to help rule out other possible infections.

Treatment
- Miconazole nitrate or clotrimazole vaginal suppositories or cream may be prescribed. Creams and suppositories are oil based and may weaken latex condoms and diaphragms.
- Diflucan, fluconazole 150 mg PO one time can be prescribed.
- Recurrence is common.

Chancroid and Genital Ulcer Disease
Chancroid has been identified as a cofactor in HIV transmission. Serologic testing for HIV should be conducted. Of those infected, 10% also have syphilis or herpes. Serologic testing and a DNA probe or culture should be obtained.[2]

Symptoms
- Lesions on external genitalia. The lesions begin as small papules and break down into painful exudative ulcers with ragged edges.
- Inguinal lymph nodes may be painful when palpated.
- Rectal bleeding may be present.
- Dyspareunia is common.

Diagnosis
- Diagnosis is based on clinical presentation. A culture may be obtained, but sensitivity is poor.
- Usually four or fewer lesions are present.
- The condition may be diagnosed by default when a herpes culture or probe result is negative.

Treatment
- Medication: Treatment is administration of ceftriaxone, azithromycin, ciprofloxacin, or erythromycin.

***Chlamydia* Infection**
Chlamydial infections often are associated with gonococcal infections, and distinguishing one from the other can be difficult. Most people are treated for both gonorrhea and chlamydia.

Symptoms
Most cases are asymptomatic and are detected by routine screening.
- If the condition is left untreated, a female patient may complain of[1,4]:
  ○ Abdominal pain (pelvic inflammatory disease; PID)
  ○ Vaginal pain
  ○ Dysuria
  ○ Postcoital pain and bleeding
  ○ Purulent vaginal discharge

  ○ Burning during urination from inflammation of the urethra
  ○ Fever
- Male patients complain of:
  ○ A thick, cloudy penile discharge if the urethra is infected
  ○ Dysuria
  ○ Epididymitis; testicular pain, swelling, tenderness, fever
  ○ Prostatitis; discharge from urethra, discomfort during or after urination, pain during or after intercourse, and/or vague lower back pain
  ○ Anal infections may be without symptoms or may cause irritation around the anus and pain with bowel movements.

Diagnosis
- Culture exudate
- DNA probe
- Obtain RPR and VDRL to rule out other sexually transmitted diseases.

Treatment
- Sexual partners should be screened and treated.
- Drugs of choice include azithromycin 1 g PO in a single dose or doxycycline 100 mg PO twice a day for 7 days. Erythromycin 500 mg PO four times a day for 7 days or amoxicillin 500 mg PO three times a day for 7 days may be used for pregnant patients.[2]

Gonorrhea
Mucosa of the genitalia (urethra in men and cervix in women), the rectum, and the oropharynx are susceptible. Gonorrhea is spread by direct physical contact (including to neonates if delivered through an infected birth canal).

Symptoms
- Females: Most exhibit mild symptoms that can be overlooked or are asymptomatic. If symptomatic, the following may be present:
  ○ Yellow and white discharge
  ○ Swollen and congested cervix; dysuria or frequency
  ○ Abnormal menses
  ○ Dyspareunia
  ○ Abdominal pain
  ○ Frequent or painful urination
- Males
  ○ Urethral discharge
  ○ Dysuria
  ○ Testicular tenderness
  ○ Rectal discomfort

- Males and females: Gonorrhea that has spread to other parts of the body may cause:
  ○ Rash
  ○ Fever
  ○ Painful, swollen joints
  ○ Other symptoms are specific to the body part that is infected, such as rectal pain and discharge if anorectal gonorrhea is present or possible gonococcal pharyngitis after oral sexual exposure.
  ○ Disseminated gonococcal infection may be present in untreated cases, usually in women. A sparse pustular or blister-type rash may be present on the extremities in addition to the above symptoms.

Diagnosis
- Gram stain smear of exudate
- Culture of exudate
- DNA probe

Treatment
Gonorrhea is often resistant to penicillin.[2]
- Cephalosporins (cefixime), ciprofloxacin (quinolones), or tetracycline is administered. Ciprofloxacin is not recommended for person under 17 years of age because it inhibits cartilage development; it also is not approved for use in pregnancy; use a cephalosporin if patient is pregnant.
- *Chlamydia* and gonorrhea often infect people simultaneously. If a chlamydial infection not been ruled out, azithromycin or doxycycline may be added to the regimen.
- Pregnant women should be treated only with cephalosporins or spectinomycin IM.
- Children weighing less than 45 kg should be treated with ceftriaxone 125 mg IM.
- Cultures should be taken from sexual partners, and the partners should be treated. Partners also may need rectal and pharyngeal cultures depending on mode of transmission.
- Reculture is recommended in 4 to 7 days.

Hepatitis B Virus
Sexual contact is the most frequently reported method of hepatitis B viral transmission. About 30% of persons have no signs or symptoms. (See Chapter 6 for more information.)

Symptoms
- Malaise
- Fatigue

- Jaundice
- Abdominal pain
- Loss of appetite
- Nausea and vomiting
- Joint pain

Diagnosis

Diagnosis is based on the results of serologic testing.

Treatment

- No specific treatments; employ rest, avoid alcohol and drugs detoxified by the liver, maintain good nutrition
- Prevention is key. A single dose of hepatitis B vaccine can be administered if treatment occurs within 24 hours of exposure, but a full series of three IM injections is still needed for protection.

Herpes Simplex Virus

Herpes is transmitted through direct physical contact with the infected secretions produced by the blisters that are characteristic of the disease. Two strains of the herpes simplex virus (HSV) have been identified. HSV1 generally affects the skin, eyes, gums ("cold sores"), mouth, or pharynx. HSV2 generally affects the genitalia and surrounding tissue. However, either type of HSV can occur in any area. There is no cure for either type, and there is a 50% chance of reoccurrence three to four times yearly. Although rare, babies can become infected during childbirth, and the disease can be life threatening.

Symptoms

- Tingling or itching at the site of inoculation.
- Clusters of tiny blisters on the penis, scrotum, vulva, perineum, vagina, cervix, thighs, buttocks, or near the anus.
- Ruptured blisters form ulcerations that eventually form a crust.
- Fever
- Headache
- Enlarged inguinal lymph nodes
- Chills
- Nausea and vomiting
- Malaise
- Dysuria may result in urinary retention.

Diagnosis

- Diagnosis usually is based on clinical presentation or viral culture.
- Herpes simplex antigen by direct fluorescent antibody technique (DFA). Recombinant technology can identify

HSV-type specific IgG antibodies, making it possible to identify the type of HSV responsible for the infection.

Treatment

- Acyclovir accelerates healing, particularly in first occurrences and particularly when it is started within 48 hours of the outbreak, but its efficacy decreases with recurrent episodes. Cases also may be treated with famciclovir and valacyclovir.
- Warm compresses, sitz baths, and aspirin may help during outbreaks.

Human Papillomavirus

Human papillomavirus (HPV) causes genital warts and is one of the most common causes of STI in the world. Health experts estimate that there are more cases of genital HPV infection than of any other STI in the United States.[2] HPV has been linked to cervical cancers and other genital cancers. Like many STIs, genital HPV infections often do not have visible signs and symptoms. Genital warts are very contagious and are spread during oral, genital, or anal sex with an infected partner. HPV infection has been linked with cervical and vulvar cancer in women and anorectal and squamous cell carcinoma of the penis in men.

Symptoms

Warty growths (condylomata) that have a cauliflower-like appearance. The growths appear in moist genital areas where coital friction occurs. In women, the warts occur on the outside and inside of the vagina, on the opening (cervix) to the womb (uterus), or around the anus. In men, genital warts are less common but usually will be seen on the tip or shaft of the penis, on the scrotum, or around the anus.

- Painless
- Often occur in clusters
- May be very tiny or can spread into large masses in the genital or anal area.
- Rarely, genital warts also can develop in the mouth or throat of a person who has had oral sex with an infected person.

Diagnosis

- Diagnosis is based on clinical presentation.
- Cervical HPV infections usually are detected by Pap smear.
- Because of the possibility of neoplasia, biopsy should be performed on all warts with atypical appearance and on warts that are pigmented or located on the cervix.
- No culture method is available.

Treatment

This virus is difficult to treat, and recurrences are frequent. Treatment is most successful when warts are small. Consider concurrent STIs as well.

- Imiquimod 5% (Aldara) cream may be prescribed. Do not use for urethral, intravaginal, cervical, or rectal lesions.
- Podophyllin (Condylox), a cytotoxic agent, or trichloroacetic acid also may be used to remove the wart. Podophyllin is contraindicated during pregnancy because it can cause spontaneous abortion.
- Liquid nitrogen may be applied.
- Lesions are removed by laser therapy in severe cases.

Pelvic Inflammatory Disease

Pelvic inflammatory disease (PID) is an infection of the uterus, fallopian tubes, and adjacent pelvic structures. It may be called salpingitis. It ranges in severity from mild to life threatening. Infertility or ectopic pregnancy may result from tubal scarring and occlusion. PID can lead to infertility.

Symptoms

Symptoms are not always apparent.

- The most common symptom is bilateral lower abdominal pain. Look for patients to be hunched over and have a shuffling gate because of the abdominal pain.
- Bleeding or pain with intercourse and spotting between periods
- Pain with manipulation of the cervix and bimanual examination of the ovaries.
- Pain also occurs with walking, urination, and sexual intercourse.
- Abnormal vaginal discharge is thick, creamy, and foul smelling and varies depending on the type of organism(s) involved.
- *Neisseria gonorrhoeae* and *Chlamydia trachomatis* are most common.
- Fever
- Elevated WBC count and ESR
- Complications can include septic shock.

Diagnosis

Diagnosis is based on clinical presentation.

Treatment

- Treatment is initiated on suspicion of the condition.
- A pregnancy test should be performed to minimize the possibility of missing an ectopic pregnancy.[3]

- Antibiotics are the drug of choice (cefoxitin, Cefoxitin, doxycycline, clindamycin, gentamicin, ofloxacin, and levofloxacin are used most often).
- Heat to the abdomen or sitz baths
- Analgesics
- Hospitalization is indicated when the possibility of a surgical emergency cannot be excluded, when a pelvic abscess is suspected, when the patient is pregnant, when an adolescent is unable to follow outpatient therapy or return for follow-up, or when a patient is HIV positive.
- Outpatient therapy is used for mild cases (WBC less than 11,000/mm^3 with no evidence of peritonitis).[4]

Syphilis

Syphilis is a disease that affects the blood vessels and is caused by the spirochete *Treponema pallidum*. The disease has four stages, and symptoms vary according to the stage. The patient moves through these stages if the disease is untreated. Syphilis can be contracted by contact with contaminated body fluids during sexual activity, through the sharing of needles, or by contact with fluid from the lesions. Syphilis is highly contagious whenever an open sore or skin rash is present.

Symptoms

Symptoms of syphilis can mimic other diseases. Syphilis is described in terms of its four stages. Each stage has a different set of symptoms.

Primary stage

A sore (chancre) that is usually painless develops at the site where the bacteria entered the body. In women, a chancre may go unnoticed if it occurs inside the vagina or at the opening to the uterus (cervix). Swelling of the lymph nodes may occur near the area of the chancre.

Secondary stage

Secondary syphilis is systemic and is characterized by a rash that appears from 2 to 8 weeks after the chancre develops. The rash usually consists of reddish brown, small, solid, flat or raised sores that are less than 2 cm (0.79 in) wide and usually affects the hands and soles of the feet. Small, open sores may be present on mucous membranes. Flu-like symptoms, weight loss, patchy hair loss, and swelling of the lymph nodes may be present. Nervous system symptoms of secondary syphilis include headaches, irritability, paralysis, unequal reflexes, and irregular pupils.

Latent (hidden) stage
If untreated, an infected person will progress to the latent (hidden), symptom-free stage and remain contagious.

Tertiary (late) stage
This is the most destructive stage of syphilis. Complications of this stage include:

- Gummas, which are large sores inside the body or on the skin.
- Cardiovascular syphilis: aneurysms, heart failure
- Neurosyphilis: affects the brain and the meninges

Diagnosis

- In stages one and two, genital scrapings are viewed under darkfield microscopy, or fluorescent antibody techniques are used.
- RPR and VDRL titers detect the organism.

Treatment

- Penicillin remains the treatment of choice.
- For penicillin-allergic individuals, doxycycline, tetracycline, or erythromycin is recommended.
- Certain antibiotics prescribed for other STIs (antibiotics with beta-lactam resistance and tetracycline) also are effective against syphilis.
- Patients treated for an STI with antibiotics other than beta-lactams or tetracycline should be tested for syphilis 1 month later.

Trichomoniasis
Trichomoniasis is considered a sexually associated, but not a sexually transmitted, disease. It is caused by protozoa.

Symptoms
An odorous, frothy, yellow-green discharge is present and is associated with vulvar irritation.

Diagnosis
Motile organisms are identified on a normal saline smear of the discharge.

Treatment

- Metronidazole is the drug of choice.
- Sexual partners should be treated simultaneously.

Vaginal Bacteriosis (VB)
Vaginosis is caused by an overgrowth of anaerobic organisms.

Symptoms
Patients have a malodorous (fishy odor), gray-white, watery discharge associated with vulvar itching.

Diagnosis

Diagnosis is based on the presence of an amine (fishy) odor to the vaginal discharge when mixed with 10% KOH (whiff test).

Treatment

- Treatment is initiated with metronidazole.
- Clindamycin may be used if the patient is pregnant.

NURSING SURVEILLANCE

1. Monitor patient for response to fluid administration.
2. Monitor patient's pain level and any changes.
3. Monitor the trend of fever, vital signs, and urine output if the abdomen is rigid.

EXPECTED PATIENT OUTCOMES

1. Pain decreases in intensity.
2. The patient understands the differences in contraceptive methods and methods for preventing STIs.

NURSING ALERT

Avoid using terms that assume marital status and sexual preference when conducting patient teaching. The term "partner" is preferred.

PATIENT/FAMILY DISCHARGE IMPLICATIONS AND EDUCATION

1. Sexual partners of the previous 60 days should be examined.
2. Follow-up cultures (test of cure) should be obtained from infected sites. The time at which this follow-up test is performed varies from 3 to 7 days after the completion of therapy, to 2 weeks after the initial diagnosis, to 4 to 6 weeks after therapy.
3. Remind the patient to avoid intercourse until he or she is cured or adequately treated.
4. When discussing birth control options and STI prevention, warn patients that some diseases are not prevented by proper and consistent use of male condoms. Herpes, syphilis, HPV, and chancroid may be transmitted, despite condom use, depending on the site of the lesions. Hepatitis B virus can be transmitted through natural skin condoms.
5. Encourage the use of condoms.

6. Teach the female patient about the need for Pap smears to detect dysplasia. All women, beginning with the onset of sexual activity or at age 21, should have regular Pap smears. Pap smears should be performed annually if the woman is sexually active. If the patient has known HPV disease, more frequent Pap smears are recommended because of the high risk for cervical cancer. Table 18-2 summarizes information about contraception and protection of the partner and patient against STIs.

Candida
Treatment of male partners is not recommended unless the man has balanitis or the woman has recurrent infections. Balanitis may be treated with topical antifungal agents.[2]

Chancroid
Sex partners who have contact with a patient who has had a case of chancroid (genital ulcer disease) diagnosed within the last 10 days should be treated. All patients should be tested for HIV and syphilis at the time of the initial diagnosis and 3 months later. Uncircumcised and HIV-infected patients may not respond to initial treatment and may require retreatment.

Chlamydia
Pregnant women should be retested for cure because erythromycin and amoxicillin are not as effective against the organism.

Gonorrhea
Sex partners who have contact with a patient who has had a case of gonorrhea diagnosed within the last 60 days should be treated.

Herpes
Barrier methods should be used at all times during sexual activity. The condom must cover all infected areas. Female condoms cover more genital area than male condoms. Sexual contact should be avoided during prodromal and symptomatic stages of the disease. Warn the patient about cross-transmittal between oral and genital lesions if the patient engages in oral sex.

Pelvic Inflammatory Disease
Coitus should be avoided until inflammation and pain subside. Intrauterine devices should be removed. Follow-up should be arranged 24 to 48 hours after ED discharge. Male sexual partners should be examined and treated if they had sexual contact during 60 days before onset of symptoms.

TABLE 18-2   The Relationship Among Contraceptive Method, STI Protection, and Patient Education[1]

Disease	Contraceptive Method That Provides Protection	Information for Follow-Up Care
Chlamydia infection	• Contraceptive sponge • Spermicide • Condom (male and female) • Diaphragm	• Refer partner(s) for evaluation
HPV	• Condom (female better than male)	• Have annual Pap smear. • Examine partner(s) for warts. • Weekly treatment until lesions resolve • Use condoms or abstain during treatment. • Emphasize relationship between HPV and cervical cancer; no evidence that treatment of visible warts affects the development of cervical cancer.
Gonorrhea	• Condom (male and female) • Spermicide • Contraceptive sponge	• Abstain until cured. Return for evaluation 2-3 days after treatment. • Have partner(s) treated.
Herpes	• Condom (female better than male)	• Abstain when lesions are present. • Have an annual Pap smear. • May transmit virus when asymptomatic; use condoms during sexual activity.
Syphilis	• Condom (male and female)	• Return for follow-up at 3-mo, 6-mo, 12-mo, and 24-mo intervals. • Refer partner(s) for evaluation.

Oral contraceptives and IUDs may increase risk of some STIs.

Vaginal Bacteriosis

Treatment of male partners is not recommended. The consumption of larger amounts of complex carbohydrates and less simple sugars has been helpful in some cases.[1,2]

REFERENCES

1. Fisher JF: Candiduria: when and how to treat it, *Curr Infect Dis Rep* 2:523-530, 2000.
2. Centers for Disease Control and Prevention: Sexually transmitted diseases treatment guidelines, *MMWR* 51:RR-6, 2002.
3. Zefer W and Holt K: Gynecological infections. In Coppola M, ed: *Emergency Clinics of North America*, Philadelphia, 2003, Saunders, pp 630-648.
4. Wiesenfeld HC, Hillier SL, Krohn M, et al: Lower genital tract infection and endometritis: insight into subclinical pelvic inflammatory disease, *Am Coll Obstet Gynecol* 100:456-463, 2002.

chapter *19*

Surface Trauma

Pam Talbert
Julia Fultz
Patty Ann Sturt

CLINICAL CONDITIONS

Abrasions
Avulsions
Contusions
Lacerations
Mammalian Bites
Puncture Wounds

INTRODUCTION

Surface trauma is any disruption or damage that causes an open wound or a closed contusion in the continuity of the skin layers. The goals of wound care are to relieve discomfort, minimize the risk of infection, restore function, and repair the wound.

FOCUSED NURSING ASSESSMENT

Perfusion

- Evaluate for ongoing blood loss.
- Monitor the trend of peripheral pulses, skin color, skin temperature, capillary refill, sensation, movement, and the degree and character of pain. Abnormal findings may indicate decreased perfusion. Perfusion may be altered if there is damage or compression to underlying vascular structures.

Skin/Tissue Integrity
General Observations

Assess and document the characteristics of the wound. A forensic ruler may help in the measuring of the wound. Document the color and shape of the wound.

- What is the location of the wound? Wounds involving the foot, lower extremity, hand, or face have a higher rate of infection.

- Is the wound open or closed? Open wounds include lacerations, avulsions, punctures, and mammalian bites. Contusions are closed wounds.
- Is there bleeding from the wound? Assess the amount of bleeding to determine whether there is uncontrolled bleeding or oozing from the site.

History

Injury information and a medical history should be obtained from the patient, family, and prehospital personnel. A high index of suspicion must be maintained for surface trauma that may have been caused by abuse, assault, or self-inflicted injury.

- Time of injury: The greater the time between the injury and delivery of care, the greater the risk of wound complications such as infection.
- Blood loss before arrival at the ED: Wounds to the head and face may result in profuse bleeding.
- Tetanus immunization status: *Clostridium tetani* is found in soil and in the gastrointestinal tracts of many domesticated animals. The incubation period for tetanus is 7 to 21 days but can range from 3 to 56 days.[1]
- Allergies: Although uncommon, determine whether the patient has an allergy to local anesthetics.
- Medical conditions: Patients with a history of cardiac or respiratory disease, diabetes mellitus, or peripheral vascular disease may be at greater risk for infection and delayed healing.
- Medications: Patients using anticoagulant or antiplatelet medications may have prolonged bleeding times and greater blood loss. Individuals using immunosuppressive medication, corticosteroids, or chemotherapy are at greater risk for infection.
- Consider abuse when the surface trauma does not correlate with the history given by the patient and family or caregiver (see Chapter 2).
- Alcohol dependence: Alcohol dependence is associated with nutritional deficits and delayed healing.

Mechanism of Injury

- What was the wounding object? The mass and velocity of the object should be considered. Increases in mass and velocity result in greater amounts of kinetic energy that must dissipate within the tissue, thereby increasing the amount of injury.
- What was the environment in which the injury occurred? Knowing the environment in which the injury occurred can provide information on possible wound contamination.

Wounds contaminated by foreign matter are at increased risk for infection. Saliva and feces contain a concentration of bacteria greater than the numbers needed to produce infection. The presence of soil particles with organic components or inorganic clay particles markedly raises the infective potential of bacteria.

Mobility

- Evaluate range of motion and sensation to identify damage to nerves, tendons, and ligaments.

LIFE SPAN ISSUES

1. Infants and toddlers have a greater head size relative to overall body size. Wounds to the head and face may bleed profusely.
2. Toddlers are at increased risk for surface trauma because of lack of coordination during ambulation.
3. School-age children often are involved in recreational and sports activities that increase the risk of surface trauma.
4. Wound healing may be delayed because of age-related diseases and skin changes. Aging skin becomes less vascular and thinner and contains fewer elastin fibers.
5. The geriatric patient may have reduced mobility and sensation, thus increasing susceptibility to injury.
6. Limited financial resources may be an obstacle to obtaining dressing supplies and medications. A social services consultation should be considered.

INITIAL INTERVENTIONS

1. Control bleeding.
2. Supply supplemental oxygen to patients who have indicators of hypovolemia secondary to blood loss
3. Initiate crystalloid infusion (Ringer's lactate or normal saline) by large-bore IVs.
4. Remove all constrictive clothing and jewelry.
5. Assess and document neurovascular status in the affected extremity.
6. Irrigate the wound with normal saline, and cover the wound with gauze.
7. Elevate the affected extremity.
8. Apply a cold pack to the area if it is edematous. Place a thin cloth between the ice pack and the skin to protect the skin from cold injury.
9. Administer tetanus toxoid as ordered (see Reference Guide 23).

10. Administer pain medication as ordered.
11. Perform steps necessary to obtain diagnostic tests.
12. Assist with wound debridement, wound irrigation, and wound closure (see Procedure 37, Wound Care). Closing wounds within 8 to 12 hours of the injury can reduce the risk of infectious complications. Lacerations more than 8 to 12 hours old may not be sutured but instead allowed to heal by secondary intention and dressing changes.[1] Fine linear facial lacerations may be sutured 24 hours after the injury because of the greater risk of disfigurement and the good vascularity of the face.[1]
13. Nursing care priorities are listed in the table on pp. 630-633.

PRIORITY DIAGNOSTIC TESTS

Laboratory Tests

Complete blood count (CBC): A CBC may be obtained to monitor blood loss by recording the trend of changes in hematocrit and hemoglobin. WBC count may be elevated if an infection is present, especially with old or contaminated wounds.

PT and PTT: Obtain these tests for patients who have multiple injuries that are associated with blood loss or patients who have a history of anticoagulant use or blood dyscrasia.

Type and crossmatch: A type and crossmatch is obtained if there are multiple injuries with hypovolemia, or if there is a possible need for surgical intervention.

Compartment pressure readings: Record readings in severe cases of surface trauma with associated edema that is limb threatening (see Chapter 11).

Culture and sensitivity: Obtain these tests on the wound exudate if the wound is infected.

Radiographs: A radiograph aids in assessment of bony structures and in identification of foreign objects. Pieces of glass greater than 1 mm thick are visible with appropriate views.[1] Organic substances such as wood are not easily seen on radiographs.

Xerograms: A xerogram will identify most organic substances (e.g., wood, seeds, and beans). This test will miss some plastics.[1]

Computed tomography scan: A CT scan is useful in identifying all foreign substances; however, the test is expensive.[1]

Ultrasonogram: This test is useful in identifying almost all substances. Air, pus, and edema may cause puzzling echoes.[1]

CLINICAL CONDITIONS

Abrasions

An abrasion is a wearing, grinding, or rubbing away of the outer layer of the skin, leaving the underlying dermis exposed (e.g., "road rash" from falls on pavement or rug or rope burns).

Symptoms

- Minimal bleeding occurs. The wound may be moist because of oozing from the capillaries.
- Pain is usually localized to the injured area.
- Localized edema may be present as a result of capillary vasodilation.
- Erythema is related to the inflammatory response.
- Dirt and debris may be embedded in the skin.

Diagnosis

- Diagnosis is based on a clinical examination.

Treatment

- Anesthetize the area (see Procedure 37, Wound Care). Use a topical anesthetic for small abrasions. Anesthetic injections may be necessary to achieve pain control for large areas of abrasion.
- Cleanse the skin around the wound (not the wound itself) with povidone-iodine (Betadine) or chlorhexidine (Hibiclens). These cleansers are noxious to the wound's defensive process.
- Clean the abrasion using aseptic technique. All foreign bodies must be removed (rock, grit, or fibers often will be embedded in the wound). High-pressure irrigation with saline, using a 19-gauge IV catheter (with the needle removed) connected to a 25-ml to 35-ml syringe, is suggested.[1] If debris is not removed from an abrasion by high-pressure irrigation, it may be necessary to cleanse the abrasion with saline and a fine-pore sponge[1] or a soft sterile brush in a circular motion. Care must be taken not to increase tissue damage with a sponge or soft brush. Objects such as glass must be removed from the wound before a brush or sponge is used.
  Failure to remove dirt and debris from the wound will result in a permanent tattooing after the wound has healed.
- Cover the abrasion with a topical antibiotic. This will prevent the wound exudate from becoming dry and crusted and from thereby interfering with wound healing.
- Leave the wound open or consider applying either a dry, sterile dressing or a vapor-permeable membrane.

NURSING CARE PRIORITIES

Potential/Actual Problem	Causes	Signs and Symptoms	Interventions
Inadequate fluid volume	Bleeding	• Active blood loss • Ecchymosis • Thirst • Decreased blood pressure • Increased hematocrit • Tachycardia	• Apply pressure to the site and pressure points. • Insert a large-bore (16-gauge or larger) IV and administer Ringer's lactate or normal saline solution as needed for hypovolemia. • Obtain blood specimens for a type and crossmatch. • Elevate the affected extremity.
Altered tissue perfusion	Damage to or compression of underlying neurovascular structures	• Decreased or diminished peripheral pulses • Pale or cyanotic color • Decreased capillary refill • Cold temperature • Decreased blood pressure in extremity	• Elevate the affected extremity to the level of the heart. • Provide supplemental oxygen. • Determine cause of altered perfusion and correct.
Altered skin/tissue integrity	• Friction • Shearing • Sharp or hard objects	• Exposed subcutaneous tissues • Erythema	• Prepare the patient and equipment for skin closure by sutures, stapling, tape closures, or tissue adhesive (Table 19-1).

		• Induration • Edema • Exudates • Bleeding • Pain • Ecchymosis	
Impaired mobility	• Damage to muscles, tendons, or ligaments • Pain • Splints, crutches, casts, slings	• Decreased muscle strength • Limited range of motion	• Splint and elevate the injured area. • Continue to monitor neurovascular status because edema may progress and impinge on neurovascular structures. • Initiate definitive measures to restore mobility. • Teach patient to use mobility aids (e.g., crutches, walker, cane).
Pain	Surface trauma and treatment	• Complaints of pain • Blood pressure and heart rate changes • Protective, guarding behavior • Restlessness/Irritability • Moaning.	• Immobilize the injured extremity. • Apply a cold pack to the area if it is edematous. • Prepare the patient for infiltration of a local anesthetic agent or nerve block (see the nursing care priorities table on pp 610–611).

Continued

NURSING CARE PRIORITIES—cont'd

Potential/Actual Problem	Causes	Signs and Symptoms	Interventions
		• Crying • Anger/Hostility	• Consider the use of EMLA. EMLA is a topical cream that contains lidocaine and prilocaine. EMLA should be applied to the site with an occlusive dressing 30 to 60 minutes before the wound is closed. • Apply LET as prescribed by the physician. LET is a topical anesthetic solution of lidocaine, epinephrine, and tetracaine. LET is considered safer than and as effective as TAC, which contains tetracaine, adrenalin, and cocaine. Application of TAC near or to the mucous membranes has resulted in serious complications, including seizures and death. • Consider the use of distraction techniques to relieve discomfort. Music and visual imagery may be helpful. • Explain procedures and sensations to expect.

| Potential for infection | • Contamination of wounds
• Preexisting medical conditions (e.g., diabetes, peripheral vascular disease) | • Increased pain
• Redness
• Swelling
• Pus
• Fever
• Presence of red streaks moving up an extremity
• Enlarged lymph nodes | • Monitor vital signs after pain medication.
• Reassess pain with a pain scale.
• Cleanse the wound (Procedure 37). Irrigation with 7 lb psi reduces the number of bacteria and the incidence of infection.[1]
• Assist with debridement. Debridement is the removal of foreign matter and devitalized tissue from the wound. The presence of devitalized tissue in the wound significantly increases the risk of infection. |
| Anxiety | • Precipitating event
• Pain
• Potential for disfigurement
• Lack of control over events | • Self reports of apprehension
• Narrowed perceptual field
• Hypervigilance
• Changes in vital signs
• Increased muscle tension | • Utilize patient's support systems.
• Explain all procedures.
• Employ distraction and relaxation techniques.
• Offer patient choices. |

Avulsions

An avulsion is a forcible separation or detachment of skin. An avulsion may be as significant as an amputation (Chapter 11), or it may be the tearing away from the body of a piece of skin and possibly the underlying tissue in varying degrees (e.g., eyelid, nose, ear, or a degloving injury).

Symptoms

- Bleeding is common.
- Pain
- Underlying structures (e.g., subcutaneous tissue, muscle, tendons, and bone) are exposed.
- Loss of function is possible.

Diagnosis

- An examination reveals obvious tissue loss. Tissue may be partially attached.

Treatment

- Apply direct pressure to control bleeding and use pressure points if bleeding continues.
- Evaluate the patient for fluid loss and the need for fluid replacement if the injury is large.
- A local anesthetic or IV sedation with analgesia (Procedure 30) for wound care may be administered before cleansing and irrigation of the wound.
- Cleanse the skin around the wound (not the wound itself) with povidone-iodine (Betadine) or chlorhexidine (Hibiclens). These cleansers are noxious to the wound's defensive process. Cleanse the wound with high-pressure irrigation with saline as described in the section Abrasions. Cleansing of the avulsed tissue is necessary if it is to be reattached. Ensure that all debris has been removed. When a person's head strikes a vehicle windshield, multiple small avulsions in which glass is embedded may result. Careful evaluation is necessary to ensure that all of the glass has been removed. Tweezers or the point of a #11 blade may be helpful in removing glass from wounds.
- Debridement of damaged tissue from the injury by the physician may be necessary.
- Closure of the wound will depend on the wound's severity. A skin flap still attached is cleaned and debrided and then undergoes primary closure. If the tissue loss is extensive, cleaning and irrigation may be performed in the operating room and skin grafting may be required.

Contusions

Contusions are characterized by bleeding within the dermis and epidermis from the disruption of small blood vessels, usually caused by blunt trauma.

Symptoms
- Swelling
- Discoloration from blood leaking into the tissue
- Pain
- Potential damage to underlying structures (e.g., swelling may cause vascular compromise; a left-upper-quadrant contusion may involve a splenic injury; a right-upper-quadrant contusion may involve a liver injury; a lower-leg contusion may involve compartment syndrome).

Diagnosis
- Diagnosis is based on a clinical examination.

Treatment
Treatment is aimed at providing comfort and preventing further edema and tissue damage.
- Cold pack is applied for the first 24 to 48 hours.
- Elevate the injured area at or above the level of the heart.
- Immobilization (e.g., with Ace bandage, splint, or sling) of the affected extremity for 24 to 48 hours after the injury may be helpful, depending on the location and severity of the injury.

Lacerations

A laceration is a cut or tear into the dermal layer of the skin that may involve the underlying structures. A laceration may be the result of either sharp or dull forces. The wound edges may be smooth and even or jagged.

Symptoms
- Bleeding; amount depends on the depth, location, and involvement of structures.
- Edema, erythema, crusting, and purulent drainage may be present, depending on the amount of time since the injury.
- The patient may exhibit sensory or motor deficits.

Diagnosis
- Diagnosis is based on a clinical examination.

Treatment
- Control the bleeding by direct pressure and by use of pressure points if bleeding continues.
- Premedicate the patient with anesthetics or analgesics for wound care, cleansing, and closure.

- Clean the wound with a high-pressure saline irrigation described in the section Abrasions.
- After the wound has been debrided, wound closure can be accomplished in one of three ways: primary closure, delayed closure, and open closure.[1] If primary closure is used, the wound is debrided, cleaned, irrigated, and closed immediately with sutures, tape, staples, or a tissue adhesive (Table 19-1). If delayed closure is used, the wound is cleaned, debrided, irrigated, and packed to prevent it from closing on its own. The patient has wound checks and a packing change in 24 hours, and in 48 hours definitive repair is performed. If the wound is to be left open to heal on its own, it is debrided, cleaned, irrigated, and dressed. More information can be found in Procedure 37, Wound Care.
- Lacerations that have been closed are dressed with an antibiotic ointment and covered with a microporous polypropylene dressing for the first 24 hours. The wound will be sealed by then and a dressing will no longer be necessary.[1]
- If the laceration is over a joint, immobilize the extremity to prevent stress on the wound.

Mammalian Bites

Mammalian bites are bites from humans or animals that cause puncture wounds but that may have associated abrasions, avulsions, contusions, and lacerations. Dog bites are the most commonly seen and tend to be lacerations, avulsions, or crush-type injuries. Cats have sharp, pointed teeth, so the bite tends to be a deep puncture wound that may penetrate deeper structures, including joints and bones.[2]

Symptoms

- Bleeding and ecchymosis may be present.
- Edema, erythema, and pain usually occur.
- Signs and symptoms of infection may be present. Many patients bitten by their own animals do not seek treatment immediately. The age, type, and location of the wound, in addition to the health of the individual, contribute to the potential for infection.
- Fever may be present.
- The patient may have a reduced range of motion if a joint is involved.

Diagnosis

- Diagnosis is based on the patient's history and a clinical examination.

TABLE 19-1   Wound Closure Methods

Method and Use	Advantages	Disadvantages
Steri-Strips		
May be used for partial-thickness lacerations or small superficial lacerations without signs of adjacent tension. Approximate the wound edges, applying Steri-Strips uniformly; use benzoin or Mastisol on adjacent skin to ensure adhesiveness of Steri-Strips.	• Eliminates the need for an anesthetic • No suture scars • Does not require medical visit for removal • Reduces tissue trauma • Reduces risk for infection	• Potential for wound edge inversion • Less strength than sutures
Sutures		
• May be used for simple and more involved lacerations; closure of deep wounds is performed in layers; suture selection is a matter of individual choice. • Absorbable suture is used for deeper layers; examples are plain or chromic catgut and the synthetics Dexon and Vicryl. • Nonabsorbable suture is used for skin closure and must be removed; examples are silk or synthetics (nylon, polypropylene) • NOTE: Synthetics have a lesser wicking action that reduces scarring potential.	• Used to close wounds with high tension • Definite closure of wound edges • Patient able to shower, and dressing is not always needed after 24 hr.	• Local anesthetic used • Follow-up appointment needed for suture removal

Continued

TABLE 19-1   Wound Closure Methods—cont'd

Method and Use	Advantages	Disadvantages
Staples May be used for linear lacerations to scalp, trunk, and extremities	• Less painful • Less risk of infection • Eliminates exposure to sharp needles • Time to closure is less • More acceptable to some patients for cosmetic reasons	• Provides less precise approximation • Should not be used when magnetic resonance imaging of the affected part may be conducted
Tissue Adhesive (e.g., Dermabond) Used for closure of traumatic laceration; may be used in closure of clean, simple facial laceration; thin film of adhesive is applied to the edges, and manual approximation is maintained for 30 seconds to 2 minutes.	• Less painful • Eliminates exposure to sharp needles • Time to closure is less • More acceptable to some patients for cosmetic reasons • Does not require medical visit for removal	• Cannot be used near the eyes • Cannot be used close to wounds under tension unless used in conjunction with subcutaneous or subcuticular sutures • Not recommended for use across joints • Wound should be kept relatively dry; avoid swimming. Blot wound dry if it gets wet.

Data from Simon B and Hern HG: Wound management principles. In Marx J, Hockenberger R, and Walls R, eds: *Rosen's emergency medicine, concepts and clinical practice,* ed 5, St Louis, 2002, Mosby.

Treatment
- Control bleeding.
- Analgesics or anesthetics may be administered for wound care, cleansing, and possible closure.
- Obtain cultures of the wound and exudate if infection is present.
- Infection is of significant concern because bite wounds are contaminated with oral flora.[2,3] Meticulous cleansing and irrigation are needed. Cat bites have a significantly higher infection rate than dog bites, and human bites are considered more serious than dog or cat bites. The wound should be evaluated for injuries to underlying structures and for foreign bodies. High-pressure saline irrigation should be performed (as described in the section Abrasions).
- Closure is controversial because of the high incidence of infection.
- If the wound is sutured, a wound check within 24 hours should be scheduled.
- Cold packs and elevation may be necessary for treating edema until improvement is noted.
- Antibiotics may be prescribed for patients with bites, as these wounds are prone to infection.
- Notify the health department to report animal bites according to local policy.
- Rabies vaccination, as well as a tetanus shot, may be required.

Puncture Wounds
Puncture wounds are penetrating wounds caused by an object forced through the skin and into the underlying tissue. Most puncture wounds occur to the extremities and involve such substances as nails, glass, or wood.

Symptoms
- Bleeding
- Pain
- Signs and symptoms of infection (e.g., erythema, warmth, edema, and drainage) may be present, depending on the age of the puncture wound.
- Embedded foreign body (pain on deep palpation over the wound is indicative of an embedded foreign body)
- Superficially, the wound may seem minor; evaluate the patient for signs of underlying tissue damage.

Diagnosis
- Diagnosis is based on clinical examination and history.

Treatment
- Control bleeding with pressure and the use of pressure points if bleeding continues.
- Obtain appropriate diagnostic studies as described in Priority Diagnostic Tests if a foreign body is suspected.
- Administer analgesics or anesthetics as necessary for wound care, cleansing, and possible exploration.
- Irrigate the wound well as the infection rate for puncture wounds is high. Anesthesia and excision of the area may be necessary to allow an adequate cleansing and exploration of the wound.
- Apply a dressing as indicated after wound exploration and closure.

NURSING SURVEILLANCE

Patient Observation
- Monitor the wound for continued bleeding or drainage. Monitor dressings for occult bleeding.
- Evaluate contusions for expansion.
- Monitor skin color, temperature, and capillary refill.
- Evaluate sensory function distal to the injury.
- Evaluate the effectiveness of pain control measures.
- Evaluate the wound for signs and symptoms of infection (e.g., erythema, edema, warmth at the wound site, purulent drainage, or unexplained temperature elevation).

Family or Significant Other Support
- Inform family members of the procedure. Place a chair by the patient's bed so the family members may sit down if desired.
- Involve family members in learning wound-care procedures and discharge instructions.

EXPECTED PATIENT OUTCOMES

1. The bleeding is controlled, and neurovascular status remains intact.
2. The patient reports relief from pain.
3. No further tissue damage results from cleansing or irrigation.
4. The patient demonstrates an understanding of wound cleansing and closure.
5. The wound is approximated or protected by dressing before discharge.
6. The patient understands the signs and symptoms of infection and the need to return to the ED or a primary care physician if infection occurs.

7. The patient or significant other understands the care of the wound.
8. The patient or significant other demonstrates knowledge of medications (e.g., analgesics, antibiotics, and immunizations) and potential side effects.
9. The patient understands follow-up instructions for wound checks and suture or staple removal.

DISCHARGE INSTRUCTIONS

Socioeconomic factors that may affect compliance with wound care at home and follow-up care should be assessed. Money for supplies and medications, the availability of running water or electricity in the home, the availability of follow-up care, and transportation to receive care should be discussed before discharge.

Wound-care instructions vary according to the type of wound, the location of the wound, and the type of closure (if any) used. The following are general instructions and must be adapted according to the type of wound:

1. Keep the dressing clean and dry for 24 hours.
2. Keep the area elevated for 24 to 48 hours with a cold pack application, if needed, to reduce edema or pain. If a laceration is over a joint, immobilization should be maintained until the sutures are removed.
3. Wash hands thoroughly with soap and water before and after wound care.
4. After the first 24 hours, remove the dressing. Cleanse the wound gently of medication residue and wound exudate with soap and water. (The patient must have his or her own bar of soap in the home designated for wound care.) Half-strength hydrogen peroxide may be used to clean the wound debris and clots that form between the sutured edges of the wound until the scab separates. (Hydrogen peroxide should not be used after the scab has separated because it is toxic to the epithelium.)[1]
5. Advise the patient that it is safe to get the wound wet after 24 hours; however, prolonged immersion of the wound in water (e.g., tub bath, swimming pool, or long showers) should be avoided. Dry the wound after getting it wet.
6. The wound may be redressed or left open to the air as appropriate. Factors to consider for redressing are the location of the wound (e.g., joints, hands, or feet), the severity of the wound, wound drainage, and the potential for contamination.

7. Reapply a thin layer of antibiotic ointment if necessary. Antibiotic ointment protects the wounded area and reduces scarring.

8. Describe the signs of infection: increased pain, redness, swelling, pus (thick white or yellow liquid as opposed to serous drainage), fever, and red streaks moving up an extremity. High-risk injuries (e.g., animal and human bites or highly contaminated wounds) should be rechecked in 24 to 48 hours regardless of their appearance.[1]

9. Take the complete dose of antibiotics as prescribed. If a rabies vaccination is indicated, the patient should be instructed to return for follow-up injections.

10. Return for wound check and suture removal as appropriate. Sutures usually are removed in 5 to 14 days (Procedure 33).

11. Cover the affected area with clothing and sunscreen for 1 year to minimize discoloration and scarring.

REFERENCES

1. Simon B and Hern HG: Wound management principles. In Marx J, Hockenberger R, and Walls R, eds: *Rosen's emergency medicine, concepts and clinical practice*, ed 5, St Louis, 2002, Mosby.

2. Weber EJ and Callaham M: Mammalian bites. In Marx JA, Hockberger RS, Walls RM, eds: *Rosen's emergency medicine concepts and clinical practice*, ed 5, St Louis, 2002, Mosby.

3. Bunzli WF, Wright DH, Hoang AD, et al: Current management of human bites, *Pharmacotherapy* 18 (2):227-234, 1998.

chapter 20

Toxicologic Conditions

Patty Ann Sturt

CLINICAL CONDITIONS: SPECIFIC OVERDOSES

Acetaminophen (Tylenol)
Anticholinergic and Antihistamine Drugs
Alcohol (Ethanol) and Alcohol Agents
   (Methanol, Ethylene Glycol)
Benzodiazepines
Calcium Channel Blockers and Beta-Blockers
Cardiac Glycosides
Cocaine
Hydrocarbons
Iron
Opioids (Codeine, Heroin)
Organophosphates
Salicylates (Aspirin)
Street Drugs
Tricyclic Antidepressants

INTRODUCTION

Acetaminophen, alcohol, antihistamines, aspirin,
benzodiazepines, beta-blockers, calcium channel blockers, and
tricyclic antidepressants (TCAs) are substances often encountered
in overdoses. The initial priority is to ensure that the patient's
airway, breathing, and circulation are intact. Suspect an overdose
with anyone who arrives with an abrupt onset of multiple
symptoms. Table 20-1 presents an overview of common overdose
substances, the symptoms, and the treatment.

FOCUSED NURSING ASSESSMENT

History
Route of Exposure (Skin, IV, or PO)
The route of exposure determines where the patient is placed
in the ED (e.g., decontamination versus resuscitation room).
If exposure is through the skin (e.g., organophosphates),

TABLE 20-1 Common Overdoses in the Emergency Department

Drug	Symptoms	Treatment
Acetaminophen	None initially; right upper quadrant pain, nausea/vomiting, pallor, diaphoresis 48-72 hr later	Acetylcysteine, activated charcoal
Alcohol	Tachycardia, hypoventilation, confusion, diplopia	Hemodialysis, lavage
Anticholinergic drugs (antihistamines, decongestants, sleeping pills)	Blurred and double vision, nonreactive dilated pupils, inability to sweat, hyperthermia, tachycardia	Physostigmine in cases of cardiac instability, lavage, activated charcoal
Benzodiazepines	Hypotension, tachycardia, respiratory depression	Flumazenil
Beta-blocking agents	Bradycardia, conduction blocks	Atropine, glucagon, whole-bowel irrigation
Calcium channel blockers	Bradycardia, conduction blocks	Calcium, dopamine, pacemaker
Cocaine	Tachycardia, hypertension, dilated pupils, dyspnea, chest pain,	Whole-bowel irrigation for body packets, sodium bicarbonate, alpha-blocking

	thrombosis, hyperthermia, hallucinations	and beta-blocking agents, vasodilators, angiotensin-converting enzyme (ACE) inhibitors, calcium channel blockers, activated charcoal, lavage
Iron	Bloody vomit and stools	Deferoxamine chelating agent
Methanol and ethylene glycol	Delayed symptoms (coma, acute rheumatic fever), tachycardia, confusion	Ethanol IV, hemodialysis
Opiates	Constricted pupils, hypotension, bradycardia	Naloxone
Organophosphates	Salivation, lacrimation, urination, defecation, nausea/vomiting, constricted pupils, muscle weakness	Pralidoxime chloride IV, atropine, skin and eye irrigation
Salicylate	Nausea/vomiting; rapid, deep respirations; tinnitus	Sodium bicarbonate, hemodialysis, whole-bowel irrigation
Tricyclic antidepressants	Bradycardia conduction blocks, hypotension, seizures	Lavage, activated charcoal, sodium bicarbonate, physostigmine

the patient's skin requires flushing, and the health-care providers are at risk for exposure.

Drugs Ingested

Determine the names of the drugs ingested. Some drugs are absorbed slowly (e.g., digoxin, aspirin, and phenytoin). Slow-release forms of drugs are treated differently.

Ingestion History

- Determine how much earlier and over what period drugs were ingested. Emptying preferably should be initiated within 2 hours of ingestion.[1]
- Determine whether the medication container or bottle is available. Calculate the number of pills or amount of fluid missing from the initial amount prescribed.
- Determine whether the patient's occupation involves possible exposure to chemicals (e.g., lead or organophosphates).

Medical History

- Determine the patient's age, weight, height, medical history, and current medications. This information helps in drug calculations and with anticipating the patient's ability to metabolize drugs.
- Determine whether there is a history of depression, schizophrenia, or suicide attempts. Patients with these conditions will need to be placed in a room where they can be closely monitored.

Patient's Last Meal

Determine the amount and time of the patient's last meal. The presence of food in the stomach may delay absorption.

Treatment Before Arrival

The use of ipecac in the home setting is no longer recommended by many poison control centers. If ipecac has been given, emesis should occur within 30 minutes. The administration of ipecac may delay the administration of oral antidotes. Vomiting may produce a vagal response and further reduce the heart rate of a patient who has ingested cardiotoxic drugs.

> **NURSING ALERT**
>
> All overdoses are potentially life threatening and should be treated as such. Patients should be triaged immediately to the ED treatment area. Symptoms occur later in patients who have ingested acetaminophen, sustained-release drugs, and methanol or ethylene glycol. These are considered acute agents. A patient may present without symptoms but deteriorate in the ED waiting area. The ED nurse or physician should call the poison control center to determine definitive treatment.

Ventilation
Breath Sounds
Pulmonary edema occurs often with hydrocarbon and opiate ingestion. Coarse or fine rales (crackles) may be auscultated. Wheezing may occur with inhalation of organophosphate insecticides.

Breathing Pattern
Opiate overdoses produce respiratory depression. Respirations may be slow and shallow. Hydrocarbons vaporize at low temperatures. They enter the pulmonary tree easily, producing bronchospasm, pulmonary edema, and aspiration pneumonitis. Salicylates, methanol, and ethylene glycol (antifreeze) produce metabolic acidosis. In cases of salicylate overdose, respirations are deep and rapid, related to direct stimulation of the respiratory center in the brainstem.

Perfusion
Apical Heart Rate
Obtain an apical heart rate for 1 minute and compare this rate and rhythm with a peripheral pulse. Many of the commonly ingested drugs produce cardiovascular effects. Calcium channel-blocking and beta-blocking agents reduce the heart rate and precipitate conduction blocks and ectopy. Anticholinergic drugs and cocaine produce tachyarrhythmias.

Blood Pressure
Peripheral vasodilation and/or myocardial depression may produce hypotension in ingestion of opioids, benzodiazepines, beta-blockers, and calcium channel blockers. Patients with cocaine toxicity often experience hypertension.

Skin
Assess skin color, temperature, and peripheral pulses. Severe iron ingestion can produce gastric hemorrhage and hypovolemic shock. Anticholinergic agents produce hyperthermia. A cocaine overdose may produce diaphoresis.

Cognition
Mental Status
Perform a neurologic assessment. Seizures and an altered level of consciousness (LOC) ranging from lethargy to confusion to coma may occur at any time if the ingested amount is great enough. The Glasgow Coma Scale (GCS) (Reference Guides 10 and 17) should be used to document eye, motor, and verbal response.

Pupil Size and Reactivity

Constricted pupils may indicate organophosphate exposure or ingestion of an opioid or benzodiazepine. Dilated pupils often are seen in cocaine use.

Hallucinations

Hallucinations are common with cocaine and lead poisoning.

Unresponsive Patient

If the patient is unresponsive, a coexisting traumatic injury (e.g., from a fall) may be present (see Chapter 20). Assess the patient for evidence of trauma such as abrasions, bleeding, ecchymoses, edema, and deformity. Keep the patient flat with the spine immobilized until spine injury has been ruled out.

Elimination

Bowel Sounds

Decreased or absent bowel sounds may slow absorption of a drug.

Urinary Output

Assess and measure urinary output. Determine whether the patient has voided since the ingestion. Some drugs (e.g., methanol and ethylene glycol) may produce acute tubular necrosis (ATN). Organophosphates overstimulate the parasympathetic nervous system, causing urination and defecation.

Bowel Movement

Assess the patient's stools. Organophosphates cause frequent defecation. Bloody stools may result from iron ingestion.

Emesis

Assess and measure emesis. Note the presence of any pill fragments. Bloody emesis may occur with iron ingestion. If the patient has received ipecac, be sure to note the amount of emesis that occurs after administration.

Risk Factors

- Young children who have access to medicine
- Geriatric patients with failing eyesight or memory
- People who are in pain or who have chronic illness and are using drugs that may impair judgment
- People who have made previous suicide attempts

LIFE SPAN ISSUES

- Adolescents tend to overdose on over-the-counter drugs instead of prescribed drugs.
- The majority of overdoses among geriatric patients not experiencing suicidal depression result from confusion,

improper use of the product, improper storage in a container other than the original, or mistaken identity. This has implications for discharge teaching.

- Geriatric patients are more likely to have chronic intoxication secondary to daily use of an agent (e.g., aspirin) or use of multiple agents. Decreased hepatic and renal blood flow associated with aging reduces drug metabolism and excretion.

INITIAL INTERVENTIONS

1. Implement measures to protect the patient's airway. If the patient is awake and a spine injury has been ruled out, place the patient in the semi-Fowler's position. Remove pillows if the patient has decreased responsiveness. Insert a nasopharyngeal airway. If the patient is unresponsive or has no gag reflex, insert an oral airway until the patient is intubated.

2. Anticipate aspiration and have suction available. If the patient is unresponsive, place the patient in the left lateral recumbent position. This position allows the drug to remain in the curvature of the stomach and reduces drug absorption.

3. Initiate pulse oximetry to monitor the degree of oxygen saturation.

4. Initiate cardiac and blood pressure (BP) monitoring.

5. Protect the patient from injury. Seizures may result from the drug overdose, hypoxia, and hypoglycemia. Pad the side rails. Keep the bed in a low position.

6. Use a nonjudgmental approach. Establish a rapport with the patient. Do not reprimand him or her for the overdose.

7. Administer the following agents as ordered and based on agent ingested and the patient's symptoms: antiemetics, naloxone, thiamine, glucose, flumazenil, calcium, vasopressor agents, inotropic agents, and antiarrhythmics.

8. Impair drug absorption and increase drug excretion
   - *Ipecac:* Suggested doses are 30 ml for anyone over the age of 5, 15 ml for a child 1 to 5 years of age, and 10 ml for a child 6 months to 12 months of age. Ipecac is contraindicated for children younger than 6 months.[2] Infants 6 to 12 months of age should receive ipecac only in the hospital setting. Ipecac directly stimulates the brain to induce emesis and irritates the gastric mucosa. Drinking water immediately after administration dilutes the ipecac and allows it to cover a larger surface area in the gut, producing greater emesis. Eighty-eight percent of patients vomit in less than 30 minutes.[2] Administering ipecac with milk products may

delay the onset of vomiting. Large items (e.g., iron pills) and heavy metals are best removed through emesis. Ipecac is contraindicated with hydrocarbon, TCA, and multidrug ingestion. The dose may be repeated once if vomiting does not occur within 30 minutes. Oral antidote administration may need to be delayed after ipecac use because of continued emesis. If a cardiotoxic drug (beta blocker or calcium channel blocker) was ingested, the act of vomiting may cause a vagal response and further reduce the heart rate. If the overdose occurred more than $1\frac{1}{2}$ hours before the patient is treated, ipecac may not be helpful.

- *Charcoal:* Activated charcoal is created by steam or chemical activation of wood pulp. This creates a highly porous substance. Most drugs bind to the walls of the pores in activated charcoal, thereby reducing the amount of drug available for absorption into the bloodstream. In general, one dose is recommended. However, additional doses may be used in theophylline and phenobarbital intoxication, or with sustained-release medications. Charcoal does not absorb ethanol, hydrocarbons, or iron. It should be used with caution after ingestion of agents known to produce ileus. It may be administered orally or through a gastric tube. A 50-g to 100-g dose is used for adults. The suggested dose for a child is 10 to 30 g or 1 g/kg. Charcoal after ipecac does not produce greater benefits and increases the risk of complications. The use of charcoal alone is often more effective. ED stays are longer for patients receiving ipecac and charcoal.

- Charcoal is not used to treat ingestion of corrosive substances because it makes endoscopy impossible. Charcoal increases the chance of aspiration in the patient with a decreased level of consciousness. Charcoal aspiration produces prolonged, severe bronchospasm. If the charcoal splatters in the eye, a corneal abrasion may occur.

- *Gastric lavage:* Gastric lavage is not recommended in the patient with a significant decrease in the level of consciousness unless the patient is intubated. Lavage must be

---

⇒ NURSING ALERT ⇐

Activated charcoal often is mixed in sorbitol (a cathartic agent). When multiple doses of activated charcoal are given, make sure they are not administered in a sorbitol solution to prevent electrolyte abnormalities and hypovolemia.

performed within 2 hours of ingestion of most drugs to be effective. After 1 to 2 hours, there is no difference in drug retrieval between the use of lavage and charcoal and the use of charcoal alone. If vomiting occurs before ED admission, lavage may not remove any additional drug and it may force the gastric contents into the small intestine. The procedure is to administer tap water or normal saline until returns through the orogastric tube are clear (1.5 to 2 liters for adults, 10 ml/kg for children). A large orogastric tube (36 to 42 Fr for adults, 26 to 28 Fr for children) is preferred for efficient removal of pill fragments. A double-lumen tube allows for rapid fluid delivery and aspiration.

- *Cathartics:* Cathartics often are used to help remove drug packets and iron. They should be used only with the first dose of charcoal. This is especially true with children and geriatric patients because of potential electrolyte abnormalities.
- *Sorbitol:* Sorbitol is an oral cathartic. For adults, a dose of 0.5 to 2 g/kg to a maximum of 150 g is given. The dose for children is 1 to 1.5 g/kg, up to a 50-g dose. Sorbitol produces fewer electrolyte abnormalities and has the shortest gastrointestinal (GI) transit time of all cathartics. It works more quickly than magnesium citrate. Sorbitol gives charcoal a sweet taste and reduces its grittiness, making charcoal more palatable.
- *Cation exchange resins:* Sodium polystyrene sulfonate (Kayexalate) is a cation exchange resin used to increase elimination of lithium. A side effect of this treatment is hypokalemia.
- *Altering urine and serum pH:* The aim of this intervention is to change the agent into a less absorbable ionized form. Acidic agents (e.g., salicylate and phenobarbital) clear more rapidly in alkaline urine.
- *Hemodialysis:* Hemodialysis is used if the ingested drug has a low molecular weight and limited protein binding. Lithium, chloral hydrate, ethylene glycol, methanol, theophylline, salicylate, and quinidine may be removed through dialysis. Dialysis can reverse metabolic acidosis if it is used early, before the drug diffuses into the tissues. Hemodialysis necessitates anticoagulation.
- *Hemoperfusion:* This intervention is used most often in overdoses of theophylline, carbamazepine, and phenobarbital.
- *Exchange transfusion:* Exchange transfusions may be used for children with lead poisoning and drugs that produce hemolytic anemia.

- *Whole-bowel irrigation:* The aim of whole-bowel irrigation is to flush enteric-coated medications, drug packets (ingested by body stuffers or body packers), or heavy metals such as lead and mercury through the GI tract. Polyethylene glycol–electrolyte solution (Colyte, Golytely) is ingested orally or infused through a nasogastric or orogastric tube. This intervention can cause electrolyte abnormalities.

Antidotes are summarized in Table 20-2.

9. Nursing care priorities are listed in the table on pp. 656-658.

PRIORITY DIAGNOSTIC TESTS

Laboratory Tests

Urine drug screening: Urine drug screening is the preferred test to identify the ingested drug. Most drugs and their metabolites are concentrated and excreted in the urine.

Serum drug screening: Screening of acetaminophen, anticonvulsants, ethyl alcohol, ethylene glycol, isopropyl alcohol, lithium, salicylates, and theophylline is best performed on a serum sample.

Arterial blood gases: ABGs may be analyzed to check for acidosis associated with salicylate, ethylene glycol, and methanol ingestion.

Electrolyte levels: Baseline potassium, chloride, and sodium levels usually are obtained because treatments may produce electrolyte abnormalities.

Glucose level: A check of the glucose level may be ordered to rule out hypoglycemia as an associated factor in unresponsiveness.

Liver enzymes and amylase level: Liver enzyme levels may be elevated in acetaminophen overdoses as a result of hepatic necrosis.

Blood ethanol level: The blood ethanol level is elevated in cases of acute alcohol intoxication.

Cardiac enzyme and isoenzyme levels: Enzyme levels may be elevated with amphetamine, TCA, and cocaine overdoses.

Blood urea nitrogen and creatinine: BUN and creatinine levels may be obtained to confirm normal renal function.

Coagulation profile: Obtain a coagulation profile if hemodialysis is necessary.

NURSING ALERT

If metabolic acidosis is present, anticipate the administration of IV sodium bicarbonate. Metabolic acidosis is common with overdoses of TCAs, and salicylates. An initial bolus is given, followed by a continuous infusion.

TABLE 20-2   Common Antidotes in the ED Setting

Antidote	Common Dosage	Use
Deferoxamine	**Initial adult and pediatric dose:** 15 mg/kg/hr IV. Rate may be titrated upward to 25-40 mg/kg/hr.	Iron poisoning
Digoxin immune FAB (Digibind) antibody fragments	**If the amount of digoxin ingested is known, use the following calculation:** Amount ingested (mg) × (bioavailability/0.6 mg) = dose of FAB in vials. The bioavailability of digoxin tablets is 0.8, for capsules 1.0. If the bioavailability is unknown, the value of 0.8 should be used. **If a 6-hour or greater post-ingestion serum concentration is known, use the following calculation:** (Serum level [mcg/ml] × 6 L/kg × patient weight [kg])/{1000 × 0.6} = number of vials **If the amount ingested and the serum digoxin levels are unknown:** 10 vials should be administered for acute adult or pediatric overdose initially with subsequent therapy as needed.	Cardiac glycoside overdose
Flumazenil	**Adult dose:** Initial dose is 0.2 mg IV over 30 seconds. If needed, an additional 0.3 mg may be given. Repeat dosing with 0.5 mg can be given every 1-2 minutes up to a total of 3 mg. **Pediatric dose:** 0.01 mg/kg IV administered titrated to effect with a maximum dose of 1 mg.	Benzodiazepines
Glucagon	**Adult dose:** 5-10 mg IV over 1 minute. If no effect in 5 minutes, repeat at up to 10-20 mg.	Beta-blocker and calcium

Continued

TABLE 20-2   Common Antidotes in the ED Setting—cont'd

Antidote	Common Dosage	Use
	Pediatric dose: 50 mcg/kg bolus over 1 minute. If there is no effect in 5 minutes, repeat at up to 10 mg.	channel blocker overdose
N-acetylcysteine	**Adult oral dose:** 0.4 to 2 mg/kg orally. Maintenance dose is 70 mg/kg orally every 4 hours for 17 additional doses (72-hour protocol). Administration may require aggressive antiemetic therapy.	Acetaminophen overdose
Naloxone (Narcan) or nalmefene (Revex)	**Adult dose:** 0.4 to 2 mg IV initially; can be repeated if no response observed to a cumulative dose of 10 mg. A continuous IV infusion may be used for persistent or recurrent effects: Mix naloxone in D₅W and administer at a rate to deliver two thirds of the initially effective bolus dose per hour.	Opioid overdose
Physostigmine	**Adult dose:** 1-2 mg IV administered slowly over 5 minutes **Pediatric dose:** 0.02 mg/kg up to 2 mg administered slowly over 5 minutes. Adult and pediatric dose may be repeated once after a 5 to 10 minute interval.	TCAs
Pralidoxime chloride	**Adult dose:** 1-2 g in normal saline IV over 30 minutes. Maintenance dose: 500 mg/hr should be continued for 24 to 48 hours or intermittent infusions of 1 g in 250 ml of normal saline every 6-12 hours. **Pediatric dose:** 25 mg/kg (up to 1 g) in normal saline infused over 30 minutes. Maintenance dose: 10-20 mg/kg (up to 500 mg) per hour for 24-48 hours	Organophosphates

Data from Dart RC, ed: *The 5 minute toxicology consult*, Philadelphia, 2000, Lippincott Williams & Wilkins.

Radiographic Examination

Abdominal films: Undissolved tablets (e.g., enteric-coated aspirin) may accumulate in the stomach, particularly if the patient has a gastric outlet disorder. The tablets may be detected on film. Iron is radiopaque; its presence can be detected by abdominal radiographs.

CLINICAL CONDITIONS: SPECIFIC OVERDOSES

Acetaminophen (Tylenol)

Acetaminophen is an oral analgesic available over the counter and in many prescription medications. It is metabolized primarily in the liver. An acute ingestion of greater than 15 g in an adult often produces liver injury.[2] It is one of the most common pharmaceutical agents involved in overdoses.

Symptoms

- Initial symptoms are nausea, vomiting, and diffuse abdominal pain.
- Patients may arrive at the ED 24 to 48 hours after ingestion with right upper quadrant pain related to liver injury. Prothrombin time (PT) and liver enzymes begin to increase.
- Severe toxicity may produce severe liver failure 3 to 5 days after ingestion. Liver failure may produce jaundice, electrolyte abnormalities, acidosis, and hypoglycemia.

Diagnosis

- If at all possible, a serum level should be obtained 4 hours after ingestion or as soon after 4 hours as possible. At least 4 hours are required for the serum level to be reliable. A serum level of 140 mg/kg or greater is toxic.[2]
- The risk of hepatotoxicity can be determined with the Rumack Matthew nomogram (Figure 20-1).

Treatment

- N-acetylcysteine (Mucomyst) is used to prevent hepatic failure. It protects the liver by improving glutathione synthesis. Hepatic enzymes should be monitored.

A loading dose of 140 mg/kg of N-acetylcysteine is given orally if the level is within toxic range. Subsequent doses of 70 mg/kg are repeated at 4-hour intervals for 17 doses. N-acetylcysteine may be of benefit up to 24 to 36 hours after an acetaminophen overdose.[3]

When N-acetylcysteine is given PO, it can make the patient vomit because of its smell. It may be mixed with cola or orange juice to improve palatability.

NURSING CARE PRIORITIES

Potential/Actual Problem	Causes	Signs and Symptoms	Interventions
Airway compromise	• Decrease in level of consciousness resulting in obstruction caused by tongue or secretions • Laryngeal edema resulting from inhalation of toxic substance	• Decreased movement of air • Stridor • Hoarseness • Snoring respirations	• Chin lift/jaw thrust • Insert airway adjunct if unresponsive. • Suction oropharynx. • Prepare and assist with intubation.
Impaired oxygenation/breathing	• Respiratory depression • Laryngeal edema, bronchospasms • Pulmonary edema • Metabolic acidosis	• Shallow, slow respirations • Wheezing • Crackles/rales • Tachypnea • Cough • Retractions • Decreased oxygen saturation	• Ventilate with bag-valve-mask device if breathing absent or ineffective. • Tracheal suction • Administer high-flow oxygen via nonrebreather mask. • Monitor respiratory effort and rate. • Monitor oxygen saturation.
Impaired circulation	• Vasodilation • Decreased contractility	• Hypotension • Tachycardia	• Monitor vital signs. • Monitor intake and output.

	• Bradycardia • Pallor • Weak pulses • Decreased urine output • Altered mental status	• Monitor mental status • Initiate two large-bore IVs • Infuse NS or LR • Administer IV calcium as ordered for calcium channel blocker overdoses. • Titrate inotropic agents as ordered. • Titrate vasopressor agents as ordered. • Administer antiarrhythmic agents as ordered.
• Fluid/blood loss • Arrhythmias		
Altered mental status		
• Hypoxia • Sympathetic nervous system depression	• Unresponsive • Responsive only to pain or verbal stimuli	• Monitor airway and breathing. • Monitor mental status. • Provide safe environment.

Continued

NURSING CARE PRIORITIES—cont'd

Potential/Actual Problem	Causes	Signs and Symptoms	Interventions
	• Sympathetic nervous system stimulation	• Agitation • Hallucinations • Manic	• Provide safe environment with continuous observation. • Remove all potentially dangerous objects from vicinity of patient.
Safety	• Suicidal ideation • Self-harm or harm to others secondary to agitation or hallucinations • Inability to safely self-administer medications	• Verbalizes thoughts of suicide • Plan to commit suicide • Agitation • Hallucinations • Difficulty with vision and/or reading medication labels • Confusion • Altered memory	• Initiate a social worker consult. • Initiate a home health consult. • Provide patient teaching.

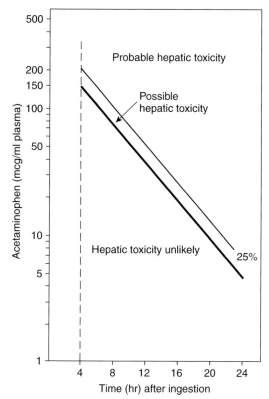

Figure 20–1   Rumack-Matthew nomogram for acetaminophen poisoning.

- Antiemetics often must be administered to ensure that the N-acetylcysteine is retained.
- Gastric lavage should be considered in patients presenting within 1 hour of ingestion and before administration of N-acetylcysteine.
- One dose of activated charcoal without a cathartic should be administered if a substantial ingestion occurred within 2 to 4 hours. Charcoal is highly effective in binding the drug. Simultaneous or alternating administration of activated charcoal and N-acetylcysteine does not reduce the effectiveness

of the N-acetylcysteine. However, administration of
N-acetylcysteine has priority over administration of charcoal.
- Beware if the patient has preexisting liver disease, because
  toxicity occurs at a lower level.
- The patient should not be discharged until a normal serum
  acetaminophen level has been identified.

Anticholinergic and Antihistamine Drugs
These over-the-counter agents often are used to relieve upper
respiratory symptoms associated with infections or allergies.
Symptoms
- Nausea and vomiting
- Altered mental status (e.g., agitation, delirium, or
  hallucinations)
- Blurred vision
- Seizures
- Dilated pupils
- Hyperthermia and inability to sweat
- Supraventricular tachycardia
- Dystonic reactions
Diagnosis
- Based on clinical presentation and history
Treatment
- Ipecac may be administered if patient arrives within 1 hour of
  ingestion.
- Activated charcoal
- Gastric lavage and activated charcoal may be useful for
  4 to 6 hours after the ingestion as a result of decreased gastric
  motility.
- Physostigmine may be administered if the patient has
  agitation or hallucinations. The adult dose is 0.5 to 2 mg slow
  IV push over 5 minutes. The dose may be repeated once after
  5 to 10 minutes if the patient's mental status does not improve.
- Benzodiazepines may be administered for the agitation.

Alcohol
Ethanol
Symptoms
Alcohol intoxication produces:
- Tachycardia
- Hypoventilation
- Confusion
- Seizures related to hypoglycemia

Diagnosis
- Diagnosis is based on the serum ethanol level. Alcohol is eliminated at a rate of 10 to 20 mg/dl/hr in the nonalcoholic.

Treatment
- Ethanol is rapidly absorbed from the stomach and small intestine. An alcohol overdose usually is treated with lavage. Lavage is most effective if the patient arrives at the ED within 1 hour of ingestion.
- Benzodiazepine may be given to prevent withdrawal side effects.
- In cases of alcohol intoxication, thiamine is administered before glucose. Thiamine is used as a cofactor to make adenosine triphosphate (ATP). If glucose is given, the only available thiamine (which is already deficient) is depleted to break down the glucose. Chronic alcohol abusers may also have gastritis, pancreatitis, and liver disease.

Methanol and Ethylene Glycol
Methanol is found in antifreeze, windshield wiper fluid, paint thinner, and "bootleg" whiskey. Ethylene glycol is found in antifreeze, solvents, and paint. Methanol is rapidly absorbed from the gastrointestinal tract, and blood levels peak 30 to 90 minutes after ingestion. Methanol metabolites produce toxicity with symptoms appearing any time from 40 minutes to 72 hours after ingestion. Ethylene glycol blood levels peak 1 to 4 hours after ingestion.

Symptoms
Symptoms are similar to ethanol intoxication.
- Slurred speech
- Ataxia
- Confusion
- Tremors
- Visual disturbances such as cloudy or blurred vision
- These substances may produce renal damage and metabolic coma.

Diagnosis
- Diagnosis is confirmed by a specific test for the serum levels of methanol and ethylene glycol.

Treatment
- Gastric lavage is indicated if the patient arrives in the ED within 1 to 2 hours of ingestion.
- Ethanol may be given IV to block the conversion of methanol into more toxic substances.
- Hemodialysis may be used for patients with severe metabolic acidosis or renal failure.

Benzodiazepines
Benzodiazepines are used as sedatives, anxiolytics, and muscle relaxants and include diazepam (Valium), lorazepam (Ativan), midazolam (Versed), and oxazepam (Serax).

Symptoms
- Hypotension
- Tachycardia
- Ataxia
- Confusion
- Slurred speech
- Respiratory depression
- Hypothermia
- Hypotension

Diagnosis
- Positive benzodiazepine serum levels confirm the overdose.

Treatment
- Flumazenil (Romazicon) reverses benzodiazepines. An initial dose of 0.2 mg IV push every 1 to 2 minutes until the desired patient response *or* 1 to 2 mg IV push is given. One mg can be repeated in 20 minutes if needed. Resedation can occur 30 to 60 minutes after administration. The maximum dose is 3 mg/hour.
- Flumazenil administration may lead to seizure activity in those with chronic benzodiazepine use and in those with concomitant tricyclic antidepressant overdose.

Calcium Channel Blockers and Beta-Blockers
These drugs (verapamil, nifedipine, diltiazem, amlodipine, felodipine, atenolol, and propranolol) reduce cardiac output and systemic vascular resistance. Individuals with preexisting pulmonary disease or asthma are at higher risk for serious complications as a result of the unopposed bronchoconstriction that occurs.

Symptoms
- Bradycardia
- Atrioventricular blocks
- Respiratory depression
- Seizures
- Coma
- Hypotension

Diagnosis
- The clinical presentation and a test of serum drug level confirm the diagnosis.

Treatment

- Do not administer ipecac.
- Administer activated charcoal if the patient is awake and alert and arrives within 1 hour of ingestion.[1]
- Administer calcium chloride IV.
- Administer IV fluids for hypotension.
- Initiate external pacing for symptomatic bradyarrhythmias.
- Titrate vasoactive agents such as dopamine, epinephrine, or norepinephrine for BP control.
- Administer glucagon in beta-blocker–induced shock. Glucagon increases intracellular calcium. The increased calcium improves contractility and increases the heart rate.

Cardiac Glycosides

These drugs include digoxin and digitalis.

Symptoms

- Anorexia and nausea
- Visual disturbances
- Life-threatening arrhythmias such as bradyarrhythmias, conduction blocks, and multifocal premature ventricular contractions
- Hyperkalemia

Diagnosis

- A test of serum drug level confirms the overdose.

Treatment

- Avoid ipecac. Emesis may increase vagal tone and produce bradycardia.
- Activated charcoal
- Digibind (digoxin-specific FAB antibody fragments) is used to counteract digoxin overdoses. These antibodies remove therapeutic, as well as toxic, amounts of the drug.
- Correct electrolyte imbalances such as hyperkalemia.

Cocaine

- Cocaine may be administered nasally (snorted), orally, through smoking, or through IV injection. Cocaine produces central and autonomic stimulation by blocking neurotransmitter uptake.

Symptoms

- Hypertension
- Chest pain
- Tachycardia
- Supraventricular arrhythmias (e.g., atrial fibrillation, atrial flutter) and ventricular arrhythmias (e.g., ventricular ectopy, ventricular tachycardia)

- Dilated pupils
- Hyperthermia
- Coronary vasospasm and thrombosis resulting in myocardial ischemia and possibly injury
- Respiratory depression
- Pulmonary edema related to an inhalation injury (freebasing) or long-term use
- Confusion
- Hallucinations, paranoia

Diagnosis
- Diagnosis is based on results of a urine drug screen and clinical findings.

Treatment
- Administer benzodiazepines as needed for supraventricular arrhythmias, hypertension, and seizure activity. Benzodiazepines modulate the stimulatory effects of the cocaine on the central nervous and cardiovascular systems.
- Administer lidocaine for treatment of ventricular arrhythmias. Lidocaine reduces the toxic cardiovascular effects of cocaine.
- Administer oxygen, aspirin, and nitrates for cocaine-related myocardial ischemia.
- Use cooling blankets, tepid water spray, and fans to cool the patient.
- Whole-bowel irrigation should be considered for patients who have ingested packets of cocaine.

Hydrocarbons
Hydrocarbons are found in petroleum, natural gas, and kerosene. Hydrocarbons vaporize at low temperatures and enter the pulmonary tree easily.

Symptoms
- Vomiting
- Wheezing (related to bronchospasms)
- Crackles (related to pulmonary edema)
- Coughing
- Tachypnea
- Confusion
- Ataxia
- Headache

Diagnosis
- A hydrocarbon overdose is diagnosed on the basis of history and symptom presentation.

Treatment
- Ipecac should not be administered.
- Remove any contaminated clothing. Wash skin with soap and copious amounts of water.
- Gastric suctioning and administration of activated charcoal may be indicated for recent ingestions. However, an endotracheal tube must be inserted first because of the aspiration potential.
- Oxygen and mechanical ventilation often are needed.

Iron
Iron is commonly found in dietary supplements such as multivitamins.
Symptoms
- Vomiting
- Diarrhea
- Abdominal pain

In major ingestions, severe effects may occur several hours after the incident and include:
- GI bleeding
- Metabolic acidosis with hyperpnea
- Tachycardia
- Hypotension
- Coagulopathies
Diagnosis
- Diagnosis is based on results of abdominal radiographs and on the serum level. The serum level should be determined 4 to 6 hours after ingestion. Serial levels are needed when iron tablets are found on abdominal radiographs.
Treatment
- Ipecac can be administered unless the patient already has vomited.
- Whole-bowel irrigation may be ordered for patients with rising iron levels or with pills evident on the radiograph.
- A serum iron level greater than 500 mcg/dl is considered toxic and often treated with chelation therapy using deferoxamine. Deferoxamine is administered at 15 mg/kg/hr per continuous IV infusion. Rapid IV administration may cause hypotension.

Opioids (Codeine and Heroin)
Symptoms
- Constricted pupils
- Vomiting

- Seizures
- Hypotension
- Bradycardia
- Pulmonary edema
- Respiratory depression
- Decreased level of consciousness and possibly coma

Diagnosis
- A urine toxicology screen is the most sensitive detection tool.
- A positive response to naloxone administration is considered diagnostic.

Treatment
- Syrup of ipecac should not be administered.
- Naloxone (Narcan) at 0.4 to 2 mg by IV push is used initially. If the patient does not respond (such as with improved respiratory rate and depth), the dose can be repeated in 2-mg increments for a total dose of 10 mg.[3] Naloxone can be administered through the endotracheal tube or by intramuscular or subcutaneous injection.

Organophosphates
Organophosphate exposure from insecticides can occur by inhalation or ingestion or through the skin.

Symptoms
Organophosphates overstimulate the parasympathetic nervous system.
- An overdose produces the SLUDGE (salivation, lacrimation, urination, defecation, gastrointestinal manifestations such as nausea and vomiting, and emesis) syndrome.
- Bradycardia
- Bronchospasms and increased bronchial secretions
- Hypotension
- Pinpoint pupils
- Muscle weakness
- Muscle fasciculations

Diagnosis
- Diagnosis is based on history and the presence of symptoms.

Treatment
- Remove contaminated clothing and jewelry. Flush contaminated skin with water.
- IV atropine. Large doses may be required, such as 2 to 5 mg every 5 minutes until control of mucous membrane hypersecretion is attained.
- Pralidoxime chloride (Protopam) is administered as an IV drip of 1 to 2 g over 30 minutes. It is most useful when

administered within 24 hours of exposure. Indications for use include muscle weakness and fasciculations. The dose is not based on heart rate or pupil size.

Salicylates (Aspirin)
Many people use salicylates regularly; therefore chronic as well as acute overdosage is possible. A single ingestion of more than 150 mg/kg often causes toxicity. Chronic ingestion of more than 100 mg/kg/day may cause toxicity.

Symptoms
- Nausea and vomiting
- Tinnitus
- Rapid, deep respirations secondary to metabolic acidosis and direct stimulation of the respiratory center in the brainstem
- Hyperthermia
- Tachycardia
- Hypotension
- Lethargy
- Confusion
- Seizures

Diagnosis
- Serum salicylate levels should be obtained every 2 hours for the first 4 to 8 hours to assess the rate of rise and to obtain a reliable level. Levels then should be obtained every 4 to 6 hours until a sustained decline in the level is noted.[3]

Treatment
- Gastric lavage should be performed in patients presenting within 1 hour of a large ingestion.
- Administer activated charcoal after or in lieu of lavage.[2]
- Urinary alkalinization should be considered for patients with toxic salicylate or rapidly increasing salicylate levels. Alkalinizing the urine traps ionized salicylate and increases excretion. Urinary alkalinization can be attained by adding 100 mEq of sodium bicarbonate to a liter of IV fluid and infusing the fluid at 200 ml/hr.
- Hemodialysis usually is initiated in patients with a severe acid–base imbalance, persistent hypotension, pulmonary edema, coma, or seizures.
- Whole-bowel irrigation may be considered when enteric-coated aspirin has been ingested.
- D_5LR or D_5NS IV solutions are given to correct dehydration.
- Glucose is administered to correct hypoglycemia.

- Monitor potassium levels. Significant potassium loss results from vomiting and increased renal excretion of potassium.

Street Drugs
See Table 20-3 for information on street drugs.

Tricyclic Antidepressants (TCAs)
TCAs such as amitriptyline, doxepin, and imipramine are oral medications commonly used for the treatment of depression and other disorders. Adults begin to develop toxic effects after ingesting three times the daily dose. Severe toxicity and death may occur in large ingestions.

Symptoms
- Respiratory depression
- Agitation
- Decreased level of consciousness that can progress to coma
- Tachycardia
- Arrhythmias including ventricular tachycardia, atrial and ventricular blocks
- Prolonged QRS and QT intervals
- Hypotension
- Seizures

Diagnosis
- Diagnosis is based on clinical symptoms and serum or urine analysis.

Treatment
- Ipecac should not be administered because the level of consciousness may decline rapidly.
- Orogastric lavage and activated charcoal should be considered for patients who present within 1 to 2 hours of overdose. The patient may need to be intubated first to prevent aspiration.
- Serum alkalinization (pH 7.5 to 7.55) is indicated for patients with QRS prolongation, ventricular arrhythmias, or hypotension that does not respond to a saline bolus of 500 ml.[1]
- Seizures are treated with benzodiazepines.
- Treat hypovolemia with isotonic crystalloids such as Ringer's lactate. Norepinephrine or dopamine may be given if hypotension persists after volume repletion.

NURSING SURVEILLANCE

1. Monitor the patient's consciousness level.
2. Monitor the trend of the vital signs and oxygen saturation.

Text continued on p. 681

TABLE 20-3   Street Drugs

Name Classification, Street Name	Effects	Overdose Indicators	Notes
Clonazepam (Clonopin) *Benzodiazepine*	• Shallow respirations • Clammy skin • Rapid pulse • Coma	• Significant CNS or respiratory depression • Hypotension and tachycardia • Hypothermia • Overdose rarely causes death unless concomitant alcohol ingestion that accentuates respiratory depression.	• Hepatic metabolism, peak plasma levels at 1-2 hours. Therapeutic serum level 20-80 mg/ml. • Administer flumazenil (Romazicon) IV over 30 seconds. • Do not induce emesis because of potential for rapid deterioration. • Gastric lavage • Charcoal • Fluid bolus NS for hypotension • Dopamine if no response to NS • Withdrawal signs and symptoms include anxiety, insomnia, tremors, and convulsions.
Cocaine *Central nervous system stimulant* Coke, snow, ready rock, French fries, teeth, blow, white, hard (base cocaine; crack or rock), soft (cocaine hydrochloride; powder)	• Strong CNS stimulant that interferes with the reabsorption of dopamine • Produces an immediate	• Paranoia • Pallor • Hypertension • Tachycardia • Chest pain, myocardial infarction	• Monitor airway. • Control agitation with benzodiazepines and environmental measures. These measures should help control the heart rate. • Benzodiazepines should help control hypertension. If hypertension is not controlled with benzodiazepines,

Continued

TABLE 20-3   Street Drugs—cont'd

Name, Classification, Street Name	Effects	Overdose Indicators	Notes
	euphoric effect, which includes hyperstimulation, reduced fatigue, and mental clarity. Effects are short term (20 min to 1 hour), and confusion, impaired judgment, and irrational, excited behaviors are seen.	• Seizures • Arrhythmias • Hyperthermia • Rhabdomyolysis caused by hyperthermia, agitation, and seizures • Dilated pupils • Bizarre, erratic, and violent behavior • Restlessness, mania • Irritability	nitroprusside can be used. • Antiseizure medication • Monitor pH for acidosis. • Maintain adequate urine output, monitor for rhabdomyolysis. • Gastric lavage generally not indicated, as the drug is not usually ingested. • Psychiatric consultation • Cocaine and alcohol mixed will produce a more intense euphoric effect. In the liver, this will produce cocaethylene, which may increase the chance of sudden death.
Ephedrine *Adrenergic agent with actions similar to epinephrine* Brigham Young weed, desert herb, Mormon tea, squaw tea,	• Peripheral vasoconstriction • Tachycardia • Diaphoresis • Decreased	• Agitation • Palpitations • Tachycardia • Hypertension • Nausea/vomiting	• Continuously monitor cardiac and respiratory function. • Control agitation with pharmaceuticals (benzodiazepine). • Monitor hypertension; if not controlled

Continued

miner's tea	appetite • Anxiety • Tremor • Weakness • Nausea	• Paranoid psychosis, hallucinations • Respiratory depression • Seizures • Coma • Concomitant use of caffeine and smoking can lead to stroke, heart attack, and seizures.	with benzodiazepines, consider nitroprusside. • Seizure precautions
Gamma hydroxybutrate (GHB) *Central nervous system depressant* Liquid ecstasy, easy lay, soap, E scoop, cherry FX bombs, cherry meth, G-riffick, grievous bodily harm	■ Similar to alcohol intoxication ■ Happiness ■ Desire to socialize ■ Nausea ■ Relaxation ■ Difficulty concentrating ■ Amnesia	• Toxicity can occur in 15-30 minutes. • Respiratory depression • Chest tightness • Agitation • Seizures • Metabolic acidosis from seizures or agitation • Loss of muscle tone • Lethargy • Labile emotions • Mild tremors • Agitation	• Prevent aspiration with vomiting. • Monitor respiratory status; intubation attempts may cause dramatic agitation and struggling. Rapid-sequence intubation may be required for success. • Pulse oximetry • Monitor cardiac rhythm. • Gastric lavage should be performed if ingestion was within the previous hour. Activated charcoal also may be administered if ingestion within previous few hours. • Check urine pregnancy test (GHB crosses the placenta)

TABLE 20-3 Street Drugs—cont'd

Name, Classification, Street Name	Effects	Overdose Indicators	Notes
			• Assess oral mucosa and lips for burns. GHB is home manufactured with lye and other strong bases.
			• GHB has a salty taste when mixed in water.
			• Symptoms usually resolve within 6 hours.
			• For small to moderate doses, withdrawal symptoms are mild to none. For heavy doses, withdrawal symptoms are similar to alcohol.
Heroin *Opiate, central nervous system depressant* Smack, H, skag, junk, Mexican black tar, China white, crank, horse	• Euphoria • After injection, drug crosses blood–brain barrier, converts to morphine, and binds rapidly to opioid receptors. • Abusers feel a "rush" and flushing of the	• Nausea and vomiting • Pruritis • Constricted pupils • Bradycardia • CNS depression • Respiratory deficiency • Noncardiogenic pulmonary edema • Seizures • Coma • Death	• Monitor for hypoxia • Continuous monitoring of cardiac and respiratory status • Antidote: Narcan for respiratory depression • Nalmefene if prolonged reversal of opioid effect is needed • Endotracheal intubation may be needed with pulmonary edema. • Benzodiazepines for seizure activity • Withdrawal symptoms will occur within a few hours of last dose: restlessness, diarrhea,

vomiting, muscle and bone pain, seizures

Inhalants *CNS depressant* *Volatile solvents* Paint thinners Paint removers Dry cleaning fluid Gasoline Glue Correction fluid Felt-tip markers **Aerosols** (Sprays that contain propellants and solvents) Spray paint Hair spray Deodorant	• ...an, dry mouth, heavy feeling extremities. • Nausea and vomiting • Rapid onset of effects • Prolonged by repeated inhalation • Euphoria heat • Exhilaration • Lowered inhibitions • Dizziness • Light-headedness • Near-normal pupil response	• Slurred speech • Incoordination • Hallucinations • Delusions • Loss of consciousness • Depressed reflexes • Prolonged abuse leads to neurotoxicity. • Cognitive abnormalities o Inability to learn new things o Inability to recognize familiar things o Inability to keep track of simple conversations • Polyneuropathy	• Will often have paint or other stains on hands, face, or clothes • Chemical odor may be noticeable. • Ensure continued airway patency. • Monitor for respiratory insufficiency. • Continuous cardiac monitoring • Chronic abusers will have liver, kidney, cerebral, and pulmonary damage. • Patients may be belligerent or violent. • Sudden sniffing death: Sniffing highly concentrated inhalants can induce irregular and rapid heart rhythms leading to cardiac failure and death within minutes of sniffing. • Asphyxiation from repeated sniffing of high concentration and inhalant displacing oxygen in lungs

Continued

TABLE 20-3 Street Drugs—cont'd

Name, Classification, Street Name	Effects	Overdose Indicators	Notes
Vegetable oil		• Inability to control movements • Loss of sensation; vision and hearing changes	• Nitrites differ in that they do not affect the CNS directly. They act primarily to dilate blood vessels and relax the muscles and are used as "sexual enhancers."
Gases Nitrous oxide (laughing gas) Whipped cream dispensers Butane lighters Propane tanks Freon			
Nitrites Amyl nitrate (poppers, snappers) NTG spray Butyl nitrite Cyclohexyl nitrate (found in room deodorizers)			
Ketamine *Dissociative anesthetic* "K," green K, special K, vitamin K, super acid **Phencyclidine (PCP)**	• Out-of-body experience • Relaxation • Euphoria • Feeling of	• Delirium • Hyperthermia or hypothermia • Hypertension or hypotension	• Mild hypoglycemia is common. • Treatment focus is on hemodynamic stability, maintaining adequate ventilation and oxygenation, and controlling agitation.

Hallucinogen PCP, angel dust, rocket fuel, mist, super weed, snorts	floating and weightlessness • Strong dissociation • Numbness • Slurred speech • Blank stare • Rapid involuntary eye movements • Amnesia • Auditory and visual hallucinations • Anxiety	• Coma • Hypoxia/apnea • Seizures	• Administer benzodiazepines for agitation. Large amounts may be needed. • Place patient in a quiet environment. • Monitor temperature and implement cooling measures if hyperthermia occurs. Hyperthermia can be significant. • Replenish fluids as necessary. • Patients can be violent.
LSD *Hallucinogen* Acid, blue, pink, window pane, sunshine, blotter, microdots, paper	Auditory and visual hallucinations Effects are unpredictable	• Daphoresis • Dizziness • Twitching • Flushing • Hyperreflexia • Hypertension • Tachycardia • Hyperthermia	• Focus on controlling airway and managing activity associated with the hallucinations. • Minimize stimulation. • Benzodiazepines for agitation • IV fluids for dehydration • Cooling measures for hyperthermia: fans, wet sheets • Complications include renal failure and CNS injury caused by prolonged seizures.

Continued

TABLE 20-3   Street Drugs—cont'd

Name, Classification, Street Name	Effects	Overdose Indicators	Notes
			• Death from overdose is unusual. Death usually results from trauma that occurs during hallucinations.
Marijuana (THC) *Central nervous system depressant* Reefer, smoke, dope, grass, weed, joint, hash, green	• Euphoria • Lowered heart rate • Lowered respiratory rate • Lethargic • Relaxed/calm • Stimulated appetite • Nausea inhibited • Exaggeration of senses • Impaired hand-eye coordination • Inability to judge distance and speed	• Hallucinations • Paranoia • Mental confusion • Panic attacks	• THC is stored in fat. It is possible for enough THC to be stored and eventually released back into the system to cause a "flashback" high.

Methamphetamine
Central nervous system stimulant

Speed, meth, chalk, ice, crystal, crank, glass, fast, grit

- Increased alertness
- Sense of well-being
- Paranoia
- Intense high
- Violent tendencies
- Dilated or constricted pupils
- Loss of appetite

- Hyperactivity
- Intense anxiety
- Extreme anorexia
- Seizures
- Arrhythmias
- Depression
- Paranoia
- Hyperthermia
- Hypertension
- Tachycardia
- Cardiovascular collapse

- Releases high levels of dopamine, which stimulates the CNS.
- Patients can be extremely violent!
- IV users are at high risk for contracting and transmitting HIV and hepatitis.
- Made in illegal labs and has a high potential for abuse and dependence; produces a severe craving
- Treatment should focus on the physiologic effects of the drug: increased temperature; increased heart rate and blood pressure that can lead to seizures, strokes, or sudden death. Antiseizure and antianxiety medications should be given.
- Gastric lavage can be used if ingestion occurred within past hour. Charcoal can be administered if ingestion occurred within the past few hours.
- Withdrawal produces headaches, dyspnea, and severe depression, and patient may be suicidal.

Continued

TABLE 20-3 Street Drugs—cont'd			
Name, Classification, Street Name	Effects	Overdose Indicators	Notes
Methylenedioxymethamphetamine (MDMA) *Central nervous system stimulant, hallucinogenic amphetamine* Ecstasy, Adam, XTC, bug, beans, love drug, roll, hug drug, dance drug, "E," "X"	• Feelings of energy • Strong feelings of well-being • Increased confidence • Colors perceived as brighter • Music sounds better • Sense of touch heightened	• Increased blood pressure • Panic attacks • Jaw clenching/teeth grinding • Paranoid thoughts • Sweating • Dehydration • Irrational behavior • Seizures • Tachycardia • Hyperthermia • Myocardial damage caused by sustained elevated heart rates	• Overdoses may result in heart attacks or extreme heat stroke and may be fatal. • Place patient in a quiet, stimulant-free environment. • Cardiac monitoring • Monitor for hypertension. • Monitor for hyperthermia. • Evaluate for hyponatremia. • Seizure precautions • Administer IV fluids for dehydration.
Methylphenidate (Ritalin) *Stimulant* Ritalin, JIF, MPH, R-ball, Skippy, the smart drug, vitamin R	• Euphoria • Increases alertness and focus • Blocks hunger and fatigue	• Hyperadrenergic state similar to amphetamine overdose • Agitation • Tachycardia	• Control agitation with benzodiazepines. • Closely monitor patient's airway patency. • Hyperthermia • Seizures: treat with benzodiazepines. • Arrhythmias

	• Hypertension • Mydriasis • Hyperthermia • Diaphoresis • Delirium • Hallucinations • Hypokalemia • Psychosis • Seizures	• Gastric lavage if ingestion was within past 1 hour • Charcoal if ingestion was within past few hours • Hypertension may respond to benzodiazepines. If not, consider a short-acting titratable agent such as sodium nitroprusside. • Beta-blockers are not suggested as treatment for tachycardias or hypertension as they may result in unopposed alpha-adrenergic receptor stimulation and worsening of hypertension.
Psilocybin *Hallucinogen* Mushrooms, shrooms, liberty caps, magic mushrooms, boomers, silly putty	• Hallucinations • Deep sense of connecting to others, nature, and the universe • Euphoria • Anxiety • Frightening hallucinations • Increased tachycardia • Psychosis • Dysesthesia • Hyperthermia	• Calm, quiet environment • Benzodiazepines for agitation • Charcoal if ingestion has been within the past hour • Antipyretics for fever • Panic attacks or agitated behavior are common reasons for ED visit. • Death from overdose is rare.

Continued

TABLE 20-3   Street Drugs—cont'd

Name, Classification, Street Name	Effects	Overdose Indicators	Notes
	• Disconnection from reality • Panic		
Rohypnol (Flunitrazepam) *Benzodiazepine* Rophies, roofies, roach, rope, "date rape drug"	• Muscle relaxation • Amnesia	• Hypothermia • Hypotension or hypertension • Bradycardia or tachycardia • Respiratory depression • Nausea • Lactic acidosis if hypoxia or hypotension occurs • Lethargy • Amnesia • Coma	• Supportive care and early airway control • Gastric lavage if ingestion has been within the past hour • Charcoal without a cathartic if the ingestion has been within the past few hours • Administer flumazenil; monitor for agitation, vomiting, confusion, seizures, arrhythmias, flushing • Normal saline (NS) bolus for hypotension. • Dopamine if inadequate response to NS.

Data from: Dart RC, ed: *The 5-minute toxicology consult*, Philadelphia, 2000, Lippincott Williams & Wilkins; Walton SC: First response guide to street drugs, Alberta, Canada, 2001, Burn and Holding; www.DEA.gov; accessed May 29, 2004.

3. Monitor intake and output to assess fluid balance and effects of interventions.
4. Monitor the patient for cardiac arrhythmia.

EXPECTED PATIENT OUTCOMES

1. The patient's level of consciousness improves compared with the time of arrival.
2. The mean arterial pressure is maintained between 70 and 105 mm Hg.
3. The airway remains patent without aspiration.
4. Drug absorption is inhibited.

DISCHARGE IMPLICATIONS

1. Check the serum level before discharge if possible.
2. Teach the family seizure precautions.
3. Teach the family the need for follow-up care to prevent later complications.
4. Teach the family about aspiration prevention because the patient may vomit at home.
5. Beware of discharging a patient with a known overdose of acetaminophen or sustained-release medications because symptoms may occur later.
6. Teach the family to keep the telephone number of the poison control center immediately available.
7. Teach the family the importance of proper storage of medications and poisonous substances.

REFERENCES

1. American Heart Association: *ACLS for experienced providers*, 2003, The Association.
2. Criddle LM: In Newberry L: *Sheehy's emergency nursing principles and practice*, ed 5, St Louis, 2003, Mosby.
3. Dart RC: *The 5 minute toxicology consult*, Philadelphia, 2000, Lippincott.

21 chapter

Trauma

Steve Talbert

FOCUSED NURSING ASSESSMENT

Care of the trauma patient begins with the primary survey. The purpose of the primary survey is to identify and correct any life-threatening conditions.[1,2] This includes assessing the airway (while maintaining spine precautions), breathing, and circulation and performing a brief neurologic examination. When the primary survey is complete, the patient is completely exposed, then covered to maintain body temperature, and a full set of vital signs is obtained. Finally, a thorough head-to-toe examination is performed to identify all potential injuries. Box 21-1, Trauma Assessment, summarizes the trauma assessment and offers a simple acronym for remembering the proper sequence.[2]

PRIMARY ASSESSMENT

Airway With Cervical Spine Precautions

1. Inspect for an actual or potential airway obstruction.
   - Foreign body
   - Blood

BOX 21-1 TRAUMA ASSESSMENT

Primary assessment: ABCD

Airway with cervical spine precautions

Breathing

Circulation

Disability (brief neurologic examination)

Secondary assessment: EFGHI

Expose (remove all clothing) and Evacuate (if necessary)

Fahrenheit (maintain body temperature)

Get full set of vital signs

Head-to-toe examination

Inspect the back

TABLE 21-1 Life-Threatening Airway Problems

Problem	Signs and Symptoms	Interventions
Airway obstruction (complete or partial)	• Dyspnea, labored respirations • Decreased or no air movement • Cyanosis • Presence of foreign body in airway • Trauma to face or neck • Edema	Airway opening maneuvers: • Jaw thrust • Chin lift • Suction Airway adjuncts: • Nasal airway • Oral airway • Endotracheal tube Surgical airway: • Cricothyrotomy • Tracheostomy
Inhalation injury	• History of inhaled steam, fire, unconsciousness, or exposure to heavy smoke • Dyspnea • Wheezing, rhonchi, and crackles • Hoarseness • Singed facial or nasal hairs • Carbonaceous sputum • Burns to face or neck	• Provide high-flow oxygen (100%) via nonrebreather mask or bag-valve device. • Prepare for endotracheal intubation as soon as possible.

- Vomitus
- Tongue
- Swelling
- Stridor
- Listen for air movement.

If the patient's airway is not patent, steps must be taken immediately to open the airway. Table 21-1 lists life-threatening airway problems, their signs and symptoms, and immediate interventions.

NURSING ALERT

A talking patient has a patent airway.

NURSING ALERT

Any patients who have blunt or penetrating trauma above the nipple line must have the cervical spine immobilized simultaneously with airway assessment.

NURSING ALERT

Intubation of the trauma patient may be difficult. Use of rapid-sequence intubation may be helpful, but application of this procedure should be reserved for practitioners with excellent airway skills.

Breathing

1. Inspect for rise and fall of the chest.
   - Asymmetry may indicate a pneumothorax or hemothorax.
   - Paradoxical movement indicates a flail chest.
2. Inspect for open chest trauma.
   - Assume that an open pneumothorax is present in the case of a sucking chest wound.
3. Inspect for work of breathing.
   - Increased work of breathing is a sign of problems with air movement or gas exchange.
   - Nasal flaring and the use of accessory muscles are classic signs of dyspnea.

4. Inspect and palpate for tracheal position.
   - The trachea may deviate away from a tension pneumothorax (usually a late sign).
5. Auscultate lung fields for the presence of breath sounds.
   - Unequal, diminished, or absent sounds may indicate a pneumothorax, hemothorax, or viscerothorax.
6. Palpate the chest for instability and subcutaneous air.
   - The presence of either bony crepitus or subcutaneous air indicates an underlying chest injury and a probable pneumothorax.

Trauma patients initially should receive 100% oxygen by a nonrebreather mask or bag-valve device. Table 21-2 lists life-threatening breathing problems, their signs and symptoms, and immediate interventions.

Circulation

1. Inspect for an obvious external hemorrhage.

NURSING ALERT

Most external hemorrhaging can be controlled with direct pressure. Clamping bleeding vessels or placing a tourniquet are measures of last resort. Direct pressure may be best applied by direct fingertip pressure to the bleeding vessel. This may require the removal of pressure dressings so that point of hemorrhage can be located.

---

2. Inspect skin color, temperature, and moisture.
   - Skin that is pale, cool, or moist indicates a poor perfusion state.
3. Palpate for central and peripheral pulse presence, rate, and symmetry.
   - Weak, thready, or absent pulses indicate a poor perfusion state.
   - Early manifestations of shock include tachycardia and cutaneous vasoconstriction.
   - Weak peripheral pulses relative to central pulses indicate a poor perfusion state.
   - Trauma patients initially should receive warm isotonic crystalloid solution (Ringer's lactate or 0.9% NaCl) through two large-bore IV lines. A large-bore IV is a 14-gauge or 16-gauge IV for adults and a 22-gauge or larger IV for pediatric patients.[1,2] A general rule of thumb to guide

TABLE 21-2   Life-Threatening Breathing Problems

Problem	Signs and Symptoms	Interventions
Tension pneumothorax (tension pneumothorax is a clinical diagnosis)	• Dyspnea, labored respirations • Decreased or absent breath sounds on affected side • Unilateral chest rise and fall • Tracheal deviation away from affected side • Cyanosis • Jugular venous distension • Tachycardia and hypotension • History of chest trauma or mechanical ventilation	• Provide high-flow oxygen (100%) via nonrebreather mask or bag-valve device. • Rapid chest decompression by needle thoracostomy on affected side • Chest tube placement on affected side
Pneumothorax	• Dyspnea, labored respirations • Decreased or absent breath sounds on affected side • May have unilateral chest rise and fall • May have visible wound to chest or back • History of chest trauma	• Provide high-flow oxygen (100%) via nonrebreather mask or bag-valve device. • Chest tube placement on affected side • Place occlusive dressing over any open chest wound and secure on three sides with tape.
Hemothorax	• Dyspnea, labored respirations • Decreased or absent breath sounds on affected side • May have unilateral chest rise and fall • Tachycardia and hypotension	• Provide high-flow oxygen (100%) via nonrebreather mask or bag-valve device. • Chest tube placement on affected side • Consider autotransfusion (Procedure 4).

Sucking chest wound (open chest wound)	• May have visible wound to chest or back • History of chest trauma (usually penetrating) • Dyspnea, labored respirations • Visible, sucking wound to chest or back • Decreased or absent breath sounds on affected side	• Provide high-flow oxygen (100%) via nonrebreather mask or bag-valve device • Cover wound with occlusive dressing and secure on three sides with tape. • Watch for signs of tension pneumothorax and remove dressing during exhalation if they are noted.
Flail chest	• Dyspnea, labored respirations • Paradoxical chest wall movement • Chest pain • Tachycardia	• Provide high-flow oxygen (100%) via nonrebreather mask or bag-valve device. • Prepare for intubation and mechanical ventilation.
Full-thickness circumferential burn of thorax	• Dyspnea, labored respirations • Shallow respirations • Obvious circumferential burns to thorax	• Provide high-flow oxygen (100%) via nonrebreather mask or bag-valve device. • Prepare for immediate escharotomy (Chapter 4).

volume replacement is the "3 for 1" rule: Each milliliter (ml) of blood loss should be replaced with 3 ml of crystalloid. Ongoing evaluation of the patient's response to fluid resuscitation is essential to ensure a good patient outcome and maintenance of end-organ perfusion status. Table 21-3 lists life-threatening circulation problems, their signs and symptoms, and immediate interventions.

Disability (Brief Neurologic Assessment)

The brief neurologic assessment consists of an assessment of level of consciousness. The Glasgow Coma Scale (GCS) assigns a number to the best eye-opening response, best motor response, and best verbal response, then combines the numbers for a total score (Reference Guides 10 [adult] and 16 [infant and pediatric]).

1. Check for the best eye-opening response.
   - The eye opening may be spontaneous or in response to voice or to pain, or there may be no eye opening.
2. Check for the best motor response.
   - The patient may obey commands, demonstrate purposeful movement (localize to pain), withdraw in response to pain, demonstrate abnormal flexion (decorticate) or extension (decerebrate), or not respond at all.

TABLE 21-3	Life-Threatening Circulation Problems	
Problem	Signs and Symptoms	Interventions
External hemorrhage	• Obvious bleeding site	• Direct pressure • Elevation
Internal hemorrhage	• Tachycardia • Weak, thready pulses • Cool, pale, clammy skin • Tachypnea • Altered mental status • Delayed capillary refill • Oliguria or anuria	• Provide high-flow oxygen (100%) via nonrebreather mask or bag-valve device. • Place two large-bore IV lines with warm isotonic crystalloid solution (Ringer's lactate or 0.9% NaCl). • Administer fluid bolus (2 L in adults or 20 ml/kg in children). • Prepare to administer blood.

3. Check for the best verbal response.
   - The patient may be oriented or confused, use inappropriate words or incomprehensible sounds, or demonstrate no verbal response.
   - Indicate a patient is intubated by placing "T" next to the total score.
4. Check for pupil size and reactivity.
   - Fixed, dilated pupils are consistent with a severe closed-head injury.
   - Unilateral dilation may indicate transtentorial herniation.
   - Constricted pupils may indicate a drug overdose or pontine damage.

The GCS evaluation should include an evaluation of motor responsiveness for all four extremities. Lateralizing motor findings are important to report and should be handled with a sense of urgency because transtentorial herniation may be imminent. When a physical examination reveals an unequal motor response, the *best* motor score should be assigned, with appropriate notation of inequality in the narrative description of the physical examination. Trauma patients who have a head injury and a GCS score of less than 15 should undergo a more detailed neurologic examination, including evaluation by a neurosurgeon.[3] Patients who have a GCS score of 8 or less should be intubated. For patients who have severe head injuries (GCS score of 8 or less), treatment goals are to maintain a systolic blood pressure (BP) of 90 mm Hg or greater and a PaO$_2$ of 60 mm Hg or greater, and avoid secondary injury resulting from hypoxemia or hypotension.[4]

SECONDARY ASSESSMENT

When the primary assessment is complete and all life-threatening conditions have been corrected, the secondary examination can be performed.[1,2] The secondary survey includes a thorough head-to-toe examination and a history of the events surrounding the injury.

Expose and Evacuate

Remove all articles of clothing. If the patient is immobilized, it is usually necessary to cut off the clothes. Exposing the patient is necessary to identify injuries quickly. Initiate plans to transfer the patient to a definitive care facility if necessary (see Procedure 27).

Optimal care for the critically injured trauma patient is often time dependent. Outcomes can be improved if the patient receives rapid, definitive care. The trauma nurse should compare the needs of the patient with resources available at the facility.

If the necessary resources are not available at the facility in which the trauma patient is receiving care, arrangements for transfer should be made as quickly as possible. Do not delay a transfer for diagnostic studies.

Fahrenheit (Maintain Body Temperature)

The patient should not be left uncovered. Hypothermia is common with the trauma patient and has detrimental effects. Measures should be taken to preserve body heat and prevent hypothermia. These measures include warm blankets, special warming blankets, an increase in the temperature of the resuscitation room, the use of warming lights, and the use of warm IV fluids. If continuous core temperature monitoring (e.g., a temperature-sensing indwelling urinary catheter) is available, it should be used to ensure prevention of hypothermia.

Get Vital Signs

A full set of vital signs should be obtained as quickly as possible. These include the heart rate, respiratory rate, blood pressure, and core body temperature. Heart monitoring and pulse oximetry should be initiated if possible. End-tidal CO_2 monitoring may be instituted with intubated patients to measure the effectiveness of ventilation and to monitor tube placement.

Head-to-Toe Examination

The head-to-toe examination is a thorough and systematic assessment of the entire body. It includes auscultation, inspection, palpation, and percussion.[1,2]

- *Head:* The head should be inspected for obvious wounds (e.g., lacerations, contusions, abrasions, or burns), external hemorrhage, deformities, impaled objects, or drainage from the nose (rhinorrhea) or ears (otorrhea). The head also should be palpated for deformities, areas of tenderness, or subcutaneous air. The stability of the midface and alignment of the teeth also should be assessed.
- *Neck:* The neck should be assessed for any obvious wounds, external hemorrhage, or impaled objects. The presence or absence of jugular venous distension (JVD) should be noted. The tracheal position should be palpated. Any areas of tenderness should be noted. Auscultation of bruits over major vessels may indicate vascular injury. The quality of the patient's voice should be evaluated for hoarseness. The patient also should be evaluated for the inability to manage his or her secretions because of pain with swallowing, which may be indicative of direct airway trauma.

┌───┐
│ ⤳ **N U R S I N G   A L E R T** ⬻ │
├───┤
│ Alignment of the cervical spine must be maintained during │
│ assessment of the neck. │
└───┘

- *Chest:* The chest should be inspected for signs of obvious injury, including the presence of a sucking chest wound, external hemorrhage, or impaled objects. The rise and fall of the chest wall should be observed for symmetry and equality. Palpate the chest wall for tenderness, crepitus, and the presence of subcutaneous air. Finally, auscultate for the depth, quality, and equality of breath sounds. The presence of bowel sounds in the chest should be noted as well.

- *Abdomen:* An abdominal assessment begins with an inspection of the abdomen for signs of obvious trauma, external hemorrhage, or impaled objects. Next, auscultate for bowel sounds or bruits in all quadrants. The abdomen should be palpated for areas of tenderness, firmness, and distension. Rigidity, distension, and pain are indicators of possible internal injury and ongoing hemorrhage or peritonitis. With any abnormal findings during the abdominal examination, a surgical abdomen should be assumed and treated accordingly with a sense of urgency.

- *Pelvis:* The pelvis should be inspected for signs of obvious trauma, external hemorrhage, or impaled objects. Next, it should be palpated for tenderness and stability. One does this by simultaneously pushing downward on the anterior aspect of the iliac crests and pushing inward on the lateral aspect of the iliac crests; then gentle pressure should be applied to the symphysis pubis. As a general rule, this assessment elicits pain or reveals instability if the pelvis is fractured. In cases of pelvic instability, repeated bony pelvic examination should be *deferred* to prevent additional blood loss caused by repeated manipulation of the pelvis.

- *Genitourinary:* The genitourinary and gynecologic assessment begins with an inspection for signs of obvious trauma, external hemorrhage, impaled objects, blood at the urethral meatus, vaginal bleeding, or a scrotal hematoma. If blood is present at the urethral meatus, insertion of an indwelling urinary catheter should be postponed until the patency of the urethra is confirmed. A vaginal exam helps to confirm or rule out internal injuries.

- *Extremities:* Inspect for signs of obvious trauma, external hemorrhage, impaled objects, or deformities. Palpate each extremity for areas of tenderness or deformity, determine capillary refill time, and assess pulse presence and quality. Pulse quality should be compared bilaterally simultaneously for equality. Likewise, sensation should be checked in each extremity and compared bilaterally for equality. Finally, the range of motion may be checked unless contraindicated.

Inspect the Back

> **NURSING ALERT**
>
> Cervical spine immobilization must be maintained while the patient is log rolled and the back assessed. Movement and sensation of extremities should be assessed **before** and **immediately after** the patient is log rolled.

The patient should be carefully log rolled onto either side. Preference should be given to the least-injured side. Inspect the back, buttocks, and dorsal side of the lower extremities for signs of obvious trauma, external hemorrhage, or impaled objects. The spine should be palpated for areas of tenderness, muscle spasms, stepoffs, or deformity. A rectal examination should be performed to determine rectal tone, the presence of blood, and direct rectal trauma. The position of the prostate also should be determined for male trauma patients before an indwelling urinary catheter is inserted. The patient should be carefully log rolled back into the supine position when the back assessment is complete.

> **NURSING ALERT**
>
> Before performing the rectal examination, the practitioner should put on a new glove. This minimizes the risk of a false-positive test for rectal bleeding.

HISTORY

Another component of the secondary assessment is the rapid obtaining of a focused history that gathers data that will be important in anticipating injuries and guiding patient care.[1,2]

This history includes an AMPLE data set: *A*llergies, *M*edications, *P*ast medical history, *L*ast oral intake, and *E*vents surrounding the traumatic event (e.g., mechanism of injury, seat belt or helmet use, type of weapon used, and loss of consciousness after the injury). The mnemonic AMPLE can serve as a reminder for the information needed. The history should include factors in the MIVT acronym: the mechanism of injury, the extent of injuries (based on prehospital assessment), vital signs in the field, and treatment in the field.

RISK FACTORS

Age

Trauma is the leading cause of death during the first four decades of life.[1,2] Although the young historically are the trauma patients, trauma is a growing problem for the geriatric population. The mechanisms of injury differ for these age-groups. Younger patients often are involved in motor vehicle crashes (driver, passenger, pedestrian, or bicyclist) or violence. Falling is the leading cause of injury for the geriatric population.

Preexisting Medical Conditions

Certain medical conditions can predispose patients to injury. These diseases create one of several conditions that increase the risk of injury, such as an altered level of consciousness, altered sensory input, or altered thought processes. Table 21-4 lists common chronic medical conditions and their mechanism for predisposing patients to traumatic injury. In addition, concurrent illnesses may alter the normal physiologic response to injury. The patient's past medical history should be carefully reviewed to determine the "expected" response to the stress of trauma.

Medications

As with preexisting medical conditions, certain medications can predispose patients to injury. Drugs that directly or indirectly alter the mental status are prime contributors. Table 21-5 lists classes of medications and their mechanism for predisposing patients to traumatic injury.

LIFE SPAN ISSUES

NURSING ALERT
Assessment and intervention priorities are the same for all patients, regardless of age.

TABLE 21-4   Common Medical Conditions That Increase Risk for Injury

Medical Conditions	Mechanism of Increased Risk	Etiology of Increased Risk
Diabetes mellitus	Altered level of consciousness	• Hypoglycemia • Hyperglycemia
Seizures	Altered level of consciousness	• Hitting head or face • Fractured extremity • Falling into path of vehicle
Cardiovascular disease	Altered level of consciousness	• Syncope
Peripheral vascular disease	Altered sensory input	• Orthostatic hypotension • Arrhythmias • Myocardial infarction • Cerebral vascular accident • Transient ischemic attack • Neuropathies
Substance abuse	Altered level of consciousness Altered sensory input Altered thought process	• Altered judgment • Altered reflexes • Unconsciousness
Psychiatric illness	Altered thought process	• Depression • Suicidal ideation • Self-destructive behavior

Pediatric Considerations
General Considerations
1. Deterioration of the child's clinical condition may be insidious; frequent reassessment of systems is critical.
2. Children have higher metabolic rates and require greater amounts of oxygen and substrates.
3. The skeletal system of a child is immature and flexible. It provides little protection for underlying structures. Consequently, serious underlying injury may be present in the absence of fractures.
4. Children, especially young children, have immature or inadequate thermoregulation. The prevention of heat loss through the use of warmed fluids, blankets, and management of the environment is critical.

TABLE 21-5   Common Medication Classes That Increase Risk for Injury

Medication Class	Etiology of Increased Risk of Injury
Antidiabetic	• Hypoglycemia
Antiseizure	• Depressed level of consciousness
Antihypertensives	• Syncope
	• Orthostatic hypotension
Antiarrhythmics	• Hypotension
	• Bradycardia
	• Arrhythmias
Antihistamines	• Central nervous system (CNS) depression
Antineoplastics	• Anemia
Antipsychotics	• Extrapyramidal symptoms
	• Hypotension
	• Arrhythmias
Barbiturates	• CNS depression
Benzodiazepines	• CNS depression
Diuretics	• Hypovolemia
	• Hypotension
	• Electrolyte imbalances
Narcotics	• CNS depression
Thyroid hormone	• Thyroid storm

5. Children have immature immune systems. The prevention of infection through the use of strict sterile technique is important.
6. The presence of the primary caregiver is important to help the child cope with the stress of a traumatic injury.
7. When assessing the child and intervening, keep the child's developmental level in mind.

Airway and Breathing

1. Children less than 4 months of age are obligate nose breathers. Nasal passages must remain clear unless an artificial airway (e.g., an endotracheal tube [ET]) is provided.
2. The trachea is shorter and more anterior in children. Intubation may be difficult.
3. Uncuffed ET use in smaller children necessitates frequent respiratory assessments to confirm placement. Securing these tubes and frequently assessing tube position are critical. Document the centimeter mark on the ET that is at the gum line for future reference in evaluating tube position.

4. Provide high-flow oxygen (100%) via nonrebreather mask, blow-by, bag-valve device, or mechanical ventilator.

Cervical Spine

1. Children younger than 8 years should have padding placed under the back and shoulders to alleviate flexion of the cervical spine. Figure 21-1 illustrates proper spinal immobilization for children.

Circulation

1. Children compensate well for hypovolemia, and symptoms of clinical shock (especially hypotension) may be masked for a prolonged period.
2. The peripheral IV selected should be as large as possible.
   - Infant: 20 gauge to 24 gauge
   - Young child: 18 gauge to 20 gauge
   - Older child: 18 gauge or larger
3. Intraosseous fluid and drug administration is an option if peripheral access cannot be obtained (see Procedure 21).
4. Fluid volume replacement is as follows:
   - Initiate 20 ml/kg of warmed isotonic crystalloid solution by rapid IV push.
   - Reassess circulatory status, and if there is no improvement, repeat 20 ml/kg bolus of warmed isotonic crystalloid solution by IV push.
   - If a shock state persists, administer 10 ml/kg warmed packed red blood cells by IV push.
   - Reassess status and repeat blood administration as necessary.

⇛ NURSING ALERT ⇚

Hypothermia has severe detrimental effects on the pediatric trauma patient. All fluids should be warmed before administration if possible. Blood should be mixed with warm saline or given via blood warmer.

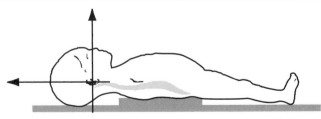

Figure 21–1 Proper spinal immobilization for children younger than 8 years. (Modified from Nypaver M and Treloar T: Pediatric spinal immobilization. *Ann Emerg Med* 23:209, 1994.)

Disability

1. When assessing mental status, keep the patient's developmental level in mind.

Geriatric Considerations
General Considerations

1. A diminished ability to compensate (loss of physiologic reserve) is a hallmark of aging.
2. Mortality is higher among the geriatric population for every body region.
3. Mortality increases with age up to 85 years.
4. Falling is the leading cause of injury in the geriatric population.
5. Geriatric patients have an increased mortality from motor vehicle crashes and burns.
6. Physiologic changes are seen in every system and vary with lifestyle and preexisting medical conditions.
7. The patient's response to medication can change with age because of altered body tissue (e.g., decreased lean body mass and increased adipose tissue), altered receptor response, altered absorption (e.g., decreased GI blood flow), or altered metabolism (e.g., decreased renal clearance).
8. The immune response is diminished. Careful attention to the prevention of infection is important.
9. Thermoregulation, especially the ability to generate heat, also is diminished. Take immediate steps to prevent hypothermia. If possible, continuously monitor the core temperature.
10. Medication use may further reduce the ability to compensate and may mask clinical signs of shock (e.g., beta-blockers blunt the tachycardic response to hypotension). Medication use also may affect the success of interventions.
11. Traditional norms that are used to guide resuscitation must be adjusted for the geriatric population. A high index of suspicion should be maintained, even with minor injuries, because of the effect of aging on physiologic reserve and the reduced ability to mount the response needed to recover from injury.

Airway and Breathing

1. There is a generalized reduction in pulmonary function.
2. Preexisting diseases (e.g., chronic obstructive pulmonary disease) may have a significant effect on compensatory mechanisms for poor oxygenation or perfusion.

Cervical Spine

1. Arthritic changes may complicate assessment and immobilization.
2. Composition changes (e.g., osteoporosis) increase the likelihood of injury.

Circulation

1. If arteriosclerosis or peripheral vascular disease is present, higher arterial pressures (hypertension) may be necessary to perfuse organs and extremities. BP may be "normal" even though patient is in a state of inadequate tissue perfusion.
2. Fluids should be administered with caution. Do not withhold needed volume, but frequently reassess the cardiovascular and respiratory systems. Watch closely for signs of fluid overload.
3. Many geriatric patients are candidates for early invasive monitoring, and the monitoring should be used to guide resuscitation efforts if indicated.

Deficit

Cognitive skills may be slowed or diminished with increasing age and certain degenerative diseases (e.g., Alzheimer's disease and dementia). Make an early effort to determine a baseline neurologic status from reliable sources.

Obstetric Considerations

General Considerations

1. Motor vehicle crashes are the leading cause of maternal injury.
2. Intravascular fluid volume, cardiac output, minute ventilation, and oxygen consumption increase during pregnancy.
3. Normal WBC counts may be as high as $25,000/mm^3$.
4. Normal hematocrit and hemoglobin levels are decreased.
5. Gastric emptying and peristalsis are slowed, resulting in an increased risk of aspiration.
6. Maternal concern may be focused on the well-being of the fetus. Reassurance is important.

Airway and Breathing

Increased oxygen consumption requires an increase in oxygen delivery. Administer high-flow oxygen to pregnant trauma patients.

Cervical Spine

Fully immobilize the pregnant patient.

Circulation

1. Increased plasma volume allows for maternal compensation, but harm may come to the fetus because of decreased oxygen.
2. Pregnant women may compensate for a prolonged period with only minimal clinical signs.

> ### NURSING ALERT
>
> The supine position, especially in later gestation, causes the uterus to rest on the inferior vena cava, causing diminished venous return, which in turn reduces cardiac output. The back board should be tilted (elevated about 4 to 6 inches using a towel roll under the right side of the backboard[2]) to make sure the uterus is not resting on the vena cava. An alternative is to manually displace the uterus by hand. Using either method, spinal immobilization should be maintained.

INITIAL INTERVENTIONS

When the primary and secondary assessments have been completed and all life-threatening conditions have been corrected (Tables 21-1 through 21-3), other initial interventions may be necessary.

1. *Gastric tube placement:* Gastric distension poses two potential problems for the trauma patient. First, distension pushes a full stomach upward into the diaphragm, reducing pulmonary capacity and, consequently, gas exchange. Furthermore, gastric distension increases the risk of vomiting and aspiration. Decompression of the stomach should be accomplished via a gastric tube as early in the resuscitation as possible. Evacuation of the stomach contents early also may minimize the degree of contamination in cases of direct trauma to the gastrointestinal tract.

> ### NURSING ALERT
>
> If a basilar skull fracture is suspected or if the midface is unstable, the gastric tube should be passed orally, not nasally.

2. *Urinary catheter placement:* A full bladder is uncomfortable for the patient, and it can increase anxiety, BP, and heart rate. An indwelling urinary catheter should be placed as soon as urethral injury has been ruled out.

3. *Pain relief:* Nonpharmacologic interventions such as positioning, ice, elevation, and splinting of musculoskeletal injuries should be initiated. For pain not controlled by nonpharmacologic interventions, intravenous opiates, anxiolytics, and muscle relaxants can be administered

---

⟩⟩⟩ **N U R S I N G   A L E R T** ⟨⟨⟨

Before an indwelling urinary catheter can be inserted, the meatus should be assessed for bleeding or signs of trauma. With males, assessment for a scrotal hematoma and prostate size and position must be performed before catheter placement.

---

judiciously and in small doses to achieve the desired effect. Care must be taken to avoid respiratory depression.

4. Other interventions include tetanus prophylaxis, dressing of wounds, and immobilization of any known or suspected fractures.

5. Trauma patients are under extreme stress and usually in a state of crisis. It is natural for them to mobilize usual coping mechanisms to adapt. However, normal coping mechanisms may be quickly overwhelmed by fear, pain, and loss of control. Interventions such as informing the patient of procedures before they are performed, maintaining eye contact, holding a hand, or taking time to listen can facilitate coping. Allowing a significant other to remain at or near the bedside may improve adaptation as well.

6. Significant others (e.g., family and friends) also may be experiencing feelings of anxiety, fear, anger, and guilt. Keeping them informed of the patient's condition and prognosis, and allowing visitation with the patient is critical to their coping.

7. Nursing care priorities are listed in the table on pp. 704-705.

PRIORITY DIAGNOSTIC TESTS

During the initial resuscitation of the trauma patient, priority diagnostic tests should be individualized based on the mechanism of injury and clinical findings. However, a number of laboratory tests, radiographic examinations, and special procedures may be anticipated. Tables 21-6 to 21-8 list common diagnostic tests and special procedures, their clinical indications, and clinical implications.

CLINICAL CONDITIONS

Although trauma may affect every body region and system, this chapter focuses on injuries to the abdomen, chest, and pelvis. Trauma to other regions is discussed in the appropriate chapters.

Abdominal Trauma

Unrecognized injuries to the abdomen are major factors contributing to preventable mortality and morbidity in trauma patients.

TABLE 21-6   Common Laboratory Tests

Laboratory Test	Clinical Implications
Complete blood count (CBC)	• Hematocrit and hemoglobin levels may be normal or above normal despite acute hemorrhage. • Normal values do not exclude hemorrhagic shock.
Electrolytes	• Baseline data • Rule out electrolyte imbalance.
Prothrombin time	• Baseline data
Partial thromboplastin time	• Rule out coagulopathies.
Amylase	• Baseline data • Elevated value may indicate possible intraabdominal injury (e.g., pancreatic injury).
Lipase	• Baseline data • Elevated value may indicate possible intraabdominal injury.
Lactate	• Baseline data • Elevated level correlates with acute hemorrhage, shock, and increased anaerobic metabolism.
Arterial blood gas	• Assess ventilatory and respiratory status. • Acidosis, especially in the presence of normal or decreased $Paco_2$ level, correlates with shock. • Base deficit of 6 or greater correlates with acute hemorrhage and shock. • Decreased Pao_2 and Sao_2 and an elevated $Paco_2$ may indicate an airway or breathing emergency.
Liver function tests	• Baseline data • Elevated values may indicate liver damage.
Type and crossmatch	• Prepare for administration of blood and blood products.

TABLE 21-7	Common Radiographic Examinations	
Radiographic Examination	**Indication**	**Clinical Implications**
Chest x-ray	• Chest trauma or pain • Shortness of breath	• Anteroposterior examination with patient in supine position if immobilized should be performed immediately upon arrival if possible. • Do not delay treatment of a suspected tension pneumothorax for a chest x-ray.
Pelvis x-ray	• Blunt trauma • Pelvic pain or instability • Blood at urethral meatus	• Anteroposterior examination with patient in supine position should be taken early in the resuscitation.
Cervical spine x-ray	• Blunt trauma • Trauma above nipple line • Neck tenderness • Neurologic deficit	• Cross-table lateral film usually obtained early in resuscitation • Immobilization should be maintained until the spine is radiographically and clinically cleared.
Thoracic and lumbar spine x-ray	• Blunt trauma • Back pain or trauma • Neurologic deficit	• Patient should be log rolled until spine is cleared radiographically and clinically.
Extremity x-ray examinations	• Extremity trauma, deformity, or pain	• Suspected fractures should be immobilized before radiographs.
Head CT scan	• Head trauma • Loss of consciousness • Focal neurologic findings • Altered level of consciousness	• Transfer to a definitive care facility should not be delayed to obtain a head computed tomography (CT) scan.

TABLE 21-7	Common Radiographic Examinations—cont'd	
Radiographic Examination	Indication	Clinical Implications
Abdominal CT scan	• Abdominal trauma or pain • Altered level of consciousness • Unreliable clinical examination	• Transfer to a definitive care facility should not be delayed to obtain an abdominal CT scan.
Abdominal ultrasound (FAST)	• Abdominal trauma or pain	• Interference in imaging may occur with obesity, bowel gas, and subcutaneous emphysema.

As many as 20% of patients with acute hemoperitoneum have benign abdominal findings when first examined in the ED. The peritoneal cavity is a major reservoir for significant occult blood loss.[1]

A high index of suspicion must be maintained with patients who have a suspected abdominal injury, especially when the suspected injury is related to occult vascular and retroperitoneal injuries. Serial abdominal examinations must be approached in a systematic and meticulous fashion, with thorough documentation of findings and changes in findings. The patient with peritoneal signs or signs of ongoing blood loss must be approached with

---

NURSING ALERT

The following is an outline for the approach to the abdominal evaluation. It is not essential to identify a specific type of injury, but it is most essential to determine whether an abdominal injury exists. The liver, spleen, and kidneys are the organs predominantly involved after a blunt injury. Essentially, the patient should be evaluated for blood loss after major solid-organ injury (liver, spleen, or kidney) or hollow viscous injury to the small or large bowel. The initial systematic evaluation of the abdomen using inspection, auscultation, percussion, and palpation is described under Secondary Assessment in this chapter. Refer to this section to review the initial approach to the abdominal examination.

NURSING CARE PRIORITIES

Potential/Actual Problem	Causes	Signs and Symptoms	Interventions
1. Impaired gas exchange	• Occluded or partially occluded airway • Chest injuries • Lung injuries • Hypoperfusion	• Increased heart and respiratory rate • Shallow respirations • Cyanosis • Restlessness • Hypercapnia • Hypoxia • Decreased hemoglobin/hematocrit	• Maintain a patent airway (jaw thrust, oral airway, nasopharyngeal airway, or intubation). • Provide suction for the patient as needed. • Provide high-flow oxygen by mask or bag-valve device. • Prepare to assist with tracheal intubation. • Monitor breath sounds and chest wall excursion and movement. • Prepare for chest tube insertion if indicated. • Monitor ABGs, blood lactate levels, and SpO_2 readings.
2. Altered tissue perfusion	• Hypoperfusion and shunting of blood	• Decreased or absent arterial pulses • Pale, cyanotic, or mottled skin color	• Initiate two large-bore intravenous lines for fluid resuscitation. • Administer warmed Ringer's lactate or 0.9% NaCl solution as indicated to

- Cool, clammy skin
- Decreased capillary refill time
- Decreased blood pressure
- Tachycardia
- Tachypnea
- Alteration in level of consciousness

maintain systolic BP greater than or equal to 90 mm Hg and urine output 0.5 ml/kg/hr in adults and 1 ml/kg/hr in children.[2]
- Apply direct pressure to external sources of bleeding.
- Monitor the patient for internal bleeding, abdominal rigidity, expanding hematomas, a decreasing level of consciousness, diminishing breath sounds, or dullness to chest percussion.

3. Pain

- Stimulation of nerve endings

- Complaints of pain
- Changes in blood pressure and heart rate
- Protective, guarding behavior

- Administer IM or IV opiates (morphine sulfate) or nonsteroidal antiinflammatory agents as ordered.
- Place the patient in a position of comfort after the spine is cleared.
- Use imagery and distraction to help the patient cope with pain.
- Allow the presence of persons from the patient's support system.

TABLE 21-8	Common Special Procedures	
Procedure	Indication	Clinical Implications
Angiography	• Suspected vessel injury • Cerebral blood flow study	• Be prepared to assess and intervene in the event of an anaphylactic reaction. • Insertion site must be watched closely for bleeding after procedure.
Diagnostic peritoneal lavage	• Abdominal trauma or pain, especially in a hemodynamically unstable patient	• Gastric and bladder decompression must be performed before a diagnostic peritoneal lavage is performed. • This procedure does not evaluate the retroperitoneal space.
Transesophageal echocardiogram	• Widened mediastinum • Significant chest trauma	• Patient is usually rolled on side for procedure. • Patient may be sedated during procedure.

a vigorous and aggressive attitude toward discovery of injury and appropriate management.

Diagnosis
- A definitive evaluation of abdominal injuries may be conducted in various ways, depending on the philosophy and resources of the institution. A protocol for evaluation of blunt abdominal trauma should be developed and followed for cases in the ED.

⤳ NURSING ALERT ⤳

The diaphragm rises to the fourth intercostal space during exhalation and extends to the sixth or seventh intercostal space, midclavicular line, or eighth or ninth intercostal space, midaxillary line, on inspiration. Level of the diaphragm at the time of injury must be considered, especially when evaluating penetrating thoracic or abdominal trauma, because the adjacent cavity also must be closely evaluated to determine the extent of the injury. With lower-chest injuries, the possibility of an abdominal injury must be considered, and chest injuries must be suspected in cases of upper-abdominal injuries.

- The evaluation of penetrating abdominal trauma usually is more straightforward than evaluation of blunt trauma.
- Nasogastric intubation and urinary catheterization are both diagnostic and therapeutic.
- The nasogastric tube decompresses the stomach, removes gastric contents, and reduces gastric volume and pressure, and thus reduces the risk of aspiration.
- The urinary catheter permits bladder decompression and evaluation for hematuria. The catheter also allows for the monitoring of urinary output that serves as a solid guide to the efficacy of fluid resuscitation.

➤ NURSING ALERT ➤

Inspection of the meatus and the rectal examination should be performed before insertion of the urinary catheter. Contraindications to urinary catheter placement, such as blood at the meatus, an inability to palpate the prostate, a high-riding prostate, or a boggy prostate, may be discovered during the examination.

Laboratory screening
Laboratory screening should be conducted per the abdominal evaluation protocol for your facility. Baseline studies typically include a CBC with differential, an amylase test, a urinalysis, and a urine pregnancy test. Alcohol and other drug screening generally is performed but depends on individual facility protocol and clinical relevance to the patient's care.

Diagnostic studies
For evaluation of genitourinary trauma, see Chapter 13.

The three major mechanisms for definitive abdominal evaluation are diagnostic peritoneal lavage (DPL), CT scanning of the abdomen, and the focused abdominal sonogram for trauma (FAST). The choice of method usually depends on the hemodynamic stability of the patient, the time available in which to determine the presence or absence of intraabdominal injury, and the individual facility's approach based on blunt abdominal trauma protocols.

1. *DPL:* The DPL is conducted to evaluate patients with hemodynamic instability. The DPL is considered 98% sensitive for intraperitoneal bleeding. DPL does not identify retroperitoneal bleeding. The only absolute contraindication to the DPL is an existing indication for celiotomy. Relative contraindications include morbid obesity, previous abdominal

operations, advanced cirrhosis, and preexisting coagulopathy. The DPL may be approached with an open or closed (percutaneous) technique. The choice of approach is dictated by the general philosophy of the department of surgery. See Procedure 12.

> ⯈ **NURSING ALERT** ⯇
>
> Before a DPL is performed, patients should have a nasogastric tube and urinary catheter in place. During the DPL, a catheter is inserted and initially aspirated. If gross bloody aspirate is obtained, this is an immediate indication for surgical intervention. If aspiration yields no blood, the patient should be lavaged with 1 L of warmed isotonic fluid. Lavage fluid drained from the abdomen then should be sent to the laboratory. Microscopic evaluation leading to celiotomy usually yields results of greater than 100,000 RBCs or 500 WBCs per cubic millimeter for patients with a blunt injury. A more sensitive indicator of bleeding (the presence of fewer RBCs) may be used as a surgical indicator for patients with a penetrating injury.[1,2]

---

2. *CT scan:* The CT scan is more specific but less sensitive than a DPL. Usually both IV and oral contrast media are administered to heighten the specificity of the examination. The CT scan provides information about specific organ injury and its extent and also can produce information about the pelvis and retroperitoneum. If the CT scan reveals free fluid, a DPL may be performed to evaluate the nature of the fluid. The advantages of CT scanning versus DPL must be weighed carefully to provide optimal care for the injured patient. Even patients with hemodynamic stability but with an abdominal examination indicative of peritoneal signs may be candidates for a DPL. Another consideration is the availability of resources in the facility and the time needed to marshal those resources for the patient instead of transferring the patient to an institution with a higher level of care. These decisions must be made collaboratively with the attending physician, receiving physician, and attending nurse based on the patient's condition and the facility with the available resources that best meet the needs of the patient.

> ### ➤ NURSING ALERT ➤
>
> When administering oral contrast, be cautious in the timing to allow for a long enough dwell time to ensure an adequate study. Examination of the lower thoracic or upper lumbar vertebrae via plain films may be obscured or equivocal with the contrast dye.

3. *Abdominal ultrasound:* The abdominal ultrasound recently has been gaining greater acceptance in many centers as another adjunct to the evaluation of both blunt and penetrating abdominal trauma. Ultrasonography equipment, as well as a trained operator to perform the examination, must be readily available. The abdominal ultrasound has many advantages in that it is portable and can be performed at the patient's bedside, it is noninvasive and relatively time efficient, and it is relatively inexpensive. Disadvantages include lower specificity for organ injury when compared with CT scanning, poor yield with obese patients or those who have extensive subcutaneous emphysema, and a learning curve for the equipment operator. Abdominal ultrasound can be repeated easily, mitigating some of the aforementioned weaknesses. The sensitivity of ultrasound ranges from 80% to 100%, the specificity from 89% to 100%, and the accuracy from 86% to 99%.

Chest Trauma
Of all patients admitted with a chest injury, only 15% require a thoracotomy for definitive management. Thus, 85% of patients with chest injuries can be managed with general resuscitative techniques, including ventilatory support, a tube thoracostomy, or other interventions for management of chest injuries.

Aortic Transection
Eighty-five percent of patients who have acute aortic transection die before reaching the hospital. The 15% who live to make it to the hospital usually are experiencing aortic dissection. The aorta has three layers of tissue: the intima, the media, and the adventitia. With dissection, the intimal and possibly the medial walls are torn. However, the adventitial layer is intact, resulting in a ballooning pseudoaneurysm or allowing for dissection down into the layers of the vessel. Patients with this condition are extremely fragile, and the condition must be diagnosed quickly and the patients transferred to a facility with cardiothoracic surgical services available immediately. The usual site of injury is

just distal to the subclavian artery at the ligamentum arteriosum that tethers the aorta posteriorly, creating a focal point for the dissipation of the shear forces in blunt injury.

Symptoms

- A conscious patient typically complains of intense and severe midscapular or low-back pain, possibly referred down into the pelvic area and lower extremities.
- Dyspnea, tachycardia, and anxiety often are evident.
- Pulse amplitude is usually magnified in upper extremities and diminished in lower extremities.
- Acute coarctation syndrome (e.g., hypertension in upper extremities and hypotension in lower extremities) may manifest.
- During auscultation, a harsh systolic parascapular murmur may be heard.
- Patients typically demonstrate a wide variability in hemodynamic parameters, especially BP variability.
- Patients' BPs usually vary from 40 to 60 mm Hg diastolic to 150 to 170 mm Hg systolic. Such wide swings in hemodynamic parameters may be caused by the stretching phenomenon on the baroreceptors contained within the walls of the injured aorta and should encourage consideration of aortic dissection in the differential diagnosis.

Diagnosis

- Diagnosis is based on a radiographic evaluation of the chest, specifically the mediastinum, with the following findings: a widened mediastinum, a loss of aortic knob shadow (may be hazy or obscured), deviation of the trachea to the right (if the patient is nasogastrically intubated, the nasogastric tube also will deviate to the right), a left apical pleural cap, and depressed or downward displacement of the left mainstem bronchus.
- The diagnosis of the aortic dissection traditionally has been confirmed via aortography; however, more studies are validating the role of transesophageal imaging for the detection of acute aortic dissection. A transesophageal echo circumvents the need for dye load, transportation off-site for special procedures, and arterial access. In the United States, aortography remains the gold standard for the confirmation of a diagnosis. Dynamic CT scanning also is being used in many institutions to confirm the diagnosis of aortic dissection.
- Consult your hospital's individual protocol for evaluation of an aortic injury.

Treatment
- Hypervolemia should be prevented to minimize additional wall stress on the already stressed or injured vessel.
- Intensive BP monitoring must be performed to evaluate hypotension as well as to treat hypertension as necessary, to avoid additional dissection and possible rupture of the aorta.
- Beta-blockers and other medications are given to reduce afterload, thereby minimizing vessel-wall stress and turbulent flow.
- A tube thoracostomy with autotransfusion may be performed for excessive blood loss.
- A resuscitative, open thoracotomy may be conducted to facilitate emergent surgical control of the aorta (Procedure 15).
- When the diagnosis has been confirmed, anticipate quick transport to the operating room with an armamentarium of blood products to minimize the potential for acute and excessive blood loss.

Blunt Cardiac Injury
Symptoms
- Anginal chest pain, dyspnea, hypoperfusion, and hypotension may be present.
- Symptoms vary depending on the extent of the injury.
- The patient may arrive in frank left ventricular failure with crackles on auscultation and with the presence of an S_3 heart sound and JVD.
- A 12-lead ECG may reveal conduction or rhythm disturbances.
- Premature atrial contractions, premature ventricular contractions, atrial fibrillation and flutter, ventricular tachycardia, and bundle branch block may occur. This is especially true of the right bundle branch block, because the right ventricle is situated to the right of the sternum, positioned anteriorly, leaving it virtually unprotected against a high-energy impact.

Diagnosis
- A 12-lead ECG and transthoracic or transesophageal imaging may be used for diagnosis.
- Some institutions use creatinine phosphokinase and lactate dehydrogenase with isoenzymes to evaluate blunt cardiac injury. However, these fail to detect injury with one third to one half of patients who have actual myocardial damage detected via transthoracic imaging and have been removed from most initial protocols for evaluation of blunt cardiac injury.
- Review your institutional evaluation protocol for blunt cardiac injury.

Treatment
- Evaluate and intervene during the primary assessment and evaluation of airway, breathing, and circulation (ABCs).
- Oxygen should be applied and vigilant ECG monitoring should ensue with early recognition and Treatment of arrhythmias.
- Potential pump failure with large contusional patterns may occur, and interventions should be initiated accordingly to maximize contractility (addition of inotropes, maximizing of filling pressures), reduce afterload (addition of vasodilators), and optimize preload (optimizing of volume status via volume infusion or diuresis, infusion of vasoactives).
- Central venous pressures should be monitored closely to guide volume resuscitation.
- Intensive-care unit or telemetry admission is likely and should be anticipated early during the patient's resuscitation if the initial ECG reveals a pattern consistent with blunt cardiac injury.

Cardiac Tamponade

Cardiac tamponade actually is an expression of the injury (blunt or penetrating); however, it occurs most often with the patient who experiences penetrating chest trauma. The manifestation is revealed by a rapid accumulation of blood in the pericardial sac, causing a restriction of myocardial pump motion and chamber filling. Stroke volume is reduced, and chamber pressures are noticeably increased.

Symptoms
- The patient has anxiety, dyspnea, and duskiness or cyanosis.
- The patient demonstrates Beck's triad: hypotension, muffled heart tones, and JVD. Beck's triad manifests all three facets in only 35% to 65% of cases. Hypovolemic patients will not show evidence of JVD.
- Kussmaul's sign (a paradoxical rise in venous pressure with inspiration when breathing spontaneously) may occur when the patient inspires deeply.
- A progression of JVD occurs with deep inspiration, instead of the normal flattening of the jugular vein.

Diagnosis
- Because cardiac tamponade and tension pneumothorax have similar symptoms, auscultation of breath sounds is crucial to a diagnosis.
- The patient with cardiac tamponade will have adequate, equilateral breath sounds.
- The patient with a tension pneumothorax, tension hemothorax, or tension viscerothorax will not have clear, equal breath sounds.

- Transthoracic or transesophageal imaging should be anticipated if the patient's condition is amenable to further diagnostic evaluation.
- With acute deterioration, prepare for pericardiocentesis.

Treatment

- Administer high-flow oxygen to maximize DO_2 (oxygen delivery).
- Prepare for pericardiocentesis. Have a basin available to evaluate the aspirated blood for coagulability and send a specimen to the laboratory for analysis of the hematocrit level.
- Inherent to the procedure is the possibility of the puncture of an uninjured chamber.
- Ongoing evaluation for the recurrence of tamponade or creation of an environment conducive to the development of tamponade (through puncture of an uninjured chamber) must be considered and remain in the decision tree for ongoing assessment.
- Should the patient experience acute deterioration, prepare for an open, resuscitative thoracotomy to decompress the pericardial effusion. Adequate technique and equipment is essential to the success of this procedure, and this procedure should be performed only in centers that have surgical backup readily available (Procedure 25).

Flail Chest and Multiple Rib Fractures

Symptoms

- Bony crepitus over fracture sites may be palpated, the patient experiences pain, and the concomitant tissue injury may be evident (e.g., pulmonary contusion, pneumothorax, and hemothorax).
- Paradoxical chest wall movement with inspiration or expiration is indicative of a flail segment.
- The patient also may experience acute oxygen desaturation because the contusional pattern may create a pulmonary alveolar capillary shunt.
- The concept of shunt implies adequate perfusion to nonventilated alveoli. Some degree of physiologic shunt (2% to 5%) occurs in healthy individuals; however, shunt resulting from conditions such as a pulmonary contusion, atelectasis, or right mainstem intubation may result in shunt as high as 40% to 50%. This will tremendously affect gas exchange (both onloading of oxygen to hemoglobin and offloading of CO_2 for exhalation).

Diagnosis

- A chest radiograph remains the hallmark in the diagnosis of rib fractures and flail segment (two or more adjacent rib fractures at two or more sites).

- The diagnosis of flail chest also can be a clinical diagnosis without the use of a chest radiograph.
- A clinical evaluation of chest wall movement may lead the clinician to the diagnosis of flail chest.

Treatment

- Tube thoracostomy is performed for pneumothoraces and hemothoraces.
- Intubation and positive pressure ventilation may be used for a pulmonary contusion with flail segment if respiratory failure occurs.
- Pain management is critical for these patients to maximize respiratory effort and gaseous exchange and to minimize atelectasis and pneumonia.
- Alternative methods of producing adequate pain management include IV analgesic administration, epidural anesthetic, traditional approaches to pain control, and other pain-management techniques such as imagery.
- Vigilant monitoring of oxygen saturation, respiratory effort, work of breathing, and CO_2 is critical in the ongoing evaluation of respiratory function.
- An arterial line may be placed to facilitate serial ABG measurement and intraarterial BP monitoring.

Hemothorax and Tension Hemothorax

The presence of blood in the pleural space represents a hemothorax. Each hemithorax can contain up to 2.5 L of blood. The capacity of the hemothorax makes acute or ongoing blood loss a possibility, a condition that would precipitate hemorrhagic shock.

Symptoms

- The patient exhibits dyspnea, hyperpnea, dullness on percussion, oxygen desaturation, diminished or absent breath sounds on the side of the injury, and, possibly, symptoms of a shock state if blood loss is excessive.
- In the case of a tension hemothorax, the clinical presentation is the same as for a tension pneumothorax, except that the causative agent is blood instead of air.

Diagnosis

- The condition usually is detected via a clinical examination.
- If the hemothorax is small (less than 250 ml), a chest radiograph may be necessary to definitively diagnose the hemothorax.
- An anteroposterior film may not delineate the hemothorax if it is small, and an upright chest film may be necessary to allow the blood to collect and become visible radiographically.

Treatment
- Perform a tube thoracostomy. Two large-bore intravenous lines should be in place before the procedure.
- Prepare for autotransfusion if the hemothorax is known or is suspected to be large (Procedure 8).
- Monitor chest drainage closely.
- If the patient has lost more than 1000 ml of blood initially or demonstrates an ongoing blood loss of more than 200 ml/hr for 3 to 4 hours (for children, greater than 5 ml/kg/hr), elective surgical thoracotomy may be pursued.

Pneumothorax and Tension Pneumothorax

A pneumothorax is manifested by the entry of air into the pleural space with the loss of negative pressure, causing partial or total collapse of the lung parenchyma on the affected side. A pneumothorax may progress to a tension pneumothorax if air continues to enter the pleural space with no mechanism for escape on exhalation. Pressure continues to rise within the thoracic cavity, resulting in the collapse of lung parenchyma on the affected side. Unrelieved, the pressure shifts the heart, great vessels, and trachea and eventually collapses the contralateral lung. Detection and treatment of a tension pneumothorax should be conducted within the context of the primary assessment.

▶ NURSING ALERT ◀

Particular concern should be given to the development of a pneumothorax or tension pneumothorax if the patient needs intubation and positive pressure ventilation for his or her injuries. Positive pressure ventilation can quickly convert a simple pneumothorax into a tension pneumothorax; thus a high index of suspicion must be maintained after intubation.

Symptoms
- The patient demonstrates dyspnea, tachypnea, hyperpnea, diminished or absent breath sounds ipsilaterally, and, possibly, diminished sounds bilaterally if a tension pneumothorax has progressed and is compressing contralateral lung parenchyma.
- Subcutaneous emphysema is possible with the development of a tension pneumothorax, as is tracheal deviation away from the involved hemithorax.

- JVD may occur, as may hypotension if severe compression of the thoracic mediastinal structures ensues.

Diagnosis

- A clinical diagnosis is more than adequate. A radiograph is not and should not be necessary to make a diagnosis.

Treatment

- Immediate decompression via needle or tube thoracostomy is indicated.
- Typically, a rush of air with either decompressive technique is heard or felt.
- The patient's condition and clinical appearance usually improve within minutes after the decompression of a tension pneumothorax.

NURSING ALERT

Remember: When a needle thoracostomy has been performed, a chest tube must follow to ensure adequate and ongoing, definitive chest management. The chest drainage system should be monitored closely for output and air leak (Procedure 8).

Pulmonary Contusion

Approximately 75% of patients with blunt chest trauma have some degree of underlying pulmonary contusion. Signs and symptoms of the contusion may take as long as 48 hours to manifest, allowing time for the contusion to blossom and create an environment of physiologic derangement, especially in children. A high index of suspicion is critical for evaluation and management of these patients. Initial lung hemorrhage occurs with interstitial and alveolar edema at the site of the contusion, followed by general inflammation. Ventilation and perfusion mismatching (shunt) develops, resulting in systemic hypoxia and hypercapnia.

Symptoms

- Surface ecchymosis over the chest wall may be present, as may hyperpnea (without subsequent auscultation of breath sounds that would be expected with the degree of hyperpnea).
- Diminished respiratory excursion, hemoptysis, and oxygen desaturation usually occur in cases of pulmonary contusion.

Diagnosis
- A chest radiograph initially may reveal a contusional pattern, and this may "fluff out" in 48 to 72 hours.

Treatment
- Supportive therapy is indicated as dictated by the patient's condition.
- Intubation and positive pressure ventilation may be necessary to minimize shunting.
- Pain control is essential to maximize alveolar insufflation for the patient with a pulmonary contusion.
- Vigilant monitoring of oxygen saturation is required.
- The judicious administration of IV fluids (crystalloid and colloid) to prevent the exacerbation of tissue edema should be the rule of thumb.
- Simultaneous independent lung ventilation may be considered to minimize barotrauma sustained by the "good" lung. Intubation with a double-lumen ET is necessary to achieve this.

Ruptured Bronchus and Trachea

The most common site of injury is at the distal trachea or proximal mainstem bronchus. This injury usually results from compressive or shear forces or a penetrating injury. The left mainstem bronchus is affected more often than the right mainstem bronchus. This is because the left bronchus is longer and more horizontal, predisposing it to the effects of shear force

Symptoms
- Respiratory distress, forceful coughing, subcutaneous emphysema, and hemoptysis often are present.
- With placement of a tube thoracostomy, a persistent large air leak usually is present.

Diagnosis
- Diagnosis is determined by bronchoscopy and clinical examination.

Treatment
- Begin resuscitation initially per primary assessment.
- A tube thoracostomy usually is necessary to optimize ventilation.
- Again, monitor for a persistent air leak, and troubleshoot accordingly.
- The ET cuff must be distal to the injury to maximize ventilation.
- Aggressive management and surgical intervention should be anticipated.

Ruptured Diaphragm (Hemidiaphragm)

A ruptured diaphragm usually results from a rapid deceleration injury. A ruptured diaphragm is more common on the left than

```
▲    N U R S I N G   A L E R T    ◄

In cases of laryngeal injuries, the patient often exhibits hoarseness,
dysphagia, and the inability to tolerate the supine position as a
result of a collapsing airway lumen with fracture. When the patient
assumes the supine position, the usual airway lumen collapses on
itself because of a fracture of the structure itself. Thus, when
patients are forced to lie supine, as they normally are to ensure
adequate spinal immobilization, the false lumen achieved with a
more upright position is collapsed and airway obstruction occurs.
Laryngeal injuries are exceedingly difficult to manage, and finding
a position of comfort and maintaining immobilization should be
the approach taken until management in a controlled environment
(e.g., the operating room) can be achieved.
```

the right. This may be because the liver protects the diaphragm on the right or because of the pattern of the kinetic energy dissipated with certain types of injuries. The diaphragm rupture allows herniation of the abdominal contents into the chest, compressing the lungs and possibly the mediastinum. If this condition is left untreated, a tension viscerothorax may result.

Symptoms
- The patient exhibits dyspnea, Kerr's sign (sharp, relentless left shoulder pain as a result of irritation of the phrenic nerve), and diminished breath sounds.
- Bowel sounds may be auscultated in the thoracic cavity in an extreme case with severe herniation.
- Hamman's crunch may be appreciated with mediastinal emphysema. This is a crunching sound heard best over the anterior chest wall at the apex. The crunching sound is synchronous with the cardiac cycle and can be auscultated in conditions leading to the presence of mediastinal air.

Diagnosis
- A chest radiograph may reveal the herniation.
- Nasogastric intubation with a radiopaque nasogastric tube supports the diagnosis by the tube's presence in the thoracic cavity on radiograph.
- A diagnostic peritoneal lavage also may be performed to evaluate for additional intraabdominal injury.

Treatment
- Nasogastric intubation and gastric decompression may lessen the effects of the herniation on chest structures.

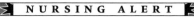

> **NURSING ALERT**
>
> A ruptured diaphragm produces a communication between the abdominal and thoracic cavities. When lavage fluid is instilled, monitor for lavage fluid drainage from the chest tube; a chest tube may need to be inserted if the fluid extravasates from the abdominal cavity to the thoracic cavity.

- Inadvertent esophageal intubation and positive pressure ventilation would be lethal because the herniated contents then would be insufflated, compounding the effects of the herniation.
- Prepare for immediate surgical intervention.

Sentinel Injuries

Some injury patterns are not particularly life threatening by themselves but should raise suspicion of other potentially life-threatening injuries. These injuries are termed "sentinel" injuries and should prompt the emergency nurse to watch for the more life-threatening associated injuries. The sentinel injuries of particular importance are outlined in the Box 21-2, Sentinel Injury and Associated Injury Pattern.

Pelvic Fractures

Pelvic fractures, especially those involving the posterior columns, can bleed vigorously, leading to exsanguination and the formation of a retroperitoneal hematoma. The hematoma can become so enlarged that it extends from the pelvis into the lower anterior abdominal wall. The DPL may be performed with an approach above the umbilicus to avoid the hematoma and prevent a false-positive finding for intraabdominal bleeding.

BOX 21-2   SENTINEL INJURY AND ASSOCIATED INJURY PATTERN

- First rib fracture: heart or great vessel injury (subclavian vein and artery), central nervous system (CNS) injury (head and neck)
- Scapula fracture: brachial plexus, pulmonary contusion, great vessel, CNS injury
- Sternal fracture: blunt cardiac injury, great vessel, pulmonary contusion
- Right lower rib fractures: liver lacerations
- Left lower rib fractures: spleen lacerations

(NOTE: Orthopedic consultation should be obtained quickly for these patients to facilitate definitive care of the pelvic fracture.)

The blood loss from the pelvic fracture should be addressed as would any blood loss precipitating a shock state. After alternative sources of blood loss have been ruled out, the pelvis should be stabilized (by external fixation, a pelvic sheet wrap [Procedure 32], or possibly a pneumatic antishock garment). This stabilization allows the retroperitoneal space to tamponade the bleeding and control ongoing blood loss.

In some instances (less than 10%), stabilization does not control blood loss from the fracture. Arteriography may be indicated to embolize ongoing arterial bleeding.

The patient's underlying renal function and physiologic condition must be considered before transport to arteriography. Management of the patient with ongoing blood loss from a pelvic fracture often requires aggressive colloid resuscitation with attention to potential coagulopathy and hypothermia.

NURSING SURVEILLANCE

The ongoing assessment of the trauma patient is a repeated primary and secondary assessment. Airway patency, adequacy of breathing and circulation, and neurologic status should be reassessed as often as needed and any time the patient's condition changes. The secondary assessment may be limited to identified injuries and known system involvement. Reassessment should be performed frequently to identify any deterioration rapidly and, consequently, to direct appropriate intervention.

EXPECTED PATIENT OUTCOMES

Expected patient outcomes vary widely from patient to patient. Generally speaking, ABCs and neurologic status should be maintained or improved. If spinal trauma is suspected or present, the preservation of function is an expected outcome. Preventing infection is important for patients with open wounds or burns. Immobilizing fractures and maintaining adequate peripheral tissue perfusion are appropriate for patients with extremity injuries.

DISCHARGE IMPLICATIONS

Trauma patients present the clinician with a unique set of challenges, both clinically and from a systems approach. Although most patients suffering from an injury are admitted to the receiving hospital, a relatively small percentage of injured patients require timely triage and transfer to a higher level of care.

Certain categories of trauma patients require transfer to a higher level of care based on the referring and receiving hospitals' capabilities. One set of guidelines for consideration of early transfer of patients has been proposed by the American College of Surgeons Committee on Trauma and is presented in Box 21-3, High-Risk Criteria for Consideration of Early Transfer.

BOX 21-3   HIGH-RISK CRITERIA FOR CONSIDERATION OF EARLY TRANSFER[2]

(These guidelines are not intended to be hospital specific.)

Central nervous system
- Head injury
- Penetrating injury or open fracture (with or without cerebrospinal fluid leak)
- Depressed skull fracture
- Glasgow Coma Scale (GCS) score of less than 14 or GCS score deterioration
- Lateralizing signs
- Spinal cord injury
- Spinal column injury or major vertebral injury

Chest
- Major chest wall injury
- Wide mediastinum or other signs suggesting great vessel injury
- Cardiac injury
- Patients who may require prolonged ventilation

Pelvis
- Unstable pelvic ring disruption
- Unstable pelvic fracture with shock or other evidence of continuing hemorrhage
- Open pelvic injury

Major extremity injuries
- Fracture or dislocation with loss of distal pulses
- Open long-bone fractures
- Extremity ischemia

Multiple-system injury
- Head injury combined with face, chest, abdominal, or pelvic injury

BOX 21-3   HIGH-RISK CRITERIA FOR CONSIDERATION OF EARLY TRANSFER[2]—cont'd

Multiple-system injury—cont'd
- Burns with associated injuries
- Multiple long-bone fractures
- Injury to more than two body regions

Comorbid factors
- Age >55 years
- Children 5 years of age or younger
- Cardiac or respiratory disease
- Insulin-dependent diabetes, morbid obesity
- Pregnancy
- Immunosuppression

Secondary deterioration (late sequelae)
- Mechanical ventilation required
- Sepsis
- Failure of single or multiple organ systems (deterioration in central nervous, cardiac, pulmonary, hepatic, renal, or coagulation systems)
- Major tissue necrosis

American College of Surgeons Committee on Trauma: Interhospital transfer. In: *Resources for optimal care of the injured patient*, Chicago, 1997, The College.

Specific issues arise with interhospital transfer to a higher level of care. Among these are the following:

1. There must be adequate communication between the referring and receiving facilities, including both written and oral communication, and between physicians and nursing personnel.
2. Interhospital transfer forms must be adequate.
3. Decisions must be made regarding transport mode (ground or air), medical evacuation, and the level of care of personnel attending the patient while in transit.
4. The patient's needs must be matched with the resources offered by the receiving facility. This "match" must be performed and the patient transferred in a timely fashion.
5. Optimal and maximal stabilization of the patient must be attained before transport, within the capabilities of the referring institution. Often physicians from the receiving

facility offer guidance in stabilization and transport procedures.

Most injured patients can be adequately treated in the initial receiving hospital. However, patients requiring a higher level of care must be promptly recognized based on the limitations and capabilities of the receiving hospital, and appropriate transfer to the appropriate higher level of care must follow.

REFERENCES

1. Emergency Nurses Association: *Trauma nursing core course*, ed 5, Des Plaines, IL, 2000, The Association.
2. American College of Surgeons Committee on Trauma: *Advanced trauma life support: course for physicians*, ed 6, Chicago, 1997, The College.
3. Cushman JG, Agarwal N, Fabian TC, et al: Practice management guidelines for the management of mild traumatic brain injury: the EAST practice management guidelines work group, *J Trauma* 51 (5):1016-1026, 2001.
4. Iacono LA: Exploring the guidelines for the management of severe head injury, *J Neurosci Nurs* 32 (1):54-60, 2000.

22 chapter

The Unresponsive Patient

Steve Talbert

INTRODUCTION

Many medical illnesses and injuries can cause an unresponsive state in a patient presenting to the emergency department (ED). Regardless of etiology, the unresponsive patient constitutes a medical emergency and should be taken immediately to an appropriate treatment area. These illnesses and injuries may include, but are not limited to, the following. For complete information, refer to the chapter associated with the condition.

- Acid–base imbalances: Conditions leading to an acid–base imbalance are either respiratory or metabolic. Regardless of the etiology, the underlying pathologic condition is an excess of either acid or base. The resulting symptoms may vary widely but usually are associated with the cardiovascular, respiratory, and neurologic systems (Chapter 17).
  - Respiratory acidosis is associated with poor gas exchange that results in hypercapnia. In contrast, respiratory alkalosis is associated with hypocapnia, usually resulting from hyperventilation.
  - Metabolic acid–base imbalances are caused by inadequate tissue perfusion (shock and lactic acidosis), renal failure, and drug ingestion.
- Alcohol intoxication (Chapter 20)
- Anaphylactic shock is a life-threatening condition caused by an antigen-antibody reaction in which chemical mediators (e.g., histamine and kinins) are released in great quantity and produce systemic effects. Tachycardia, tachypnea, respiratory distress, wheezing, hypotension, and pallor are classic symptoms.
- Cardiogenic shock has two primary types of causes: coronary causes (e.g., acute myocardial infarction [AMI]) and noncoronary causes (e.g., cardiomyopathy or valve disease). Regardless of the etiology, the underlying pathophysiology is the impaired pumping ability of the left ventricle. Poor cardiac

output and inadequate ventricular emptying are the primary characteristics of cardiogenic shock (Chapter 5).

- ○ Symptoms include hypotension, delayed capillary refill, and pale, cool, moist skin.
- ○ Other assessment findings include cyanosis and pulmonary edema.

- Electrolyte abnormalities: The symptoms associated with electrolyte imbalances are specific for the specific electrolyte involved. The neurologic, cardiovascular, respiratory, and endocrine systems are affected most often by electrolyte imbalances.

- Encephalopathy usually is associated with conditions causing hepatic or renal failure. A history of cirrhosis, liver failure, renal failure, or alcohol abuse should heighten suspicion for encephalopathy.

- Endocrine disorders: Endocrine etiologies for unresponsiveness typically involve one of the following glands: pancreas, thyroid, or adrenal (Chapter 8).

- ○ Hypothyroidism (myxedema coma) is characterized by shock, hypothermia, generalized edema, and hypoventilation and usually is seen in people over the age of 50 years.
- ○ Thyroid storm may be associated with electrolyte imbalances and hyperglycemia.
- ○ Myxedema coma can be differentiated by the presence of hyponatremia, hypoglycemia, and lactic acidosis.
- ○ Acute adrenal crisis also may be manifested by hyponatremia and hypoglycemia.

- Hypovolemic shock is a condition caused by intravascular fluid loss (internal or external). A history of traumatic injury, vomiting, or diarrhea is significant and should raise suspicion of hypovolemia.

- Hypoxia and the resultant hypoxemia can manifest themselves in a variety of ways. The underlying cause usually is related to inadequate gas exchange at the alveolar capillary membrane or to decreased minute ventilation. The diagnosis of hypoxia and hypoxemia is confirmed through arterial blood gas analysis that confirms a decreased PaO_2 and SaO_2. Other findings may include hypercapnia and acidosis (Chapter 17).

- Infection: Systemic symptoms (sepsis) include hypotension; cool, mottled, clammy skin; petechiae and purpura; and weak, thready pulses. Patients with a history of immunosuppression (e.g., AIDS or chemotherapy) and cancer patients are at increased risk for infections (Chapter 6).

- Insulin: Clinical symptoms associated with insulin shock (hypoglycemia) are hypotension, diaphoresis, tachycardia, seizures, and pale, clammy skin. Patients using insulin usually are known diabetics who have missed meals, have an acute illness, or have recently exercised (Chapter 8).

- Intracranial lesions: Symptoms include seizures, focal neurologic findings (e.g., hemiplegia), elevated mean arterial pressure, tachypnea, and bradycardia. Significant history includes hypertension, recent trauma, previous intracranial lesions, known mass, old CVA or transient ischemic attack, history of a cerebral aneurysm, sudden onset of headache, or behavioral changes. The patient may have obvious head trauma (Chapter 15).

- Overdose: Symptoms associated with overdoses vary, depending on the agents ingested. A description of the scene in which the patient was found or a recent history by family or friends often is the best clue. The patient may have a history of suicide attempts. Systems often affected by overdoses are the cardiovascular system (tachycardia or bradycardia; hypertension or hypotension), the respiratory system (tachypnea or bradypnea), and the neurologic system (abnormal pupil size or reaction, or seizures) (Chapter 20).

- Psychogenic disorders: A psychiatric history and known psychiatric medication use should raise the index of suspicion for this etiology. Other life-threatening causes for unresponsiveness must be ruled out. A history of similar behavior, depression, and mental illness increases the likelihood of a psychiatric cause (Chapter 3).

NURSING ALERT

Psychiatric patients eventually die of an organic disease or process. Life-threatening problems must be identified or ruled out first even in the presence of a psychiatric history and medication. Assessment findings vary widely from patient to patient.

- Seizure: The postictal patient may have been seen having a seizure or may have a history of seizure, thermoregulation, trauma, and uremia. Associated symptoms with seizures are tachycardia and warm, flushed, moist skin. The patient also may be hyperthermic. Incontinence of both bladder and bowel is common. Identification of certain traumatic injuries such as lacerations to the tongue, mouth, or head and abrasions or fractures in the extremities, face, or skull also may suggest a seizure etiology (Chapter 15).

- Thermoregulation can cause unresponsiveness through either extreme hyperthermia or hypothermia. Symptoms are different for each condition (Chapter 9).
  - Early hyperthermia is characterized by hot, dry skin and by hypertension. Late hyperthermia is characterized by cool skin, hypotension, arrhythmias, and seizures.
  - Hypothermia is associated with a core body temperature of less than 35° C (95° F). The skin is cool or cold to the touch. Cardiac manifestations include hypotension, arrhythmias, and weak, thready pulses. Bradypnea and dilated pupils also are common findings.

FOCUSED NURSING ASSESSMENT

The initial assessment focuses on the airway, breathing, and circulation (ABCs), a brief neurologic examination, and a critical history. It is followed by a detailed secondary assessment that focuses on the risk factors for unresponsiveness.[1-6] One can use the mnemonic "AEIOU TIPS HAT" to remember risk factors leading to unresponsiveness (Box 22-1).[1-9] One begins the secondary assessment by exposing the patient, taking measures to maintain the body temperature, and obtaining a complete set of vital signs, including a rectal temperature. The secondary assessment then should proceed with a complete head-to-toe assessment, which may reveal clues to help identify the cause of unresponsiveness.

Oxygenation and Ventilation

- Examine the airway for patency by using a modified jaw-thrust maneuver. Observe the airway for any source of potential or actual obstruction, listen for breath sounds, and feel for air movement.
- If the airway is compromised, it is essential to establish a stable, patent airway through the removal of any obstruction or the placement of an artificial airway before continuing the assessment.
- Care must be taken to protect the cervical spine if the etiology of the patient's unresponsiveness is either traumatic or unknown.
- Assessment of breathing includes the respiratory rate, depth, pattern, and work of breathing. Respiratory rates vary with age, anxiety, acid–base balance, and other physiologic and psychologic factors.

BOX 22-1   RISK FACTORS FOR UNRESPONSIVENESS

A	Alcohol
E	Electrolytes, encephalopathy, endocrine
I	Insulin, intracranial lesion
O	Overdose
U	Uremia
T	Trauma
I	Infection
P	Psychogenic
S	Seizure, shock
H	Hypoxia
A	Acidosis, alkalosis
T	Thermoregulation

- Respirations that are continuously deep or shallow may be symptoms of an underlying respiratory, metabolic, or central nervous system disorder.
- Tachypnea or bradypnea, especially when prolonged, are signs of respiratory distress and metabolic problems.
- Abnormal respiratory patterns such as Biot's respiration, Cheyne-Stokes respiration, and Kussmaul breathing are classically associated with various medical conditions (Table 22-1).
- Work of breathing or respiratory effort should be assessed. Signs of increased work of breathing include nasal flaring, retractions, and the use of accessory muscles.
- Inspect for symmetrical chest rise and fall. Unequal chest rise and fall may indicate a pneumothorax or hemothorax. Paradoxical chest wall movement suggests a flail chest segment.
- Auscultate lung sounds bilaterally. Diminished, absent, or abnormal breath sounds (e.g., wheezing, rales, or rhonchi) may indicate the presence of a pneumothorax, hemothorax, pulmonary edema, or airway constriction.

Perfusion

- Note the pulse rate and quality, skin color, temperature, moisture, and capillary refill. Palpation for the presence and quality of carotid, femoral, brachial, or radial pulses is the first step.
- A weak, thready pulse or absence of distal pulses is indicative of poor perfusion and hypotension. Other significant assessment

TABLE 22-1   Respiratory Patterns and Associated Clinical Conditions

Respiratory Pattern	Description	Associated Clinical Conditions
Biot's respiration	Fast, deep inspirations interrupted by sudden periods of apnea	Increased intracranial pressure (late sign)
Cheyne-Stokes respiration	Gradual rhythmic transition, going from hyperventilation to apnea, with the cycle continuously repeating	• Increased intracranial pressure • Encephalopathy • Overdose of narcotics, barbiturates, or hypnotics
Kussmaul breathing	Fast, deep respirations that may be labored	• Metabolic acidosis • Ketoacidosis • Renal failure

findings consistent with poor perfusion are cool and pale or mottled and clammy skin.

- As a general rule, a prolonged capillary refill time (3 seconds or more) is associated with poor perfusion. However, capillary refill time may increase with aging and hypothermia.
- If perfusion is compromised, steps should be taken to augment circulatory volume. Current recommendations are the placement of two large-bore (e.g., 18-gauge or larger) IV lines and administration of an isotonic crystalloid solution (Ringer's lactate or 0.9% NaCl). Unresponsive patients should have at least one IV line inserted during the initial assessment.

Neurologic

- Assess pupillary size and reactivity. (See Chapter 15, Figure 15-1, and Box 15-1.)
- Calculate a Glasgow Coma Scale score, which assesses best motor response, best verbal response, and best eye-opening response (Reference Guides 10 and 16).[4,5] This initial examination provides critical baseline data for later comparison.
- Table 22-2 lists some common neurologic findings and their associated clinical conditions.

TABLE 22-2 Neurologic Findings and Associated Clinical Conditions

Associated Clinical Conditions	Neurologic Finding
Dilated, nonreactive pupils, unilateral or bilateral	• Increased intracranial pressure • Overdose of barbiturates • Anticholinergic drugs (e.g., atropine sulfate)
Constricted pupils	• Overdose of narcotics • Cholinergic activity
Sluggish pupil reactivity	• Metabolic process (e.g., drug ingestion) • Structural problem (e.g., closed-head injury)
Flaccid extremities	• Spinal cord injury • Closed-head injury
Spasticity of muscles	• Seizure disorder • Electrolyte imbalance
Abnormal flexion or extension of extremities	• Closed-head injury • Increased intracranial pressure
Unilateral flaccidity or weakness	• Closed-head injury • Intracranial lesion (bleed, mass, ischemia)

Odor
- The smell of ethanol on the breath of the unresponsive patient is a good indicator that alcohol may be involved.
- A ketone odor to the breath may indicate ketoacidosis.

History
- Obtain a focused history as quickly as possible from EMS personnel, family, friends, bystanders, or medical alert devices.[2-7] Searching through pockets, wallets, purses, and bags may provide valuable information about medications, regular physicians, and preexisting medical conditions. Table 22-3 lists the questions asked during a focused history and their clinical application.
- Family, friends, or bystanders also may confirm ingestion of alcohol.
- Drugs, medications, or pill bottles at the scene could indicate ingestion and should be brought to the ED.

TABLE 22-3   Patient History and Clinical Implications

Question	Clinical Implication
Events surrounding the unresponsive episode	• If traumatic, suspect closed-head injury or shock. • If ingestion, suspect overdose and alcohol. • Note any patient complaints before unresponsiveness occurred (e.g., chest pain, nausea, and headache).
When the unresponsiveness occurred	• If after trauma, suspect closed-head injury or shock. • If after medication (e.g., insulin), suspect adverse drug reaction or overdose.
Associated symptoms	• Patient complaints such as dizziness, chest pain, shortness of breath, or headache may indicate a cardiovascular or neurologic etiology. • Symptoms such as vomiting, diarrhea, or bleeding point toward hypovolemia. • Fever may indicate an infectious process.
Regular medications	• Insulin use may lead to hypoglycemia. • Diuretics may cause hypovolemia or electrolyte imbalances. • Patients taking antihypertensive medication are prone to intracranial problems such as cerebrovascular attack (CVA) and bleeding.
Medical history	• Endocrine disorders may cause unresponsiveness. • Renal failure may cause uremia/encephalopathy. • Liver failure may cause encephalopathy. • Patients with a history of CVA, transient ischemic attack (TIA), cerebral aneurysm, or hypertension are more prone to intracranial problems. • Patients with cardiovascular disease are prone to cardiogenic shock. • Immunocompromised patients are more susceptible to infections.
Allergies	• Exposure to a known antigen may result in anaphylaxis.

LIFE SPAN ISSUES

⋙ NURSING ALERT ⋘

Regardless of the patient's age, priorities of care begin with airway, breathing, and circulation (ABCs) and reduction of the neurologic deficit. The mnemonic "AEIOU TIPS HAT" is valid for patients of all ages.

Pediatric Patients[1]

1. Intraosseous infusion may be used with children if the nurse is unable to obtain peripheral IV access.
2. Common etiologies of unresponsiveness include the following:
   - Infection
   - Trauma
   - Seizure
   - Overdose
3. Reye's syndrome also must be considered with children. Look for the following signs:
   - A history of recent viral illness (e.g., cold or flu symptoms). Reye's syndrome usually occurs during the recovery period of a viral illness and often is associated with aspirin administration during the illness. Reye's syndrome affects the liver and brain, causing cerebral edema and fat accumulation in the liver. Delayed diagnosis is associated with increased mortality.
   - Diarrhea, abnormal respiratory patterns, seizures, and hypoglycemia may be sequelae of Reye's syndrome.
   - A progression from confusion and lethargy to unresponsiveness
   - Abnormal liver enzyme studies and ammonia levels without associated jaundice
   - Abnormal posturing or respiratory arrest

Geriatric Patients[7]

1. Common etiologies of unresponsiveness include the following:
   - Trauma
   - Overdose or medication interaction
   - Infection
   - Endocrine causes
   - Acidosis or alkalosis
   - An intracranial lesion (cerebrovascular attack [CVA], subdural hematoma [SDH], mass)
   - Hypoxia

Obstetrics

1. Common causes of unresponsiveness include the following:
    - Infection (e.g., sepsis)
    - Shock (etiologies: ruptured uterus or abruptio placenta)
    - Overdose (suicide attempt or attention-seeking behavior; takes available medication [iron pills are common])
    - Seizure
    - Endocrine abnormalities
    - Trauma

INITIAL INTERVENTIONS

1. A patent airway should be established and maintained throughout the resuscitation.
2. Breathing and ventilation should be supported through the administration of 100% oxygen. If the patient is breathing adequately, a nonrebreather mask may be applied. However, if ventilation is inadequate or there are no spontaneous respirations, the patient should be ventilated via a bag-valve-mask device. Placement of an endotracheal tube should be considered for any unresponsive patient.
3. Circulation is supported through the establishment of two large-bore IV lines (14-gauge or 16-gauge for adults) with administration of warm crystalloid solution (0.9% NaCl or Ringer's lactate).
4. A neurologic deficit should be addressed through proper positioning of the patient (e.g., do not occlude venous return from the head), special precautions (e.g., padded side rails), and repeated neurologic assessments to rapidly identify any changes.
5. Unresponsive patients initially should receive 100% oxygen via an appropriate route (e.g., nonrebreather mask, bag-valve device, or ventilator) until deemed unnecessary based on the history and physical examination.
6. Reversal agents such as naloxone (Narcan) and flumazenil (Romazicon) should be administered when appropriate.
7. The universal administration of $D_{50}W$ to the unresponsive patient is not recommended. If a bedside glucose level is readily available, it should be checked before the administration of $D_{50}W$.[6]
8. In patients with alcohol toxicity or chronic alcoholics, it is common to administer thiamine, multivitamins, folic acid, and magnesium IV to reverse electrolyte imbalances and malnutrition.

9. Treatment for electrolyte disturbances focuses on correcting the imbalance through supplemental administration of the electrolyte that is lacking (e.g., potassium chloride infusion) or measures to reduce the concentration of an electrolyte (e.g., dialysis).

10. A neurosurgery or neurologic consultation should be obtained as quickly as possible if an intracranial mass or lesion is suspected.

11. Therapies specific to cardiogenic shock are directed at correcting the underlying cause and improving cardiac output. These include pharmacologic therapy to augment contractility (e.g., dobutamine) and mechanical adjuncts such as intraaortic balloon pumps or ventricular assist devices. Thrombolytic therapy and angioplasty are probable interventions if the shock is cardiogenic.

Nursing care priorities are listed in the table on pp. 735.

PRIORITY DIAGNOSTIC TESTS

As a general rule, diagnostic testing for the unresponsive patient may be described as the "safety-net" approach, which screens for a multitude of potential etiologies in the shortest possible time.[2,4,6]

Common Laboratory Diagnostic Tests

Alcohols: Alcohol toxicity is confirmed through blood sample testing. Note that the level of ethanol needed to induce unresponsiveness varies considerably.

NURSING ALERT

Chronic drinkers may have high blood alcohol levels and still be conscious.

Ammonia level: Hepatic failure allows toxins (e.g., ammonia) to build up in the blood, causing neurotoxicity that is manifested by an altered level of consciousness.

Anion gap: An elevated anion gap indicates acidosis.

Arterial blood gas (ABG): Changes in acid–base balance can result in changes in mental status.

Blood urea nitrogen (BUN)/creatinine: Renal failure allows the buildup of nitrogenous wastes, which is reflected by an increase in BUN and creatinine.

NURSING CARE PRIORITIES

Potential/Actual Problem	Causes	Signs/Symptoms	Interventions
1. Injury			• Keep the bed in a low position with side rails up. • Maintain a patent airway. • Administer high-flow oxygen. • Administer neuromuscular blocking agents and anticonvulsants per physician order.
2. Altered cerebral perfusion			• Avoid increases in intracranial pressure. • Suction only as necessary. • Elevate the head of the bed. • Avoid hip flexion. • Avoid neck flexion. • Administer IV fluids at keep-vein-open rates unless hypovolemia coexists.

Complete blood count (CBC): An increase in WBC may indicate an infectious process. Decreased hemoglobin and hematocrit is indicative of anemia.

Drug (toxicology) screen: Assists in identifying the presence of medications and the specific levels.

Electrolytes (Na, K, Cl, Ca, Mg, PO₄): Increase or decrease in electrolyte levels can cause unresponsiveness or an alteration in LOC.

Glucose: Hyperglycemia or hypoglycemia can cause altered LOC.

Hepatic enzymes: Elevated liver enzymes often manifest with changes in LOC.

Medication levels: Overdosage or undermedication can cause alterations in mental status.

Common Radiographic Tests

Cervical spine x-ray examination: To determine the presence of cervical spine fractures or abnormalities.

> **➤ NURSING ALERT ➤**
>
> All seven cervical vertebrae and the top of the first thoracic vertebrae must be visualized for the cervical spine to be cleared.

Chest x-ray examination: To identify the presence or absence of pneumonia, pneumothorax, and traumatic injury.

Computed tomography (CT) scan of head: Performed to identify structural abnormalities, such as masses, lesions, or bleeding. The exam first is performed without contrast then is performed again with contrast if needed.

Other Diagnostic Tests

Electrocardiogram (ECG): Abnormalities may be seen with acute coronary syndromes, myocardial ischemia, or electrolyte disturbances.

Lumbar puncture: Identifies the presence of an infectious process in the spinal fluid.

NURSING SURVEILLANCE

In general, ongoing surveillance of the unresponsive patient is a continuation of the primary assessment combined with the safety-net approach to diagnosis. Regardless of etiology, every unresponsive patient should have his or her ABCs and any neurologic deficit reassessed and documented on a regular basis. If a significant change is noted in the patient's condition, the primary assessment should be repeated, with any changes from the initial assessment noted.

Components of Primary Assessment

1. Airway patency and cervical spine control
2. Effectiveness of breathing and ventilation
3. Adequacy of perfusion
4. Mental status and neurologic checks
5. Exposure of all body surface areas, including extremities and back
6. Vital signs, including core body temperature

Focused Assessments

Each specific cause of unresponsiveness is associated with characteristic assessment and diagnostic findings. After an etiology has been determined, those specific parameters should be reassessed for any improvement or worsening of the patient's condition.

EXPECTED PATIENT OUTCOMES

1. The airway remains patent.
2. Breathing and ventilation are effective.
3. Circulation and perfusion are adequate.
4. Mental status improves or remains the same.
5. Known underlying causes are corrected.

DISCHARGE IMPLICATIONS

Few patients treated for unresponsiveness in the ED are discharged home from the ED. Exceptions may include patients who have had an alcohol overdose, patients with chronic seizures, hypoglycemic patients who are holding down orally ingested food, and psychiatric patients. Such patients should go to a safe environment when they leave the ED. When they are discharged, the reason for their unresponsiveness must be clearly explained to them. Timely follow-up with a primary care provider or clinic is essential.

REFERENCES

1. Ashwal S and Cranford R: The minimally conscious state in children, *Semin Pediatr Neurol* 9 (1):19-34, 2002.
2. Ferrera PC and Chan L: Initial management of the patient with altered mental status, *Am Fam Physician* 55 (5):1773-1780, 1997.

3. Kanich W, Brady WJ, Huff JS, et al: Altered mental status: evaluation and etiology in the ED, *Am J Emerg Med* 20 (7):613-617, 2002.
4. Limmer D and Monosky K: Assessment of the altered mental status patient, *Emerg Med Serv* 31 (3):54-58, 81, 2002.
5. Malik K and Hess DC: Evaluating the comatose patient: rapid neurologic assessment is key to appropriate management, *Postgrad Med* 111 (2):38-46, 49-50, 2002.
6. Sulkowski JA and Judy KD: Acute mental status changes, *AACN Clin Issues* 8 (3):319-334, 1997.
7. O'Keefe KP and Sanson TG: Elderly patients with altered mental status, *Emerg Med Clin North Am* 16 (4):701-715, 1998.
8. Sagarin MJ, Brown DF, and Nadel ES: Altered mental status in alcoholism, *J Emerg Med* 19 (3):271-274, 2000.
9. Cartlidge N: States related to or confused with coma, *J Neurol Neurosurg Psychiatr* 71 (suppl 1):i18-19, 2001.

unit four

Procedures

1 procedure

Advanced Airway Management

John W. Isfort

The ability to achieve and maintain a patent airway is essential to cerebral function and life. In most cases, basic or advanced airway management can be achieved without difficulty or complications. However, on occasions, the airway "nightmare" can occur. Therefore it is imperative to have a plan of action to minimize the risk of airway failure.[1]

TRACHEAL INTUBATION

Tracheal intubation is used for definitive airway control. It can be accomplished orally for patients of all ages either with or without chemical sedation and paralysis, or nasally for adult and adolescent patients. Certain patient situations may require modifications of the basic principles of tracheal intubation presented in this section.

Description

A tracheal tube (TT) is a clear, hollow, flexible tube with openings at each end (Figure P1-1). The proximal end has a standard 15-mm adapter that connects to ventilatory devices. The distal ends of TTs (sizes 5 to 6 or larger) have a cuff that is designed to fill the void space in the adult trachea past the vocal cords. Air is injected into the cuff by way of a pilot balloon. The amount of air in the pilot balloon is reflective of the amount of air in the cuff. The seal created by the inflated cuff does not prevent aspiration, but it does help somewhat to protect the patient in the event of aspiration. Centimeter markings on the proximal half allow quick determination of the depth of the tube in the trachea. Tracheal tubes range in size from 2 to 9 mm. The number correlates to the internal diameter of the tube.

The pediatric TT does not have a cuff. Uncuffed tracheal tubes are placed in children 8 years of age or younger. The trachea of the pediatric patient is less rigid than the adult's and narrows at

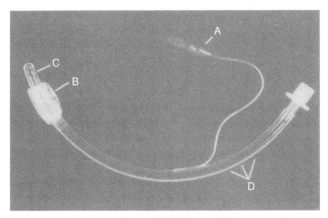

Figure P1-1 Tracheal tube. A, Pilot balloon with a one-way valve connected to the cuff by a small hollow tube. B, Cuff: low pressure, high volume. C, Murphy's eye allows air passage if the larger distal opening becomes occluded. D, Centimeter markings of tube length from distal tip. (From Dailey R, Simon B, and Young G: *The airway: emergency management,* St Louis, 1992, Mosby.)

the cricoid cartilage just past the vocal cords. This allows a "seal" to be created when a correctly sized TT is properly placed in the trachea, negating the need for a cuff. In addition to centimeter markings on the tube for depth reference, a pediatric uncuffed TT has black rings around the distal end of the tube for determining depth as the tube is placed.

Adult and pediatric tracheal intubation usually is achieved orally via direct visualization of the glottic opening and vocal cords with a laryngoscope blade and handle. The blade is either straight (Miller) or curved (MacIntosh) and varies in length, from size 0 for neonates and infants to size 4 for large adults. Laryngoscopes are battery operated and have a source of light in the distal end of the blade that facilitates visualization of the glottic opening.

Nasotracheal intubation is used in situations where direct laryngoscopy cannot be performed, such as cases of oral airway obstruction or glossal edema. Nasotracheal intubation is a "blind" intubation, as the glottic opening is not visualized during placement of the tube. The TT is passed through the nasal passage, past the pharynx and vocal cords, and into the trachea. The use of a flexible-tip TT such as the Endotrol may improve tracheal placement. The tip of an Endotrol can be flexed via a pull ring at the proximal end. The pull ring is attached to a monofilament line that runs the length of the TT through the wall and is anchored to the end, allowing for manipulation of the end of the tube.

Indications, Contraindications, and Cautions

Indications, contraindications, and cautions for orotracheal and nasotracheal intubation are listed in Table P1-1.

Equipment

- Protective eyewear, mask, and gloves
- Stethoscope
- Oxygen source
- Functioning suction equipment
- Magill forceps (foreign body removal)
- Rigid tonsillar-tip suction device
- Suction catheters properly sized for the TT being used
- Airway adjuncts and equipment
  - Bag-valve device and a properly fitting mask
  - Oral and nasal airways
- Two properly sized TTs (Table P1-2)
- 10-ml syringe for filling the TT cuff with air
- Laryngoscope handle with two differently sized blades, curved and straight
- Appropriately sized stylet
- Anesthetic (lidocaine jelly), lubricating water, and soluble topical agents
- Phenylephrine hydrochloride (Neo-Synephrine) spray for nasal intubation
- Monitors:
  - Esophageal detection device (EDD) (Figure P1-2)
  - Exhaled CO_2 detection devices (Figure P1-3)
  - Pulse oximeter
  - Cardiac monitor
- Rapid sequence intubation medications:
  - Premedication: atropine, lidocaine, fentanyl
  - Defasciculation medication: vecuronium (Norcuron), rocuronium (Zemuron)
  - Sedation (induction) agents: midazolam (Versed), etomidate (Amidate), ketamine (Ketalar), thiopental (Pentothal)
  - Neuromuscular blocking agents: succinylcholine (Anectine, Quelicin), rocuronium

TABLE P1-1   Considerations for Tracheal Intubation

	Orotracheal Intubation	Nasotracheal Intubation

Indications	• Establishment, maintenance, or protection of the airway
	• Increase in the physiologic benefits of oxygenation and ventilation
	• Intubation requiring a larger tube than one that can be advanced through the nasal passage
		1. When RSI is contraindicated or unavailable
		2. Dyspneic patients whose condition (e.g., chronic obstructive pulmonary disease, asthma, and pulmonary edema) could worsen or who cannot tolerate the supine position
		3. Oral cavity not sufficiently accessible to permit orotracheal intubation
		  • Wired jaws
		  • Anatomic problems (e.g., small mouth or temporomandibular joint ankylosis)
		  • Trismus (e.g., tetanus and intraoral infections)
		  • Actively seizing
		  • Obstructing lesions of the anterior oropharynx (e.g., tumors, Ludwig's angina, lingual swelling or hematoma, and dental abscesses)
		4. Inability to attain proper sniffing position.
		  • Decerebrate rigidity
		  • Tetanus
		  • Severe degeneration joint disease or rheumatoid arthritis of the cervical spine
		5. Comatose, breathing patients (e.g., sedative overdose, cerebrovascular attack, or head injury)

Continued

TABLE P1-1 Considerations for Tracheal Intubation—cont'd

	Orotracheal Intubation	Nasotracheal Intubation
Contraindications	There are no absolute contraindications for orotracheal intubation in patients who need definitive airway control.	1. Apnea 2. Nasal or posterior pharynx obstruction 3. Children under 10 years of age (relative to size)[2] 4. Thrombolytic therapy within 12 hours
Cautions	There are some relative contraindications in which orotracheal intubation may be difficult or could worsen or complicate an existing condition: 1. Anticipated surgical access through the mouth 2. Major maxillofacial fractures or trauma 3. Significant bleeding in the supraglottic area 4. Possible unstable cervical spine injuries 5. Epiglottitis 6. Rheumatoid arthritis or ankylosing spondylitis	1. Facial fractures 2. Basilar skull fractures 3. Cribriform plate fractures (Battle sign, raccoon's eyes, fluid from the nose or ears, and crepitus when palpating the facial bones may be indicative of the above fractures.) 4. Clenched teeth that limit access to the oral cavity for suctioning 5. Anticoagulation 6. Neck trauma with the potential for dislodging a blood clot 7. Suspected foreign body obstruction, including epiglottitis

TABLE P1-2   Proper Sizes of Endotracheal Tubes

Age	Average Weight (lb) (kg)	ET Size	Blade Size
Premature	3 (1.5)	2.5, 3.0	0
Term	7.5 (3.5)	3.5	0
6 mo	15 (7)	3.5	1
1 yr	22 (10)	4.0	1
3 yr	33 (15)	4.5	1 or 2
6 yr	44 (20)	5.5	2
8 yr	55 (25)	6.0	2
11 yr	77 (35)	6.5	2 or 3
14 yr	99 (45)	7.0	3
Adult females	120 lb (54.5) and up	7.0-8.0	3
Adult males	160 lb (72.5) and up	8.0-9.0	3 or 4

- 10-ml and 1-ml syringes for medication administration
- Rescue airways
  - Laryngeal mask airway (LMA)
  - Combitube
- Tape, cloth ties, or commercial device to secure the TT
- Surgical cricothyrotomy tray: may be needed if the patient cannot be successfully intubated or ventilated.

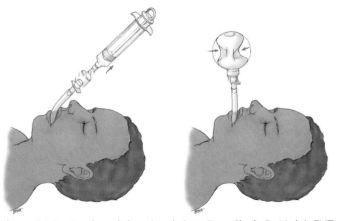

Figure P1-2   Esophageal detection devices. From Shade B: *Mosby's EMT intermediate textbook*, St Louis, 1997, Mosby.

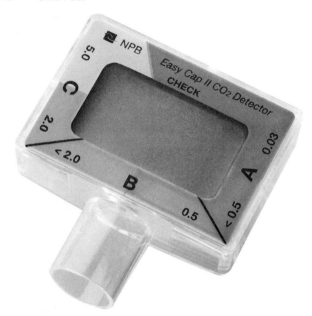

Figure P1-3 Colormetric CO_2 detector. (Courtesy Tyco Health Care.)

INITIAL NURSING ACTIONS

General Endotracheal Intubation
1. Discuss the procedure thoroughly with the conscious patient.
2. Preoxygenate the patient with 100% O_2.
3. Ensure patent IV line.
4. Ensure that proper noninvasive monitors are in place (e.g., electrocardiogram, blood pressure, pulse oximeter) and an exhaled CO_2 detection device if available.
5. Gather all the needed equipment and personnel.
6. Check the laryngoscope and blades to ensure that the batteries and light source are functional.
7. Prepare the TT while keeping the distal two thirds sterile.
   - Check the patency of the TT cuff.
   - Lubricate the stylet with xylocaine jelly or another water-soluble lubricant to allow for easy removal. For the oral intubation procedure, insert a malleable stylet into the TT, making sure that it does not extend past Murphy's eye or the distal end of the tube. When the stylet is in the appropriate

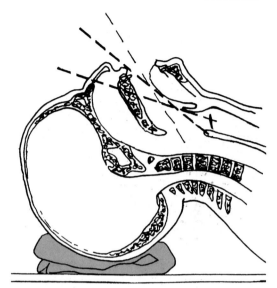

Figure P1-4 Intubating or "sniffing" position. Note approximation of three critical axes. (From Dailey R, Simon B, and Young G: *The airway: emergency management,* St Louis, 1992, Mosby.)

position, the top of the stylet usually is bent over the top of the 15-mm adapter to make sure it does not inadvertently advance and cause injury to the patient during the procedure. Bend the TT and stylet to create a gentle curve in the tube with a sharp upward turn of the distal 2 to 3 inches at approximately a 30-degree angle.

- Lubricate the cuff and distal aspect of the TT with xylocaine jelly or another water-soluble lubricant.

8. Ensure that standard precautions are being maintained (protective eye wear, mask, and gloves).

9. Place the patient in the proper position; this is very important.
   - Sniffing position with head resting on a folded towel. Obese patients may need padding under the shoulders to facilitate the sniffing position (Figure P1-4).
   - Infants may need a towel under the shoulders to compensate for the large occiput when positioning for a neutral sniffing position. Do not hyperextend an infant's neck.
   - If there is a possibility of a cervical spine injury, the patient is kept in neutral alignment with manual stabilization.

10. When the TT is in place, inflate the cuff with a 10-ml syringe. Place only enough air in the cuff to stop exhaled air from leaking around the cuff.
11. If tracheal intubation cannot be achieved within 30 seconds, stop the procedure. Reoxygenate and ventilate the patient for 15 to 30 seconds, monitoring oxygen saturation, and then reattempt intubation.[3]
12. Confirm tracheal placement of the tube.

⚔ NURSING ALERT ⚔

No one method of evaluating placement of the tracheal tube is 100% accurate. Confirmation of tracheal tube placement should consist of multiple confirmation techniques.

- Visualization of the TT passing through the vocal cords
- Auscultate over the epigastrium with the first ventilated breath. Gurgling or burping sounds are suggestive of esophageal placement of the tube. Breath sounds may be faintly heard over the epigastrium, but they should be less audible than those heard over the anterior chest. It is possible for coarse basilar rales to mimic air bubbling in the stomach.
- Note equal, bilateral rise and fall of the chest.
- Auscultate breath sounds over the anterior and lateral aspect of the chest. Breath sounds should be present and equal bilaterally.
- Note fogging of the TT.
- Aspirate air using an esophageal detection device (EDD) (Figure P1-2). If the tube is in the esophagus, there will be very little if any air to aspirate.
- Detection of exhaled CO_2 by a CO_2 detector (e.g., Colormetric) (Figure P1-3) or a measurable reading of CO_2 on a continuous end-tidal CO_2 monitor. Results of this technique will be unreliable in the patient without a perfusing rhythm as pulmonary blood flow stops and the level of CO_2 will be so small it will be undetectable.[3]
- Improved signs of oxygenation and ventilation:
  - Improved skin color, capillary refill, heart rate
  - Improved pulse oximeter readings (this may take several minutes)
- Note lung compliance when ventilating the patient. Is the patient easy to ventilate? If the TT is in the esophagus, the patient will become difficult to ventilate as the stomach fills with air.

> ### NURSING ALERT
>
> **When in doubt, pull it out.** If tracheal placement of the tube is at all questionable after the above confirmation checks, the tube should be removed and the patient reoxygenated before reintubation is attempted.

13. Note the centimeter marking at the teeth/gums or the naris and document. In the average adult, this will be 19 to 23 cm orally and approximately 26 to 28 cm nasally. In children, the depth orally will depend on the size of the child (see Reference Guide 18).
14. Secure the TT, making sure it cannot be moved by activity such as suctioning, ventilating, and patient movement. Have someone secure the TT by hand until the tube has been secured.
    - Secure the TT in place with adhesive tape.
      - Clean and dry the surface of the face.
      - Apply Mastisol or other adhesive to the skin surface of both cheeks beside the mouth.
      - Wrap the middle portion of a 6-inch strip of 1-inch cloth tape around the TT at the level of the teeth, and secure the ends to the previously prepared skin surface.
    - Follow the manufacturer's directions for commercially prepared TT holders.
15. Insert a gastric tube, and attach it to suction to evacuate and deflate the stomach.
16. Continue to ventilate and oxygenate the patient; place the patient on a ventilator.

Orotracheal Intubation

1. Visualize the glottic opening and vocal cords (Figure P1-5)
   - With the left hand, insert the blade of the laryngoscope into the right side of the mouth and sweep the tongue to the left.
   - Advance the tip of the blade:
     - The straight blade is placed under the epiglottis to lift it up.
     - The curved blade is advanced into the vallecula to lift the epiglottis.
   - Lift the lower jaw with the laryngoscope and displace it up and forward at a 30-degree to 45-degree angle.
     - Keep the blade off and away from the teeth.
     - Do not pull back on the handle; instead, push it forward and up with a lifting motion. Displace the mandible up and away from the patient.

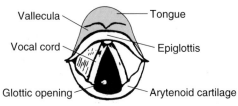

Figure P1-5   Anatomic structures seen during direct laryngoscopy.

- ○ Use **B**ackward, **U**pward, **R**ightward **P**ressure (BURP) to manipulate the thyroid cartilage and increase visualization of the glottic aperture.
2. With the right hand, insert the TT into the mouth and through the glottic opening and vocal cords. An assistant can retract the right side of the mouth to widen the area to pass the tube under direct visualization.
   - Advance the TT until the cuff completely disappears through the vocal cords or one or more of the black rings on the distal end of the pediatric uncuffed TT passes through the vocal cords.
   - Grasp the TT at the level of the lips with the left hand after setting down the laryngoscope, and carefully pull out the stylet.
3. Inflate the cuff as described under Initial Nursing Actions.
4. Confirm tracheal placement of the TT and secure as described in Initial Nursing Actions.

Nasotracheal Intubation
1. Prepare the naris and nasal passage with phenylephrine (for vasoconstriction) and with 2% xylocaine jelly. A nasal pharyngeal airway may be placed and then removed to spread the topical anesthetic agent evenly.
2. Generously lubricate the distal end of the TT with a water-soluble lubricant or 2% xylocaine jelly.
3. Gently introduce the distal end of the TT into the naris, parallel to the floor of the nasal cavity (90-degree angle to the face), with the bevel facing toward the septum. Advance it along the floor of the nasal passage into the posterior oropharynx. A slight, gentle twisting motion may help. If passage on one side cannot be achieved, try the opposite side. A slightly smaller tube (0.5 to 1 mm smaller) may be needed for nasotracheal intubation.

4. Advance the TT until it reaches the glottis. This usually stimulates a cough in patients with an intact cough reflex.

5. Advance the TT to the glottic opening. Listen with your ear at the distal end of the TT tube for breath sounds. Condensation should appear on the tube. Application of cricoid cartilage pressure (Sellick's maneuver) may move the glottic opening to a more posterior position, facilitating placement of the tracheal tube.

6. During patient inhalation, gently but quickly advance the TT 5 to 6 cm through the glottic opening.

7. Confirm tube placement as described under Initial Nursing Actions.

8. Note the depth of the tube at the naris. Secure the TT with a commercial holding device or adhesive tape, making sure that the tube cannot be moved by activity such as suctioning and ventilating.

Rapid Sequence Intubation

Rapid sequence intubation (RSI) is an orotracheal intubation procedure facilitated by administration of an IV sedative (induction) agent and short-acting neuromuscular blocking agents (NMBA) (paralytic). The specific drugs selected for RSI are tailored to fit the patient and the situation. The goal is to achieve orotracheal intubation rapidly after airway reflexes are lost. RSI increases the chance of successful intubation on the first attempt because of complete muscle paralysis and absence of breathing and the gag reflex. It has become the "gold standard" for airway control in the emergency setting. RSI has six stages: preparation, preoxygenation, pretreatment, paralysis, placement, and postintubation management.[4] These stages are described in Table P1-3. See Figure P1-6 for an example of an RSI medication algorithm.

⋙ NURSING ALERT ⋘

The use of RSI to facilitate endotracheal intubation is not without risk. Patients who cannot be successfully intubated must be ventilated by bag-valve-mask device with 100% oxygen until the paralysis resolves. **The ability to produce a good seal on the face with the mask is of paramount importance for effective ventilation. This should be determined before an RSI protocol is initiated.** Preparations for a surgical cricothyrotomy should be made in case tracheal intubation is unsuccessful.

TABLE P1-3   Steps for Rapid Sequence Intubation

Preparation	• Prepare the patient, gather necessary items, formulate a plan. • Explain the procedure to the patient if possible. Assess the patient for difficulty of intubation and bag-mask ventilation. • Ensure adequate intravenous access. • Test suction. • Load the tracheal tube with a lubricated stylet, and test the cuff. • Initiate preoxygenation. • Assemble all necessary equipment. • Calculate medication dosages and draw up drugs. • Establish cardiac and blood pressure monitoring. • Initiate pulse oximetry. • Establish a backup plan in case of an unsuccessful intubation.
Preoxygenation	Apply 100% oxygen by nonrebreather mask for 5 minutes of normal tidal volume breathing. • This crucial step replaces the nitrogen reserve in the lungs with oxygen and allows for at least 3 minutes of apnea without significant desaturation in a reasonably healthy adult. This step allows the administration of a sedative and succinylcholine to a spontaneously breathing patient, allowing paralysis and unconsciousness to ensue, then intubation without interposed mechanical ventilation. • If time does not permit 5 minutes of preoxygenation, approximately 80% of the effect can be achieved through the administration of 100% oxygen for 8 vital capacity breaths (largest breaths that the patient can take).
Pretreatment	Pretreatment medications are administered to counteract some of the physiologic effects of the procedure. LOAD is a useful tool when determining the need for pretreatment medication[6]:

Lidocaine: 1.5 mg/kg IV for patients with an increased ICP or reactive airway disease (status asthmaticus and asthmatic patients). Onset of effect occurs 2-3 minutes after administration.

- May blunt the increase in ICP that occurs in response to intubation, which would be beneficial in patients with a proven or presumed elevation in intracranial pressure.
- Helps to prevent bronchospasm and laryngospasm in patients with reactive airway disease and to suppress the cough reflex.

Opioid (fentanyl): 3 ncg/kg for patient with an increased ICP; ischemic heart disease, intracranial aneurysm, vascular dissection.

- Reduces the sympathetic response (heart rate, blood pressure) to intubation, which may be beneficial in patients with the above conditions.

Atropine: 0.02 mg/kg for children <10 years old and for repeat doses of succinylcholine in adults.

- In all children less than 10 years of age, administer atropine to prevent the bradycardia induced by succinylcholine in this age-group.
- Redosing of adults with succinylcholine is known to produce bradycardia and, although rare, asystole.

Defasciculation: vecuronium 0.01 mg/kg or rocuronium 0.06 mg/kg for patients >5 years old (or 20 kg) who will be receiving succinylcholine and have a proven or presumed increased ICP or have an open globe injury/increased ocular pressure.

- Fasciculations (fine chaotic contractions) occur with administration of succinylcholine, which may increase ICP, intragastric pressure, and intraocular pressure. A defasciculating dose of a nondepolarizing NMBA limits the effect of the fasciculations. This step often is omitted if the airway procedure is being performed on an emergency basis.
- Reducing the intragastric pressure helps to prevent regurgitation.

Continued

TABLE P1-3   Steps for Rapid Sequence Intubation—cont'd

NOTE: Nondepolarizing agents such as vecuronium and rocuronium do not produce fasciculations, so administration of a defasciculating dose is not necessary if either of these two drugs is used for paralysis.

Paralysis

Approximately 2 minutes after the administration of the last pretreatment drug, administer a sedative agent (etomidate or midazolam) followed quickly by succinylcholine or rocuronium.

- The choice of sedative agents is highly individual and might include etomidate 0.3 mg/kg or midazolam 0.1 to 0.3 mg/kg IV. In general, only a single sedative agent should be used, and the agent should be administered rapidly.
- Immediately after the sedative administration, as the patient begins to lose consciousness, have an assistant apply cricoid pressure (Sellick's maneuver), which is firm posterior displacement of the cricoid cartilage. Sellick's maneuver occludes the esophagus and helps to prevent passive regurgitation. Sellick's maneuver should be performed until placement of the tracheal tube has been confirmed.

NOTE: If active regurgitation should occur, release cricoid pressure. Maintaining cricoid cartilage pressure during active regurgitation could increase intragastric pressure and cause esophageal rupture. After the appropriate dose of a neuromuscular blocking agent has been administered, active regurgitation is no longer possible.

- Administer succinylcholine 1.5 to 2 mg/kg IV. This potent, depolarizing neuromuscular blocking agent induces intubation-level paralysis universally in 45 to 60 seconds. Administer rocuronium 1 mg/kg if succinylcholine is contraindicated.
- Do not ventilate the lungs during this brief phase of paralysis unless the patient was severely hypoxic before the intubation sequence was begun or the SPO$_2$ reading is <90% and the benefits of oxygenation are believed to outweigh the risks of aspiration.

Placement	• Position the patient for intubation. Approximately 45 seconds after administration of the succinylcholine, check the mandible for flaccidity and proceed with intubation.
	• After the tube has been placed, confirm tracheal placement using multiple confirmation techniques. When tracheal placement has been confirmed, release the Sellick's maneuver and secure the tube.
	• If the intubation attempt is unsuccessful, continue with the Sellick's maneuver, and ventilate and oxygenate the lungs with a bag and mask for 30 to 60 seconds before undertaking a second attempt.
	• If neither intubation nor ventilation can be successfully achieved, placement of a rescue airway device (LMA or Combitube) or a surgical airway or needle cricothyrotomy should be performed.
Postintubation	• Obtain a chest radiograph.
	• Administer long-acting neuromuscular blocking agents (e.g., pancuronium, vecuronium) and sedatives (e.g., benzodiazepines) to facilitate ongoing therapy if necessary.
	• Initiate mechanical ventilation.

From Walls RM: Rapid sequence intubation. In Walls RM, ed: *Manual of emergency airway management*, ed 2, Philadelphia, 2004, Lippincott Williams & Wilkins; and Walls RM: Airway. In Marx JA, Hockberger RS, and Walls RM, eds: *Rosen's emergency medicine: concepts and clinical practice*, ed 5, St Louis, 2002, Mosby.
Warning: Do not use a paralyzing agent if you cannot bag-mask ventilate a patient and are not prepared to surgically manage the patient's airway!

**University of Kentucky
Emergency Transport Services
Rapid Sequence Intubation (RSI)
Medication Administration Algorithm**

Time (Minutes)	Medication or Action
−5.00	**Preoxygenate and prepare medications**
−3.00	**Lidocaine** (1-1.5 mg/kg)
−2.00	**Atropine** (0.02 mg/kg if patient <10 y/o) or if administering repeat dose of succinylcholine in adults and pediatrics **Vecuronium** (0.01 mg/kg) *Or* **Rocuronium** (0.06 mg/kg)
−1.50	**Etomidate** (0.3 mg/kg) *Or* **Midazolam** (0.1-0.3 mg/kg Sellick's maneuver (until ETT is placed)
−1.00	**Succinylcholine** (1.5-2 mg/kg for adults) (2 mg/kg for pediatrics) *Or* **Rocuronium** (1 mg/kg)
−0.00	Insert endotracheal tube, confirm placement (visually, breath sounds, $ETco_2$, EDD), secure tube with commercial device

Courtesy of the University of Kentucky Air Medical Service

Figure P1-6 RSI medication algorithm. (Courtesy of the University of Kentucky Air Medical Services.)

>≥ **NURSING ALERT** ⩾<

Succinylcholine is the NMBA used most often because of its rapid onset and short duration. However, succinylcholine administration has been associated with severe hyperkalemia when given in certain patient conditions within certain time frames. The hyperkalemia can be severe enough to produce death. Succinylcholine should not be given to patients in the following circumstances[4,5]:

- Burns over 10% of the body surface area (BSA) from 48 hours to 6 months after burn or before complete healing of the burn.
- Spinal cord injury from 3 days to 6 months after paralysis
- Denervation syndrome until inactive for 6 months (multiple sclerosis)
- Crush injuries for 3 days to 6 months after crush injury
- Abdominal sepsis for longer than 3 days
- Stroke patient or a patient with a spinal cord injury from 3 days to 6 months after injury
- Patients known or suspected to have significant hyperkalemia (renal patient who has missed dialysis or a patient in acute renal failure)
- History or family history of malignant hyperthermia

>≥ **NURSING ALERT** ⩾<

Hyperkalemic arrest secondary to succinylcholine administration consists of:

- *Calcium chloride 10%:* adult: 5-ml IV bolus of a 10% solution over 5 minutes. Child: 0.2 to 0.3 ml/kg of a 10% solution over 5 to 10 minutes.
- *Sodium bicarbonate:* adults and children: 1 to 2 mEq/kg IV bolus
- *Insulin and glucose:* adult: 5 to 10 units regular insulin IV bolus with 100 ml D_{50}. Child: 0.5 to 1 g/kg dextrose as D_{25} or D_{10} followed by 1 unit of regular insulin for every 4 g of dextrose given.
- *Kayexalate retention enema:* adult: 15 to 60 g. Child: 1 g/kg.
- Hemodialysis

RESCUE AIRWAYS (LARYNGEAL MASK AIRWAY AND COMBITUBE)

When tracheal intubation is unsuccessful and the patient is in a "can't intubate, can't ventilate" condition, one must have an alternative plan for achieving oxygenation and ventilation.[3-5,7-11,13] Two of the rescue airway devices used most often are the laryngeal mask airway (LMA) and the Combitube. In the emergency setting, these two devices are temporary measures until a definitive airway can be obtained.[1,10]

Laryngeal Mask Airway (LMA)

The LMA (from the Laryngeal Mask Company) consists of an inflatable silicone mask and rubber connecting tube (Figure P1-7, *A*). It is inserted blindly into the pharynx, and when it is inflated, it forms a low-pressure seal around the laryngeal inlet, permitting gentle positive-pressure ventilation. It is for use in the unconscious patient without a gag reflex. The LMA is not a replacement for endotracheal intubation.[8,10,12]

Indications

1. For temporary use in the difficult-airway situation when tracheal intubation is not possible
2. For airway control during routine and emergency anesthetic procedures
3. As an alternative to the use of a face mask with bag-valve-mask ventilations

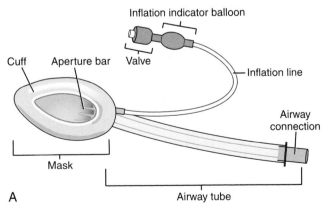

A

Figure P1-7 **A,** Laryngeal mask airway.

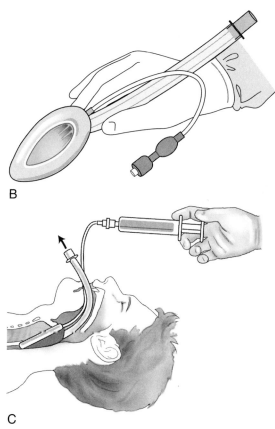

B

C

Figure P1-7 cont'd B, Method for holding the LMA. C, Correct placement of a laryngeal mask airway.

Contraindications/Cautions

1. The LMA should not be placed in a patient with an intact gag reflex. Patients should be significantly obtunded before the LMA is inserted.
2. Use with caution if it is unknown whether the stomach is empty and in patients with conditions that cause delayed gastric emptying. The LMA does not protect from aspiration.[9,11-13] In the "can't intubate, can't ventilate" scenario, the use of the LMA must be evaluated against the inability to oxygenate and ventilate and the risk of aspiration.

3. In situations in which the patient requires high peak airway pressures for effective ventilation, the inflated mask may not support the increased pressure needed to ventilate the patient.
4. The LMA is not effective if there is a laryngeal airway obstruction.

Nursing Actions

1. Preoxygenate the patient with 100% oxygen.
2. Select the appropriate size (Table P1-4).
3. Check cuff patency, then remove air completely; maximum deflation will facilitate correct placement.
4. Lubricate the posterior portion of the cuff with only water-soluble lubricant.
5. Hold the LMA like a pen at the junction of the cuff and the tube (Figure P1-7, *B*).
6. Insert the LMA into the oral cavity with the mask opening facing toward the tongue and the black line oriented toward the upper lip. Press the tip of the cuff against the hard palate (visualize to confirm tip placement).
7. Using the index finger as a guide, advance the tube into the hypopharynx until resistance is felt. Do not use force. The tip of the cuff should be pressed against the upper esophageal sphincter. The black line should be oriented toward the upper lip.
8. Inflate the cuff with enough air to obtain a seal. (See Table P1-4 for maximum volumes.)
9. As the cuff is inflated, the tube may adjust its position slightly as it settles into the correct position (Figure P1-7, *C*).
10. Ventilate the patient and assess placement:
    - Ventilate the patient with slow controlled breaths to prevent the leaking of air around the cuff.
    - No cuff should be visible in the oral cavity.
    - A slight swelling will be seen in the neck around the thyroid and cricoid areas.
    - The chest will rise and fall with ventilations.
    - Bilateral breath sounds will be present.
    - Confirm acceptable oxygen saturation.
11. The LMA cuff will not prevent aspiration. Suction the oropharynx as necessary
12. Prepare for definitive airway control.

Combitube

The Combitube (Kendall Co.) is a double-lumen tube through which the patient can be ventilated whether the tube enters the

TABLE P1-4	Laryngeal Mask Airway Size Approximation	
Weight	Size	Maximum Inflation Volume
Up to 5 kg	Size 1	Up to 4 ml
5-10 kg	Size 1½	Up to 7 ml
10-20 kg	Size 2	Up to 10 ml
20-30 kg	Size 2½	Up to 14 ml
30-50 kg	Size 3	Up to 20 ml
50-70 kg	Size 4	Up to 30 ml
70-100 kg	Size 5	Up to 40 ml
Over 100 kg	Size 6	Up to 50 ml

April, 2004. The Laryngeal Mask Company Limited. Reprinted with permission from LMA North America, Inc.

esophagus (most likely) or the trachea. The shorter lumen (clear tube) resembles a tracheal tube and has a distal opening. The longer lumen (blue tube) is occluded at the end and has holes situated in the pharyngeal area between the occluded end and the large cuff. The tube has two cuffs, a larger distal cuff that will occlude the oropharynx and permit ventilations should the tube enter the esophagus (Figure P8-1, A) and a smaller distal cuff that will occlude the trachea and permit ventilations should tracheal placement occur (Figure P1-8, B). Insertion of the Combitube is a blind procedure. The Combitube is used in people greater than 5 feet tall. The Combitube SA (small adult) is used for people between 4 feet and 5 feet tall. There are no pediatric sizes.

Indications

- Emergency airway situation in which endotracheal intubation and ventilation is not possible

Contraindications and Cautions

- The Combitube is contraindicated in a patient with an intact gag reflex and in people less than 4 feet tall.
- The Combitube is not effective in patients with a glottic or subglottic airway obstruction (laryngeal spasm, edema, tumors, foreign bodies) or epiglottitis.[13]
- Use cautiously in patients with known esophageal disease or inhalation burns, or those who have ingested a caustic substance. In the "can't intubate, can't ventilate" scenario, the use of the Combitube must be evaluated against the inability to oxygenate and ventilate.

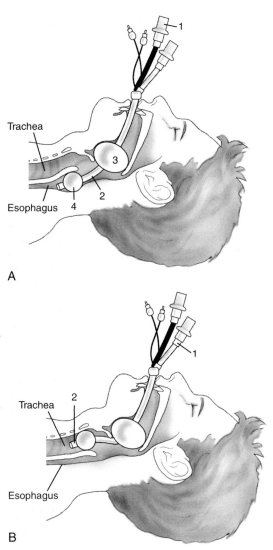

Figure P1-8 **A,** Combitube: For esophageal placement: (1) the blue port connects with fenestrations to indirectly ventilate the lungs; (2) ventilations through the blue port exit the Combitube through fenestrations just above the trachea; (3) the large latex cuff seals the pharynx and prevents ventilations from exiting; (4) small cuff at the distal end. **B,** Combitube: For tracheal placement: (1) the clear port connects with the distal lumen and provides direct ventilation; (2) the distal end of the Combitube has an opening. (Blanda M, Gallo UE: Emergency airway management, *Emerg Med Clin North Am* 21(1):1-26, 2003.)

Nursing Actions

1. Select appropriate size (see Table P1-5).
2. Test the cuffs for leaks, and completely deflate the cuffs.
3. Lubricate the tube with a water-soluble lubricant.
4. Position the patient with the head in a neutral position. The anterior portion of a cervical collar must be removed while in-line cervical stabilization is manually maintained.[13]
5. Insert the thumb of your left hand into the patient's mouth and grasp the tongue and jaw; pull forward.
6. Insert the Combitube midline along the tongue until the incisors (or gums) rest between the two black rings. If resistance is met, withdraw the tube, reposition, and reattempt. Do not force the tube.
7. Inflate the larger proximal cuff (oropharyngeal cuff) with air by way of the blue pilot balloon marked with a number 1. Inflate the smaller distal cuff (tracheal cuff) with air by way of the white pilot balloon marked with a number 2. For air amounts see Table P1-5. The tube may move slightly as the balloon seats itself on the oropharynx.
8. Determine esophageal versus tracheal tube placement. Most tubes are placed in the esophagus; in this case the esophageal (blue) port is ventilated first. Using a bag-valve device, ventilate through the blue tube (tallest) and observe for chest rise and fall. With chest rise and fall, continue to ventilate through the blue tube and evaluate breath sounds bilaterally over the midaxillary lines and the epigastrium and test with an exhaled CO_2 detector or EDD[13] (Figure P1-8, *A*). If no chest movement is noted, ventilate through the clear tube (tracheal placement) (Figure P1-8, *B*). Observe for chest rise and fall and assess breath sounds bilaterally over the midaxillary lines

TABLE P1-5	**Combitube Sizes**		
Height of Patient	**Tube Size**	**Large Cuff (Blue Pilot)**	**Small Cuff (White Pilot)**
4 to 5 feet	37 French	85 ml of air	5-12 ml of air
5 feet or taller	41 French	100 ml of air	5-15 ml of air

From Rich JM, Mason AM, Bey TA, et al: The critical airway, rescue ventilation, and the Combitube: part 1, *AANA J* 72 (1):17-27, 2004.

and the epigastrium, and test with an exhaled CO_2 detector or EDD.[13] The tube is secured by the large pharyngeal cuff, eliminating the need for additional fixation.[13]

9. An inability to ventilate through either tube may indicate the Combitube has been inserted too deeply. Deflate the cuffs and pull the tube out 2 to 3 cm. Reinflate the cuffs, and attempt ventilations again via the blue tube.[10,11]

10. Monitor pulse oximetry.

11. Replace the cervical collar when oxygenation and ventilation have been established.

12. With the tube in the esophageal position, the unused tracheal lumen can be used to suction out gastric fluid and small particles if necessary.[14]

13. Prepare for definitive airway.

PATIENT CARE MANAGEMENT

1. Potential complications from tracheal intubation include:
   - Oral trauma to the lips, tongue, teeth, and oral mucosa
   - Laryngeal trauma to the epiglottis, vocal cords, and tissues surrounding the glottic opening
   - Tracheal trauma
   - Epistaxis during nasal intubation
   - Vomiting and aspiration
   - Bradycardia from vagal stimulation, particularly in the pediatric population

2. Assess and reassess the patient's ventilation, oxygenation, and perfusion status. Evaluate for cyanosis, dyspnea, tachycardia, anxiety, agitation, restlessness, decreasing oxygen saturation, or hypotension.
   - Pneumothorax: diminished breath sounds on the affected side, may have unilateral chest wall rise and fall, pain.
   - Tension pneumothorax: diminished or absent breath sounds on the affected side, unilateral chest rise and fall, jugular vein distension, hyperresonance on the affected side, and tracheal deviation away from the affected side (late sign), pain.
   - Dislodgment of the TT from the trachea:
     - TT migration into the esophagus (most common)
       - Causes increasing difficulty in providing the appropriate tidal volume
       - Stomach expansion
       - Decreased breath sounds bilaterally or absent breath sounds if the patient has no spontaneous effort
       - The patient may be able to talk or make noises.

- ○ TT migration into the oropharynx:
  - ◆ The patient may be able to talk or make noises.
  - ◆ Air will be heard escaping with ventilations.
  - ◆ The TT depth will have changes from the initial centimeter markings.
- ○ Inadvertent advancement of the TT into the right mainstem bronchus:
  - ◆ Diminished or absent breath sounds on the left side
  - ◆ Unilateral chest wall rise and fall with ventilations
- ○ Occluded TT: inability to ventilate, no breath sounds bilaterally, inability to pass a suction catheter
- ○ Air leaks around the TT associated with a ruptured or leaking TT cuff: inability to provide an adequate tidal volume, deflated pilot balloon that will not reinflate adequately when air is added, ventilating the patient causes air to escape from the mouth with bubbling of secretions.
- ○ A pediatric TT tube that is too small to provide an adequate seal: inability to provide an adequate tidal volume, air leaking from the mouth, bubbling of secretions in the mouth.
- ○ Oxygen source that is not functioning correctly
- ○ Ventilator malfunction
- ○ Airway needs suctioning.

3. Suction the oropharynx and TT as needed. The cuffs do not seal well enough to completely protect the patient from aspiration. Suctioning of the oropharynx is still required.

4. Be prepared to implement the alternative airway management plan should intubation efforts be unsuccessful.
   - Continue to ventilate the patient with 100% oxygen. Ensure proper bag-mask technique: two hands using E/C clamp technique to make an effective mask seal. The use of an oral airway and two nasal airways will facilitate effective ventilations.
   - Consider "rescue" airway device (LMA or Combitube).
   - Prepare and set up for surgical cricothyrotomy.

REFERENCES

1. Levitan RM: Patient safety in emergency airway management and rapid sequence intubation: metaphorical lessons from skydiving, Ann Emerg Med 42 (1):81-88, 2003.
2. Luten RC and Goodwin SA: Pediatric airway techniques. In Walls RM, ed: *Manual of emergency airway management*, ed 2, Philadelphia, 2004, Lippincott Williams & Wilkins, pp 228-235.

3. American Heart Association: *Textbook of advanced cardiac life support,* Dallas, 2000, the association.

4. Walls RM: Airway. In Marx JA, Hockberger RS, and Walls RM, eds: *Rosen's emergency medicine concepts and clinical practice,* ed 5, St Louis, 2002, Mosby, pp 2-21.

5. Schneideer RE and Caro DA: Neuromuscular blocking agents. In Walls RM, ed: *Manual of emergency airway management,* ed 2, Philadelphia, 2004, Lippincott Williams & Wilkins, pp 200-211.

6. Thompson Micromedex Healthcare Series, vol 120, Succinylcholine, 0.4 treatment overview, Greenwood Village, CO, 2004, July, 2004, www.micromedex.com.

7. Butler KH and Clyne B: Management of the difficult airway: alternative airway techniques and adjuncts, *Emerg Med Clin North Am* 21 (2): 259-289, 2003.

8. Murphy MF and Walls RM: Identification of the difficult and failed airway. In Walls RM, ed: *Manual of emergency airway management,* ed 2, Philadelphia, 2004, Lippincott Williams & Wilkins, pp 70-81.

9. Davis DP, Valentine C, Ochs M, et al: The Combitube as a salvage airway device for paramedic rapid sequence intubation, *Ann Emerg Med* 42 (5):697-704, 2003.

10. Blanda M and Gallo UE: Emergency airway management. In Peth HA, ed: *Emerg Med Clin North Am* 21 (1):1-26, 2003.

11. Idris AH and Gabrielle A: Advances in airway management. In Thakur RK, ed: *Emerg Med Clin North Am* 20 (4):843-857, 2002.

12. The Laryngeal Mask Company: *Laryngeal (LMA) mask airway*, San Diego, November, 2001, the company.

13. Rich JM, Mason AM, Bey TA, et al: The critical airway, rescue ventilation, and the Combitube: part 1, *AANA J* 72 (1):17-27, 2004.

14. Rich JM, Mason AM, Bey TA, et al: The critical airway, rescue ventilation, and the Combitube: part 2, *AANA J* 2 (2):115-124, 2004.

procedure 2

Airway Suctioning

Patty Ann Sturt
Jeff Sotski

DESCRIPTION

Nasotracheal, endotracheal, and tracheostomy tube suctioning
serves as a mechanism for removing secretions from the trachea.
Removing accumulated secretions helps to maintain a patent
airway, maximize oxygenation, and prevent clinical deterioration
secondary to hypoxia.

INDICATIONS

1. Nasotracheal:
   - To clear secretions from the pharynx and trachea in
     nonintubated patients with a:
     - Weak or ineffective cough
     - Decreased level of consciousness
   - To stimulate a cough reflex to mobilize secretions to larger
     airways
   - To obtain a sputum specimen for laboratory analysis
2. Endotracheal/tracheostomy
   - To maintain patency of the endotracheal or
     tracheostomy tube
   - To clear secretions from the trachea
   - To stimulate a deep cough for the purpose of mobilizing
     secretions to the larger airways
   - To obtain a sputum specimen for laboratory analysis

CONTRAINDICATIONS/CAUTIONS

1. Hypoxia may occur or become pronounced during airway
   suctioning.
2. Never force the suction catheter through an obstructed naris.
   An obstruction may result from a deviated septum, a nasal
   polyp, or enlarged turbinates.
3. Relative contraindications for nasotracheal suctioning include
   patients:
   - With recent upper airway surgery

- With increased intracranial pressure
- With a significant coagulopathy or bleeding disorder
4. Do not perform nasotracheal suctioning in patients with severe facial and/or head trauma.

EQUIPMENT

1. Portable or wall suction unit with regulator
2. Suction canister
3. Suction connector tubing
4. Appropriate-size sterile suction catheter with intermittent suction port or a closed catheter suction device for endotracheal tube suction. For nasotracheal suctioning, choose a catheter that is no more than one half the internal diameter of the naris.
   - Adult: 12 to 14 French
   - School-age: 8 to 10 French
   - Small child: 6 to 8 French
   - Infant: 5 to 6 French
5. Sterile gloves
6. Sterile saline solution

NOTE: Commercially prepared suction kits with saline, gloves, and catheters are available.

7. Sputum trap if specimen to be collected

INITIAL NURSING ACTIONS

1. Preoxygenate the patient with high-flow oxygen for 2 minutes before suctioning.
2. Assemble suction canister and attach to portable or wall suction source.
3. Attach suction tubing to canister.
4. Set suction regulator gauge between 80 and 100 mm Hg.
5. Elevate head of bed to 45 degrees for nasotracheal suction. The head should be midline and placed in "sniffing position." Assess the nares to identify any obstruction or narrowing. Choose the most open naris.
6. Open catheter package, maintaining sterility of catheter.
7. If performing nasotracheal suctioning, apply small amount of water-soluble lubricant onto the sterile field from opened catheter package.
8. Don sterile gloves.
9. Maintain sterility of catheter by keeping catheter in dominant hand. The dominant hand must remain sterile. Use the nondominant, or "clean hand," to connect the suction tubing to the end of the catheter.

10. Lubricate catheter:
    - Use water-soluble lubricant for nasotracheal suction catheter. Excessive lubricant can occlude the catheter.
    - Use sterile saline for endotracheal tube or tracheostomy tube suction catheter.

➤ N U R S I N G   A L E R T ◄

Instillation of saline should not be routinely performed as part of the suctioning procedure. It is not effective in thinning or loosening secretions.[1,2]

---

11. Remove oxygen-delivery device with nondominant hand.
12. Encourage patient to take deep, slow breaths. Insert catheter without suction applied. Advance catheter during inspiration.
    - Nasotracheal: Introduce the catheter into the naris parallel to the floor of the nasal cavity (at a 90-degree angle to the face). Advance along the floor of the nasal passage into the posterior oropharynx. Advance the catheter to the glottic opening, which will make the patient cough. As the patient inhales, advance the catheter through the glottic opening to a total depth of approximately 20 cm for adults, 14 to 20 cm for older children, and 8 to 14 cm for younger children.
    - Endotracheal or tracheostomy tube suction: Gently insert catheter until resistance is met or patient coughs.
13. Withdraw suction catheter over 10 to 15 seconds while intermittently applying suction and rolling the catheter between the thumb and the index finger.
14. Assess the need to repeat the suctioning procedure. If another pass with the suction catheter is necessary, reoxygenate the patient before repeating the procedure.
15. Replace oxygen-delivery device with the prescribed amount of oxygen.

➤ N U R S I N G   A L E R T ◄

If the patient is being suctioned nasotracheally and another pass is necessary, the suction catheter can be withdrawn only as far as the posterior pharynx. If the patient tolerates the catheter in this position, allow the patient to recover and then suction again. This will avoid additional trauma to the nasal mucosa.

PATIENT CARE MANAGEMENT

1. Monitor the patient's color, heart rate, and oxygen saturation during and after suctioning.
2. Monitor the oxygen saturation and discontinue suctioning if the O_2 saturation decreases below 90%, or 5% below baseline value.[3]
3. Monitor the heart rate for variability. Discontinue the procedure if the heart rate increases by 40 beats per minute or decreases by 20 beats per minute.[3]
4. Assess lung sounds.
5. Monitor for arrhythmias.
6. Assess for changes in mental status, which could be indicative of hypoxia.

REFERENCES

1. Ridling DA, Martin LD, and Bratton SL: Endotracheal suctioning with or without instillation of isotonic sodium chloride solution in critically ill children, *Am J Crit Care* 12 (3):212-220, 2003.
2. Ackerman MH and Mick DJ: Instillation of normal saline before suctioning in patients with pulmonary infections: a prospective randomized controlled trial, *Am J Crit Care* 7:261-266, 1998.
3. Perry A and Potter P: *Clinical nursing skills and techniques*, ed 5, St Louis, 2002, Mosby.

procedure 3

Arterial Blood Gas Sampling

Mary Rose Bauer

DESCRIPTION

Arterial blood gas specimens (ABGs) are obtained by direct aspiration of blood from an artery. Although this procedure may be performed through aspiration of blood from an indwelling arterial line, this procedure focuses on percutaneous arterial puncture.

INDICATIONS

ABGs are useful:
- To evaluate oxygenation, ventilation, and perfusion.
- To evaluate acid–base balance.
- To document a baseline for future reference.
- To evaluate the effectiveness of interventions.

CONTRAINDICATIONS

The risk versus benefit of ABGs should be considered in the presence of the following:
- Previous surgery or injury at the intended puncture site
- Ongoing anticoagulant therapy
- History of a blood dyscrasia
- Altered skin integrity or infection at the intended puncture site
- A decrease in collateral circulation
- Fibrinolytic therapy within 24 hours

EQUIPMENT

- Antiseptic swab
- Alcohol swab
- 2 × 2 gauze pads
- Gloves
- Heparinized syringe (usually available in a prepackaged kit): 1 ml for pediatrics, 3 ml for adults
- 25-gauge, ⅝-inch needle

- 20-gauge to 22-gauge, $1\frac{1}{2}$-inch needle (for deeper arteries)
- Butterfly catheter for pediatric patients
- Adhesive tape
- Specimen label
- Container of ice

NURSING ACTIONS

1. Explain the procedure to the patient.
2. Select the arterial puncture site. Any accessible artery may be used; however, the radial, brachial, and femoral arteries are used most often. Hospital policy may dictate sites from which arterial samples may be taken (see Table P3-1). One should consider the following factors when choosing an arterial puncture site:
   - The site must be easily accessible.
   - The pulse must be easily palpable.
   - The artery must be easily compressible.
   - In children, the brachial artery may be easier to palpate.

   In the absence of palpable peripheral pulses, the femoral artery is the recommended site for an arterial puncture. One may estimate the location of the femoral artery by drawing an imaginary line between the anterosuperior iliac spine and the symphysis pubis. The midpoint of that line over

TABLE P3-1   **Recommendations for Arterial Site Selection**

Site	Considerations
Radial artery	• Safest site • Most accessible • Site not adjacent to large veins • Usually has adequate collateral circulation
Brachial artery	• More difficult to palpate and stabilize • Has less collateral circulation • Increased risk for venous puncture • Should be used when radial artery cannot be accessed
Femoral artery	• Requires more specialized training to access • No adequate collateral flow if obstructed • Located directly adjacent to the femoral vein • May be considered in emergency situations

the inguinal area should be the femoral artery. The puncture should be made distal to the inguinal ligament. Before selecting the radial artery as the puncture site, the Allen test should be performed to evaluate collateral circulation to the hand (see Figure P3-1). Ask the patient to make a fist, and compress the patient's ulnar and radial arteries with your fingers. After a few seconds, ask the patient to open his or her hand. The hand should appear pale and blanched. Release the ulnar artery and observe the palm or hand for flushing. Rapid flushing indicates good collateral circulation through the ulnar artery. If the hand remains blanched, collateral circulation may be compromised and another site should be selected. If the patient is unable to make a fist (e.g., if the patient is unconscious), tightly close the patient's hand manually until blanching occurs.[1] Note that the necessity of performing the Allen's test is somewhat controversial. Practice should be dictated by your institution's policy.[2,3]

3. Cleanse the area with an antiseptic swab. Allow the area to dry.

4. Wipe the area with an alcohol swab. Povidone-iodine leaves a sticky residue on the skin and may interfere with subtle finger movements.

5. Palpate the pulse with the middle and index finger or the index finger only of the nondominant hand. You may then perform an arterial puncture by inserting the needle between the two fingers or by inserting the needle just distal to the index finger.

6. The angle of insertion varies depending on the site selected. For a radial artery puncture, the syringe should be held at a 45-degree angle with the bevel of the needle turned upward. A brachial artery puncture may be performed at a 45-degree to 60-degree angle. A femoral artery puncture should be performed at a 90-degree angle.

7. Slowly insert the needle over the point of maximal pulsation. Observe closely for the appearance of blood within the needle hub. Arterial pressure should be sufficient to fill the syringe without manual aspiration. However, with patients who have decreased peripheral perfusion or hypotension, gentle aspiration may be necessary. The amount of blood required for ABG analysis may vary among institutions; 0.5 to 1 ml usually is sufficient.

8. During insertion, the needle may inadvertently puncture both sides of the artery, resulting in a small flash of blood into the

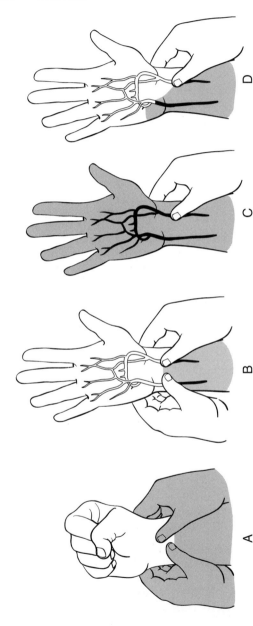

Figure P3-1 Allen's test. **A,** Elevate the hand above the level of the heart and have the patient make a fist. Compress the radial and ulnar arteries. **B,** Ask the patient open the fist. The hand should be pale and blanced. **C,** Release the ulnar artery. Rapid flushing indicates good collateral circulation, **D,** The hand will remain blanced with inadequate circulation. (From May JL: *Emergency medical procedures,* New York, 1984, John Wiley & Sons.)

needle hub but no further flow into the syringe. If this occurs, slowly withdraw the needle until blood return is noted. If no blood return occurs and the pulse remains palpable, withdraw the needle until the bevel is almost visible and redirect it toward the point of maximal pulsation.

9. Loss of arterial pulsation during puncture attempts may indicate arterial spasm or formation of a hematoma. If this occurs, withdraw the needle, apply manual pressure for 5 to 10 minutes, and select another site.

10. After the arterial blood sample has been obtained, withdraw the needle and apply manual pressure for 5 to 10 minutes.

11. Follow the manufacturer's directions and institutional policy regarding needle safety. Remove air bubbles from the specimen and cap the syringe as soon as possible. One can remove air from the specimen by holding the syringe upright, tapping the sides of the syringe to direct air bubbles upward, and expelling the air by gently pushing upward on the plunger.

12. Apply a dressing to the site.

13. Label the specimen. Be sure to include the patient's temperature and the type and concentration of supplemental oxygen.

14. Place the specimen in a sealed container and then place the container on ice. Zip-locking bags work well. Place one bag inside another. Put the labeled specimen in the inner bag and seal it. Pour ice into the outer bag around the specimen and seal it. Pushing the specimen into a prefilled ice container may result in inadvertent expulsion of the syringe contents.

PATIENT CARE MANAGEMENT

1. Assess the puncture site for bleeding after manual pressure is released.

2. If the patient is alert and oriented, instruct him or her to notify you if bloody drainage is noted on or around the dressing or if visible bruising occurs around the puncture site.

3. Assess the site for bleeding and hematoma formation every 15 minutes for approximately 1 hour.

4. Assess the circulatory status distal to the puncture site by evaluating skin color and temperature, capillary refill, and distal pulses.

5. Document the arterial puncture site on the nursing record.

> ### ⇒ NURSING ALERT ⇐
>
> All arterial puncture sites require manual pressure for a **minimum** of 5 minutes. Larger, higher-pressure arteries such as the femoral artery may require 10 minutes of manual pressure to establish hemostasis. Clotting times vary depending on the presence of preexisting diseases that alter clotting factors, medical and surgical interventions that deplete clotting factors, the reduction of clotting factors resulting from hemorrhage and multiple blood transfusions, and the use of anticoagulants. The duration of application of manual pressure should be increased accordingly. Patients receiving IV fibrinolytics require the application of manual pressure followed by a pressure dressing.

> ### ⇒ NURSING ALERT ⇐
>
> To improve the accuracy of blood gas results, wait 30 minutes after suctioning or ventilator changes.

REFERENCES

1. Perry AG and Potter PA: *Clinical nursing skills*, St Louis, 2002, Mosby.
2. Durbin CG: Radial arterial lines and sticks: what are the risks? *Respir Care* 46 (3), 2001.
3. Lanni HA and Smith SG: Allen's test: fact or myth? *Respir Care* 46 (3), 2001.

procedure 4

Arterial Line Insertion and Monitoring

Theresa M. Glessner

DESCRIPTION

Indwelling arterial pressure lines are cannulas inserted into peripheral arteries. These lines allow continuous monitoring of the patient's pulse and blood pressure and frequent arterial blood draws.

INDICATIONS

1. Continuous hemodynamic monitoring and frequent assessment of arterial blood gases
2. Significant respiratory compromise
3. Diabetic ketoacidosis
4. Shock
5. Acute respiratory distress syndrome
6. Titration of vasopressor agents
7. Determination of the mean arterial pressure and cerebral perfusion pressure in patients with a ventricular catheter device

EQUIPMENT

- 500-ml IV bag of normal saline (flush solution)
- Pressure bag
- 20-gauge, $1\frac{1}{2}$-inch or 2-inch angiocatheter
- Antiseptic solution
- Tincture of benzoin
- 2-0 silk sutures
- Lidocaine 1%, 10-ml vial
- Needles (25-gauge for skin and 18-gauge for withdrawing solution from vials) and syringes of different sizes
- Sterile towels
- Sterile scissors
- Sterile needle holder
- Sterile gauze

- Sterile gown
- Sterile gloves
- Male Luer-Lok cap
- Pressure tubing with flush device, transducer, stopcock, and extension set
- Central or deep-line dressing kit, or bio-occlusive dressing
- Armboard
- Monitor with hemodynamic capabilities
- Transducer cable

INITIAL NURSING ACTIONS

1. Explain the procedure to the patient.
2. Gather equipment.
3. Determine from the physician which site is to be cannulated. Preferred sites of cannulation are the radial, femoral, dorsalis pedis, and axillary arteries. The radial artery usually is used because it usually has good collateral circulation and is easily accessible. If the radial artery is to be used, perform Allen's test (Procedure 3).
4. Position the extremity properly. Expose the ventral surface of the forearm, dorsiflex the wrist, and place a rolled washcloth under the dorsal surface of the wrist. The hand can be taped to an armboard or other firm surface to maintain this position.
5. Prepare a flush solution with normal saline. A heparinized solution may be used, as determined by institutional policy and procedure. If used, heparin 1 to 4 units per milliliter may be added to the 250-ml or 500-ml bag of normal saline. The flush solution should be mixed according to hospital protocol.
6. Attach the flush solution to the pressure tubing. If the tubing is not fully assembled, connect the transducer to the pressure tubing proximal to the flush device. Attach a stopcock to the end of the pressure tubing and add a pressure extension set.
7. Place the flush solution into the pressure bag and hang the bag on an IV pole.
8. Clear all air from the pressure tubing and transducer by opening the roller clamp and activating the flush device according to the manufacturer's directions.
9. Inflate the pressure bag to 300 mm Hg and clamp the pressure bag to maintain the pressure.
10. Connect the transducer to the transducer cable. Attach the cable to the monitor.

11. Place the transducer at the level of the catheter tip.[1,2]
12. Turn the stopcock off to the patient side. Open the transducer to air and zero the system. The exact mechanism used to zero the system depends on the manufacturer. When the system is zeroed, close it to air. Zeroing the system negates other pressure influences.
13. When the physician has cannulated the artery, firmly attach the pressure tubing to the catheter.
14. Activate the flush device to clear the line and catheter of any blood.
15. After the catheter is sutured in place by the physician, clean the site with antiseptic solution. Apply benzoin around the area. Place sterile gauze or bio-occlusive dressing over the site. Tape the gauze and the pressure setup securely to the patient's arm.

PATIENT CARE MANAGEMENT

1. For accidental dislodgment of the catheter, apply pressure to the site for 10 to 15 minutes.
2. Monitor the color, temperature, sensation, and movement of the area distal to the catheter. Complications include hematoma formation, intraluminal clotting, arterial spasm, thrombosis, and nerve injury. Report all complications to the appropriate physician because limb loss can result from long-standing ischemic problems.
3. Withdraw blood for arterial blood gas analysis and other laboratory tests as ordered by the physician and based on the patient's clinical condition.
   - Attach a 5-ml syringe to the stopcock port closest to the catheter.
   - Turn the stopcock off to the monitor and on to the patient. For an adult-size patient, withdraw 3 to 5 ml of blood to clear the line of flush solution and blood. Turn the stopcock off to the port and discard the syringe.
   - Coagulation studies usually are drawn last to ensure a nonheparinized specimen.
   - Attach another syringe to obtain needed blood specimens. Use a heparinized syringe to obtain blood for an ABG. Turn the stopcock off to the monitor and on to the patient. Withdraw the necessary blood. Turn the stopcock off to the port. Remove the syringe.
   - Flush the line to the patient. Turn the stopcock off to the patient and flush the access port. Turn the stopcock on to

the patient and monitor. Recap the stopcock port with a Luer-Lok cap.

4. Dampening of the waveform often is caused by air in the tubing or transducer, by clot formation, or by a kink in the catheter.
5. The transducer should be zeroed every 4 to 8 hours and each time the patient is repositioned.
6. Change the arterial line site dressing every 48 hours or per hospital protocol.

REFERENCES

1. Lynn-McHale DJ and Preuss T: Pulmonary artery catheter insertion (assist) and pressure monitoring. In Lynn-McHale DJ and Carlson KK, eds: *2001 AACN procedure manual for critical care*, ed 4, Philadelphia, 2001, WB Saunders, pp 439-456.
2. Rossoll LW: Arterial line insertion and monitoring. In Proehl J, ed: *Emergency nursing procedures*, ed 3, Philadelphia, 2004, WB Saunders, pp 413-421.

procedure 5

Burn Dressing

Julia Fultz

DESCRIPTION

There are two types of burn dressings, open and closed.

- Open dressings are used on areas that are hard to dress, such as the head, neck, and perineum. An antibacterial agent is applied to the wound, and the wound is not covered. In some cases, a layer of fine mesh gauze may be applied to the wound.
- With closed dressings, an antibacterial agent or a nonstick layer of gauze is placed over the wound, and the wound is covered with a bulky dressing. Closed dressings are used most often on patients treated on an outpatient basis, ambulatory patients, those who must work specifically with their hands, children, and patients with burns in areas that will be covered by clothing.

INDICATIONS

1. Provide an optimal environment for healing
2. Help prevent infection
3. Protect the wound from further damage
4. Absorb exudate
5. Assist in debridement of burned tissue
6. Protect uninjured skin from excretions and secretions
7. Reduce pain from air currents passing over the wound in the initial stages of healing
8. Reduce evaporative heat loss

CONTRAINDICATIONS/CAUTIONS

Patients who are being transferred to a burn facility within 24 hours of injury do not need their wounds debrided or covered with antibacterial agents. Wounds can be gently cleaned with a mild soap, then covered with a clean sheet or a nonstick dressing to prevent pain from air currents passing over the wound. If the transfer will not take place within 24 hours of the injury, contact the receiving facility for directions regarding wound care.[1] Any antibacterial agents applied will have to be fully removed for evaluation of the burn wound on arrival at the receiving facility, at considerable discomfort to the patient.

EQUIPMENT

- Pain medication
- Personal protective equipment
  - Sterile gloves, hats, masks, gowns, and eye protection
- Wound-cleaning equipment
  - Sterile saline solution (warmed to body temperature)
  - Sterile basin
  - Mild soap or antiseptic solution
  - 35-ml syringe attached to an 18-gauge IV catheter (needle removed) for irrigation
  - Soft sterile surgical brush
  - Sterile, curved scissors
  - Sterile forceps
- Antibacterial agent (see Table P5-1)
- Sterile tongue blades
- Appropriate dressing material
  - Temporary wound covering such as Biobrane or Omiderm
  - Nonadherent porous mesh gauze
  - Sterile 4 × 4 gauze sponges
- Securing material
  - Semielastic coarse mesh gauze such as Kerlix
  - Tubular net-type bandage
- Good light source

NURSING ACTIONS

1. Administer pain medication before the procedure, allowing enough time for effective analgesia.
2. Wear sterile hats, gowns, masks, and eye protection during irrigation of the burn (to prevent splash back into eyes); and sterile gloves before initiation of care.
3. Fill a sterile basin with warmed sterile saline. Using the 35-ml syringe and the 18-gauge catheter, irrigate the burn to remove gross debris.
4. Gently cleanse the burned area with mild soap or antiseptic solution and thoroughly rinse with warmed sterile saline. Gentle use of a soft surgical brush also may be beneficial in cleaning the wound. Hair immediately around the wound may need to be shaved.
5. If permitted by your institution's nursing policies and procedures, remove any loose, nonviable skin, debris, and

TABLE P5-1   Topical Burn Injury Antibacterial Agents

Drug	Dose/Route	Considerations
Mafenide acetate (Sulfamylon): excellent antibacterial activity against a broad range of microorganisms. Good eschar and cartilage penetration.	Spread topically over burned area using a gloved hand or a tongue blade twice daily.	• Used on deep partial-thickness and full-thickness burns • Causes considerable pain on application to sensate burn wounds. • Hyperchloremic metabolic acidosis is frequent when used on extensive burns. Moderate to severe hyperventilation occurs to compensate. • Rash is a rare side effect. • Do not use if patient is allergic to sulfa drugs.
Petroleum-based or mineral-based (Bacitracin, Polysporin, Neosporin): effective against gram-positive and limited gram-negative organisms; limited eschar penetration.	Spread thin layer topically; reapply as needed.	• Used on superficial burn wounds, facial burns, superficial partial-thickness wounds. • Nonpainful when applied
Silver nitrate 0.5% solution: effective against most strains of *Staphylococcus* and *Pseudomonas*; many gram-negative aerobes that commonly colonize burn wound.	Dressings are saturated with silver nitrate and rewet every 2 hours.	• Stains everything it touches brown or black. Wound evaluation difficult because of discoloration. • Monitor for hyponatremia, hypokalemia, hypochloremia, and hypomagnesemia (leached from the wound).

Continued

TABLE PS-1   Topical Burn Injury Antibacterial Agents—cont'd

Drug	Dose/Route	Considerations
Concentrations above 5% are histotoxic. Poor eschar penetration.		• Methemoglobinemia is possible. • Painless upon application • Not effective on established infections • Do not allow to dry; may cause a hyperpyrexia.
Silver sulfadiazine (Silvadene): broad antimicrobial activity. Prophylactic agent used most often in burn patients. Poor eschar penetration.	Spread topically over burned area using a gloved hand or a tongue blade twice daily.	• Used on deep partial-thickness and full-thickness burns. • Painless to apply • Penetrates eschar poorly. • Transient leukopenia occurs; spontaneous resolution within a few days. • Hemolysis in patient with glucose-6-phosphate dehydrogenase (G-6-PD) deficiency. • If renal function impaired, do not apply to more than 20% of body surface area. • Rash is a rare side effect. • Do not use if patient is allergic to sulfa drugs. • Do not use if patient is pregnant or nursing, and on infants under 2 months of age.

From Kagan RJ and Smith SC: Evaluation and treatment of thermal injuries, *Dermatol Nurs* 12 (5):334-349, 2000. Hartford CE: Care of outpatient burns. In Herndon DN, ed: *Total burn care*, Philadelphia, 2002, Saunders; and Heggers JP, Hawkins H, Edgar P, et al: Treatment of infection in burns. In Herndon DN, ed: *Total burn care*, Philadelphia, 2002, Saunders.

blisters (broken, tense, or infected) if appropriate, using sterile forceps and scissors. If you are not permitted to debride tissue, request that the physician perform the debridement. Blister care is controversial[2] (see Chapter 4). The physician responsible for the patient will determine care.

6. Cotton-tipped applicators dipped in sterile saline can be used to gently remove loose skin from the lips and from around the eyes, ears, and nose. Do not vigorously debride the eyelids because the skin is very thin. Cotton-tipped applicators should be used only on the outer ear, and never in the ear canal.

7. Dress the wound. There are many opinions about the appropriate dressing for burn wounds. The physician in charge and/or hospital policy will dictate what dressing will be used. Some methods of dressing burn wounds follow. Dressings often are not applied to the face, head, neck, and perineum because of difficulty securing them. If the patient or caregiver will have to change dressing at home, explain each step as it is performed.

    a. Antibiotic ointments such as Neosporin, Polysporin, and Bacitracin usually are applied to small or superficial wounds. Deep partial-thickness and third-degree burns usually are covered with an antibacterial burn cream such as silver sulfadiazine, mafenide acetate, or silver nitrate.[3] If ordered, apply antibacterial cream using a sterile tongue blade or a sterile gloved hand. (If using a jar of antibacterial cream, do not dip the tongue blade or gloved hand back into the jar after it has come into contact with the wound, or the cream will become contaminated.)

    b. Cover the antibacterial cream with fine mesh gauze (e.g., Telfa). If no antibacterial agent is used, apply mesh gauze that contains a water-soluble lubricant to prevent sticking.

    c. Temporary wound coverings such as Biobrane or Omiderm may be used on well-cleaned, non-infected, partial-thickness burns as an alternative to antimicrobial agents. These coverings adhere to the wound and are left in place until the wound heals. As the wound heals, the covering will separate from the healed skin. Separated dressing edges can be trimmed. If an infection develops, the covering must be removed and the wound treated with antibacterial agents.[4,5]

    d. For wounds that will drain, cover the mesh gauze, antibacterial agent, or temporary wound covering with multiple layers of absorbent padding, about 1 to 2 inches thick, to absorb drainage. The goal is to prevent drainage from soaking through to the outside layers, thereby providing a tract down to the wound for microorganisms.

e. Secure the bulky dressing with semielastic mesh gauze (e.g., Kerlix), wrapping extremities distally to proximally, or use a tubular net-type bandage.

f. Hands must be wrapped in a functional position (fingers slightly flexed with the thumb abducted away from the palm with a roll of gauze such as Kling or Kerlix in the patient's palm to support the position). Wrap fingers and toes individually to allow for range of motion. Leave the tips of the fingers and toes exposed for evaluation of circulation.

g. Hydrocolloid dressings absorb fluid. As a result, a gel forms either within the dressing or on the surface of the wound, providing a moist environment for wound healing. These dressings usually are used on small-area partial-thickness burns, and they may be left in place for several days. Secondary bulky dressings are not required.[4,6]

PATIENT CARE MANAGEMENT

Potential Complications

1. Infection
2. Diminished perfusion distal to a circumferential dressing
3. Further wound damage
4. Reaction to cream/ointment (rare)

Patient Care

1. Check circulation distal to any circumferential dressing.
2. Administer tetanus toxoid as ordered.
3. Elevate the extremity above the level of the heart to minimize swelling.
4. Encourage movement of an extremity to help reduce edema.

Discharge Considerations

- Itching: antipyretics, cool compresses, and alcohol-free lotions may help reduce discomfort.
- Patient will need to drink plenty of water and increase protein intake to promote healing.[3]
- Inform the patient the wound may produce copious exudate in the initial stages and may become dry and itchy as it heals, all of which is normal.
- Burn injuries produce an inflammatory response, so inflammation caused by infection can be more difficult to detect. Some mild redness, pain, tenderness, and edema can be normal.

Inflammation or redness extending away from the burn, a bad odor, a greenish exudate, swelling beyond the initial baseline amount, increased pain, and fever are indications of infection. Localized infections often will produce an elevated temperature only in the afternoons.[4]

- If the patient is to be discharged, teach about dressing changes. Advise the patient that if the dressing sticks to the wound, the wound can be soaked in cool, clean tap water to help remove the dressing. At each dressing change, antibacterial ointments or creams must be removed as completely as possible through gentle cleaning techniques. As the wound heals, moisturizing the area with lotion will help reduce the dryness and itching.

- Plans for follow-up care, usually within 24 hours (with a private physician or with the emergency department) must be made before discharging the patient.

- Elevate an affected extremity for 24 hours if possible.

- Keep the dressing clean and dry.

- Superficial wounds usually heal within 5 to 10 days. Medium-depth wounds usually heal within 10 to 14 days. Deep partial-thickness burns take 4 to 6 weeks to heal.[3] Full-thickness burns smaller than 2 cm heal from the wound edges; larger full-thickness burns require skin grafting.

REFERENCES

1. American Burn Association: *Advanced burn life support provider manual,* Dallas 2001, The Association.
2. Flanagan M and Graham J: Should burn blisters be left intact or debrided? *J Wound Care* 10 (2):41-45, 2001.
3. Kagan RJ and Smith SC: Evaluation and treatment of thermal injuries, *Dermatol Nurs* 12 (5):334-349, 2000.
4. Hartford CE: Care of outpatient burns. In Herndon DN, ed: *Total burn care,* Philadelphia, 2002, Saunders.
5. Turner DG: Ambulatory care of the burn patient. In Carrougher G. ed: *Burn care and therapy,* St Louis, 1998, Mosby.
6. Jones V and Milton T: When and how to use hydrocolloid dressings, *Nurs Times* 96 (4):5-7, 2000.
7. Heggers JP, Hawkins H, Edgar P, et al: Treatment of infection in burns. In Herndon DN, ed: *Total burn care,* Philadelphia, 2002, Saunders, pp 120-169.

6 procedure

Capillary Blood Sampling

Naomi North

DESCRIPTION

Capillary blood sampling, more commonly know as heel stick, finger stick, or microcapillary blood collection, is the process of puncturing the patient's skin at the capillary bed with a lancet to collect small volumes of blood for testing. This procedure may be used in the emergency department when serum laboratory and bedside glucose tests are ordered. This form of collection can be used to minimize the amount of blood taken from pediatric and adult patients with decreased blood volumes. It is also helpful when intravenous access is not needed and venipuncture is difficult to obtain.

INDICATIONS

A capillary blood collection should be performed when intravenous access is not needed or considered unobtainable, and laboratory/bedside tests are ordered. Heel sticks should be performed only on pediatric patients less than 1 year of age or in those who are not yet walking. Finger sticks can be performed on adults and pediatric patients greater than 1 year of age.

CONTRAINDICATIONS

Capillary blood sampling should be avoided when:
- Large amounts of blood or multiple tubes are needed.
- Blood cultures, coagulation studies, and/or ESR are ordered.
- Extremities have signs of compromised blood flow, or fractures, casts, or splints are present on the extremity.
- The area has bruising, puncture sites, nodules, burn, rash, edema, or other skin or tissue damage.

EQUIPMENT

- Gloves
- Alcohol (povidone-iodine should not be used, as it may alter some lab values)

- Heel warming device when performing heel sticks (a warm towel or diaper with warm water may be used)
- Appropriate-size lancets
- Sterile gauze or sterile cotton balls
- Collection tubes/devices

NURSING ACTIONS

1. Gather the needed equipment.
2. Identify the patient, and explain the procedure.
3. Identify the appropriate area for puncture (Figures P6-1 and P6-2) and apply a warming device as needed. If a warming device is used, it should be left in place for 3 to 5 minutes.
4. Clean the area, prep with alcohol, and allow to air dry.
5. The medial or lateral aspect of the heel is the site of choice for capillary puncture in infants (Figure P6-1). When collecting heel-stick specimens, it may be helpful to hold the patient's foot with your thumb on the plantar surface, with the first finger under

---

➤ NURSING ALERT ◄

If warming devices are used, caution should be taken to avoid burning the skin.

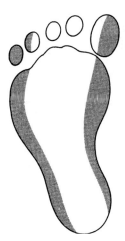

Figure P6-1 Shaded areas represent areas on infant's foot used for obtaining blood specimen.

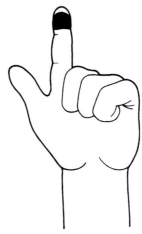

Figure P6-2 Shaded area represents area commonly used for obtaining blood specimen from finger.

the heel, and with the remaining fingers on top of the foot surface.

6. When performing finger sticks, it is considered best to use the second or third finger as a collection site. The tip or side of the finger never should be punctured because of the small distance between skin and bone (Figure P6-2).

7. Wipe away the first drop of blood with either sterile gauze or a cotton ball, as the first drop contains interstitial fluids and may contaminate the specimen.

8. Apply gentle pressure with thumb and first finger to elicit blood flow; do not squeeze or milk area because of the increased risk of contamination of specimen and trauma to the site.

9. Collect blood into appropriate containers, allow blood to drip into tubes to reduce contamination from skin.

10. When blood collection is completed, place gauze or a cotton ball on the puncture site and hold it in place until bleeding has stopped, bandages and tape are contraindicated because of the risk of trauma to the skin and can be a choking hazard in pediatric age-groups.

11. Label specimen containers according to your department's regulations; be sure to note the source as "heel," "finger," or

"capillary" because normal values are adjusted with consideration of the source.

PATIENT CARE MANAGEMENT

1. If possible, allow a familiar person hold a child during the procedure. This helps to reduce the stress and anxiety for the patient and helps maintain immobility for the collector.
2. Although the use of a warming device is not required for regular serum values, its use is suggested to improve blood flow. A warming device must be used when collecting a capillary blood gas to increase arterial flow.
3. If possible, choose a lancet designed for the type of stick being performed. Automatic finger-stick lancets should not be used for heel sticks, as the puncture is a crescent shape; the manual and automatic heel lancets make lateral cuts.
4. If using manual lancets for puncture, use caution not to insert too deeply to avoid excess tissue damage. The puncture should be no deeper than 2 mm; thus automatic heel-stick devices are preferred for heel sticks.
5. If unable to obtain a sufficient amount of blood from the puncture site, apply gauze or a cotton ball and try again at a different site. Never repuncture the site because of the risk of soft-tissue damage and the potential for specimen contamination.

REFERENCE

1. McCall RE and Tankersley CM: Skin puncture principles. In Goucher J, Linkins E, and Ruppert K, eds: *Phlebotomy essentials,* ed 3, Baltimore, Philadelphia, 2003, Lippincott Williams & Wilkins.

7 procedure

Central Venous Pressure Management

Billie Jean Walters

DESCRIPTION

Central venous pressure (CVP) or right atrial pressure (RAP) monitoring:

- Refers to the measurement of pressure within the right atrium, which serves as an estimate of the volume status of the right heart.
- The normal range is 3 to 10 cm H_2O or 2 to 6 mm Hg.

INDICATIONS

1. To guide fluid administration or replacement, or to assess the effectiveness of diuretic administration:
   - A low CVP often occurs in patients who are hypovolemic.
   - An elevated CVP occurs in cases of fluid overload or retention.
2. To assess right heart function:
   - The CVP may be increased in right-side heart failure.
3. The CVP is not a reliable indicator of left ventricular failure. Left ventricular failure increases filling pressure of the left side of the heart, resulting in a backup of blood into the pulmonary vasculature. Pulmonary edema is present by the time the CVP becomes elevated.

EQUIPMENT FOR CATHETER PLACEMENT AND MONITORING

These supplies are available in commercially packaged kits.

For Catheter Placement
- Single-lumen, double-lumen, or triple-lumen infusion catheter
- 1% lidocaine
- 5-ml and 10-ml syringes and different-size needles for injection of lidocaine
- Antiseptic skin solution, such as povidone-iodine solution
- Sterile towels

- Needle introducer
- 10-ml to 20-ml syringe
- Guide wire

For CVP Monitoring With a Manometer
- CVP water manometer with three-way stopcock
- Extension tubing
- IV fluid and administration set
- Indelible marker

For CVP Monitoring With a Transducer and Monitor
- Transducer
- Pressure tubing
- Pressurized flush bag
- Monitor
- Indelible marker

NURSING ACTIONS

1. If using a manometer:
   - Attach the stopcock to the end of the manometer.
   - Attach the extension tubing to one port of the stopcock and the IV administration set to the other port.
   - Turn the stopcock off to the manometer, and flush the entire length of tubing with IV solution.
2. If using a pressure monitoring system:
   - Attach a 500-ml bag of 0.9 normal saline to the pressure tubing.
   - Apply a pressure bag to the 0.9 normal saline and inflate to 300 mm Hg.
   - Flush the tubing by pulling or depressing the flushing mechanism on the tubing.
   - Connect the tubing to the monitor transducer cable.
   - Calibrate, zero, and level the transducer to the phlebostatic axis (the intersection of the midaxillary line and the fourth intercostal space).
3. Explain the procedure, and obtain informed consent.
4. Prep the catheter insertion site with antiseptic solution.
5. Position the patient supine and in a slight Trendelenburg position (if tolerated by the patient).
6. The physician will inject the patient with a local anesthetic and drape the area. Insertion sites include:
   - Subclavian
   - Internal jugular vein

7. A needle is inserted and a guide wire is threaded through the needle. A catheter is placed over the guide wire, and then the guide wire is removed and the catheter sutured into place.
8. The catheter tip usually is placed into the superior vena cava just above the right atrium.
9. Obtain an order for a chest x-ray examination to confirm accurate placement.
10. Connect the end of the extension tubing to the catheter.
11. Adjust the IV rate as prescribed by the physician.

CVP Measurement

1. Position the patient supine or with the head of the bed elevated 30 to 45 degrees.
2. Identify the phlebostatic axis, which approximates the level of the atria located at the intersection of the midaxillary line and the fourth intercostal space.
3. Mark the phlebostatic axis with an indelible marker.
4. If using a manometer, position the zero mark of the water manometer or the transducer at the phlebostatic axis.
5. To obtain a CVP reading with a transducer, the transducer must be connected to a monitoring system. The CVP reading will be recorded in mm Hg if a transducer is used.
6. Turn the stopcock off to the patient and open to the IV solution and manometer.
7. Allow IV solution to slowly fill the manometer to the 25-cm level.
8. Do not let fluid overflow from the top of the manometer.
9. Turn the stopcock off to the IV solution, and open it to the patient and manometer.
10. The fluid level will fall and fluctuate with respirations; allow the fluid level to stabilize and read during end expiration.
11. The measurement should be recorded at the lowest point of the water meniscus.
12. Turn the stopcock off to the manometer and on to the patient (catheter) and IV solution.
13. Infuse IV solution through the central venous line as prescribed.
14. Document the CVP reading in cm H_2O.

PATIENT CARE MANAGEMENT

Complications of CVP line insertion include:
- Dysrhythmias

- Pneumothorax
- Air embolism

Nursing responsibilities after insertion include:

- Note the trend of the CVP readings.
- Observe for disconnection of tubing.
- Monitor insertion site and dressing for bleeding.

8 procedure

Chest Tube Management and Autotransfusion

Maggie Borders

DESCRIPTION

Chest tubes are inserted to remove air and fluid from the pleural cavity, to restore negative intrapleural pressure, and to achieve full reexpansion of the lung. The fourth or fifth intercostal space (or nipple line) slightly anterior to the midaxillary line often is used as the insertion site. The area is cleansed with a povidone-iodine solution, draped, and locally infiltrated with anesthetic solution. A small incision is made along the rib, a curved hemostat is inserted, and a small tunnel is formed through blunt tissue dissection until the parietal pleura can be palpated. A larger curved hemostat often is then used to puncture the parietal pleura. The surgeon then enlarges the puncture site by opening the hemostats and pulling them back out of the chest. At this point, a gloved finger is placed into the pleural space to ensure a clear passage for the tube. The chest tube is guided into the opening with a curved clamp, and then the tube is connected to a drainage system. The tube is sutured into place. Placement is confirmed by noting fogging in the tube, feeling air movement from the tube, and taking a chest x-ray to confirm proper placement and position.

INDICATIONS

- Pneumothorax
- Hemothorax
- Pleural effusion
- Empyema
- Severe blunt chest injuries, such as a flail chest or a pulmonary contusion necessitating positive pressure ventilations

EQUIPMENT

- Povidone-iodine solution
- 4 × 4 gauze sponges
- 1% lidocaine hydrochloride (optionally with epinephrine) for local anesthesia

- Syringe and needles
- Sterile gloves
- Sterile towels
- #10 scalpel
- Large and small curved hemostats
- Suture material (O silk) /needle holder
- Petroleum jelly–impregnated gauze dressing
- 3-inch to 4-inch tape
- Chest drainage system (with autotransfusion device if needed)
- Chest tube of appropriate size as follows:

Age	Chest Tube Sizes
Newborn	8-16 Fr
6 months	14-20 Fr
1 year	14-24 Fr
3 years	16-28 Fr
5 years	20-32 Fr
8 years	24-32 Fr
12 years	28-36 Fr
Adult	28-40 Fr

Smaller sizes can be used for removal of air; larger sizes are needed for fluid removal. Anticipate the need for a 36 to 40 Fr tube in an adult trauma patient.

NURSING ACTIONS

1. Assemble the chest drainage system. Fill the water-seal and suction-control chambers as specified by system instructions.
2. Place the patient in the semi-Fowler's position if the situation allows, and provide 100% oxygen.
3. Monitor the patient throughout the procedure. Provide verbal support and comfort measures.
4. Administer analgesia as prescribed.
5. After insertion, connect the chest tube to the collection chamber and the suction-control chamber to the suction source.
6. Apply a dressing with occlusive gauze, 4 × 4 sponges, and 3-inch to 4-inch tape.
7. Secure tubing connections with adhesive tape or plastic banding to avoid inadvertent disconnection. Coil the extra tubing from the drainage system flat on the bed to prevent dependent loops where blood can collect.

PATIENT CARE MANAGEMENT

- Monitor the patient's vital signs, skin color, and breath sounds before and after the procedure.
- Note blood or fluid in the collection chamber. Mark the level of drainage hourly on the collection system. Surgical intervention usually is required if blood loss:
  - ○ In adults is 1000 to 1500 ml immediately or 200 to 300 ml/hr[1]
  - ○ In children is greater than 20% of the child's estimated circulating blood volume immediately or greater than 1 to 2 ml/kg/hr[2]
- Observe for fluctuation, or "tidaling," of the fluid level in the water-seal chamber. The fluid level rises when the patient inhales and drops when the patient exhales. If the patient is mechanically ventilated, the opposite occurs: the fluid level drops on inspiration and rises on expiration because intrapleural pressure increases with positive-pressure ventilation. Fluctuation indicates system patency. Lack of fluctuation may indicate an obstruction or kink in the system.

NURSING ALERT

It may be difficult to assess "tidaling" and breath sounds when suction is in use. Suction may be turned off momentarily to obtain an accurate assessment. The purpose of the suction is to facilitate the removal of air and fluid. The water seal remains intact even when suction is not in use.

- If blood clots or tissue obstruct the tubing, gently knead the tubing between your fingers to facilitate clearance (chest tube "milking" or "stripping" may increase negative pressure enough to damage lung tissue and is not routinely recommended).
- Do not clamp the chest tube unless absolutely necessary because clamping may lead to an accumulation of air in the pleural space and result in a tension pneumothorax. Clamping a tube briefly may be necessary to change the drainage system or to evaluate the system for air leaks.
- If the patient is to be transported or if suction is not being used, leave the suction tubing connector open to air. Do not clamp it. One-way valves such as the Heimlich valve may be used instead of the larger drainage system when transporting patients. One-way valves allow air to escape and fluid to drain but are much smaller than the typical drainage system.

- If the chest tube is accidentally pulled out, immediately cover the site with an occlusive dressing taped on three sides and notify the physician.

NURSING ALERT

Constant bubbling in the water-seal chamber indicates an air leak. A small air leak may be present as long as there is air in the pleural space (until the lung heals completely). Notify the physician if you notice a large air leak or a new air leak. To determine the origin of an air leak, momentarily clamp the chest tube close to the insertion site. If the bubbling in the water-seal chamber stops, the air leak originates from the patient—either at the insertion site or in the pleural cavity. If the bubbling does not stop, the leak is in the drainage system. Check to ensure tight connections. The drainage system may need to be replaced.

AUTOTRANSFUSION

Autotransfusion is the infusion of autologous blood shed by a patient with massive hemothorax or after thoracic surgery. The main benefits of autotransfusion include immediate availability of warm, perfectly matched whole blood and lack of transfusion reactions. Blood collected from patients with massive hemothorax should be transfused or discarded within 6 hours from the time collection begins. Shed blood can be depleted of the normal clotting factors, so it is important to monitor coagulation studies. Autotransfusion of more than 25% of the patient's estimated blood volume (about 2000 ml in the adult patient) is not recommended. Hyperkalemia may result from the hemolysis of red blood cells that can occur during collection and transfusion.

Contraindications
- Coagulopathy
- Suspected thoracoabdominal injury (e.g., diaphragmatic rupture). There is a significant risk of sepsis if blood becomes contaminated with gastric or intestinal contents.
- Pulmonary or systemic infections
- Malignant neoplasm
- Blood collected from injuries more than 4 hours old

Equipment
- Autotransfusion unit (many drainage systems come equipped with this)

- Suction setup
- Blood tubing with 170-micron to 260-micron filter
- IV normal saline for blood infusion
- Anticoagulant (usually citrate or heparin) is optional

Nursing Actions
1. Some companies recommend that anticoagulants be instilled into the autotransfusion chamber before transfusion. Be familiar with the equipment used in your institution, and follow the manufacturer's instructions for collecting blood from the patient.
2. Prime the blood tubing with normal saline. A 170-micron to 260-micron filter must be used to filter any clots or tissue that may be in the shed blood.
3. When enough blood has been collected (usually 500 to 1000 ml), remove the autotransfusion unit from suction, and replace suction to the chest drainage system or another autotransfusion unit.
4. Spike the transfusion unit with the blood tubing, and infuse according to your institution's protocol.
5. Use a blood tubing set for each autotransfusion.
6. Monitor the patient for coagulopathies and electrolyte imbalances.
7. Prepare patient for surgery as indicated.

⇒ N U R S I N G   A L E R T ⇐

To reduce the risk of an air embolus, remove all the air from the autotransfusion unit before transfusion.

⇒ N U R S I N G   A L E R T ⇐

Rapid infusion of blood containing the anticoagulant citrate may result in citrate toxicity and myocardial depression; this may be evidenced by arrhythmias, tingling around the mouth, and abdominal cramping.

REFERENCES
1. Mattox KL, Feliciano DV, and Moore EE: *Trauma*, ed 4, New York, 2001, McGraw Hill.
2. Kadish H: *Thoracic trauma*, In: Fleisher GR and Ludwig S, eds: *Textbook of pediatric emergency medicine*, ed 4, Philadelphia, 2000, Lippincott, Williams & Williams.

procedure 9

Crutch Walking

Lee Garner

DESCRIPTION

Crutches may be needed by emergency department (ED) patients to allow unilateral, non–weight-bearing ambulation. The crutches most commonly used are the underarm or axillary crutches with hand bars.[1]

INDICATIONS

Lower-extremity injuries such as sprains, contusions, and fractures

EQUIPMENT

Adjustable crutches with axilla pads, hand bar pads, and crutch tips

INITIAL NURSING ACTIONS

1. Measuring for crutches:
   A. Ensure that axilla pads, hand bar pads, and crutch tips are in place.
   B. Have the patient stand and bear weight on the unaffected extremity. Place the crutches 2.5 to 5 cm (1 to 2 in) or 2 to 3 fingerbreadths below the axilla. Adjust the crutches so they extend 5 cm (2 in) in front of and 15 cm (6 in) to the side of the feet.
   C. With the patient standing upright and erect, adjust the hand bars to the point where there is approximately a 15-degree to 30-degree elbow flexion.[2] The hand grips can be adjusted by removing the screws and sliding the hand grips to the appropriate level. Slide screws back into the crutches. Replace the bolts and tighten firmly. The patient's arms should never be straight (Figure P9-1).
2. Ambulating with crutches:
   A. Place weight on palms of the hands and not the axilla.
   B. Use the proper standing position, called the tripod position. In this position, the crutch tips are placed about 5 cm (2 in)

> ### ➤ NURSING ALERT ➤
>
> The radial nerve passes superficially under the axillary area. Continual pressure on the axilla can injure the radial nerve, resulting in weakness to the forearm, wrist, and hand.

  in front of the feet and out laterally about 15 cm (6 in). This creates a wide and stable base of support.

  C. Look forward (not at the feet) and advance the crutches and affected leg forward at the same time.

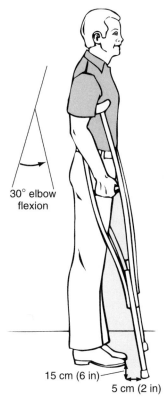

30° elbow flexion

15 cm (6 in)

5 cm (2 in)

Figure P9-1 The standing position for determining the correct length of crutches. (From Kozier B, et al: *Fundamentals of nursing: concepts, process, and practice,* ed 6, Upper Saddle River, NJ, 2000, Prentice-Hall.)

D. Move the unaffected leg forward and through to a position slightly ahead of the crutches.[3]

3. Going up stairs (Figure P9-2):
   A. Assume the tripod position at the bottom of the stairs.
   B. While balancing weight on the hands, move the unaffected leg onto the step.
   C. Shift body weight to the unaffected leg and move the affected leg and crutches up onto the step. Keep the affected leg slightly bent during this move.

4. Going down stairs (Figure P9-3)
   A. Shift body weight to the unaffected leg. Move the crutches and the affected leg onto the step. Keep the affected leg slightly in front of the body during the move.
   B. Transfer body weight to the crutches and move the unaffected leg to that step. When moving the unaffected leg to the step, land on the heel and not the toes.

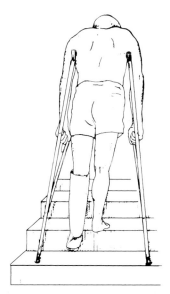

Figure P9-2   When climbing stairs, the patient places weight on the crutches while moving the unaffected leg onto a step first. (From Barber J, Stokes L, and Billings D: *Adult and child care,* ed 2, St Louis, 1977, Mosby.)

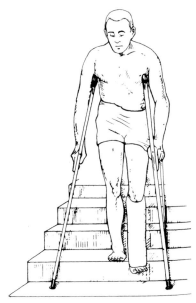

Figure P9-3   When descending stairs, the patient first moves the crutches and affected leg down to the next step. (From Barber J, Stokes L, and Billings D: *Adult and child care,* ed 2, St Louis, 1977, Mosby.)

> ### ⚡ **N U R S I N G   A L E R T** ⚡
>
> A simple way to remind patients of these steps is that the "good" (unaffected leg) goes up first toward heaven when traveling up stairs. Likewise, the bad (affected) leg goes down first when moving down the stairs.

---

5. Sitting down onto the chair or bed:
   A. Slowly turn around and back up until the back of the unaffected leg touches the chair or bed.
   B. Transfer both crutches to the hand on the same side as the affected leg. Hold onto the crutches with the hand bars. Grasp the arm of the chair with the other hand.
   C. Hold the affected leg slightly forward, and slowly lower self into a sitting position.
6. Getting out of chair or bed:
   A. Move forward to the edge of the chair or bed.

B. Grasp the crutches by the hand bars in the hand on the affected side. Grasp the arm of the chair by the hand on the unaffected side.
C. Push self up.
D. Assume the tripod position before moving.

PATIENT CARE MANAGEMENT

Instruct the patient to do the following:
1. Remove loose rugs and small objects on the floor at home.
2. Stay off wet or waxed floors, ice, and grass. These can be slippery.
3. Wipe off wet crutch tips.
4. Avoid escalators.
5. Wear sturdy, low-heeled shoes.
6. Avoid alcohol or medications that may impair balance, perception, and judgment.

REFERENCES

1. Newberry L: *Sheehy's emergency nursing principles and practice,* St Louis, 2003, Mosby.
2. Perry AG and Potter PA: *Clinical nursing skills technique,* St Louis, 2002, Mosby.
3. Perry AG and Potter PA: *Fundamentals of nursing,* ed 5, St Louis, 2001, Mosby.

10 procedure

Decontamination of a Patient

Patty Ann Sturt
Joseph Hill

DESCRIPTION

Ideally, patients should be decontaminated at the scene or before reaching the hospital. However, such decontamination of patients may not be possible. In addition, patients exposed to a hazardous substance may arrive at triage with no prior notification to the emergency department (ED). Emergency departments must have decontamination procedures and equipment readily available. Goals of patient decontamination include:

1. Removing the hazardous substance to prevent possible injury or to stop ongoing injury to the patient
2. Preventing contamination to health-care workers, other patients, visitors, and equipment

Health-care workers who may be involved in patient decontamination must receive training and demonstrate competency regarding the:

1. Institutional policies and procedures on hazardous-materials-incident response.
2. Appropriate use of personal protective equipment (PPE), including respirators.
3. Decontamination equipment location and set-up.

Documentation of training and competency should be kept in the employee's file.

INDICATIONS

- Actual or possible history of exposure to a hazardous substance and signs and symptoms suggestive of exposure.
- Specific history of exposure to a hazardous substance via vapor, dust, liquid, or visible particles.

NURSING ALERT

Emergency department staff involved in patient decontamination should have reference material readily available that describes the chemicals frequently transported via truck or rail through the community. The reference material should include the signs and symptoms associated with exposure to the chemical and the treatment.

CONTRAINDICATIONS/CAUTIONS

- Some hospitals have decontamination rooms with an outside entryway. Care should be taken to ensure contaminated patients do not enter the ED.
- Many hospitals do not have the benefit of a decontamination room. In such cases, the decontamination area may be set up outside of the ED. Care should be taken to ensure the decontamination area is far enough from the building to prevent patients from inadvertently walking into the ED before decontamination and to prevent air-borne particles from entering the hospital's ventilation system.

EQUIPMENT

1. Appropriate-level PPE based on the agent involved (if known), possibly including:
   - Chemical-resistant mask/hood
   - Two sets of impermeable and tear-resistant gloves
   - Impermeable and tear-resistant boots
   - Duct tape or chemical-resistant tape
   - Respiratory protection equipment
   - In-line air source and hoses compatible with the suit
   Or
   - Powered air-purifying respirator (PAPR) with a cartridge appropriate for the known or suspected agent
   Or
   - Respirator mask with supplied air source
2. Water source with attached water hose of a length sufficient to reach the decontamination area.
3. Water-delivery device for patient decontamination, such as:
   - Water hose with attached sprayer or nozzle to distribute water
   - Portable shower unit or commercially available portable decontamination shower

4. Containment device, such as an inflatable pool if using water hose with sprayer or nozzle. This will help to contain the water in one area and reduce the amount of water that reaches the surrounding grounds.
5. Additional equipment may be needed for holding an unconscious patient or a patient that is unable to stand:
   - Two large saw horses with a high weight capacity
   - Back board

   Or
   - Commercially available decontamination stretcher with drainage barrels or containers
6. Portable screens for patient privacy
7. Traffic cones
8. Large and small plastic bags
9. Indelible markers
10. Buckets
11. Soft sponges
12. Rolls of plastic
13. Mild liquid soap
14. Gowns
15. Disposable slippers
16. Towels
17. Blankets

NURSING ACTIONS

- Determine whether the substance is known.
- Establish a specific outside zone or sectioned-off area (hot zone) where contaminated patients are undressed and decontaminated. Only employees with appropriate PPE should enter this zone. Identify this zone and mark it with traffic cones.
- Establish a clean area well away from the hot zone and closer to the ED entrance where decontaminated patients can be placed in gowns and slippers and given blankets.
- Turn on the water source and set up the water-delivery system to be used.
- Don the suit, two gloves on each hand, and the boots.
- Secure gloves and boots to suit with tape.
- Don the respiratory protection equipment.
- Instruct the patient to remove clothing. This is one of the most important steps in patient decontamination. Most of the hazardous substance may be on the clothing. If the patient cannot remove the clothing, remove or cut the clothing from

head to toe. Attempt to keep the clothing away from the patient's face to prevent inhalation and eye contamination.

- Place clothing and personal belongings in plastic sealable bags. Using an indelible marker, label the bag with the patient's name, date, and time.
- If the patient is alert and cooperative, instruct the patient to shower or spray water over the entire body from top to bottom and wipe skin with a soapy sponge. Instruct the patient to spray water and wash the area between skin folds, under the arms, and between the legs.
- If the patient is unable to shower self, spray water on patient from top to bottom. Ensure that water reaches area between skin folds, under the arms, between the legs, and on the back.
- Instruct the patient to move to clean area and put on gown and slippers.
- A staff member should be near or at the ED entrance to escort the patient to a treatment room.
- After all patients have been decontaminated and are in the ED, the decontamination team should rinse off the suits and then remove the PPE using the following steps[1]:
    1. Remove tape used to secure gloves and boots to suit.
    2. Remove outer gloves, turning them inside out as they are removed.
    3. Remove suit, turning it inside out and folding it downward. Avoid shaking the suit.
    4. Remove boot from one foot and step over to a "clean area" away from the hot zone. Remove other boot and place that foot in the clean area.
    5. Remove the mask or respirator.
    6. Remove inner gloves.
- After removing PPE, the staff should shower and change clothing.
- The hot zone should be secured so others cannot enter it. Contact the appropriate agency or department to remove and clean the area used for decontamination.

PATIENT CARE MANAGEMENT/STAFF SAFETY

- Law enforcement agencies will determine whether patient belongings may be needed as evidence.
- Pediatric and elderly patients are more prone to hypothermia. Use warm water when possible. Cover the patient quickly after decontamination.

- Communication is challenging when staff members are wearing PPE. Consider using hand signals to indicate when a member of the decontamination team is tired or needs a break. In general, an individual with PPE and a respirator should not be in the hot zone for more than 20 to 30 minutes.
- Only individuals who are physically fit and have met the appropriate training requirements should be allowed to wear PPE and enter the hot zone.
- ED personnel must be fit-tested for respirators by personnel trained in the procedure. Information on chemicals can be obtained 24 hours a day from the Chemical Transportation Emergency Center (CHEMTREC) at (800) 424-9300.[1]
- Health-related support for hazardous-materials emergencies can be obtained 24 hours a day from the Agency for Toxic Substances and Disease Registry (ATSDR) at (404) 498-0120.[1]

REFERENCES

1. Department of Health and Human Services (DHHS), Agency for Toxic Substances and Disease Registry: *Hospital emergency departments: a planning guide for the management of contaminated patients*, Atlanta, 2001, DHHS.

procedure *11*

Defibrillation

Jo Lynn McKee

Defibrillation is the treatment of choice for ventricular fibrillation (VF) and pulseless ventricular tachycardia (VT). Until recently, this procedure has been performed only in settings equipped for advanced cardiac life support.

Both monophasic and biphasic waveform defibrillators now are available to emergency cardiac care providers. Historically, external defibrillators delivered energy in a monophasic waveform. The current in a monophasic waveform travels in one direction, delivering a high amount of current for a short period of time. The biphasic waveform defibrillator delivers the current in one direction for the first part of the shock phase and then reverses direction for the second part of the phase. Because the current reverses direction, there is a greater change in waveform amplitude with less current delivered. This may result in less damage to myocardial tissue. The amount of current delivered with biphasic defibrillators varies among manufacturers. The emergency nurse should become familiar with the type of defibrillator used in his or her setting.

With the advent of automated external defibrillators (AEDs), defibrillation now can be performed in a variety of settings by emergency cardiac care providers and laypersons. The AED and its use will be described later in this procedure.

DESCRIPTION

In defibrillation, electrical energy is delivered to the myocardium to depolarize or stun the entire myocardium.[1] With successful defibrillation, after this brief period of asystole, the pacemaker cells initiate organized electrical activity that produces effective cardiac muscle contractions and return of a pulse.

INDICATIONS

1. Ventricular fibrillation
2. Pulseless ventricular tachycardia

EQUIPMENT

- Standard defibrillator with cardiac monitor
- ECG electrodes
- Conductive gel, two gel pads, or two self-adhesive disposable defibrillator pads

INITIAL NURSING ACTIONS

Routine care of the defibrillation equipment includes inspection of the equipment every shift. Determine that ECG paper, monitoring electrodes, and defibrillator gel or pads are available. Examine the cables, connectors, paddles, and defibrillator for damage. Test the adequacy of the battery power supply and the ECG display by turning on the equipment and charging the paddles. With most models, the paddles can be safely discharged into the equipment. Clean the equipment and restock supplies after each use.

Defibrillation with Standard Defibrillator

1. Turn on the defibrillator.
2. Commercially available defibrillation pads or paddles should be placed in either the sternum-apex position or the anterior-posterior position. If defibrillation paddles are used, apply a conductive gel pad to the chest wall or conductive gel to the paddles. See Figure P11-1 for standard paddle or pad placement.
3. Select the initial energy level appropriate for the type of defibrillator available: monophasic defibrillators, 200 joules; or biphasic defibrillators, the clinical equivalent.
4. Confirm VF or pulseless VT on the monitor. The patient's rhythm can be monitored via the paddles, defibrillation pads, or monitor leads.

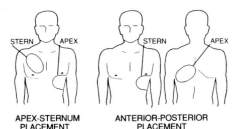

APEX-STERNUM
PLACEMENT

ANTERIOR-POSTERIOR
PLACEMENT

Figure P11-1   Recommended placement of paddles and defibrillation pads.

5. Charge the defibrillator. Make sure the defibrillator is in the "unsynchronized" mode.
6. Announce "all clear" and visually check that all team members are clear of the patient, equipment, and stretcher.
7. If using paddles, press the paddles onto the chest wall with approximately 25 lb of pressure.
8. Deliver the shock by simultaneously pressing the discharge buttons on the paddles or on the unit if using defibrillator pads.
9. Assess the patient's rhythm on the monitor. If VF or pulseless VT continues, charge the defibrillator to 300 joules (or the appropriate energy level for the biphasic defibrillators) and deliver a second shock.
10. Deliver a third shock at 360 joules (or the appropriate energy level for biphasic defibrillators) if VF or pulseless VT persists.
11. If the rhythm is not converted after three successive shocks, start CPR and follow Advanced Cardiac Life Support (ACLS) protocols.

The use of pediatric-size paddles or defibrillator pads is advised for children less than 1 year of age or weighing 10 kg or less. In the pediatric patient, the use of pediatric-size paddles (usually supplied by the defibrillator manufacturer) is advised. For the initial pediatric shock, 2 joules/kg are used, followed by successive shocks of 4 joules/kg.

NURSING ALERT

- Do not defibrillate over nitroglycerin patches or permanent pacemaker pulse generators.
- Avoid pacemaker generators and internal cardioverter defibrillators by placing paddles at least 5 inches from the pulse generator. Placing paddles or pads either too close or on these devices will reduce the chance of successful defibrillation.
- Do not allow gel to form a path between the paddles. A burn injury to the patient could result.

PATIENT CARE MANAGEMENT

Early defibrillation is the gold standard of emergency cardiac care. Every effort should be made not to delay defibrillation in favor of other treatments.

1. Continue CPR if delays in defibrillation occur. Do not perform CPR between the three initial consecutive shocks.
2. Continue monitoring and assessing cardiopulmonary status after defibrillation.

3. Other interventions before and after defibrillation may include:
   - Airway and ventilation management by intubation or cricothyrotomy
   - IV medication administration
   - Endotracheal medication instillation if rapid IV access cannot be achieved.
   - Antiarrhythmic therapy after successful conversion with the antiarrhythmic last given before conversion
   - Document the event and a code summary.
   - Patient and family education

AED

The AED is a computerized defibrillator that analyzes the patient's rhythm, recognizes a shockable rhythm, and advises when a shock should be delivered. Indications for use are a patient with signs of cardiac arrest, including unresponsiveness, absence of breathing, and absence of circulation. AEDs can be used in the adult and pediatric ($\geq$ 1 year old) populations.[2] Ideally, the device should be capable of delivering a pediatric energy dose.[2] Currently available pad and cable systems for use with pediatric patients are used with the adult device, but they reduce the level of delivered energy. Not all manufacturers make pediatric-size pads. Be familiar with the equipment available to you.

Defibrillation with the AED

1. Turn the power on.
2. Attach the defibrillation cables to the pads, and apply the pads to the patient in the same fashion as with a standard manual defibrillator.
3. Press the analyze button. Make sure that no one is in contact with the patient and that the patient is not moving.
4. If VF or pulseless VT is present, the AED will charge to 150 to 360 joules, indicate that a shock is advised, and deliver the shock automatically. The energy level of each shock is preset by the AED manufacturer.
5. Announce "All clear" and visually confirm that all team members are clear of the patient, stretcher, and equipment.
6. Press the shock button when advised to do so.
7. Repeat the steps until VF or pulseless VT is no longer present or until three successive shocks have been delivered. Reassess the patient's ABCs and proceed with CPR if necessary.

8. Postdefibrillation care should include: 12-lead ECG; vital signs; neurological checks; labs such as ABG, serum electrolytes, and serial enzymes; chest x-ray if intubated; and inspection of the chest wall for burns.

NURSING ALERT

As with standard defibrillation pads, do not place an AED electrode pad over a medication patch or an implanted device (pacemaker or implanted cardioverter defibrillator device). Place the electrode pad at least 1 inch to the side of the implanted device.[3] Remove medication patches and wipe the area clean before attaching the AED pad.

PATIENT CARE MANAGEMENT

1. If "no shock" is indicated by the AED, check for signs of circulation. If **no** signs of circulation are present, perform CPR for 1 minute, then reassess.
2. Do not touch the patient while the AED is analyzing the rhythm.
3. A hairy chest may prevent good contact between the electrode and the patient, resulting in a "check electrode" message on the AED. Press firmly on the electrode. If this does not eliminate the message, quickly pull off the electrode to remove excess chest hair, and then apply a new electrode, or clip the hair on the chest with scissors or a razor and apply a new electrode.
4. Become familiar with your equipment and how it operates. Routine care of the equipment includes inspection of the cables, connectors, and outer case. Check the AED daily by turning it on and making sure the "ready for use" indicator is on.
5. Store all the necessary supplies with the AED. At least two sets of spare defibrillator electrodes, scissors or razors for clipping hair, spare battery (if appropriate for the model), alcohol pads, and cotton sponges are helpful.

REFERENCES

1. American Heart Association: *ACLS: principles and practice*, Dallas 2003, The Association.
2. Sampson RA, Berg RA, and Bingham R: Use of automated external defibrillators for children: an update, *Circulation* 1:3250-3255, 2003.
3. American Heart Association: *Advanced cardiac life support provider manual*, Dallas 2001, The Association, p 214.

12 procedure

Diagnostic Peritoneal Lavage

Patty Ann Sturt

DESCRIPTION

Diagnostic peritoneal lavage (DPL) is an invasive procedure used to detect intraperitoneal blood, bile, bacteria, amylase, and white blood cells after abdominal trauma. DPL is considered 98% sensitive for intraperitoneal bleeding.[1,2] DPL is neither organ-specific nor injury-specific and cannot detect retroperitoneal bleeding. DPL is performed through either the closed or the open technique. In the closed technique, catheter is inserted percutaneously. In the open technique, a small incision is made below the umbilicus through the skin and subcutaneous tissue to the fascia. The catheter is then inserted through the peritoneum into the peritoneal cavity. The open technique is preferred in patients with pelvic fractures or advanced pregnancy.[3]

NOTE: Emergency medicine physicians and surgeons may prefer to use a focused assessment sonogram in trauma (FAST) of the abdomen if available rather than DPL. A FAST is noninvasive and can be used to detect the presence of intraperitoneal blood.

INDICATIONS FOR PROCEDURE

1. Multiple blunt injuries with indicators of hemodynamic instability, such as hypotension, and any of the following:
   - Unreliable abdominal examination because of an altered level of consciousness. An altered level of consciousness may occur in patients with brain injury, alcohol intoxication, or drug ingestion.
   - Decrease in sensation from a spinal cord injury
   - Injury to adjacent structures, such as lower ribs, pelvis, or lumbar spine
   - Multiple trauma requiring general anesthesia for nonabdominal surgical procedures
2. Lap belt injury (abdominal wall contusion) with suspicion of bowel injury.[1]
3. Hemodynamically stable patients with blunt abdominal trauma and pain when a FAST or CT scan is not available

4. Hemodynamically stable patient with low-velocity penetrating abdominal trauma, such as a stab wound, and questionable peritoneal penetration

CONTRAINDICATIONS/CAUTIONS

1. Any patient with a gunshot wound (GSW) traversing the peritoneal cavity will require surgery (regardless of the DPL results). DPL is not indicated.
2. Surgery should be expedited in the hypotensive patient with penetrating trauma to the abdomen. DPL is not indicated.
3. The patient with blunt abdominal trauma, indicators of peritoneal irritation, and hemodynamic instability despite fluid resuscitation will require rapid surgery (see Chapter 21). Surgery should not be delayed for a DPL.
4. Relative contraindications include:
   - Previous intraabdominal surgeries. Multiple abdominal surgeries increase the risk of adhesions. Adhesions may cause the intestines to adhere to the abdominal wall. Intestinal perforation may occur when the catheter is introduced.
   - Morbid obesity
   - Advanced cirrhosis
   - Preexisting coagulopathy

EQUIPMENT

- Gastric tube
- Urinary catheter
- Antiseptic solution
- Sterile gloves
- Mask
- Gown
- Razor
- 5-ml, 10-ml, and 20-ml syringes
- Needles of various sizes
- Sterile drapes (Four sterile towels usually are used.)
- Sterile gauze sponge
- Local anesthetic (Lidocaine 1% with epinephrine often is used.)
- Peritoneal lavage catheter and introducing stylet
- 1000 ml of warmed normal saline (NS) or Ringer's lactate solution
- IV tubing: maxidrip solution set
- Needle holder and straight scissors
- Suture material
- Sterile specimen container

• Small dressing for covering catheter entrance site
(NOTE: Preassembled kits containing much of this equipment are available.)

INITIAL NURSING ACTIONS

1. If needed, diagnostic abdominal x-rays should be taken before DPL is performed. The procedure may produce artifacts such as intraperitoneal air on the films.
2. Explain the procedure and provide verbal support to the conscious patient.
3. Insert an indwelling urinary catheter before the procedure.[4,5]

> **NURSING ALERT**
>
> Inserting an indwelling urinary catheter is extremely important, because a full bladder may be punctured during the advancement of the catheter toward the pelvis.

---

4. Pass a nasogastric or orogastric tube to decompress the stomach and prevent stomach perforation during peritoneal catheter insertion.
5. Spike the IV bag with the IV tubing set. Flush the IV tubing. Keep the end of the tubing capped and sterile.
6. Place the patient in a supine position.
7. The nurse or physician may shave the abdomen at and around the insertion site if necessary.
8. The nurse or physician should prep the abdomen with antiseptic solution from the costal margin to the symphysis pubis.

NOTE: At this point, the physician drapes the abdomen and injects the area with lidocaine. For adults, the usual site for catheter insertion is the midline, 2 to 3 cm below the umbilicus or one third of the distance from the umbilicus to the symphysis pubis. For pregnant women at greater than 12 weeks' gestation, the catheter may be inserted above the umbilicus. The catheter is directed through the peritoneum toward the pelvis. When the catheter is in place, a 10-ml or 20-ml syringe is attached. Aspiration of gross blood is considered positive, and it is not necessary to infuse NS or Ringer's lactate into the peritoneal space.

9. Attach the IV tubing to the catheter.
10. Open the IV tubing clamp and infuse 1 L. For children, infuse 10 ml/kg.[1]

11. The physician may gently massage the abdomen to distribute the fluid throughout the peritoneal cavity.
12. When the infusion is complete, lower the IV bag and allow the fluid to return by gravity. As much of the fluid as possible should be removed from the peritoneal cavity. Turning or logrolling the patient may facilitate removal of the fluid.
13. Some laboratories will accept the IV bag with the fluid. Others require the fluid in a sterile container. Hand carry the IV bag or container to the laboratory for testing as ordered by the physician. Commonly ordered tests may include a red blood cell (RBC) count, white blood cell (WBC) count, and an amylase level. The fluid also can be checked for the presence of bile and/or bacteria.
14. Report test findings to the physician. The following findings are associated with a positive lavage:
    - RBC count >100,000/mm^3
    - WBC count >500/mm^3
    - Amylase level >175 mg/dl
    - Presence of bile or bacteria (indicates intestinal perforation or injury)

NOTE: The ability to read newspaper print through the fluid in the IV bag is NOT a reliable indicator of a negative lavage.

15. When the catheter has been removed and the wound has been sutured (if applicable), place a sterile dressing over the site.

PATIENT CARE MANAGEMENT

1. Monitor the DPL site for bleeding, hematoma, and signs of infection.
2. Continue to assess the abdomen for pain, tenderness, distension, and rigidity.
3. Prepare the patient for surgery as indicated.

REFERENCES

1. Advanced Trauma Life Support Subcommittee: *Compendium of changes for seventh edition ATLS student manual*, Chicago, 2002, American College of Surgeons.
2. Moloney PA and Czerwinski SA: *Nursing care of the pediatric trauma patient*, St Louis, 2003, Saunders.
3. Herman ML: Gastrointestinal trauma. In Newberry L, ed: *Emergency nursing principles and practice*, ed 5, St Louis, 2003, Mosby.
4. Emergency Nurses Association: *Trauma nurse core course*, Chicago, 2000, The Association.
5. Proehl JA: Diagnostic peritoneal lavage. In Proehl JA, ed: *Emergency nursing procedures*, ed 3, Philadelphia, 2004, Saunders.

13 procedure

Ear Irrigation

Mark B. Parshall

INDICATIONS

Ear irrigation is commonly ordered to remove impacted cerumen or a foreign body from the external auditory canal. One or both ear canals may be impacted.

CONTRAINDICATIONS

Contraindications include a ruptured tympanic membrane (TM), myringotomy tubes, and Ménière's disease. Irrigation should not be performed if the patient has vertigo. If vertigo, nystagmus, or pain develops during the procedure, the procedure should be discontinued and the physician notified.[1-3]

EQUIPMENT

- Metal piston (Reiner-Alexander) syringe

Or

- 30-ml or 60-ml Luer-Lok syringe with a16-gauge or 18-gauge Teflon Angiocath sheath or a hub and clipped tubing from a butterfly. (A metal needle should never be used.)

Or

- Irrigation device (e.g., Water-Pik) with special ear-tip[1] (see below)

And

- Warm (body temperature) water or saline[1-3]
- Two basins: one for irrigant and one for runoff
- Otoscope
- Ceruminolytic drops (liquid docusate sodium,[4] Debrox, or Cerumenex)
- Towels and a gown to drape patient's clothing
- Examination gloves

INITIAL NURSING ACTIONS

1. Explain the procedure to the patient and ask that any discomfort, vertigo, or nausea be reported immediately.

2. Examine both ears with an otoscope, even if only one is impacted, because this will establish a baseline for subsequent inspection.

3. If a ceruminolytic agent is being used, it should be instilled at least 10 minutes before irrigation.

4. The irrigation tip should not be advanced beyond the cartilaginous portion of the ear canal. In an adult, the pinna may be pulled upward and backward, and in a small child, downward and backward to straighten the ear canal.

5. The direction of the irrigation should be toward the posterosuperior aspect of the ear canal, not at the TM (e.g., at the 1 o'clock position in the left ear and the 11 o'clock position in the right ear).[2] Irrigation can be continued until the impaction is relieved or the patient reports discomfort.

6. If a Water-Pik is used, great care must be taken to ensure that the pressure is not excessive and remains constant. A special Water-Pik–compatible tip designed for ear irrigation helps to avoid excessive pressure to the TM.[1]

PATIENT CARE MANAGEMENT

1. At times a large plug will be irrigated free. If a ceruminolytic agent was used before irrigation, the impaction may tend to break up into small pieces as irrigation progresses.

2. An otoscopic examination should be performed at intervals during the irrigation and at the conclusion of the procedure.

3. If irrigation is successful, patients generally report a marked improvement in hearing and relief from the feeling of fullness in the ear.

4. If a ceruminolytic is ordered as the sole therapy instead of irrigation, the cerumen may swell as it begins to soften, causing the patient to experience some decrease in hearing before hearing improves.[1]

5. There is often some degree of redness of the ear canal after irrigation. At times the physician may decide to treat the inflammatory reaction as an external otitis, although it often resolves spontaneously within a day or two without treatment.

6. There may even be a small amount of superficial bleeding, which should stop spontaneously.

7. Assuming the TM is intact, some sources recommend instillation of a few drops of isopropyl alcohol or other drying agent (e.g., VoSol Otic Solution or Domeboro Otic) after irrigation.[2]

8. Recommendation of ceruminolytic agents to prevent recurrence is at the discretion of the physician. Docusate sodium liquid, 1% solution (Colace liquid, 1%), and Debrox are available over the counter; Cerumenex is available by prescription only.

REFERENCES

1. Grossan M: Safe, effective techniques for cerumen removal, *Geriatrics* 55:80, 2000.
2. Zivic RC and King S: Cerumen impaction management for clients of all ages, *Nurs Pract* 18 (3):33, 1993.
3. Aung T and Mulley GP: Removal of ear wax, *Br Med J* 325:27, 2002.
4. Singer AJ, Sauris E, and Viccellio AW: Ceruminolytic effects of docusate sodium: a randomized, controlled trial, *Ann Emerg Med* 36:228-232, 2000.

procedure *14*

ECG: 12-Lead, 15-Lead, and 18-Lead ECG Monitoring

Patty Ann Sturt

DESCRIPTION

The electrocardiogram (ECG) is one of the most important noninvasive procedures performed in the emergency department. The ECG records electrical activity in the heart. The electrical current that passes through the heart also radiates to the nearby tissues. Electrodes placed on the skin can detect and transmit the current to the ECG machine, which records the activity as a series of waveforms.

INDICATIONS

1. To assist with the diagnosis and location of myocardial ischemia, injury, or infarction. This may require serial ECGs.
2. To aid in diagnosis of cardiac arrhythmias and conduction defects.
3. A 15-lead ECG is used to evaluate right ventricular myocardial infarction.
4. An 18-lead ECG is used to evaluate posterior wall myocardial infarction.

CONTRAINDICATIONS/CAUTIONS

- Shivering or patient movement may create artifact and reduce the quality of the ECG.
- The ECG does not measure the pumping ability of the heart; a patient may have low cardiac output with a normal ECG.
- The sensitivity of the ECG is controversial. Be aware that a patient may have an MI that is not detected by an ECG.

EQUIPMENT

- Multiple-lead ECG machine
- Leads
- Electrodes (prepackaged with gel) or ECG plates
- Electrical conductive paste or gel if plates are used

INITIAL NURSING ACTIONS

1. Explain the procedure to the patient.
2. Remove clothing over all areas where electrodes will be applied.
3. Center the patient on the stretcher so that the body does not touch the siderails.
4. Connect the power cord to a grounded electrical outlet.
5. Turn on the machine and enter demographic information required by the machine or your institution.
6. Apply self-sticking electrodes, or electrode paste or gel if plates are used.
7. Apply chest leads[2] (see Figure P14-1)
   - V1: Fourth intercostal space (ICS) at the right sternal border
   - V2: Fourth ICS at the left sternal border
   - V3: Fifth ICS, midway between V2 and V4 at the fifth ICS
   - V4: Fifth ICS at the midclavicular line (MCL)

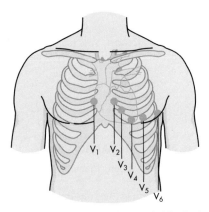

Figure P14-1   Anatomic placement of precordial leads. (From Phipps W, Sands J, and Marek J: *Medical-surgical nursing,* ed 6, St. Louis, 1999, Mosby.)

- V5: Fifth ICS, midway between V4 and V6 at the left anterior axillary line
- V6: Fifth ICS at the left midaxillary line
8. Apply an electrode and one lead to each forearm and the medial aspect of each leg.

⯈ NURSING ALERT ⯇

Shaving of the chest may be necessary if excessive hair is present.

---

9. Encourage the patient to relax and not to move or talk during the procedure.
10. For a 15-lead ECG (also known as a right-side ECG), move electrodes V4 through V6 to the right side of the chest (see Figure P14-2).
    - V4R: Fifth ICS at right MCL
    - V5R: Fifth ICS at right anterior axillary line
    - V6R: Fifth ICS at right midaxillary line
11. For an 18-lead ECG, place leads V7 through V9 on the left posterior surface.[1] These leads are added to the standard 12-lead and 15-lead electrodes (see Figure P14-2).

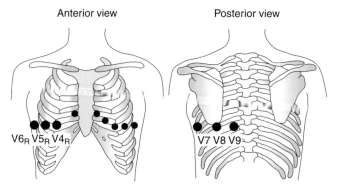

Figure P14-2   Alternate paddle placement for synchronized cardioversion and defibrillation in the patient with a permanent pulse generator. (From Boggs R, Wooldridge-King, M: *AACN procedure manual for critical care,* ed 3, Philadelphia, 1993, WB Saunders.)

- V7: Fifth ICS at the posterior axillary line
- V8: Fifth ICS at the posterior MCL
- V9: Fifth ICS at the left paraspinal border
12. Press the appropriate button to activate and record the ECG.
13. Disconnect the leads from the patient.
14. Remove electrodes and paste or gel from the skin.

PATIENT CARE MANAGEMENT

1. Serial ECGs may be ordered to monitor the trend of changes in the patient's ECG over time.
2. Loose connections, broken lead wires, patient movement, or patient contact with metal may result in an inadequate ECG tracing.

REFERENCES

1. McMahon MD: 12, 15, and 18 Lead electrocardiograms. In Proehl JA, ed: *Adult emergency nursing procedures,* Philadelphia, 2004, Saunders.
2. Perry PG and Potter PA: *Clinical nursing skills and techniques: assisting with electrocardiogram,* ed 5, St Louis, 2002, Mosby.

procedure *15*

Emergency Thoracotomy

Theresa M. Glessner

DESCRIPTION

Open thoracotomy is an emergency procedure during which the chest is opened surgically to correct exsanguinating hemorrhage or cardiac arrest from an unknown cause after blunt or penetrating trauma.

INDICATIONS

Emergency thoracotomy is indicated for cardiopulmonary arrest in the patient who has had signs of life (pulse, blood pressure, cardiac electrical activity, respiratory effort, or motor function of any type) just before or after arrival in the emergency department (ED); the patient may have suffered blunt or penetrating trauma to the chest or abdomen.

CONTRAINDICATIONS

This procedure is *not* indicated for patients who have not had signs of life since the time of the traumatic injury or have not had signs of life for greater than 15 minutes before arrival at the emergency department.

EQUIPMENT

1. Povidone-iodine solution
2. 4 × 4 Sponges
3. Sterile gowns, gloves, masks, hats, and shoe covers
4. Thoracostomy tray: Many facilities have preassembled trays with the equipment needed to perform an emergency thoracotomy. See Box P15-1 for content usually found in one of these trays.

INITIAL NURSING ACTIONS

1. The patient must be on a cardiac monitor throughout this procedure.
2. The patient's airway must be secured by endotracheal intubation before initiation of this procedure because

BOX P15-1   EQUIPMENT FOR EMERGENCY THORACOTOMY

- Finochietto-Buford rib spreader with two large blades and two small (pediatric) blades
- Tuffier rib spreader
- Two $9\frac{1}{2}$-inch DeBakey aneurysm clamps
- One medium Satinsky clamp
- Six Vanderbilt clamps
- Two 8-inch Sarot needle holders
- Curved Mayo scissors
- Two Metzenbaum scissors
- Eight large towel clamps
- One straight Liston bone cutter
- One Lebsche sternal chisel
- One mallet
- Two 9-inch DeBakey forceps
- Two $5\frac{1}{2}$-inch tissue forceps
- Four sterile towel packs (six each)
- Sterile Teflon sheet (6×6 felt)
- Four packs of lap sponges
- Two 2-0 silk sutures
- Dacron tape
- Four 4-0 Prolene sutures
- Ten 2-0 Ticron sutures
- No. 21 scalpel
- 3-0 Prolene suture
- $\frac{1}{4}$-inch pledget
- $\frac{3}{8}$-inch pledget
- Six 3-0 Prolene sutures with strung $\frac{1}{4}$-inch pledget
- Small Satinsky clamp
- Two $9\frac{1}{2}$-inch sponge forceps
- Two 8-inch Allis clamps
- Two 8-inch Gemini clamps (right-angle forceps)
- Two 6-inch Gemini clamps
- Two 8-inch standard needle holders
- Two 7-inch Sarot needle holders
- Two Duval lung clamps
- 8-inch curved Metzenbaum scissors
- $6\frac{3}{4}$-inch straight Mayo scissors
- Six curved Kelly clamps
- Large Allison lung retractor
- Small Allison lung retractor
- Medium Richardson retractor

BOX P15-1   EQUIPMENT FOR EMERGENCY THORACOTOMY—cont'd

- Small Richardson retractor
- Two $9^1/_2$-inch DeBakey forceps
- Two $7^3/_4$-inch DeBakey forceps
- Two vessel clude Neuromedics
- No. 10 scalpel
- No. 11 scalpel
- Sterile Foley catheter
- Sterile internal defibrillator paddles

---

there is little access to the head during the procedure, making bag-valve-mask ventilation difficult.

3. Assist the surgeon in donning his or her sterile gown, gloves, mask, and cap. Assist in preparing the patient for the procedure; prep the patient with 4×4 sponges and a povidone-iodine solution, and apply sterile drapes to the patient's thorax for the procedure.

4. Ensure that the thoracotomy tray is opened, using sterile technique, and is awaiting the surgeon when he or she is ready to perform the procedure. Using sterile technique, prepare yourself or an assistant to perform the duties of a scrub nurse—to hand the surgeon the instruments as needed. Another nurse must monitor the patient's vital signs and continually assess the patient during the procedure.

5. Cardiopulmonary resuscitation must be stopped during the time that the incision is made but will be continued internally after the chest has been opened.

Physician Actions

After the patient is prepped and draped, the physician makes a skin incision with the scalpel. The incision is a left thoracotomy incision made at the fourth or fifth intercostal space and can be extended to the right. Occasionally the incision is a mediastinal approach, but spreading the ribs is much easier than sawing the sternum. Next, either the sternal chisel and mallet are used to make a mediastinal opening or the fascia is cut away and the rib spreaders are used to gain access to the heart.

- Occasionally a rib must be cut away, using the bone cutter, for better visualization.
- The physician looks for the source of bleeding and will need lap sponges and 4×4 sponges to dry the area. When the source

of bleeding is found, the physician will need a variety of clamps and sutures to close the bleeding vessel.
6. Be prepared to perform internal defibrillation; be sure that the defibrillator is in working order. Have the surgeon hand the defibrillator end of the cable to someone, so it can be properly attached to the defibrillator and be ready when the chest is open.

Physician Actions
The internal defibrillator paddles are placed on each ventricle. The maximum amount of energy that can be delivered internally is 20 joules.
- Be ready to perform internal cardiac massage and internal defibrillation as ordered by the physician.
- If the surgeon is successful in resuscitating the patient, be ready to proceed to the operating room for further evaluation of the patient's injuries.
- The surgeon may place a Foley catheter in the heart to tamponade the bleeding if there is a visible hole in the heart or aorta, or it may be placed for fluid resuscitation if the heart is flat (without any circulating volume). IV fluids given through this catheter must be warmed.

Physician Actions
If the patient is successfully resuscitated, the physician will sterilely drape the patient and proceed to the operating room; the physician will not close the chest in the emergency department.

PATIENT CARE MANAGEMENT

1. Continuously assess and monitor the trend of the patient's vital signs, noting any return of pulse, blood pressure, or cardiac electrical activity.
2. Monitor the fluid resuscitation that continues throughout this procedure.
3. Note the amount of energy used with each internal defibrillation attempt (up to 20 joules).
4. Note any change in the patient's condition during this procedure. This additional data may help the surgeon in diagnosing a specific correctable problem.
5. The patient may need to be transported to the operating room while internal cardiac massage is ongoing. If this occurs, try to maintain sterility as much as possible. Cover the patient with a sterile sheet if possible.

6. If the patient has an indwelling Foley catheter in the heart to tamponade bleeding or for fluid resuscitation, make sure that the balloon is inflated and that it is not dislodged during the procedure or during transport.

POTENTIAL COMPLICATIONS

The most common outcome of this procedure is death. Complications include further injury to the thorax, exsanguination, and further myocardial and pleural injury.

16 procedure

External Jugular Intravenous Access

Elizabeth Clark

DESCRIPTION

The external jugular vein runs in a line from the angle of the jaw to the junction of the medial and middle thirds of the clavicle (Figure P16-1, *A*).[1] Intravenous cannulation of the external jugular vein provides peripheral venous access through standard IV insertion techniques.

INDICATIONS

- External jugular cannulation is indicated to obtain peripheral venous access in children and adults when no suitable sites are available on the extremities.
- External jugular access may be used for fluid, blood, and medication administration, as well as for obtaining venous specimens.

CONTRAINDICATIONS/CAUTIONS

- External jugular cannulation is contraindicated in patients who have penetrating neck wounds, significant blunt trauma to the neck, or soft-tissue damage to the neck.
- The head should not be turned if there is a possibility of a cervical spine injury. This makes insertion more difficult. One person must maintain manual in-line cervical spine stabilization throughout the procedure.
- Caution should be used in pediatric patients to ensure that the airway is not compromised during the procedure by turning of the head.
- Caution must be used in patients who may have difficulty tolerating the supine position.

EQUIPMENT

- Antiseptic solution
- Local anesthetic (optional)

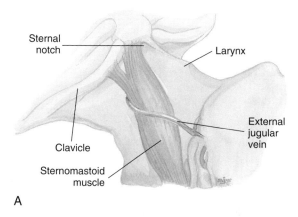

Sternal notch

Larynx

Clavicle

Sternomastoid muscle

External jugular vein

A

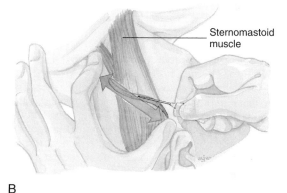

Sternomastoid muscle

B

Figure P16-1 A, Anatomy of external jugular vein. **B,** External jugular venipuncture. (From Sanders MJ: *Mosby's paramedic textbook,* ed 2, St Louis, 2003, Mosby.)

- IV tubing and fluid
- Appropriate IV catheter
- Tape
- Dressing supplies

INITIAL NURSING ACTIONS

1. Assemble the necessary equipment.
2. Place the patient in a supine, head-down position. This will promote venous filling and prevent air embolism.

3. Turn the patient's head to the side opposite the cannulation site.
4. Clean the skin with antiseptic solution.
5. To anchor the vein, place the opposite thumb over the distal portion, just under the mandible. Place the opposite index finger over the proximal end of the vein, just above the clavicle, to produce a tourniquet effect (Figure P16-1, *B*).
6. Align the cannula with the vein and puncture midway between the angle of the jaw and the clavicle.
7. When blood is returned, advance the catheter off the needle until the hub is securely against the skin.
8. Attach IV tubing and initiate fluid. Monitor for signs of infiltration.
9. Secure the catheter with tape and apply dressing. Secure IV tubing with tape to prevent accidental discontinuation.

PATIENT CARE MANAGEMENT

1. Frequently evaluate the external jugular line site for signs of infiltration, and discontinue fluid immediately if signs are present. Extravasation of fluid and vasoactive medications into the neck is a serious complication; thus diligent monitoring is required.
2. Evaluate the site daily for signs of infection and be prepared to change the IV site and administer antibiotics if signs are present.
3. Observe for the presence of a hematoma at the insertion site, especially in patients who are receiving anticoagulation therapy. Airway compromise can appear rapidly in these cases.
4. Monitor for signs of pulmonary embolism, such as dyspnea, sudden onset of pleuritic chest pain, tachypnea, and tachycardia. The patient should be placed in a supine, head-down position any time the IV tubing is disconnected from the catheter hub and when the catheter is discontinued.
5. Application of a cervical collar over the site is acceptable if there is suspicion of a cervical spine injury.

REFERENCES

1. Hasting D: Fluid resuscitation skills. In Campbell JE, ed: *Basic trauma life support for paramedics and other advanced providers,* ed 4, Upper Saddle River, NJ, 2000, Brady/Prentice Hall Health.

procedure *17*

Eye Irrigation

Mark B. Parshall

INDICATIONS

- Dilution or decontamination of chemicals or injuries
- Removal of debris (e.g., dust) from the eyes

CONTRAINDICATIONS

- Open or impaled globe

EQUIPMENT

- Eyewash fountain or eyewash/facewash fountain (if available)
- Ophthalmic topical anesthetic drops
- pH test strips (if acid or alkali exposure)
- 1 to 2 L of normal saline or Ringer's lactate per eye
- Standard drip IV tubing (e.g., 10 to 15 drops/ml)
- Hair wash tray, sink, or Chux to divert runoff
- Irrigating lens (Morgan lens) (optional)
- Lid retractors (optional)
- Towels and gloves

INITIAL NURSING ACTIONS

1. Explain the procedure to the patient.
2. Assess visual acuity (see Procedure 36) unless a corrosive chemical injury is suspected.
3. Instill a topical anesthetic as prescribed by the physician.
4. Pediatric patients may need to have hands restrained during the procedure.

EYEWASH FOUNTAIN OR EYE/FACEWASH

If an eyewash fountain is available, instruct the patient to place his or her face in the middle of the two streams so that water is flushing over the eyes and lids. Instruct the patient to blink his or her eyes in the streams and look in all directions with the eyes open. Continue for at least 15 minutes. According to the American National Standards Institute (ANSI: Standard Z358.1, 1998) an eyewash fountain should be capable of delivering at least 1.5 L/min (0.4 gal/min) to both eyes simultaneously.[1] This is a substantially higher flow than can be achieved by manual irrigation or irrigating lenses. Eyewash/facewash fountains have an even higher flow rate over a larger area.

Manual Irrigation

1. Position the patient to catch runoff, and drape clothing with Chux or towels to keep from getting wet. Topically anesthetize the eyes.
2. Gently retract the lids with your nondominant hand. If the lids are swollen, an assistant may be necessary. A Desmarres lid retractor may be used.
3. Begin the flow of irrigant through the IV tubing, holding the distal end of the tubing in the dominant hand. The irrigant should be free flowing, not dripping. The rate can be adjusted to patient comfort.
4. Direct the flow in all directions on the anterior globe. The lower conjunctival fornix can be exposed by gentle traction on the lower lid. The palpebral conjunctiva of the upper lid can be exposed by a retractor, by gentle traction, or by eversion over an applicator swab.
5. In general, a liter of irrigant to each eye that needs irrigation is sufficient, except in the case of corrosives (strong acids or alkali), for which the amount of irrigant needed depends on the conjunctival pH (see Chapter 12).

Irrigation Via an Irrigating Contact Lens (Morgan Lens)[2,3]

1. Explain the equipment to the patient and instill a topical anesthetic. Position and drape the patient.
2. Attach IV tubing to the extension on the irrigating lens.
3. Run a small amount of irrigant over the ocular surface of the lens to lubricate.
4. Ask the patient to look down. When the patient looks down, grasp the extension tubing of the lens and slip the lens under the upper lid. The lens should go into the upper portion of the eye without resistance.
5. Ask the patient to look up. With your free hand, gently retract the lower lid until the lower lid is outside the margin of the lens. Release the lid so that it covers the lower part of the lens.
6. Open the flow clamp and adjust the rate to patient comfort. Irrigate with 1 to 2 L of Ringer's lactate or saline per eye.

7. To remove the lens, ask the patient to look up. Retract the lower lid gently. The lens will pop off the ocular surface. Ask the patient to look down. When the patient looks down, slide the lens out from under the upper lid.

PATIENT CARE MANAGEMENT

1. An eye shower achieves much higher volumes at relatively lower pressure than other methods. If the ED does not have an eye shower, often the hospital laboratory does. Use of the shower may be followed by use of an irrigating lens or by manual irrigation.
2. Apart from the eye shower, other methods of irrigation are safest if the patient is supine.
3. Y-connectors are available for the Morgan lens so that the nurse can irrigate both eyes simultaneously from one bag of irrigant and one infusion set. When the Y-connector is used, the volume of irrigant should be doubled (e.g., a minimum of 2 L should be used if 1 L per eye is desired). Independent setups also can be used for each eye if needed.
4. Most patients tolerate the Morgan lens well, but a few do not. The nurse should remain with the patient or close at hand in case the patient becomes restless or frightened.
5. The Morgan lens comes with clear instructions in each lens packet. It is a good idea to post the package insert wherever eye irrigation is regularly performed in the ED.

REFERENCES

1. Cameron M: Guide to emergency eyewashes and showers, *Occup Health Saf* 71 (5):112, 2002.
2. Quigley MT: Eye irrigation. In Proehl JA: *Emergency nursing procedures,* ed 3, St Louis, 2004, Mosby.
3. Ramponi D: Go with the flow during an eye emergency, *Nursing 2000* 30 (8):54-56, 2000.

18 procedure

Fluid Administration

Donna Arvin Isfort

DESCRIPTION

Intravenous fluid administration may be required for volume resuscitation, administration of maintenance fluids, or possible administration of drugs.

INDICATIONS

1. Potential for administration of IV medications
2. History or physical exam findings consistent with hypovolemia related to illness or injury
   - History
     - Vomiting and diarrhea
     - Bleeding
     - Poor oral intake
   - Physical exam
     - Fever
     - Tachycardia and hypotension are signs of reduced vascular volume.
     - Orthostatic blood pressure and pulse may indicate hypovolemia when a change occurs in heart rate (greater than 20 beats/min) or systolic blood pressure (greater than 20 mm Hg) between position changes.
     - Skin color, temperature, and turgor
     - Cool, clammy skin indicates vasoconstriction and the need to shunt blood to core organs (e.g., heart and brain).
     - Poor skin turgor and dry mucous membranes suggest dehydration.
     - Capillary refill greater than 2 seconds may indicate hypovolemia (unless the patient is a geriatric individual noted to have peripheral vascular disease or hypothermia).
     - Altered level of consciousness
     - Restlessness and irritability are the first indications of decreasing blood volume. Lethargy and decreased

responsiveness occur later related to decreased cerebral oxygenation.

EQUIPMENT

- Protective gear for the caregiver
- Appropriate sizes of IV catheters (consider the size of the patient and the reason for fluid administration)
- IV fluids chosen according to need (Table P18-1)
- IV tubing and extension set chosen according to need
- Antiseptic solution
- Dressings for IV site
- IV additives: drugs and electrolytes
- Blood tubes if serum specimens are needed

INITIAL NURSING ACTIONS

Fluid Resuscitation

1. Initiate two large-bore IV lines (14-gauge to 16-gauge, 1.25-inch–long catheter for adults, 22-gauge catheter or greater for pediatric patients) with Ringer's lactate or normal saline.
2. For maximizing fluid administration, use the largest diameter tubing available. Trauma tubing is preferable. If trauma tubing is not available, blood-infusion tubing may be used. If regular IV tubing is used, use a Maxi-drip set.
3. Obtain a specimen for a complete blood count, coagulation studies, electrolyte levels, and possible type and crossmatch simultaneously.

⋙ NURSING ALERT ⋘

Attempts to gain IV access must not interfere with efforts to correct problems with airway or breathing.

---

4. Consider placement of an intraosseous needle in a child if you are unable to access a vein (Procedure 21). The usual site for intraosseous infusion is the proximal tibia. The distal femur can be used in infants. Colloids, crystalloids, and medications can be administered through the intraosseous line. An intraosseous infusion site should be considered a temporary measure for use during emergencies and resuscitation. When the patient is stabilized, venous access should be obtained and the intraosseous infusion

TABLE P18-1 IV Fluids

Solution Type	Examples	Uses	Cautions
Isotonic (Similar to osmolarity of serum. Remains in intravascular compartment.)	0.9% normal saline (NS) Lactated Ringer's (LR) or Ringer's lactate	• Volume expander used in hypovolemia • Packed red blood cell administration • Volume expander used in hypovolemia and acute blood loss	• Risk of fluid overload, especially in CHF and hypertension. • Lactate is equivalent to bicarbonate, so it should not be used if the patient has a preexisting alkalosis.
Hypotonic (Less osmolarity than serum. Pulls water from the intravascular space into the interstitial space.)	NS 0.45% NS 0.2% Dextrose 5% in water (D₅W)	• Shifts water into intracellular spaces • Used for maintenance fluid if patient is at risk for free water loss • May be used for adult patients for IV admixture	• D₅W can cause increased ICP due to the shift of fluids. • D₅W may cause hyperglycemia and electrolyte dilution if used for fluid resuscitation. • 0.45% NS can cause increased ICP and fluid overload.
Hypertonic (Higher osmolarity than serum. Pulls fluid from the intracellular and interstitial spaces into the intravascular space.)	Dextrose 5% in NS Dextrose 5% in 0.45% NS 3% Saline Dextrose 10% in NS Dextrose 10% in water Dextrose 20% in water	• Shifts fluid from intracellular space to extracellular space • Used for maintenance fluid • Increases sodium osmolality • Used to treat hyponatremia • Use in water intoxication states created by too much hypotonic fluid administration • To promote diuresis	• D10% and D20% solutions may irritate the vein and should be given through a central line if possible. • 3% saline should be infused slowly as it can cause pulmonary edema due to increased intravascular volume.

Reference: Smeltzer SC and Bare BG: *Brunner & Suddarth textbook of medical surgical nursing*, ed 6, Philadelphia, 2004, Lippincott Williams & Wilkins, p 259.

line should be removed. This will help reduce the possibility of osteomyelitis.
5. Anticipate the need for administering blood products. Set up IV blood administration tubing and prime with normal saline (Reference Guide 3). Obtain a blood warmer or rapid infusion device. The shortest possible IV tubing should be used to ensure that fluid remains warm upon entry at a slower infusion rate.

Maintenance Fluid and IV Drug Administration
1. Insert a 20-gauge or larger IV catheter in the adult and a 24-gauge or larger IV catheter in infants and children with appropriate IV fluid as ordered.
2. See Reference Guide 5 for medication administration formulas and Reference Guide 9 for fluid administration formulas.

PATIENT CARE MANAGEMENT
1. Ensure IV lines remain patent.
2. The level of consciousness improves or remains at baseline. A Glasgow Coma Scale score (see Reference Guide 10 for adults and Reference Guide 16 for children and infants) should be documented and monitored throughout the emergency department (ED) stay.
3. Monitor hemorrhage. Facilitate patient transport to the OR if necessary.
4. Monitor arterial blood gas results.
5. The patient must be reassessed frequently because subtle and rapid changes may occur. Areas that should be reassessed include: vital signs and orthostatic vital signs; pulses; capillary refill; skin color, temperature, and condition; and breath sounds.
6. As the patient becomes normovolemic, urine output should improve. Normal urinary output varies by age as follows: infants (2 to 3 ml/kg/hr), toddlers, (2 ml/kg/hr), school age (1 to 2 ml/kg/hr), and adults (0.5 to 1 ml/kg/hr).
7. Specific gravity should be checked to assess the concentration of urine. A specific gravity of greater than 1.015 may be indicative of decreased fluid volume or an increase in solutes causing osmotic diuresis.
8. Monitor for signs of fluid overload (see Box P18-1). Symptoms of fluid overload may not appear immediately after IV fluid administration. The development of edema, dyspnea, and

tachycardia may indicate the decreased ability of the heart to manage the circulating blood volume.

9. Monitor hemodynamic readings, if available.

BOX P18-1   SIGNS OF FLUID OVERLOAD

- Dyspnea, crackles on auscultation
- Tachycardia, distended neck veins
- Diaphoresis, edema
- Increased central venous pressure and pulmonary wedge pressure

procedure *19*

Gastric Tube Insertion and Lavage

Ronald Stewart Gray

DESCRIPTION

Gastric intubation is a procedure performed often in the emergency department. In gastric intubation, a tube is inserted through either the nose or the mouth into the stomach for gastric evacuation or lavage. Lavage removes blood and clots in patients who have upper gastrointestinal bleeding.

INDICATIONS

1. Remove gastric contents and suppress vomiting. Assess for presence of blood.
2. Remove toxic substances
3. Prevent gastric dilation and aspiration
4. Instill radiopaque contrast media
5. Perform therapeutic or diagnostic gastric lavage

CONTRAINDICATIONS

1. Insertion of a gastric tube in patients who have ingested a caustic substance (e.g., acid or lye) may cause further esophageal damage.
2. Nasogastric tubes should not be inserted in patients who have massive facial trauma or a basilar skull fracture. In such cases, the tube should be inserted orally.

EQUIPMENT

Gastric tubes are also known as Levin, Salem-sump, Ewald, and Levacuator tubes. The Salem-sump tube has a vent lumen that allows for controlled suction force at the drainage openings. The sump tube also is less likely to become lodged against the stomach wall.

- Water-soluble lubricant
- 60-ml piston syringe, irrigation bulb syringe, or Toomey syringe

---

NURSING ALERT

The size and type of tube used depend on the reason for placement. For adult patients who have active upper gastrointestinal bleeding, a large-bore tube (32 to 36 Fr) should be inserted through the mouth.

- Emesis basin
- Tape
- Stethoscope
- Suction equipment
- Gloves
- Normal saline

INITIAL NURSING ACTIONS

1. Explain the procedure to the patient.
2. If the patient is alert, place the patient in a high Fowler's position.

NURSING ALERT

Maintain spinal immobilization in trauma patients. Have suction readily available. Be prepared to logroll the patient if vomiting occurs.

Nasogastric Placement

1. Measure the distance of insertion by placing the tip of the tube at the patient's nose and following the length of the tubing to the ear and then from the ear to the xiphoid process. Mark the tubing at this point.
2. Examine the nose and select the larger naris. If the patient is alert, ask whether he or she has any history of nasal fracture. Use the unaffected side if possible.
3. Lubricate the end of the tube with a water-soluble lubricant. Lidocaine jelly may be used to lubricate the tube and anesthetize the nasal tract if the patient is not allergic to lidocaine.
4. Insert the tube into the nostril at a 60-degree to 90-degree angle to the plane of the face.
5. When the tube is in the oropharynx, have the patient flex the head forward slightly and swallow several times. If possible,

have the patient swallow a few sips of water through a straw. Advance the tube (while the patient swallows) to the previously marked point.

NURSING ALERT

If the tube slips into the trachea, violent coughing will ensue. Withdraw the tube into the oropharynx and try again to advance the tube into the esophagus and stomach.

Orogastric Placement

1. If the patient is alert, place the patient in a high Fowler's position. Once placed, if a lavage is to be performed, place the patient on the left side in a slight Trendelenburg position to promote the return of lavage fluid and to prevent aspiration.
2. Measure the distance of insertion by placing the tip of the tube at the lips. Follow the length of the tubing to the angle of the jaw and then from the jaw to the xiphoid process. Mark the tubing at that point.
3. If the patient is uncooperative, place a bite block in the mouth to prevent the patient from biting the tube.
4. Lubricate the tip of the tube, and pass it gently over the tongue, aiming down and back toward the pharynx.

NURSING ALERT

For toxic ingestions, a size 36 to 40 French gastric tube should be considered.

---

5. Flex the patient's head forward, and advance the tube when the patient swallows.

NURSING ALERT

Do not flex the head if there is a possibility of a cervical spine injury.

Confirmation of Tube Placement

1. Verify proper placement by aspirating gastric contents or by injecting 20 to 30 ml of air (with a piston, bulb, or Toomey syringe) into the tube while listening over the stomach with a stethoscope for a pronounced gurgling sound.

2. Secure the tube with tape or a gastric tube holder. Do not tape the tube to the forehead because this places pressure on the nares.

PATIENT CARE MANAGEMENT

1. Connect the tube to low wall suction, usually described as 40 to 60 mm Hg or as prescribed by the physician.
2. Lavage may be needed for patients who have upper gastrointestinal bleeding or who have ingested a toxic substance.
   - Pour normal saline solution into a container. For patients who have GI bleeding, the use of iced saline is controversial. Some clinicians prefer using room-temperature tap water on the grounds that it breaks up clots better and does not reduce core body temperature as much.
   - Instill 150 to 200 ml (the actual volume is controversial) of fluid in an adult patient by a piston or catheter-tip syringe. Gently withdraw the fluid with the syringe and discard the fluid into a measured basin. For pediatric patients, 10 ml/kg of lavage solution is used.
   - Continue the lavage until the fluid returns clear or an endoscopy is performed. Prepackaged gastric lavage kits that can be connected to suction are commercially available.
3. Consider giving the patient anesthetic throat lozenges or spray to relieve throat discomfort caused by the tube.

► NURSING ALERT ◄

Verify placement of the nasogastric tube every 4 hours, after each transfer, and before administration of medication, contrast media, or fluid through the tube.

REFERENCE

1. Rossoll LW: Insertion of orogastric and nasogastric tubes. In Proehl JA, ed: *Emergency nursing procedures*, ed 3, Philadelphia, 2004, WB Saunders, pp 469-473.

procedure 20

Intracranial Pressure Monitoring

Linda Murray
Lisa Fryman

DESCRIPTION

Intracranial pressure (ICP) monitoring produces continuous
data about the pressure exerted within the cranial vault.
The most common tools for measuring ICP are the
intraventricular and the intraparenchymal catheters. Measurement
of ICP is best achieved by use of an intraventricular catheter
placed into the anterior horn of the lateral ventricle of the
nondominant hemisphere (right hemisphere in most humans).
An advantage of intraventricular catheter placement is that
cerebrospinal fluid (CSF) can be withdrawn to help control
the patient's ICP.

The normal ICP is 0 to 15 mm Hg. Cerebral perfusion
pressure (CPP) can be calculated if the ICP is known. CPP is an
indirect measurement of cerebral blood flow and is calculated by
subtracting the ICP from the mean arterial pressure (MAP).
Normal CPP is considered 60 to 100 mm Hg. Maintaining a
CPP above 70 mm Hg in the brain-injured patient may reduce
mortality and improve quality of survival.[1]

INDICATIONS

ICP monitoring is appropriate in:
1. Patients with a severe head injury (Glasgow Coma Scale score
   of 8 or less) and an abnormal admission CT scan (contusions,
   hematomas, edema, compressed basal cisterns)[1]
2. Patients with a severe brain injury (Glasgow Coma Scale score
   of 8 or less) and a normal admission CT scan if two or more
   of the following apply:
   - Age over 40 years
   - Motor posturing (unilateral or bilateral)
   - Systolic blood pressure of less than 90 mm Hg[1]

CONTRAINDICATIONS/CAUTIONS

1. ICP monitoring is not routinely indicated with mild to moderate brain injury.[1]
2. Coagulopathies, such as an elevated PT/PTT, should be corrected before the procedure is initiated.
3. Generalized cerebral edema resulting in small, compressed ventricles may preclude the use of a ventricular catheter.

EQUIPMENT

- Sterile gloves and gowns, masks, caps, and sterile drapes
- Razor
- Antiseptic solution
- Local anesthetic
- 5-ml to 10-ml syringes and different sizes of needles
- Transducer cable, module, and monitor
- Pressure transducer and tubing for appropriate monitoring system
- Nonbacteriostatic normal saline (NS)
- Suture material, needle holder, and pickups
- Antibiotic ointment and a dressing with an occlusive covering
- ICP insertion tray; commercially prepared trays are available and usually include:
  - ○ Twist drill and bits
  - ○ Needle holder
  - ○ Sharp, blunt scissors
  - ○ Knife handle and scalpel (no. 11 blade)
  - ○ 4 × 4 sponges
  - ○ ICP catheter: intraventricular catheter or an intraparenchymal catheter
  - ○ CSF drainage system
- IV pole for drainage system. Pole should be stationary (i.e., attached to the bed) to prevent inadvertent dislodgment of catheter.
- Sedatives and/or analgesics

INITIAL NURSING ACTIONS

1. Document a preprocedure neurologic assessment.
2. Prepare the patient. Explain the procedure; administer analgesics, sedatives, and neuromuscular blocking agents as ordered.
3. Prepare the transducer and monitoring system according to the manufacturer's instructions using strict aseptic technique. If a system requires flushing, a preservative-free

(nonbacteriostatic) 0.9% sodium chloride solution should be used.

4. Elevate the head of the bed 20 to 30 degrees.[2] The neck should be kept in a neutral position. Place a protective barrier under the head.

5. Maintain the position of the transducer at the level of the top of the ear, which corresponds to the foramen of Monro (Figure P20-1). Set the system to zero. If the system is a fluid-coupled system, the transducer can be zeroed either before insertion or after insertion of the monitoring device as long as it is zeroed before ICP pressure monitoring begins.

≥ NURSING ALERT ≤

The sterility of the system must be preserved at all times. Aseptic technique must be maintained throughout the procedure.

≥ NURSING ALERT ≤

Never place a transducer with a flushing device in an ICP monitoring set-up, such as one that would be used for an arterial line or a pulmonary artery (PA) catheter.

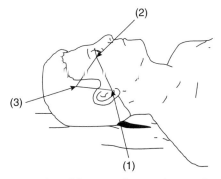

Figure P20-1 Location of foramen of Monro for transducer placement. Map an imaginary equilateral triangle from (1) the external auditory meatus, to (2) the outer canthus of the eye, to (3) behind the hairline. Point 3 is the location of the foramen of Monro. (From Stillwell S: *Mosby's critical care nursing reference,* St Louis, 2002, Mosby.)

Fiberoptic and sensor systems must be zeroed before insertion of the monitoring device.[3]

6. Ensure monitoring systems have been correctly connected and calibrated.

7. Don sterile attire and drape the patient as needed.

8. The physician will shave the patient's hair and prep the insertion site with an antiseptic solution. Depending on the patient's condition and the urgency of the situation, lidocaine may be injected to anesthetize the insertion site. Utilizing sterile technique, a twist drill is used to make a burr hole anterior to the coronal suture at the level of the mid-pupillary line, and the catheter is inserted. The distal end of the catheter is sutured to the scalp after a good waveform has been obtained.

9. Assess waveform and record the opening pressure. Calculate CPP.

10. Place antibacterial ointment around the insertion site as directed by the physician. Cover the site with a sterile occlusive dressing.

11. Reassess the patient's neurologic status.

12. Document the neurologic assessment, type of procedure performed, location of the catheter, and patient's response.

If a CSF drainage system is to be used, these additional actions must be performed:

1. After the intraventricular catheter is inserted, the distal end is connected to the transducer and the CSF drainage system (Figure P20-2).

2. A cord attached to the drainage bag allows for the external CSF drainage collection system to be suspended from the IV pole. Ideally, the IV pole should be attached to the bed to reduce the possibility of accidental dislodgment if the IV pole is moved.

3. A drip chamber, which is similar in appearance to the drip chamber on IV tubing, is found on the external CSF drainage system. The drip chamber should be placed 10 to 20 cm above the level of the foramen of Monro, or as ordered by the physician.

4. CSF can be drained intermittently or continuously, as prescribed. With intermittent drainage, the system is turned for drainage when the ICP reaches a certain level. The physician usually orders drainage of CSF when the ICP is 20 mm Hg or greater.[1] The system should be turned off to drainage when the prescribed level of ICP has been reached.

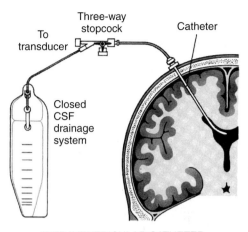

INTRAVENTRICULAR CATHETER

Figure P20-2   Intraventricular catheter (IVC) monitoring system with a closed CSF drainage system. (From Barker E: Intracranial pressure and monitoring. In Barker E, ed: *Neuroscience nursing, a spectrum of care*, ed 2, St Louis, 2002, Mosby, p 394.)

⋙ NURSING ALERT ⋘

Lowering the external CSF drainage bag below 10 to 20 cm above the level of the foramen of Monro can cause free flow of CSF and can result in vascular collapse and subdural hematoma.

---

5. Document characteristics of CSF (clarity, color, and amount of drainage).

PATIENT CARE MANAGEMENT

1. Elevate the head of the bed to 15 to 30 degrees (unless contraindicated) and maintain the head and neck in a neutral position to promote venous drainage. Avoid extreme flexion of the hips, which can increase intraabdominal pressures and impede drainage from the brain.
2. Evaluate and record a mean intracranial pressure hourly unless otherwise prescribed. The mean ICP reading should be

obtained at end expiration to avoid the intrathoracic pressure effects on the cerebral venous system.[4]

3. Avoid kinks in the drainage system.

4. Evaluate and document the clarity, color, and amount of CSF drainage.

5. Ensure the integrity of the system to prevent the entrance of air and infection-causing organisms. Keep all stopcocks capped and use Luer-Lock connections. Air bubbles in the system will affect the displayed pressure reading.

6. Assess CSF system drainage patency. Notify the physician if there is no CSF drainage in the presence of elevated ICP.

7. Maintain the transducer at the level of the foramen of Monro (Figure P20-1).

8. Monitor the ICP waveform and document the mean pressure. The ICP waveform consists of three major peaks (Figure P20-3, Table P20-1). Additional peaks may be present in some patients. If P_2 is higher than P_1, suspect decreased compliance. Compliance is the ability of the brain to accommodate changes in volume (brain tissue, blood, or CSF). If volume continues to increase and the brain can no longer make alterations to accommodate the increased volume, compliance decreases and the pressure within the cranial vault rises. Pressure rising in the cranial vault affects arterial and venous pressures, which is reflected in the ICP waveform.

9. Notify the physician if loss of waveform occurs or if abnormal waveforms are noted on a waveform trend (Table P20-2 and Figure P20-4).

10. If the patient needs suctioning, make sure the ICP drainage system is closed to the patient before initiating the suctioning procedure to prevent unnecessary drainage of CSF.

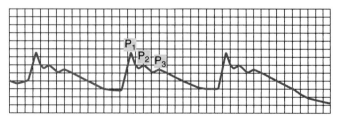

Figure P20-3 Intracranial pressure waveform components. (From Stillwell S: *Mosby's critical care nursing reference,* ed 3, St Louis, 2002, Mosby.)

TABLE P20-1   Three Peaks of the ICP Waveform: P_1, P_2, and P_3

P_1: Percussion wave	Reflective of arterial pressure: myocardial systole	• Sharply peaked • Consistent in amplitude • Changes with extreme hypotension and hypertension
P_2: Tidal wave	Reflective of cerebral compliance	• Terminates at the dicrotic notch • More variable • Considered the most clinically significant wave. As ICP increases, P_2 will increase until it becomes taller than P_1, which is indicative of a loss of cerebral compliance.
P_3: Dicrotic wave	Reflective of venous pressure	• Immediately follows the dicrotic notch and slopes into the diastolic baseline

From Barker E: Intracranial pressure and monitoring. In Barker E. ed: *Neuroscience nursing, a spectrum of care*, ed 2, St Louis, 2002, Mosby; and Sullivan J: Intraventricular catheter insertion (assist), monitoring, care, troubleshooting and removal. In Lynn-McHale DJ and Carlson KK, eds: *AACN procedure manual for critical care*, ed 4, Philadelphia, 2001, WB Saunders, pp 561-569.

11. Set the fluid-coupled transducer system to zero at the level of the foramen of Monro every shift (or as the manufacturer recommends), after position changes, or when there is a sudden change in the ICP reading or waveform. (Fiberoptic and sensor systems cannot be re-zeroed after catheter placement.)

12. See Table P20-3 for troubleshooting of the ICP monitor and appropriate nursing actions.

13. Assess for signs and symptoms of rising intracranial pressure (see Chapter 15) and manage as indicated.

14. Prophylactic antibiotics may be ordered by the physician to prevent brain infection.

TABLE P20-2 Waves that May Be Seen With Trending of the ICP Waveform (5-min to 60-min Time Frames)

A waves: plateau waves	• Produced by secondary changes in cerebral blood volume • Sudden transient elevations of 50 to 100 mm Hg from an already elevated ICP	• The most life-threatening and dangerous waves; indicative of worsening intracranial hypertension • Correlate with a patient who has cerebral hypoxia/ischemia • Often accompanied by neurologic deterioration or herniation • Last 5 to 20 minutes
B waves	• Correspond to fluctuations in arterial blood pressure related to respiratory cycle • Sharp spikes of 20 to 50 mm Hg	• Occur every 30 to 60 seconds • Intermittent elevation in pressure that is not sustained • Tend to be associated with a decrease in LOC • May precede A waves
C waves	• Low-amplitude fluctuations associated with changes in arterial pressure • Pressure up to 20 mm Hg	• Occur at intervals of 4 to 8 minutes • Significance unknown

From Barker E: Intracranial pressure and monitoring. In Barker E, ed: *Neuroscience nursing, a spectrum of care*, ed 2, St Louis, 2002, Mosby; and Sullivan J: Intraventricular catheter insertion (assist), monitoring, care, troubleshooting and removal. In Lynn-McHale DJ and Carlson KK, eds: *AACN procedure manual for critical care*, ed 4, Philadelphia, 2001, WB Saunders, pp 561-569.

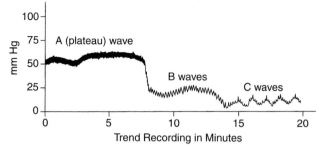

Figure P20-4 Intracranial pressure waves. Composite diagram of, **A**, plateau waves; **B**, sawtooth waves; and **C**, small, rhythmic waves. (From Barker E: *Neuroscience nursing, a spectrum of care*, ed 2, St Louis, 2002, Mosby, p 395.)

TABLE P20-3	Troubleshooting for ICP Monitoring
Problem	**Action**
No waveform or dampened waveform	• Check all connections, power source, and gain setting. • Assess for air bubbles, clots, or debris in the system.

High-pressure reading	• Ensure transducer level placement.
	• Check calibration and repeat zeroing procedure.
	• Evaluate the patient, and implement measures to perform the following:
	  • Assess airway, ventilator settings, and ABGs for hypoxemia and hypercarbia.
	  • Ensure elevation of the head of the bed by 15 to 30 degrees or as indicated by the physician.
	  • Maintain neutral position of head (avoid extreme rotation).
	  • Limit flexion in lower extremities and hips.
	  • Monitor for excess muscle activity, and if present administer muscle relaxants and/or paralytics as ordered.
	  • Assess for abdominal distention, and decompress as necessary.
	  • Observe for sources of noxious stimuli, and remove if noted.

Continued

TABLE P20-3	Troubleshooting for ICP Monitoring—cont'd
Problem	**Action**
	• Avoid hyperthermia; administer antipyretics as needed.
	• Monitor pulmonary artery pressure, cardiac output, Svo_2 (pulmonary artery oximetry), and blood pressure for elevation and treat as indicated.
	• Prevent electrolyte imbalance.
Low-pressure reading	• Check transducer level placement (Figure P20-1).
	• Assess for the presence of otorrhea or rhinorrhea.
	• Check for dislodged or kinked catheter and notify physician if present.

REFERENCES

1. Brain Trauma Foundation: *Management guidelines of severe traumatic brain injury*, 2000, retrieved July, 2004, www2.braintrauma.org/guidelines/.
2. Barker E: Intracranial pressure and monitoring. In Barker E, ed: *Neuroscience nursing, a spectrum of care*, ed 2, St Louis, 2002, Mosby, pp 379-408.
3. Sullivan J: Intraventricular catheter insertion (assist), monitoring, care troubleshooting and removal. In Lynn-McHale DJ and Carlson KK, eds: *AACN procedure manual for critical care*, ed 4, Philadelphia, 2001, WB Saunders, pp 561-569.
4. Stillwell SB: *Critical care nursing reference*, ed 3, St Louis, 2002, Mosby, pp 501-506.

procedure *21*

Intraosseous Infusion

Elizabeth Clark

DESCRIPTION

Intraosseous infusion (IO) is used for emergent fluid and medication administration in patients of all ages when attempts at venous access have been unsuccessful. In critical situations, an attempt is considered unsuccessful after two failed punctures or 90 seconds. Traditionally, IO access has been reserved for children, but it is becoming used more widely in the management of adults. Currently, there are no formal guidelines for the use of intraosseous access in adult patients. Additional research is needed before its efficacy can be definitively determined. There is minimal risk of complications if the procedure is performed properly and appropriately. Colloids, crystalloids, and medications that can be administered intravenously can be administered intraosseously. Intraosseous access is a temporary measure and should be replaced with venous access as soon as possible.[1,2]

INDICATIONS

Intraosseous cannulation is indicated in any critical situation in which fluid and/or medications must be administered immediately to a patient with no venous access.

CONTRAINDICATIONS/CAUTIONS

- An IO should not be placed in an extremity with an acute or recent fracture.
- Bone disorders such as osteoporosis and osteogenesis imperfecta are contraindications for establishment of IO access.
- Marrow-toxic drugs should not be infused via an IO site.
- An IO catheter should not be placed through infected or burned skin.

COMPLICATIONS

Potential complications associated with IO insertion are tibial fractures, puncture through the posterior cortex, fat embolism, infection, and clot formation.

EQUIPMENT

- Appropriate IV administration set and IV fluid
- Specifically designed IO needles, such as the Cook or Sur Fast brands, bone-injection guns, or Jamshidi-type bone-aspiration needles (spinal needles and standard hypodermic needles may be used but are not recommended because they bend easily and are easily clogged with bone marrow).
- Antiseptic solution
- Syringe for aspiration
- Tape
- Gauze
- Dressing supplies

INITIAL NURSING ACTIONS

1. Assemble the necessary equipment.
2. Prepare the site with antiseptic solution. The most common site is 1 to 2 cm or approximately two fingerbreadths below and medial to the tibial tuberosity (Figure P21-1). Alternative sites include the distal femur, medial malleolus, and anterior superior iliac spine. The distal tibia may be used in older children and adults. A specifically designed commercial device for sternal placement may be used in adults in the absence of a sternal fracture.
3. Stabilize the leg and insert the needle into the anterior-medial aspect of the leg perpendicularly or pointed slightly inferiorly to avoid the epiphyseal plate (Figure P21-1).
4. Advance the needle until the bone is reached. With firm pressure and control, use a twisting motion to advance the needle through the bone and into the bone marrow cavity. This is identified by the feel of a "pop" as the needle enters the bone marrow cavity.
5. Remove the stylet, if applicable, and attempt to aspirate marrow (this does not always occur). Follow the aspiration with a normal saline flush of the needle to prevent an occlusion by the bone marrow. Placement is correct if the cannula flushes without signs of infiltration and fluids flow freely. The needle also should stand upright without support if it is firmly planted in the marrow.

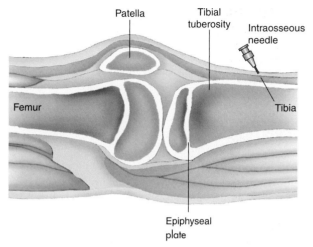

Figure P21-1 Obtaining intraosseous access. (From Sanders MJ: *Mosby's paramedic textbook,* ed 2, St Louis, 2003, Mosby.)

6. Attach the appropriate IV administration set and fluid.
7. Secure the leg to a padded board or splint and apply a bulky dressing around the IO cannula to prevent dislodgment.

PATIENT CARE MANAGEMENT

1. Ensure patency by assessing for the free flow of fluids and by evaluating the intraosseous site frequently for signs of infiltration. Be alert for symptoms of compartment syndrome secondary to extravasation.
2. Anticipate and prepare for the need to gain venous access as soon as the patient's condition has stabilized or resuscitation is complete. This minimizes the chance of developing osteomyelitis.
3. Assess the IO site for the development of infection and administer antibiotics as ordered.
4. Prevent excessive movement of the leg that may cause dislodgment.

REFERENCES

1. Hazinski MF, ed: *Pediatric advanced life support,* Dallas, 2001, American Heart Association.
2. American Heart Association: ACLS principles of practice. In Cummins RO, Filed JM, and Hasinski MF, eds: Dallas, 2003, The Association.

22 procedure

Lumbar Puncture

Erin Chiswell

DESCRIPTION

In a lumbar puncture (LP), a hollow needle with a stylet is inserted into a subarachnoid space below the L3 vertebrae, usually between L4 and L5, to obtain cerebrospinal fluid (CSF) for diagnostic purposes, to measure pressures, or to instill medications.

INDICATIONS

1. To test CSF for diagnosis of one of the following:
   - Meningitis
   - Subarachnoid hemorrhage
   - Central nervous system (CNS) infection of pathology
2. To measure CSF pressure (CSF may be removed to reduce pressure if necessary)
3. To instill blood, medications, anesthetics, or radiopaque contrast media

CONTRAINDICATIONS

- An infection in the lumbar area
- A patient who is receiving coagulopathy or anticoagulation therapy
- Signs of elevated intracranial pressure such as papilledema, head trauma, or focal neurologic deficits. If this is suspected, a CT scan should be performed before the LP is performed.

EQUIPMENT

Prepackaged sterile, disposable adult and infant LP trays are commercially available. If a tray is not available, gather the following:
- Sterile gloves
- 1% lidocaine (or 1% lidocaine with epinephrine, depending on physician preference)
- Antiseptic solution (such as povidone-iodine solution)
- Sterile towels and gauze sponges

- Four sterile collection tubes
- 3-ml to 5-ml syringe
- 22-gauge or 25-gauge needle, 1 ½ inches in length
- Pressure manometer with a three-way stopcock
- Spinal needles with stylet
  - Adults: 20-gauge to 22-gauge, 1 ½ inches
  - <1 year: 22-gauge, 1 ½ inches
  - >1 year: 22-gauge, 2 ½ inches
- Small adhesive dressing

INITIAL NURSING ACTIONS

1. In accordance with hospital policy, obtain informed, written consent after the physician explains the procedure to the patient.
2. Gather the equipment and place it at the bedside.
3. Properly position the patient in one of the following positions:
   - Adults:
     - *Lying position:* Assist the patient to the lateral decubitus position with his or her back close to the edge of the stretcher. Instruct the patient to lie on his or her side with back bowed, bringing knees and chin in toward chest. Place a pillow under the head and between the knees to maintain spine alignment. Assist the patient in maintaining this position during the procedure by placing your hands or arms behind the neck and knees (Figure P22-1).
     - *Sitting or upright position:* Have the patient sit on the edge of the stretcher and curl his or her back out by placing the head and arms over a padded bedside table.
   - Infants:
     - Place infant upright with thighs flexed up toward abdomen and neck flexed forward. Stabilize the infant against your upper torso and immobilize the extremities with your hands (Figure P22-2).

NURSING ALERT

Avoid hyperflexion of the neck in infants and children to avoid airway obstruction. Observe for signs of respiratory distress and monitor pulse oximetry during the procedure.

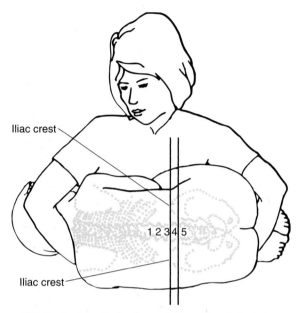

Figure P22-1   Position for lumbar puncture. The desired sites are the interspaces between L3 and L4, or L4 and L5. (From Kelley SJ: *Pediatric emergency nursing,* ed 2, 1994, Appleton & Lange.)

Iliac crest

Iliac crest

1 2 3 4 5

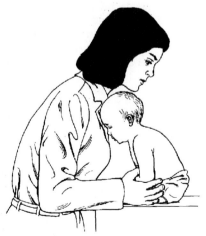

Figure P22-2   Position for lumbar puncture of an infant.

4. The physician will do the following:
   - Cleanse the skin with antiseptic solution.
   - Place a sterile towel under the patient and across the back.
   - Inject the area with lidocaine.
   - Insert and advance the needle until the subarachnoid space is entered.
   - Remove the stylet to observe CSF flow.
   - Attach a stopcock and manometer to the needle to measure CSF pressure. Normal pressure is 50 to 200 mm H_2O.[1] The patient should relax the legs and neck to prevent falsely elevated readings.
   - Remove the manometer and collect CSF in the collection tubes. The tubes and the corresponding laboratory tests are[2]:
     - #1: Culture and sensitivity, Gram stain, and red blood cell count
     - #2: Protein and glucose determinations
     - #3: Cytology
     - #4: Cell count
     - Reinsert the stylet and remove the needle.
5. Place the small adhesive dressing over the puncture site.
6. Cleanse antiseptic solution from the patient's back.
7. Send specimens to the laboratory for studies ordered by the physician.

PATIENT CARE MANAGEMENT

1. Document the patient's reaction to the procedure, the specimen disposition, and the appearance of the CSF.
2. Instruct the patient to lie prone for 2 to 4 hours, or per physician's instructions, to reduce the chance of a spinal headache.
3. Encourage oral fluids to increase CSF volume.
4. Observe puncture site for swelling, hematoma, or CSF leakage. If CSF leakage is noted, notify the physician immediately.
5. Observe the patient for neurologic changes, such as altered level of consciousness, pupil changes, elevated blood pressure or temperature, irritability, numbness, tingling, or decreased mobility in lower extremities.
6. If spinal headache results from CSF leakage, a blood patch (injection of autologous blood into the epidural space) may be required.

REFERENCES

1. Lavoie FW and Saucier JR: Central nervous system infections. In Marx JA Hockberger RS, and Walls RM, eds: *Rosen's emergency medicine: concepts and clinical practice,* ed 5, St Louis, 2002, Mosby, pp 1527-1541.
2. Fischbach FT: *A manual of laboratory and diagnostic tests,* Philadelphia, 2000, Lippincott Williams & Wilkins.

procedure 23

Medicolegal Evidence

Patty Ann Sturt

DESCRIPTION

Forensic laboratories have been established to serve a vital need in the criminal justice system. Their purpose is to scientifically analyze physical evidence that may be used in a court case. However, analysis of the evidence is possible only when the evidence has been collected and preserved in the correct manner. Emergency department nurses play a vital role in the collection and preservation of evidence from patients.

"Physical evidence" includes hair, fibers, blood, body secretions, glass, bullets, or almost anything that can be collected or deposited. Physical evidence helps in proving that a crime has been committed.

INDICATIONS

Indications for the collection and preservation of medicolegal evidence may include cases of suspected suicide, homicide, physical assault, sexual assault (Procedure 27), and driving under the influence of alcohol or illegal drugs.

EQUIPMENT

The equipment needed will depend on the medicolegal specimen to be collected and can include the following. Most state crime labs or law enforcement agencies have specific kits for blood alcohol specimens and urine drug screens.

- Gloves. Wear gloves when touching or packaging evidence.
- Povidone-iodine (Betadine) prep or swab. Never prep the patient's skin with a product that contains alcohol when obtaining a blood alcohol specimen.
- Dry paper. Place a piece of dry paper over stains to prevent the transfer of the stain from one area to another as the clothing is folded.
- Paper bag(s). Dry any blood-stained or wet clothing at room temperature and place each item of clothing to serve as evidence in a separate paper bag. *Do not use plastic bags* for

clothing or shoes. Plastic retains moisture and permits fungal and bacterial growth, which may destroy valuable evidence. Plastic bags may be used for collection of hair samples.
- Padded envelope. Bullets and blood tubes should be placed in a padded envelope.
- Labels. Each bag, envelope, or container with evidence must be labeled.
- Tape. Each bag and envelope must be sealed with tamperproof tape.

NURSING ACTIONS

1. Medicolegal evidence should be collected and preserved according to specific state laws and following the hospital's policies and guidelines.
2. *Always* maintain the chain of evidence. The chain of evidence is simply documentation of who has possession of the evidence at all times. Transfer of evidence from one health-care professional to another should be documented. This documentation should include the name and signature of the person receiving the evidence and the time. The number of health-care professionals with possession of the evidence should be kept to a minimum to maintain the integrity of the evidence. In most cases, the evidence is handed over to a police officer or law enforcement officer. The law enforcement officer should sign a document that states that he or she received the evidence and the time of receipt. This chain of evidence should be kept in the patient's medical record (chart). Some institutions use a specific form for documenting chain of evidence. Evidence may be rendered invalid in court if the chain of evidence is not maintained and recorded.
3. If the evidence is placed in a lock box or refrigerator, document the name of the individual who placed the evidence in the lock box and the time.
4. The following principles should be followed in the collection and preservation of clothing:
   - Articles of clothing may provide useful information about the weapon and help distinguish entrance wounds from exit wounds. Clothing fibers will deform in the direction of the passing projectile. Gunpowder residues and soot will deposit on clothing. Residue that is invisible to the naked eye may be seen with forensic laboratory staining techniques. Do not cut or rip through bullet holes when cutting clothing for removal. Allow the garment to air dry (if wet) before packaging.

Place paper over and under the bullet hole and fold the garment over twice. Place the garment in a paper bag.

- Stains on clothing (such as semen, blood, grass, or soil) may provide crucial evidence. Blood stains may help to identify the assailant. If the stain is wet, it must be air-dried. Package each item of clothing separately to avoid contamination.
- A law enforcement officer may request clothing for analysis of fibers. Fibers on clothing may be microscopically examined for the type, dye content, or weave content. This may produce useful evidence if the fibers found match the fibers of the suspected assailant's clothing or fibers from carpet or other objects at the scene of the crime. Handle the garment gently to avoid removal of loose fibers.

5. A bullet can be examined in a forensic laboratory to determine whether it was fired from a specific firearm through comparison of striated marks or microscopic marks. Bullets should be handled with gloves or rubber-tipped forceps to ensure the preservation of microscopic markings. Do not scratch or place a mark on the bullet. Place each dried bullet in a separate padded envelope or wrap each one in clean, soft tissue paper and place in a separate rigid container. Document the anatomical location from which the bullet was removed.

6. Syringes and other drug paraphernalia occasionally are found on a patient. In general, if you cannot see residue in the syringe or paraphernalia, there is not enough residue to identify the substance. Mark the container with "Contains Syringes" in bold lettering.

7. Follow these principles when collecting blood for determining alcohol or drug levels for medicolegal purposes:
   - Follow the hospital policy regarding the collection of blood for medicolegal purposes. Many state forensic laboratories have specific kits for the collection of blood.
   - Use nonalcoholic swabs when prepping the skin.
   - Place tubes in a plastic bag, and then place the plastic bag in a padded envelope.
   - Do not remove the stopper from the blood collection tube. The introduction of air may result in degradation of the alcohol within the specimen.

8. Knives or sharp metallic objects should be air dried and placed in a paper bag or cardboard box.

9. Each bag, envelope, blood tube, and other container with evidence should be labeled with the following:
   - Patient's name

- Hospital identification number
- Date and time
- Name of the person sealing the evidence
- Description of the item, such as bullet, article of clothing, or swabbed location

10. Seal each envelope, bag, tube, or container with a tamper-proof seal or tape.

PATIENT CARE MANAGEMENT

Never leave evidence unattended or in an area where others can tamper with it.

procedure *24*

Nebulizer Treatment

Bruce W. Walters

DESCRIPTION

A nebulizer sprays a fine, liquid mist of medication directly into the respiratory tract by using oxygen or air under pressure.

INDICATIONS

1. Bronchospasm related to asthma, COPD, or croup, or other airway diseases.
2. To promote expectoration of mucus.

EQUIPMENT

- Nebulizer set (nebulizer cup, mouthpiece or mask, and tubing to connect to gas inlet or nebulizer machine)
- Compressed gas source with oxygen or air
- Medication to be administered. Commonly used medications include:
  - Bronchodilators
    - Albuterol (Proventil)
    - Alupent
    - Xopenex
  - Sympathomimetic bronchodilator
    - Racemic epinephrine
  - Anticholinergic bronchodilator
    - Atrovent
  - Mucolytics
    - Mucomyst

INITIAL NURSING ACTIONS

1. Verify the physician order and gather equipment.
2. Explain the procedure to the patient.
3. Ascertain known hypersensitivity to the ordered medication.
4. Position the patient upright if possible to facilitate deep breathing.

> ### NURSING ALERT
>
> Atrovent is contraindicated in patients with a severe allergy to peanuts or soya lecithin. Soy lecithin is an ingredient in Atrovent.[1]

5. Perform a respiratory assessment, including respiratory rate, work of breathing, and lung sounds. A peak expiratory flow rate (PEFR) should be obtained in the asthmatic patient.

6. Assess the heart rate. Nebulizer medications can increase the heart rate and may precipitate dysryhthmias. Administer nebulized medications with caution in the patient with a rapid heart rate or underlying heart disease.

7. Place the medication and appropriate amount of diluent into the nebulizer cup and screw the cap on securely. The normal diluent is 2.5 ml of normal saline. Some medications are premixed with saline solution and do not require further dilution.

8. Connect one end of the air tubing to the oxygen or air source and the other end of the air tubing to the nebulizer cup (Figure P24-1).

9. Connect the mouthpiece or face mask to the nebulizer cup.

10. Turn on the oxygen or air flow meter and adjust the flow until a fine mist of medication is coming through the face mask or mouthpiece.

11. To ensure optimal absorption of the medication when the nebulizer is being administered through a mouthpiece, instruct the patient to seal the lips tightly around the mouthpiece and to take slow, deep breaths through the mouth. The mist should "disappear" with each inhaled breath.

12. If the nebulizer is to be administered through a face mask, place the mask over the patient's mouth and nose. Encourage the patient to take deep breaths in and out for the duration of the treatment.

13. Encourage the patient to continue slow, deep breaths until all the medication in the nebulizer cup is gone. You may need to tap the sides of the nebulizer cup to ensure that all medication is given.

14. If the patient is an infant or child who will not tolerate a mask, the nebulizer treatment may be administered via blow-by; hold the nebulizer circuit approximately 6 inches away from the patient's face. The caregiver may assist by holding

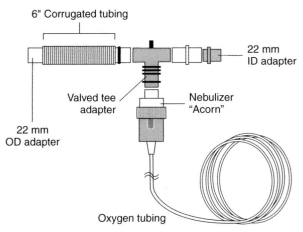

Figure P24-1   Nebulizer.

the circuit to help keep the infant or child calm. The nurse should stay with the patient for the duration of the nebulizer treatment.

15. Assess the patient's heart rate throughout the procedure. If the heart rate increases by 20 beats per minute, the treatment should be discontinued and the physician should be notified.

16. If the patient vomits or experiences a severe coughing episode during the treatment, stop the treatment and allow the patient to rest for a few minutes before continuing the treatment.

17. Obtain peak flow measurements when the nebulizer treatment is concluded.

18. If the patient will be receiving nebulizer therapy at home, instruct the patient to wash the circuit with warm, soapy water and rinse well after each use.

REFERENCES

1. Cohen MR: Medication errors, *Nursing 99* 29 (1):12, 1999.

25 procedure

Pediatric Intramuscular Injections

Terry Nalle

DESCRIPTION

Intramuscular injection is a method of drug administration in which medication is deposited under the muscle fascia below the fatty subcutaneous layer.

INDICATIONS

Medications administered intramuscularly are taken up relatively quickly by the body and are absorbed more quickly because of the vascular nature of deep muscle tissue.[1]

CONTRAINDICATIONS/CAUTIONS

1. Intramuscular injections should be avoided in the presence of muscle atrophy because of the reduced absorption.[2]
2. Using the same site repeatedly can result in fibrosis of muscle tissue.[3]

EQUIPMENT

- Alcohol swab
- Gloves
- Anesthetic agent if indicated
  - Dermal anesthetic
  - Wrapped ice cube for approximately 1 minute before injection
- Syringe
- Medication in the volume intended for injection
- Appropriate gauge of needle (consider the amount of medicine, viscosity, and tissue to be penetrated)
- Adhesive dressing

INITIAL NURSING ACTIONS

1. Explain procedure and purpose of the medication to the patient and/or parent.

2. Gather equipment. Select the appropriate needle and syringe, keeping in mind the amount of fluid (syringe size), viscosity of fluid (needle gauge), and amount of tissue to be penetrated (needle length).

3. Identify an appropriate site. Make certain the muscle is large enough to accommodate the volume and type of medication (Figures P25-1 through P25-4). If possible, allow older children to help select injection site.

➤ NURSING ALERT ➤

Select a site where skin is free of irritation and danger of infection.

---

4. Expose the injection site to produce an unobstructed view of the landmark (Figures P25-1 through P25-4).

5. Obtain sufficient help in restraining the child, as behavior is often unpredictable and the child may be uncooperative.

6. Place the infant or child in a lying or sitting position.

7. Stabilize the muscle for disposition of medication.

8. Prep skin appropriately and allow skin to air dry before injection.

9. Insert the needle quickly at a 90-degree angle, using a dart-like motion, and aspirate for blood.

➤ NURSING ALERT ➤

If blood appears on aspiration, withdraw the needle and discard the medication. Blood in the syringe indicates insertion into a vein.

---

10. If no blood appears on aspiration, slowly inject the medication.

11. Remove the needle quickly and apply firm pressure to the site after injection.

12. Place a small adhesive bandage on the puncture site.

14. Discard the syringe and needle into a sharps container.

15. Record the time of injection, drug, dose, injection site, and patient tolerance of the procedure.

TABLE P25-1 Sites, Volume and Needle Sizes for Intramuscular Injections

Site	Landmark	Maximum Injection Volume	Needle Size	Comments
Vastus lateralis (Figure P25-1)	Middle third of thigh between the greater trochanter and the knee	• Infants: 0.5 to 1 ml • Children: up to 2 ml	22-gauge to 25-gauge 1-inch to 1.5-inch needle	• Preferred site for infants and children under 3 years old • Large muscle that is free of important nerves or blood vessels
Ventrogluteal (Figure P25-2)	Make a "V" with the palm on the greater trochanter, index finger over the anterior superior iliac crest, and middle finger over the posterior iliac crest.	• Infants: up to 0.5 ml • Children: up to 2 ml	22-gauge to 25-gauge 1-inch to 1.5-inch needle	• Can tolerate large injection volumes • Area free of important nerves and blood vessels • Easily accessible

Dorsogluteal (Figure P25-3)	Draw an imaginary line between the greater trochanter and the posterior superior iliac spine; injection site is above and lateral to this line.	Children: up to 2 ml	20-gauge to 25-gauge 1-inch to 1.5-inch needle	• Contraindicated in children younger than 3 years or children who have not been walking longer than 1 year • Danger of injury to sciatic nerves • Can tolerate large injection volumes • Exposure of site may cause embarrassment in older children
Deltoid (Figure P25-4)	Two fingerbreadths below the acromion process of the humerus	0.5 to 1 ml	22-gauge to 25-gauge 1/2-inch to 1-inch needle	• Small muscle mass • Easily accessible site • Rapid absorption rate • Danger of radial nerve injury in young children; use in older children and adolescents

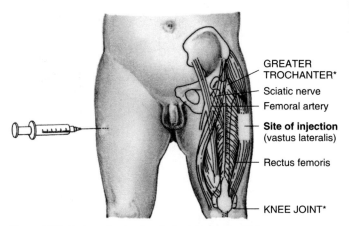

Figure P25-1   Locating landmarks for injection in thigh.

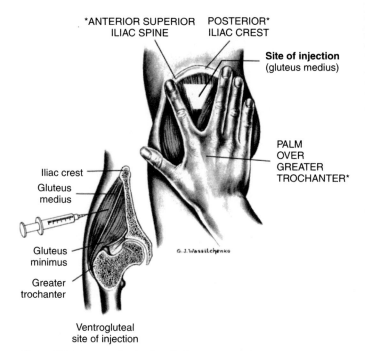

Figure P25-2   Locating landmarks for injection in hip.

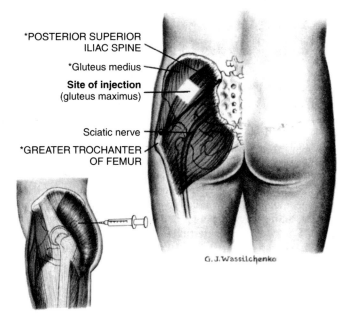

*POSTERIOR SUPERIOR
    ILIAC SPINE

*Gluteus medius

Site of injection
(gluteus maximus)

Sciatic nerve

*GREATER TROCHANTER
    OF FEMUR

G.J.Wassilchenko

Figure P25-3   Locating landmarks for injection in gluteus maximus.

PATIENT CARE MANAGEMENT

1. Observe patient for 15 to 20 minutes after injection for signs or symptoms of an allergic reaction.
2. Instruct caregiver to watch for signs and symptoms of infection, such and redness, swelling, increased pain or tenderness, red streaks, or unexplained fever.

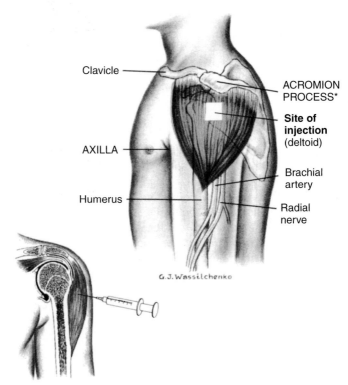

Figure P25-4   Locating landmakrs for injection in upper arm.

REFERENCES

1. Rodger M: Drawing up and administering intramuscular injection: a review of the literature, *J Adv Nurs* 3:574-582, 2000.
2. Perry A and Potter P: *Clinical nursing skills and techniques,* ed 5, St Louis, 2002, Mosby.
3. Hockenberry D, Wilson M, Winkelstein M, et al: *Wong's nursing care of infants and children,* ed 7, St Louis, 2003, Mosby.

procedure 26

Pericardiocentesis

Maggie Borders

DESCRIPTION

In pericardiocentesis, a catheter is placed into the pericardial space and fluid is aspirated from the pericardial sac. Removing excess fluid that has accumulated within the pericardial sac allows for improved filling of the heart, increased contractility, and improved cardiac output.

INDICATIONS

- Cardiac tamponade
- Pericardial effusion
- Aspiration of fluid for cytology and microbiology evaluation

EQUIPMENT

- Cardiac monitor
- Povidone-iodine solution
- Sterile gowns, gloves, and drape
- Masks and hair covers
- Three-way stopcock
- 60-ml syringe
- Suture material
- Hemostat
- Sterile IV tubing and drainage collector
- Catheter adapter
- Occlusive dressing
- Sterile alligator clamp
- ECG machine
- A 16-gauge to 18-gauge pericardiocentesis needle, 6 inches or longer (may use a spinal needle or an over-the-needle catheter per physician's preference)
- Ultrasound machine (some physicians prefer to perform pericardiocentesis using echocardiography for better visualization of cardiac structures; the nursing expectations remain the same)

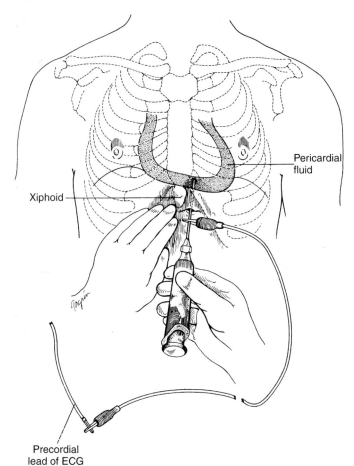

Figure P26-1 Pericardiocentesis guided by ECG. (From Wilkins EW, Jr [Ed.], *Emergency medicine: scientific foundations and current practice,* Baltimore, 1989, Williams & Wilkins, p 1017.)

NURSING ACTIONS

1. Position the patient with the head of the bed elevated approximately 45 degrees.[1] In the trauma patient, the reverse Trendelenburg position may be used.
2. Explain the procedure to the patient, and provide emotional support.

3. Initiate cardiac monitoring and 100% oxygen.
4. Establish a large-bore peripheral IV for fluid, blood, or medication administration as ordered.
5. Monitor the patient throughout the procedure. Observe closely for changes in cardiac rhythm and ST segment or T wave elevation, which may indicate that the catheter is contacting the epicardium. Electrical conduction from the epicardium is most accurately assessed by attaching a sterile alligator clamp to the needle and connecting it to the V lead on an ECG (see Figure P26-1); this is recommended if time permits.
6. If the catheter is left in place for potential reaspiration, attach it to the collection device using the sterile IV tubing and a stopcock. Secure all connections with tape, and place caps over the stopcock openings.
7. Cover the insertion site with an occlusive dressing after the catheter has been secured or removed.

> **NURSING ALERT**
>
> If CPR is in progress, continue chest compressions until needle insertion is initiated.

> **NURSING ALERT**
>
> Pericardial fluid is usually defibrinated and will not rapidly clot, while blood inadvertently aspirated from within the cardiac chambers will clot rapidly. Clotting times may vary depending on preexisting disease states, medical interventions that reduce clotting factors, hemorrhage, and the use of anticoagulants. Traumatic cardiac tamponade resulting from rapid hemorrhage into the pericardial space may clot within the pericardial sac, making aspiration impossible.

PATIENT CARE MANAGEMENT

- Assess vital signs, peripheral perfusion, heart sounds, and cardiac rhythm at least every 15 minutes for 1 hour, and then advance according to the patient's condition. If invasive monitoring has been initiated via a pulmonary artery or central venous catheter, the pressures obtained from these devices also should be documented. Notify the physician if symptoms of pericardial tamponade reoccur (e.g., jugular vein distension, respiratory distress, hypotension).

- Monitor and record blood and fluid drainage within the collection system every 15 minutes for 1 hour, then continue hourly.
- If clots develop in the collection tubing, gently knead the tubing to advance the clots into the collection chamber.
- Monitor for complications, including arrhythmias, pneumothorax, myocardial laceration, and esophageal injury.

REFERENCES

1. Emergency Nurses Association: *Trauma nursing core course,* ed 5, Chicago, 2000, The Association.

procedure 27

Preparation for Interfacility Patient Transfer

Edward Crews

DESCRIPTION

The transfer of a patient with an emergency medical condition to another facility must follow the federal regulations set forth by the Emergency Medical Treatment and Active Labor Act (EMTALA). These regulations list the obligations that the referring and receiving facilities must meet before a transfer is initiated[1] (see Box P27-1). The decision to transport a patient to another facility must be made only after the potential benefits are weighed against the potential risks.[2] The referring physician ultimately is responsible for the decision to transfer a patient; however, the transfer may be a collaborative effort between the referring and receiving physicians. After a decision has been made to transfer, the applicable policies and procedures for performing a transfer must be followed. The patient must be stabilized while the plan to transfer is being implemented.

INDICATIONS

- The patient's medical needs require a higher level of care than the referring facility is capable of providing
- The patient or family request transfer to another facility

CONTRAINDICATIONS/CAUTIONS

There are no absolute contraindications to interfacility transport, but there are cautions that must be considered. The referring facility is responsible for selecting a safe and appropriate mode of transport.

- Weather can be a major factor for both air and ground transportation. The risk that inclement weather will interfere with the transfer should be considered early in the process.
- The transport crew must be proficient and capable of caring for the patient being transported, and must have the necessary equipment available.

Box P27-1   EMTALA Transfer Mandates

- The physician certifies in writing that the medical benefits of the transfer outweigh the risks of the transfer based on information available at the time of the transfer.
- The transferring hospital provides medical treatment within its capabilities to minimize the risks of the transfer to the patient and unborn child.
- The receiving facility has available space and qualified personnel for treatment of the patient.
- A physician at the receiving facility has agreed to accept and care for the patient.
- Copies of all medical records related to the emergency condition for which the patient is being seen are sent to the receiving hospital.
- The transfer is effected through qualified personnel, appropriate vehicle, and transportation equipment needed to provide care during the transfer.

- Space constraints make the transport of some equipment difficult (e.g., interior configuration of some aircraft may preclude transport of a hare traction splint).
- The inability to secure a device (e.g., intraaortic balloon pump) may present safety issues.

Patient cautions:

- *Pregnant patient:* The transport crew must have appropriate access to the patient and the ability and equipment to care for the newly born patient should a precipitous delivery occur.
- *Violent patients:* Patients who are actively combative or have the potential to become actively combative cause concern for safety. Consideration of a sedative or a paralytic agent may be needed to ensure a safe transport.
- *Patient weight and girth:* Stretcher weight limitations, aircraft cabin configurations, and aircraft weight restrictions may affect the choice of mode of transport.
- *Patients who are prisoners:* The ability to transport prisoners will depend on the transport service. Details should be communicated to the transporting agency early in the process.

EQUIPMENT

Equipment needed during transport varies according to the patient's needs. Transport vehicles must have the necessary

transport equipment available to care for the patient populations
served.

NURSING ACTIONS (TO INITIATE THE TRANSFER)

1. Be familiar with the hospital's transfer policies and procedures
   before the need arises to transfer a patient. The capabilities
   of hospitals (e.g., designated trauma, stroke, pediatric, or
   burn centers and hospital specialties such as neonatal ICU,
   replantation centers, or hyperbaric chamber facilities) in the
   surrounding area and the capabilities of transport services
   and specialized transport teams should be identified. Safe
   helicopter landing zones should be identified and
   appropriately marked.

> ### ▶ NURSING ALERT ◀
>
> The physician is responsible for identifying and contacting a
> receiving physician to confirm acceptance of the patient and
> to transmit patient information. The referring physician, after
> consultation with the accepting physician, is responsible for
> choosing the mode of patient transport.

---

2. The patient's primary nurse must give report to a nurse at the
   accepting hospital.
3. Make copies of appropriate medical records and send them
   with the patient. These may include:
   - Prehospital records
   - Physician and nursing assessments and notes
   - Discharge summaries
   - Physician certification for transport (stating that the benefits
     of transport outweigh the risks of the transport)
   - Informed consent to transport signed by the patient or a legal
     guardian
   - Copies of radiographs, CT scans, laboratory study results,
     electrocardiograms, and test interpretations
   - List of the patient's valuables and clothing, and
     documentation of their disposition.
4. Identify the patient and family wishes. For example, a patient
   with a fear of flying may agree to transport by ground only.
5. Give the patient report to the transport crew.

> ### ⋙ NURSING ALERT ⋘
>
> If a patient cannot sign informed consent for the transfer because of the severity of the illness and the family or a legal guardian cannot be located, the patient can be transferred under an implied consent, the belief that any prudent person would agree to a transfer that was deemed necessary for the well-being of the patient.

> ### ⋙ NURSING ALERT ⋘
>
> Transfer should not be delayed for the completing or copying of medical records when the patient has a time-dependent injury or illness (e.g., stroke, myocardial infarction, trauma). Accurate and complete verbal communication of patient information to the receiving facility in these circumstances is of critical importance. Documentation can be sent by facsimile or by courier to the receiving facility after it is completed.

PATIENT CARE MANAGEMENT

Stabilizing treatment should be provided to the best of the referring facility's capabilities:

1. Assurance of a patent airway and adequate respiratory status. The patient should be intubated before transport if there is an indication that the patient may be unable to maintain the airway independently.
2. Trauma patients should be appropriately immobilized on a long backboard with a cervical collar, head immobilization device, and straps.
3. Circulatory support to maintain hemodynamic stability. This may be achieved through the administration of crystalloid fluid boluses, blood products, or vasopressors such as dopamine and Levophed.
4. Control of external bleeding
5. Intravenous access with at least one and preferably two IV catheters of appropriate size. Trauma patients should have two large-bore (14-gauge or 16-gauge) catheters.
6. The patient's neurologic status should be assessed, and intervention should be initiated to reduce increased intracranial pressure and stop seizures if at all possible before transport.

7. Assist with the placement of a chest tube or tubes in a patient who has a pneumothorax. Air volume expands with increased altitude, so a pneumothorax will expand as altitude increases and can become a life-threatening injury.

8. Nasogastric or orogastric tubes should be placed in patients who are immobilized (as a way to minimize the risk of aspiration) or patients who are being transported by air (because the expansion of air within the stomach and upper intestines as altitude increases can cause discomfort to the patient and may interfere with ventilation).

9. Urinary catheters should be placed if monitoring of urinary output is necessary.

10. Wounds should be dressed if time permits. Continue to monitor for occult bleeding. Do not delay transport for wound care unless the wound is life or limb threatening.

11. Fractures should be splinted. If air splints are in place, they often must be removed for air transport because the air within the splint will expand as altitude increases. Resplint the extremity with an alternative device. The stabilization provided by splinting will minimize damage to broken bones resulting from movement caused by vibration.

12. Administer antiemetics to prevent motion sickness or antianxiety medications as ordered.

13. Provide care for the family and significant others:
    - Explain the reason for transfer, destination, mode of transport, expected length of time required for the transport, and who will be caring for the patient during the transport.
    - Provide information about the patient's condition.
    - Give the family directions to the receiving facility and pertinent telephone numbers.
    - Allow the family to visit the patient before transport.

REFERENCES

1. Emergency Medical Treatment and Active Labor Act (EMTALA), suppl 1995, 42 USCA section 1395dd.
2. Warren J, Fromm RE, Orr RA, et al: Guidelines for the inter- and intrahospital transport of critically ill patients, *Crit Care Med* 32 (1):256-262, 2004.

28 procedure

Pulmonary Arterial Catheter Insertion and Monitoring

Theresa M. Glessner

DESCRIPTION

Pulmonary artery (PA) catheters are vascular-access catheters inserted through a large central vein (femoral, internal jugular, or subclavian) into the right side of the heart with the tip of the catheter extending into the PA. The purpose of the catheter is to directly measure pressures in the right side of the heart, indirectly measure pressures in the left side of the heart, and measure cardiac output.

INDICATIONS

1. Monitoring of fluid status
2. Right or left heart failure
3. Shock states
4. Titration of vasoactive drugs

CONTRAINDICATIONS

The presence of a bleeding or coagulation disorder is a reason to consider the risk versus the benefit of using a pulmonary arterial catheter. There are no absolute contraindications to this procedure.

EQUIPMENT

- PA catheter (Figure P28-1)
- Introducer kit
- Local anesthetic
- Sterile gloves
- Povidone-iodine solution
- Transducer setup with pressure bag and pressure tubing. Two transducers or a cardiac bridge device will be needed to monitor CVP readings. A bridge is a stopcock device that is placed between the distal lumen hub and the proximal injectate lumen hub. It is used to direct the flow of the pressurized fluid through the proximal injectate lumen hub to

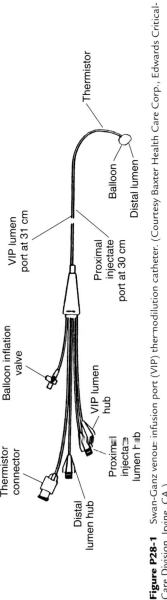

Figure P28-1 Swan-Ganz venous infusion port (VIP) thermodilution catheter. (Courtesy Baxter Health Care Corp., Edwards Critical-Care Division, Irvine, CA.)

Thermistor

Balloon

Distal lumen

VIP lumen port at 31 cm

Proximal injectate port at 30 cm

Balloon inflation valve

VIP lumen hub

Thermistor connector

Distal lumen hub

Proximal injectate lumen hub

obtain CVP readings. Pressurized fluid and tubing is required to overcome the higher pressures in the pulmonary artery.

- Monitor with pressure capability and appropriate cables
- Cardiac output monitor with appropriate cable and cardiac output setup. Cardiac output may be monitored manually or with a continuous cardiac output machine. If cardiac output is to be monitored manually, will also need: IV solution, tubing, and 10-ml syringe.
- 4 × 4 gauze
- Sterile normal saline for flushing of ports, and 10-ml syringes and needles for each port

INITIAL NURSING ACTIONS

1. Ensure that this procedure is thoroughly explained to the patient and his or her family before it is initiated and that informed consent has been obtained.
2. Ensure appropriate functioning of the monitoring equipment.
3. Assemble the transducer, and prepare the flush system. Normal saline, 500 ml, is the solution of choice for the flush system. One should pull the air from the flush bag by inserting an 18-gauge needle into the port and expressing the air out. The pressure tubing should be completely flushed through each stopcock to eliminate all air bubbles. Air bubbles in the pressure tubing can cause dampening of the PA waveform.[1] After flushing the pressure tubing, inflate the pressure bag to 300 mm Hg.
4. Assemble and flush the cardiac output measurement system. Ensure that the computation constant for the cardiac output computer is appropriate for the size of the catheter used and the temperature of the diluent.
5. To avoid errors in pressure readings, the system must be "zeroed" to the atmosphere. The stopcock should be turned off to the patient, which opens the system to air. The "zero" button on the monitor then should be depressed. When "zero" appears on the monitor, turn the stopcock off to air.
6. Level the transducer at the phlebostatic axis, which is the reference point for the atria when the patient is in a supine position. The phlebostatic axis is at the level of the fourth or fifth intercostal space, midaxillary line.
7. Connect the pressure tubing to the end of the distal lumen hub of the PA catheter and flush the catheter. Use the enclosed syringe to inject air through the balloon inflation

valve on the PA catheter to assess patency. A patent balloon should inflate after the injection of no more than 1.5 ml of air and deflate passively.

8. The physician will identify the landmarks for insertion and anesthetize the area with a local anesthetic such as 1% lidocaine. The catheter then is placed through strict sterile technique.

9. When the physician has advanced the catheter approximately 10 to 15 cm, the nurse will be asked to inflate the balloon.

10. The electrocardiogram (ECG) should be continuously monitored for ventricular arrhythmias, such as ventricular tachycardia, PVCs, and ventricular fibrillation, which can occur during insertion through the right ventricle. Remain with the patient throughout the procedure, providing verbal support and comfort measures.

11. After the catheter is floated to an occlusion or wedge position, the physician will ask for the balloon to be deflated.

12. Immediately after insertion of the catheter, a portable chest x-ray examination should be performed to verify line placement and to rule out a pneumothorax caused by insertion of the introducer. When catheter placement is confirmed, it is sutured in place.

13. After the catheter is sutured in place, a sterile dressing should be applied through strict aseptic technique. Dressing requirements may vary, and institutional policy should be followed. Secure the catheter to the patient with tape to prevent catheter dislodgment from the weight of the catheter or accidental pulling on the catheter.

14. Continuously monitor the PA pressure.

15. Record all hemodynamic parameters—CVP, pulmonary artery pressure (PAP), pulmonary capillary wedge pressure (PCWP; also known as pulmonary capillary occlusion pressure, PCOP), cardiac output/cardiac index (CO/CI), systemic vascular resistance (SVR), and other parameters—according to department protocol.

PATIENT CARE MANAGEMENT

1. Assess and monitor the trend of the patient's vital signs and hemodynamic parameters, noting improvement or deterioration.

2. Record hemodynamic parameters every hour or per department protocol, and notify the physician of any significant changes in the patient's condition.

3. Ensure that transducer(s) are zeroed to atmosphere at least every shift or per department protocol.

4. Monitor PA waveform for signs of catheter migration. If the catheter floats in (distally), the waveform may change to a permanent wedge or occlusion waveform. If the catheter floats out (proximally), the waveform may show a right ventricular tracing (Figure P28-2). Notify the physician if the catheter migrates, as either condition can be life threatening.

5. Continuously monitor the patient's ECG. Ventricular arrhythmias may indicate catheter migration into the right ventricle. Notify the physician, as the catheter may need to be floated back into the pulmonary artery.

6. Ensure that all stopcocks have sterile Luer-Loks on each unused port.

7. If blood specimens are being withdrawn through the PA catheter system, ensure that the system is thoroughly flushed after each blood draw to prevent clot formation in the catheter.

8. The pressure bag always should be inflated to 300 mm Hg to prevent blood from backing up into the pressure tubing, and to ensure a crisp waveform.

9. The balloon should be allowed to passively deflate after each PCWP (PAOP) reading. If the balloon does not deflate, attempt to manually deflate the balloon with the syringe. If abnormal resistance is felt when inflating the balloon, and the balloon does not passively deflate, the balloon is probably ruptured and should not be reinflated at any time until the catheter is replaced.

11. If an SVO_2 or Oximetrix PA catheter is used (Figure P28-3), ensure the following:
    - The SVO_2 monitor and cables are available and functional.
    - The optical connector is attached to the cable and monitor, and is calibrated before the catheter is removed from the package.
    - The SVO_2 system is calibrated with the in vivo method every 24 hours or per department protocol.

POTENTIAL COMPLICATIONS

1. Pneumothorax resulting from deep-line insertion
2. Bleeding at the site
3. Life-threatening arrhythmia
4. Puncture of a great vessel or the heart with the catheter
5. Poor catheter placement
6. Balloon breakage during insertion
7. For troubleshooting of problems, see Table P28-1.

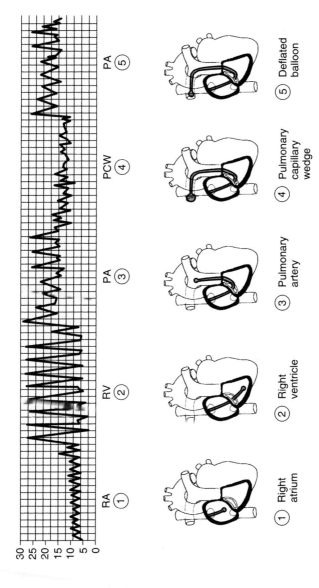

Figure P28-2 PA waveforms: RA, RV, PA, wedge. (Courtesy Abbott Critical Care Systems, Mountain View, CA.)

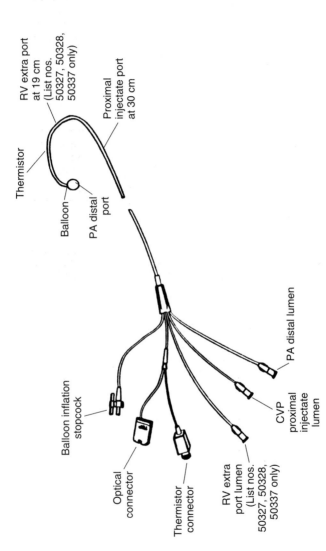

Figure P28-3 SVo₂ PA catheter. (Courtesy Abbott Critical Care Systems, Mountain View, CA.)

TABLE P28-1   Troubleshooting

Problem	Cause	Solution
Bleed back	• Loose connections • Open stopcock • Crack in transducer or connection	• Check connections • Check system
Dampened waveform	• Air bubbles • Clot • Loose connections	• Check connections • Flush system • Check system
False readings	• Transducer not properly zeroed or not at the phlebostatic axis	• Zero transducer; always zero at the phlebostatic axis
No waveform	• Transducer not properly connected to monitor	• Check system

REFERENCES

1. Lynn-McHale DJ and Preuss T: Pulmonary artery catheter insertion (assist) and pressure monitoring. In Lynn-McHale DJ and Carlson KK, eds: *2001 AACN procedure manual for critical care,* ed 4, Philadelphia, 2001, WB Saunders, pp 439-456.

29procedure

Rehydration

Jill Ann Dinsmore

DESCRIPTION

Dehydration is a condition of negative fluid balance that results when fluid loss is greater than fluid intake. This condition can result from many disease processes. Rehydration to restore a normal fluid balance must be achieved in patients who are dehydrated.

INDICATIONS

1. Reduced fluid intake
2. Loss of body fluids through sensible fluid losses, such as vomiting and diarrhea; insensible losses, such as diaphoresis, fever, and hyperventilation
3. Compartmentalization of fluids

CONTRAINDICATIONS/CAUTIONS

There are no absolute contraindications to rehydration; however, patients who are elderly, have a history of renal failure, or have a history of congestive heart failure require careful monitoring of vital signs and urine output to reduce the likelihood of fluid overload.

EQUIPMENT

1. Oral rehydration solution (ORS), such as Pedialyte, or glucose/electrolyte solution
2. Cup or bottle
3. IV catheters (22-gauge to 24-gauge for children, 16-gauge to 20-gauge for adults)
4. IV tubing
5. Normal saline

INITIAL NURSING ACTIONS

Children With Mild to Moderate Dehydration (See Table P29-1)

1. Administer a challenge of an oral rehydrating solution (ORS), such as Pedialyte, in small amounts, ($^1/_2$ ounce every

TABLE P29-1   Assessment of Pediatric Dehydration

Assessment Parameter	Minimal or No Loss of Body Weight)	Mild to Moderate (3%-9% Loss of Body Weight)	Severe (More Than 9% Loss of Body Weight)
Mental status	Well; alert	Normal; fatigued; restless; irritable	Apathetic; lethargic; unconscious
Thirst	Drinks normally; might refuse liquids	Thirsty; eager to drink	Drinks poorly; unable to drink
Heart rate	Normal	Normal to increased	Weak, thready or nonpalpable
Breathing	Normal	Normal; fast	Deep
Eyes	Normal	Sunken orbits	Deeply sunken orbits
Tears	Present	Decreased	Absent
Mouth and tongue	Moist	Dry	Parched
Skin fold	Instant recoil	Recoil in less than 2 seconds	Recoil in greater than 2 seconds
Capillary refill	Normal	Prolonged	Prolonged; minimal
Extremities	Warm	Cool	Cold; mottled; cyanotic
Mucous membrane	Slightly dry	Dry	Parched
Urine output*	Normal to decreased	Decreased	Minimal

Managing acute gastroenteritis among children oral rehydration, maintenance, and nutritional therapy, *MMWR* 52 (RR-16):1-20, 2003.
*Normal urine output for infants is 2 ml/kg/hr and for children is 1 ml/kg/hr.

15 minutes) initially. If tolerated, 50 to 100 ml/kg of an ORS may be given over 2 to 4 hours.
2. If the vomiting or diarrhea persists and the patient is unable to retain the oral fluids, IV fluids are needed, and admission may be considered.

Children With Moderate to Severe Dehydration (See Table P29-1)
1. Establish a 22-gauge to 24-gauge IV and administer a 20-ml/kg bolus of normal saline or Ringer's lactate.

2. If unable to obtain IV access, in cases of severe dehydration, intraosseous access may be needed (see Procedure 21).
3. Reassess, and if the child continues to be symptomatic (decreased level of consciousness, irritability, weak peripheral pulses, poor capillary refill, or tachycardia) a additional boluses of 20 ml/kg may be given.

NURSING ALERT

All children with severe dehydration require IV fluids and most likely an admission to the hospital.

Adults With Mild Dehydration
An oral fluid challenge with clear fluids such as Seven-Up or ice chips.

Adults With Moderate to Severe Dehydration
1. If the patient is vomiting, antiemetics and antidiarrhea medications may be given.
2. Establish a 16-gauge to 20-gauge IV and administer a fluid bolus. The initial bolus consists of 1 L of an isotonic solution such as normal saline (NS) over 30 to 45 minutes.
3. Reassess the patient, and further 1-L boluses may be given if needed.

PATIENT CARE MANAGEMENT
Discharge Information for Infants and Children
1. Give clear fluids such as Pedialyte or other ORS solutions in small, frequent amounts, and advance to larger amounts as tolerated. If the infant is breast-feeding, offer the ORS or Pedialyte between feedings.
2. For children over 2 years of age, Pedialyte, Popsicles, Jell-O water, or noncaffeinated clear soda such as Seven-Up can be offered in small, frequent amounts. Sports drinks do not have an adequate electrolyte concentration to treat diarrhea, and the use is discouraged by the American Academy of Pediatrics.[1]
3. Avoid fruit juices, as these may increase the amount and frequency of diarrhea.
4. Return to the emergency department if the following symptoms occur or worsen:
   • Decreased tearing
   • Decreased urine output

- Change in activity or increased lethargy
- Inability to tolerate oral intake of clear fluids
- Excessive diarrhea

5. Follow up with your pediatrician in 24 to 48 hours.

Discharge Information for Adults

1. Drink plenty of fluids (clear preferred).
2. If vomiting, start with clear diet and advance as tolerated.
3. Return to the emergency department if you experience:
   - Dizziness with position changes
   - Dark urine with a strong odor
   - Decrease in urine output
   - Inability to tolerate PO
   - Excessive diarrhea

REFERENCES

1. Managing acute gastroenteritis among children: oral rehydration, maintenance, and nutritional therapy, *MMWR* 52(RR-16):1-13, 2003.

*30*procedure

Sedation for Procedures

Patty Ann Sturt

DESCRIPTION

In procedural sedation, sedatives or dissociative agents are administered with or without analgesics to induce a state that allows the patient to tolerate unpleasant procedures while maintaining cardiorespiratory function.

The two levels of sedation used for procedures in the emergency department (ED) are moderate (formerly known as conscious sedation) and deep.

Moderate Sedation
Moderate sedation is a drug-induced depression of consciousness during which patients respond purposefully to verbal commands, with or without light tactile stimulation. The patient independently maintains a patent airway and adequate ventilation. Cardiovascular function usually is maintained.[1]

Deep Sedation
Deep sedation is a drug-induced depression of consciousness during which patients cannot be easily aroused to verbal stimuli, but respond purposefully to repeated tactile or painful stimulation. There is a greater risk of the patient losing the ability to independently maintain a patent airway and effective ventilations. Thus patients may require airway and ventilatory assistance.[1]

> ### ⋙ NURSING ALERT ⋘
>
> It is not always possible to predict how an individual patient will respond to medication intended to produce moderate or deep sedation. Thus the RN must be prepared to assist with airway measures and ventilatory assistance for any patient requiring procedural sedation.

INDICATIONS

Procedural sedation may be used in ED patients requiring the following:

1. Closed manipulation or reduction of dislocations and/or fractures
2. Suction curettage
3. Extensive laceration repairs
4. Incision and drainage
5. Foreign body removal
6. Endoscopic procedures
7. Invasive diagnostic procedures

CONTRAINDICATIONS/CAUTIONS

- Recent alcohol ingestion. Alcohol can compound the actions of many of the medications used for procedural sedation.
- Severe renal dysfunction
- Patients receiving monoamine oxidase (MAO) inhibitors or tricyclic antidepressants
- Hemodynamic instability
- Significant respiratory distress
- The elderly may have a prolonged response to medications used for sedation with analgesia because of delayed metabolism of drugs.
- The absorption, metabolism, and excretion of medications in pediatric patients is variable, so pediatric patients should be monitored closely.

EQUIPMENT

- IV fluid, tubing, and catheter
- Procedural medications and their antidotes
- Pulse oximeter
- Emergency cart with airway equipment, bag-valve-mask device, resuscitation drugs, and a monitor/defibrillator
- Oxygen and oxygen-delivery devices such as a nasal cannula and nonrebreather mask
- Suction
- Automatic blood pressure (BP) device or BP cuff and stethoscope

NURSING ACTIONS

1. Follow hospital policies and procedures and state board of nursing regulations regarding the administration of procedural sedation and analgesic medications, and patient monitoring.

2. The RN providing procedural sedation and analgesia must:
   - Have an understanding of the drugs administered
   - Understand and follow the laws set forth by the state Board of Nursing regarding administration of medications for sedation and analgesia
   - Have the ability and training to monitor the patient's response to the procedure and the procedural medications
   - Have the skills necessary to manage potential complications
3. Explain the procedure and purpose of procedural medications to patient and family.
4. Ensure a consent form for the procedure and procedural sedation has been obtained and signed by the patient or caregiver.
5. Obtain a history and baseline assessment data, including the following:
   - Current medications and drug allergies
   - Medical and surgical history; should include information about previous experiences with sedation and analgesia
   - History of substance abuse
   - Blood pressure, heart rate, respiratory rate, level of consciousness, skin color, and oxygen saturation
   - Planned method of transport home
   - Food or fluid intake within the past 8 hours
6. Establish IV access. Use an 18-gauge or larger needle if significant blood loss is a possibility.
7. Initiate continuous pulse oximetry.
8. Initiate cardiac monitoring in patients with one or more of the following:
   - Deep sedation planned or expected for the procedure
   - History of respiratory disease
   - History of cardiac disease
   - Elderly
9. Administer and titrate the medications in small incremental doses based on the physician's order, hospital policies, and the individual's response.
   - The medications ordered most often for sedation include:
   - Benzodiazepines such as midazolam (Versed), diazepam (Valium), and lorazepam (Ativan)
   - Opiates such as meperidine (Demerol), morphine, and fentanyl (Sublimaze)
   - Dissociative agents such as ketamine HCl[2]
   - Barbiturates such as phenobarbital are used more often with children.[3]

10. Reversal agents should be readily available. Naloxone (Narcan) is the agent for reversal of opioids such as Demerol and fentanyl. Flumazenil (Romazicon) is the reversal agent for benzodiazepines.

NURSING ALERT

Narcan and Romazicon have short half-lives, and thus the patient is at risk for deterioration in level of consciousness and respiratory status, which may necessitate subsequent doses. The patient should be monitored for at least an hour after a reversal agent is administered.

PATIENT CARE MANAGEMENT

1. A patent IV must be continuously maintained during the procedure.
2. The RN managing the care of the patient receiving procedural sedation should not leave the patient unattended.
3. Oxygen saturation must be continuously monitored during the procedure. Supplemental oxygen should be given if the oxygen saturation decreases from the patient's baseline.
4. Anticipate the need to administer oxygen to any patient with a baseline SpO_2 of 95 mm Hg or less.
5. The blood pressure, heart rate, respiratory rate, level of consciousness, and pulse oximeter values should be obtained and recorded every 5 to 15 minutes during the procedure. The patient's respiratory status, including respiratory rate, depth, and skin color, should be continuously monitored.
6. Continuously monitor the cardiac rhythm and rate of patients receiving deep sedation and those with a history of cardiac or respiratory disease.
7. Vital signs, oxygen saturation, cardiac rhythm (as appropriate), and level of consciousness should be evaluated and documented at the completion of the procedure and at least every 15 minutes until the patient's values return to baseline. Consider the use of a sedation scoring system to monitor the level of sedation.
8. Before discharge from the ED, the patient and significant others should receive verbal and written instructions to include signs and symptoms of complications, restrictions on diet and activity, and a follow-up appointment as needed.

Documentation should reflect that the patient and significant others received, repeated, and understood the instructions.

9. The patient should not be allowed to drive when discharged from the ED.

REFERENCES

1. Smith DF: *Sedation, anesthesia, and the JCAHO,* ed 2, Marblehead, MA, 2001, Opus Communications.
2. Glickman A: Ketamine: the dissociative anesthetic and the development of a policy for its safe administration in the pediatric emergency department, *J Emerg Nurs* 21:116-124, 1995.
3. Krauss B: Management of acute pain and anxiety in children undergoing procedures in the emergency department, *Pediatr Emerg Care* 17:115-122, 2001.

procedure *31*

Sexual Assault Evidence Collection

Erin Chiswell

DESCRIPTION

Rape and sexual assault continue to be common crimes in our society. Emergency department (ED) nurses must understand their role in the care of these patients. The primary role of the nurse includes (1) minimizing further physical and psychologic trauma to the victim and (2) collecting and preserving medicolegal evidence for potential use in the legal system.

Sexual assault nurse examiners (SANEs) are utilized in many states. SANEs are nurses trained and licensed to assess, care for, and collect evidence from sexual assault patients.

INDICATIONS

Patients who come to the ED reporting a sexual assault.

CONTRAINDICATIONS

The chances of finding physical evidence decrease in direct proportion to the time that has elapsed between the assault and examination. Generally, if the assault took place more than 72 hours before the examination, it is unlikely that trace evidence will still be present on the patient. However, evidence may still be gathered by documenting any findings obtained during the examination, such as lacerations, bruises, bite marks, and statements about the assault. In addition, counseling on prophylaxis for sexually transmitted infections (STIs) and community support services should be provided.

EQUIPMENT

Sexual assault evidence collection kits (rape kits) usually are available. If a kit is not available, obtain the following:

- Three consent forms (separate consent forms for each of the following: medical treatment, evidence collection, and release of evidence collection and medical record to the police)

- Large paper bags for clothing
- 8 to 10 envelopes
- Tape
- Sterile comb
- 8 to 12 packages of cotton-tipped applicators
- Microscopic slide with slide cover and container
- Two blood tubes with an anticoagulant
- Labels with the patient's name, hospital identification number, date, time of evidence collection, specimen collected, and name of collector
- Speculum (Have different sizes available. If vaginal trauma is present, a small speculum may be needed to prevent additional discomfort.)
- Chlamydia and gonorrhea cultures
- Personal care items such as toothbrush, toothpaste, and soap for the patient's use after the exam

INITIAL NURSING ACTIONS

1. Some sexual assault victims suffer life-threatening injuries. Always assess and treat life-threatening injuries first.
2. Place the patient in a private area away from other patients and visitors. The sexual assault victim should never be allowed to wait in the lobby.
3. Approach the patient in a nonjudgmental manner, conveying empathy and concern. Sexual assault victims experience psychologic trauma. Although this may be more difficult to recognize than the physical trauma, these patients should be treated with special consideration. Each person has his or her own way of coping with sudden stress. Victims may appear calm, indifferent, submissive, jocular, angry, withdrawn, or even uncooperative and hostile toward those who are trying to help, all of which are within the range of anticipated reactions.
4. Explain the plan of care, which includes identification of injuries, collection of medicolegal evidence, STI and pregnancy prophylaxis, and support service referrals. Use terminology that the patient will understand. Avoid medical terminology.
5. Offer to call a friend or family member if there is no one with the patient. Offer to call the rape crisis center that serves the area to send a counselor to the ED.
6. Obtain consent on the three forms described in the equipment section. If adult victims are reluctant to sign a consent form for the collection of evidence, they should be assured that

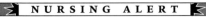

> ## NURSING ALERT
>
> Every effort should be made to have one primary nurse assigned to the patient. Sexual assault victims often experience shame, guilt, and fear. *The patient is more likely to express his or her concerns and cooperate with the examination if a rapport is established with one nurse.*

    evidence will *not* obligate them to pursue prosecution of their case.

7. Notify police per hospital policy and state laws. Sexual assault victims should be gently encouraged to report the assault and cooperate in the police investigation. However, they may refuse to do so and maintain this right.

8. Follow the hospital policy regarding the collection of sexual assault medicolegal evidence. In many institutions, the nurse, or SANE, may collect the appropriate clothing, saliva swabs, and hair and blood specimens.

> ## NURSING ALERT
>
> All specimens must be dry before they are placed in an appropriate bag or envelope. If the specimen is wet, allow it to air dry, and then put it in the appropriate container. Each bag (paper only) or envelope must be sealed with tape and labeled appropriately as described in the equipment section. **Never use plastic bags, and never lick envelopes to seal!**

9. Have the patient undress and put on a hospital gown while standing on a sheet or pad. Hair, grass, fibers, or other evidence *may fall from the clothing while the patient undresses.* Carefully fold the pad (or sheet), and place it in a paper bag with a label. Collect the underwear and place them in a small paper bag. Seal the bag with tape, and attach a patient label to the outside of the bag. *The underwear can be analyzed for seminal fluid, spermatozoa, and foreign debris.*

10. Other pieces of clothing should be collected if damaged or torn, or have stains.

11. Observe the patient's entire body to locate all injuries. Document any injuries in great detail. Photographs may help in recording injuries. If photographs are to be taken, a separate

consent form must be obtained. Contact the police department to send a photographer trained in taking evidence pictures. If one is not able to respond, take the pictures in a well-lit area. First, take a picture of a plain paper with the time, date, patient's name, identification number, and photographer's name on it. Begin and end the roll with pictures of this paper. Take pictures of injuries, first showing the location of the injury on the body, and then showing the injury in close-up shots. Position the camera perpendicular to the body surface, and include a size reference, such as a ruler, near the injury.

12. Scrape underneath the fingernails and then clip all 10 nails over paper towels. Fold these paper towels in on themselves and place in an appropriate container. *These may contain skin, blood, hair, and fibers of the assailant.*

13. Pull (or have the patient pull) at least 15 head hairs from different locations on the scalp. *Rationale: Hair may have been transferred from the suspect to the victim. Hair from different parts of the scalp has different colors, textures, and components. Having all these hairs and their roots allows them to be compared with other hairs collected, possibly from the suspect.*

NURSING ALERT

When obtaining any hair specimen, grasp the hair near the root when pulling it out to obtain the root for DNA testing. **Never cut hairs or pluck with tweezers!**

---

14. Place either the pad provided in the evidence kit or paper towels under the patient's bottom and perineal area. Thoroughly comb the pubic hair with downward strokes. Place the comb on the paper and gently fold the paper, wrapping the comb up in it and placing it all in an envelope.

15. Pull (or have the patient pull) at least 15 pubic hairs from different locations. *The pulled pubic hairs are used for comparison with hairs found at the crime scene or on the assailant's body.*

16. Obtain blood in two tubes containing an anticoagulant for medicolegal purposes. If a kit is being used that contains a special blood card or blotter to determine DNA status, use a

sterile dropper or syringe to fill the area as directed by the kit. *The purpose of this step is to determine the victim's blood type, group, and properties. This may be useful in identifying the victim's blood if it is found on the suspect or at the crime scene.[1]*

17. Other blood should be obtained at this time, if ordered by the physician. (Blood and urine screens for toxicology should be performed if the victim feels that he or she may have been drugged by the assailant or if the victim's medical condition warrants toxicology screening for optimal patient care. For patients at risk for pregnancy, a urine or blood test should be performed to rule out preexisting pregnancy.)

18. If a vaginal assault occurred, assist the physician with the collection of evidence during the pelvic examination. A water-lubricated sterile speculum of appropriate size should be used, as other lubricants can interfere with interpretation of forensic materials. Collect four vaginal swabs. Place three in an envelope as usual and use the other one to smear on the slide. (The slide should not be fixed or stained.) Place the vaginal smear in a slide holder, tape it closed, and label it. Write "vaginal" on the frosted end of the slide. *The vaginal swabs and smear are analyzed for spermatozoa and properties of blood groups. The alleged assailant (if known) will have blood drawn to test for his blood groups. If there is a match between the swabs and his blood groups, it can serve as medicolegal evidence in court.*

19. If anal assault occurred, collect four anal swabs.

20. If oral-genital assault occurred, collect four buccal swabs. Swab along the buccal area and gum line.

PATIENT CARE MANAGEMENT

1. The physician or nurse should document the patient's description of the assault. This should include any oral, vaginal, or rectal penetration. Quote the patient as much as possible. Never use speculation in the medical record. Even if medical findings are consistent with patient's statements, do not imply this. Document factually only what is observed in the exam or what is said by the patient.

2. Document and describe any bruises, lacerations, bite marks, or other signs of trauma. Describe color, shape, size, and body location of each injury. Body diagrams are useful in showing the location and type of injury.

3. The date of the patient's last menstrual period, name of any sexual partner in the last week, and contraceptive history should be recorded.

4. Administer antibiotics for STI prophylaxis as ordered by the physician.

5. Treatment for the prevention of pregnancy should be discussed with the patient. If a urine or blood pregnancy test is negative, birth control pills may be prescribed. Initially two birth control tablets should be given orally with instructions to repeat in 12 hours. Inform the patient that nausea and vomiting may occur. Small, frequent meals may reduce the nausea. The patient should be informed that the menstrual period or breakthrough bleeding will start within a few days.

6. Refer the patient to a rape crisis center or sexual assault counselor for counseling.

7. Refer the patient to a gynecology clinic for follow-up STI, HIV, and pregnancy testing. Currently, HIV testing of sexual assault victims in the ED is controversial. Emergency departments do not routinely provide confidential individual HIV counseling. For this reason the patient can be referred to a health department, clinic, or office that performs the test and provides counseling.

8. Provide clean clothing and a private area for cleansing after the exam. Assist the patient in finding transportation home.

9. Maintain the chain of evidence at all times. If at all possible, one nurse should assist with the evidence collection and maintain possession of the evidence until it is signed over to a law enforcement officer. Anyone who takes possession of the kit must document his or her name and time of the possession until the officer takes it to the police department. When this occurs, document the officer's name and the time the officer collected the evidence. (Refer to Procedure 23.)

REFERENCE

1. Patel M and Minshall L: Genitourinary emergencies: management of sexual assault, *Emerg Med Clin North Am* 19 (3), 2001.

procedure 32

Splint Application

Carlos Coyle
Ronald Stewart Gray
Kathy Blanton

DESCRIPTION

Splinting is a technique used to temporarily immobilize or stabilize an injured extremity. Immobilization reduces pain, swelling, muscle spasm, bleeding into the tissue, and the risk of fat emboli. Immobilization also can prevent a closed fracture from converting to an open fracture.

INDICATIONS

Splinting is indicated any time there is trauma to an extremity with evidence of deformity, angulation, bony crepitus, edema, ecchymosis, significant pain, open soft tissue injury, an impaled object, or neurovascular compromise.[1]

EQUIPMENT

- Select the appropriate type of splint. The are four general categories of splints, which are outlined in Table P32-1:
  1. Soft nonrigid splints
  2. Hard rigid and semirigid splints
  3. Pneumatic-inflatable splints
  4. Traction splints
- Padding material
- Elastic bandages (Ace wraps)
- Tape

INITIAL NURSING ACTIONS

1. Explain the procedure to the patient.
2. Consider pain-control measures.
3. Prepare the patient for splinting:
   - Remove clothing over the injury site.
   - Dress open wounds.
   - Remove jewelry.

TABLE P32-1 Four General Categories of Splints

Type of Splint	Examples	Uses/Comments	Application
Soft nonrigid	• Pillows • Blankets	Foot and ankle injuries	• Position the pillow around the area to be splinted, secure the splint with cravats or tape.
	• Bed sheet wrap	Splinting pelvic fracture	• Wrap a folded bed sheet around the pelvis at the level of the greater trochanters of the femurs. Tighten the sheet by twisting the ends anteriorly. To secure, tie or clamp the ends (Figure P32-1).
	• Sling and swathe	Stabilizing clavicle and scapular fractures	• Place the extremity across the chest in a position of comfort. • Place a cravat under the affected extremity with the top of the triangle at the patient's elbow. • Tie the pointed end at the elbow to form a cradle. • Tie the other two ends at the side of the patient's neck. • Tie two wide cravats together and wrap them around the patient's upper torso and affected side to secure the sling to the body.
Hard rigid and semirigid	• Aluminum • Wood • Plastic • Plaster • Fiberglass	Support, compression, and alignment of sprains and fractures	• Pad the splint and ensure that it is long enough to extend above and below the joints of the suspected fracture site. • Apply gentle traction above and below the fracture site. • Place the splint under the extremity and secure with an elastic bandage.
	• Leatherette splints with Velcro	Support, compression, and alignment to the	• Place the wrist in the splint, making sure the splint is below the palmar crease.

Continued

	sprained wrist	• Mold the splint for a snug fit, close the thumb strap, close the loop-lock compression strap around the wrist, and finally close the remaining strap.
Vacuum splints	• Full-body immobilization • Dislocated shoulders, joints, arms, and legs	• Applied in a manner similar to other splints and often secured with straps that are connected to the splint • Attach the pump to the valve to remove air and make the splint rigid. • To remove the splint, the valve should be opened and the allowed to fill with air.
Pneumatic-inflatable	Air splints	• Fractures of the forearm and lower leg • Observe the extremity for compartment syndrome.	• Apply gentle traction above and below the suspected fracture site, and slide the splint under the extremity. • Secure and inflate the splint until finger pressure can dent only slightly. • Release the gentle traction only after the splint has been inflated. • Observe the splint for loss of pressure.
	Pneumatic antishock garments (PASG)	• Stabilization of pelvic and femur fractures • Contraindications include head injuries, pregnancy, CHF, penetrating abdominal trauma,	• For splinting the pelvis, apply the garment in the usual manner and inflate all three compartments to approximately 20 mm Hg. • For femur fractures, only the affected leg sections should be inflated.

TABLE P32-1 Four General Categories of Splints—cont'd

Type of Splint	Examples	Uses/Comments	Application
Traction	• Thomas half ring • Hare traction splint • Sager traction splint	tension pneumothorax, cardiac tamponade. • To stabilize femur fractures and to reduce muscle spasms • Traction splints should not be used for fractures of the fibula, tibia, ankle, foot, or upper extremity, or if a knee or hip injury is present.	• Generally, two clinicians (and optimally three) are needed to apply a traction splint. • The first clinician applies manual traction by holding the lower leg and pulling with both hands. • Manual traction must be maintained until the splint is in place. **Hare or Thomas half ring traction splint application** 1. Assemble the equipment (Figure P32-2). 2. Adjust the length of the splint, using the patient's uninjured leg as a guide. Place the padded ischial bar (Hare) or padded ring (Thomas) next to the patient's iliac crest, and extend the distal end of the splint by loosening the sleeve-locking device. The end of the splint should be approximately 10 inches past the heel of the foot (Figures P32-3 and P32-4). 3. Tighten the sleeve-locking device. 4. Open all support straps (those that support the thigh and lower leg) or tie four cravats with overhand knots spaced evenly throughout the splint.

5. With manual traction still being applied, slide the splint under the affected extremity until the padded ischial strap or ring is against the ischial tuberosity.

6. Pad the groin area with gauze or other suitable material. Secure the ischial strap.

7. Place the ankle hitch.

8. Pull the release ring on the traction ratchet and release the traction strap. Connect the D rings of the ankle hitch to the S hook of the traction strap.

9. Apply mechanical traction by turning the ratchet knob until the splint equals manual traction. The clinician holding traction should feel the gentle release of pressure as the splint assumes the traction.

10. Extend the heel stand into place to elevate the leg.

11. Secure the Velcro straps or cravats, two above and two below the knee. Do not place straps over the suspected fracture site (Figure P32-5).

12. Assess the pedal pulses, skin color and temperature, capillary refill, sensation, and movement in the foot of the splinted extremity.

Sager traction splint application

1. Assemble equipment

2. Place the splint medial to the injured extremity with the padded bar resting against the inner aspect of the thigh (Figure P32-6).

Continued

TABLE P32-1 Four General Categories of Splints—cont'd

Type of Splint	Examples	Uses/Comments	Application
			3. Adjust the length until the wheel of the pulley is level with the heel of the patient.
			4. Secure the thigh strap.
			5. Wrap the ankle harness snugly above the ankle, and secure the strap under the heel.
			6. Shorten the loop of the ankle harness by threading the strap through the D buckle.
			7. Release the lock on the splint, and pull the shaft out until the desired amount of traction tension is noted on the marking of the pulley wheel. The amount of traction should equal approximately 10% of the patient's body weight.
			8. Secure straps at the thigh, knee, and lower leg (Figure P32-7).
			9. Strap ankle and foot together to prevent rotation of the injured extremity.
			10. Reassess pedal pulses, skin color, temperature, capillary refill, sensation, and movement in the foot of the injured extremity.

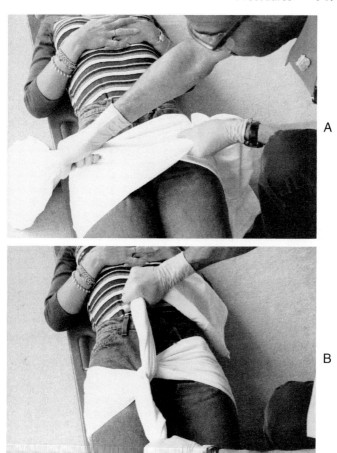

A

B

Figure P32-1   **A,** The smoothly folded sheet is wrapped around the pelvis and centered on the greater trochanters of the femur. **B,** The ends of the sheet are then crossed and tightened to produce pressure to stabilize the pelvis. Defining appropriate stability or pressure is difficult. Providers must use their judgment, trying to return the pelvis to the normal anatomic position. (Ramzy AI, Murphy M, and Long W: Splinting pelvic fractures, *JEMS* May, 2003, pp 68-78.)

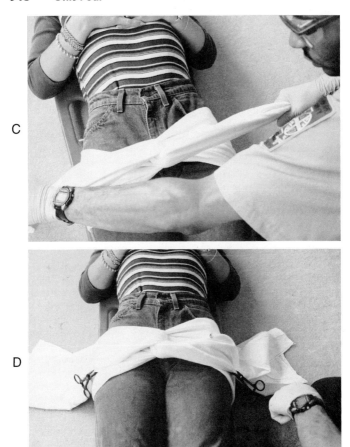

Figure P32-1—cont'd   C, After the sheet is tightened, the sheet wrap ends are crossed so friction helps lock it in place. **D,** Secure the ends of the sheet with clamps (or the ends can be tied in a secure knot). (Ramzy AI, Murphy M, and Long W: Splinting pelvic fractures, *JEMS* May, 2003, pp 68-78.)

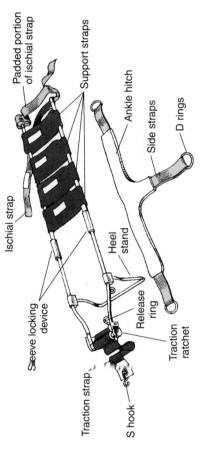

Figure P32-2   Hare traction equipment.

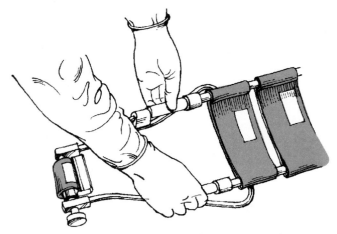

Figure P32-3 Adjusting length of splint with sleeve-locking device.

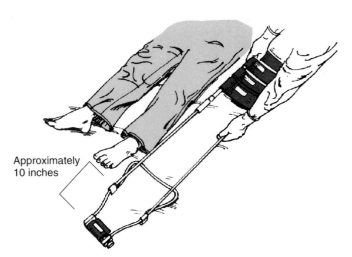

Approximately
10 inches

Figure P32-4 Extending Hare traction splint 10 inches past foot.

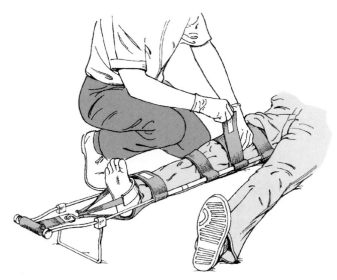

Figure P32-5   Application of strap.

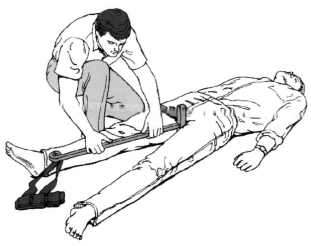

Figure P32-6   Application of Sager traction splint to medial aspect of injured leg.

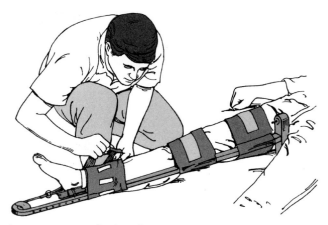

Figure P32-7   Application of straps.

- Complete a baseline neurovascular assessment (distal and proximal pulses, color, temperature, movement, sensation, and capillary refill of the digits).
4. Apply padding over bony prominences.
5. For nonjointed areas, immobilize the injured area along with the joint above and the joint below the site.
6. Splint the joint in the position found unless the distal pulse is diminished or absent.

⇒ NURSING ALERT ⇐

When no pulse is palpable, apply sustained and gentle traction along the long axis of the extremity, distal to the injury, until the pulse can be palpated. If any resistance is encountered, discontinue the process and splint in the position found.

---

7. Assess the neurovascular status before and after splinting, if the splint is removed or reapplied, or if the extremity is repositioned. Splints should not be constrictive, and fingers and toes should be left out of the bandage to aid in circulation checks.
8. The **F-A-C-T-S** formula can be used to monitor the patient's neurovascular status[2]:
   - **F**unction
   - **A**rterial pulse

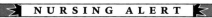

> ### NURSING ALERT
>
> If neurovascular status worsens after splint application, the splint
> should be removed and neurovascular status should be
> reassessed. The splint then can be replaced.[1]

- Capillary refill
- **T**emperature (skin)
- **S**ensation

9. Elevate the extremity above the level of the heart unless there is a potential compartment syndrome, in which case place the limb at the level of the heart.

APPLICATION OF COMMON SPLINTS

See Table P32-2.

TABLE P32-2 Application of Common Fiberglass/Plaster Splints	
Type of Splint	**Application**
Posterior short leg splint (ankle)	1. Measure (from the toes to below the knee) and cut a 4-inch or 6-inch–wide roll (Figure 32-8, *A*).
	2. Place the foot at a 90-degree angle to the leg.[3]
	3. Apply the roll to the back of the leg, and fold the plaster at the toes toward the heel (Figure P32-8, *B*).
	4. Tuck in the fold at the heel area. Secure the fold with an elastic bandage (Figure P32-8, *C*).
	5. Flare back the plaster below the knee, secure the plaster with an elastic bandage, and position and hold the foot at a 90-degree angle to the leg until the plaster is set (Figure P32-8, *D*).
Stirrup (ankle)	1. Measure (from medial to lateral and under the heel of the foot) and cut a 2-inch, 3-inch, or 4-inch–wide roll (Figure P32-9). This measurement should begin and end approximately 2 inches below the patella. You may reduce the length for sprains that are less severe.[2]
	2. Flex the foot at a 90-degree angle to the leg.[2]
	3. Apply the stirrup, centering on medial and lateral side of leg.

Continued

TABLE P32-2 Application of Common Fiberglass/Plaster Splints—cont'd

Type of Splint	Application
	Anchor the stirrup with an elastic bandage just above the ankle. Wrap around the heel and across the talus bone in a figure-eight several times, and then proceed up the leg.
Volar cock-up splint	1. Measure from the base of the fingers to midforearm and cut a 3-inch or 4-inch–wide roll.
	2. Apply and secure the roll to the volar side (inner aspect) of the arm and palm, positioning the wrist in a 15-degree to 30-degree dorsiflexion[3] (Figure P32-10).
Ulnar gutter (boxer) splint	1. Use a template to cut a 3-inch or 4-inch roll, measuring from the fingertips to midforearm.
	2. Fold the roll to form the desired gutter, and place the flap in the palm of the hand (Figure P32-11).
	3. Pad between fourth and fifth fingers. Position the hand with the fingers in "position of function" at a 50-degree flexion at the metacarpophalangeal joint, a 15-degree to 20-degree flexion at the interphalangeal joint, and the wrist in a neutral position.
Sugar tong splint	1. Measure for the splint: Forearm: Measure from the knuckles over the flexed elbow and around the back to the hand at the midpalmar crease.
	2. Using a 3-inch or 4-inch–wide roll, apply the splint with the elbow at 90-degree flexion, and secure the splint with an elastic bandage (Figure P32-12).

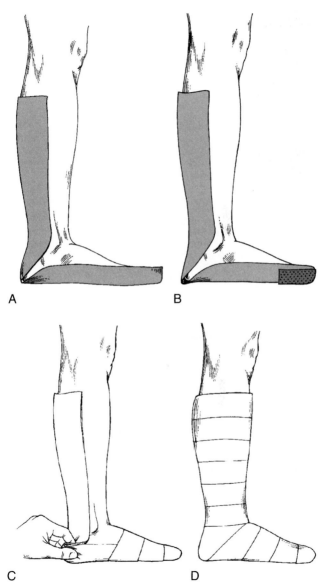

Figure P32-8   A-D, Application of posterior short leg splint.

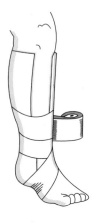

Figure P32-9 Application of stirrup (ankle) splint.

PATIENT CARE MANAGEMENT

1. Instruct the patient to keep the splint clean and dry.
2. Plaster requires 12 to 24 hours to dry. If plaster becomes wet, it will crumble and not harden again. Prevent impression of the plaster during this time as it may become misaligned, causing pressure sores to develop. Instruct the patient that the splint may feel warm as it is being applied but that any burning sensation should be reported.
3. Instruct the patient to assess the fingers and toes for signs of decreased neurovascular status—coolness, dusky color, swelling, or a decrease in sensation. If any signs are noted, the patient should notify appropriate medical personnel.
4. Report pain that increases and does not respond to pain medication.
5. Review **RICE** (rest, ice, compression, elevation) instructions with the patient. Elevate the limb to reduce swelling and pain, and apply cold packs as directed.
6. Instruct the patient that if neurovascular compromise is experienced, he or she should loosen the elastic wrap and observe for improved circulation.
7. The patient should be instructed to avoid placing sharp objects inside the splint for scratching.
8. Instruct the patient in crutch walking as needed (Procedure 9).
9. Pneumatic antishock garments (PASGs) should be deflated only under the direct supervision of a physician. The release of the PASG reduces peripheral vascular resistance, expands the

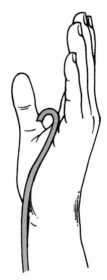

Figure P32-10 Application of volar cock-up splint.

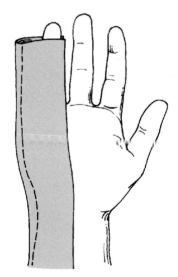

Figure P32-11 Placement of ulnar gutter splint to form desired gutter.

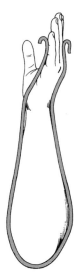

Figure P32-12   Application of sugar tong splint.

size of the vascular space, and removes about 250 ml of blood from active circulation. Deflating the garment too quickly or prematurely on someone who is compensating for shock could have devastating effects.[4]

10. Temperature and altitude changes can affect pressure inside an air splint. Observe the extremity for signs of neurovascular compromise.

PATIENT CARE MANAGEMENT OF TRACTION SPLINTS

1. Monitor the neurovascular status of the injured extremity at frequent intervals.
2. Maintain traction until definitive stabilization, such as Steinmann pin insertion, is initiated.
3. If pedal pulses are absent or there are other significant changes in neurovascular status, inform the physician. The amount of traction may need to be slightly decreased or increased.

REFERENCES

1. Emergency Nurses Association: *Trauma nurse core course,* ed 5, Chicago, 2000.

2. *Ortho-Glass splinting course manual,* Charlotte, NC, 2001, BSN Medical.
3. Davis DP: Splinting. In Rosen P, Chan TC, Vilke GM, et al: *Atlas of emergency procedures,* St. Louis, 2001, Mosby, pp 272-284.
4. Bledsoe BE, Porter RS, and Cherry RA: *Paramedic care: principles and practice in trauma emergencies,* Upper Saddle River, NJ, 2001, Prentice-Hall.

33 procedure

Suture and Staple Removal

Ellen Williams

DESCRIPTION (SUTURE REMOVAL)

In this procedure, nonabsorbable sutures are removed from a wound that shows signs of healing with no gaps in skin integrity. The risk of infection increases if sutures remain in place too long.

INDICATIONS

The amount of time stitches stay in place depends on several factors, including the type of laceration, type of wound closure, age and health of the patient, and presence of infection (see Table P33-1).

CONTRAINDICATIONS

The presence of gaping wound edges or signs of infection are indicative of poor wound closure. If such signs are present, the physician should be notified to determine whether the sutures should be removed or additional wound care is required.[1] Patients who are prone to delayed healing of wounds include those with diabetes, obesity, immunosuppression, and vascular disease, and those receiving chronic steroid therapy.

EQUIPMENT

- Suture removal kit (forceps, scissors, 4 × 4 gauze)
- Normal saline or an antiseptic solution
- Hydrogen peroxide
- Dressings as needed
- Skin tape closures (if needed)

INITIAL NURSING ACTIONS

1. Explain the procedure to the patient.
2. Gently clean the suture line with normal saline or an antiseptic solution; use hydrogen peroxide to remove dried blood or dried drainage.
3. Note the type of sutures placed (see Figure P33-1). Most sutures removed in the emergency department are intermittent sutures.

TABLE P33-1   Timing of Suture Removal

Location	Time (Days)
Eyelid	3
Cheek	3-5
Nose, forehead, neck	5
Ear, scalp	5-7
Trunk	7-10
Arms and legs	7-10
Hands and feet	7-14
Joints	10-14

The above time frames are general guidelines. These recommendations should be tailored to individual needs. Older patients or patients with a chronic illness may have longer healing times. Leaving sutures in place too long increases the risk of abscess and scar formation. Premature removal of sutures may result in wound disruption and delayed healing.

▶ NURSING ALERT ◀

Exposed suture material on the skin surface is considered contaminated. This technique (see Nos. 5 and 7 on p. 924) avoids pulling contaminated suture through the underlying tissue. **Do not** cut the suture on both sides. This would leave no way to remove the suture material remaining below the skin surface.

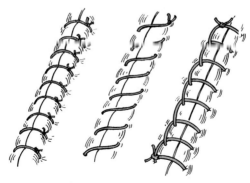

Figure P33-1   Types of sutures: *Left,* intermittent; *middle,* continuous; *right,* blanket.

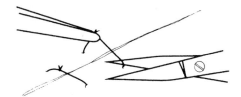

Figure P33-2   Technique for removing intermittent sutures.

4. To remove intermittent sutures, grasp the suture knot securely with the forceps and gently pull upward (see Figure P33-2).
5. Cut the stitch as close to the skin as possible, and pull the stitch out.
6. Document the number of stitches removed.
7. When removing continuous sutures, including blanket stitch sutures (see Figure P33-1), snip the sutures on one side of the suture line and remove them through the opposite side, thereby avoiding pulling contaminated suture through the healing wound.
8. Clean the site as before. Examine the wound for separation of wound edges. If noted, apply skin tape closures (e.g., Steri-Strips or Shur-Strips butterfly closure) to keep the wound edges in contact.
9. Apply a small dressing if there is any bleeding or per physician order.

PATIENT CARE MANAGEMENT

1. Instruct the patient to watch for signs and symptoms of infection, such as redness, swelling, pus, red streaks, increased pain or tenderness, and unexplained fever.
2. Remind the patient to keep the wound clean until it is completely healed and not to pick at crusts or scabs; they will fall off naturally.

DESCRIPTION (STAPLE REMOVAL)

In this procedure, staples are removed from a wound that shows signs of healing with no gaps in skin integrity. Premature removal may cause delayed healing, scar widening, or wound dehiscence. Delayed removal of staples can increase the risk of infection.

INDICATIONS

The amount of time staples stay in place depends on the part of the body affected (e.g., head and neck, 3 to 5 days; chest and abdomen, 5 to 7 days; lower extremities, 7 to 10 days).

CONTRAINDICATIONS

Notify the physician if the wound shows signs of inadequate healing, such as opening of the wound, signs of infection, redness, drainage, inflammation, pain, or tenderness. The presence of the above symptoms may indicate the need to keep staples in place or initiate additional wound care. Some conditions can increase the risk of infection. These conditions include diabetes, immunosuppression, chronic steroid medication, vascular compromise, and obesity.

EQUIPMENT

- Staple removal kit (staple extractor and gauze)
- Normal saline or an antiseptic solution
- Hydrogen peroxide
- Dressings as needed
- Skin tape closures (if needed)

INITIAL NURSING ACTIONS

1. Explain the procedure to the patient.
2. Gently clean the staple line with normal saline or antiseptic solution; use hydrogen peroxide if dried blood or dried drainage is present.
3. Place the nose of the extractor device beneath the center of the staple (Figure P33-3).
4. Squeeze the handles of the extractor together to lift the edges of the staple up until it is reformed
5. When the extractor is fully closed and the staple reformed, lift the extractor gently from the skin.
6. Examine the wound for any separation of the wound edges. If separation is noted, apply skin tape closures (e.g., Steri-Strips or Shur-Strips butterfly closure) to keep the wound edges in contact.

PATIENT CARE MANAGEMENT

1. Instruct the patient to watch for signs and symptoms of infection, such as redness, swelling, pus, red streaks, increased pain or tenderness, and unexplained fever.

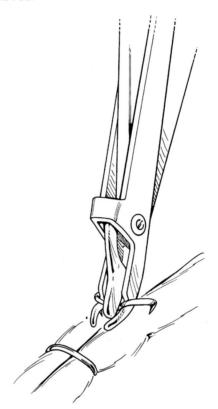

Figure P33-3   Staple removal.

2. Remind the patient to keep the wound clean until it is completely healed and not to pick at crusts or scabs; they will fall off naturally.

REFERENCES

1. Perry AG and Potter PA: *Clinical nursing skills techniques*, ed 5, St Louis, 2002, Mosby.

procedure *34*

Thoracentesis and Paracentesis

Mary Rose Bauer

THORACENTESIS

Thoracentesis is a procedure used to evacuate air or fluid and to obtain sterile fluid specimens from the pleural space. This procedure can be performed at the bedside with sterile technique.

INDICATIONS

1. Accumulation of fluid (pleural effusion) because of an inflammatory or infectious process
   - Fluid may be removed from the pleural cavity for therapeutic or diagnostic purposes.
2. Accumulation of air (tension pneumothorax) resulting from chest trauma or trauma of the visceral pleura
   - Removal of air will facilitate lung expansion. However, tube thoracostomy is the treatment of choice.
3. Need to instill medications intrapleurally

CONTRAINDICATIONS

1. The patient's respiratory status is compromised because of certain conditions, such as ruptured diaphragm or emphysema. (These patients have a higher incidence of a pneumothorax secondary to lung perforation)
2. Coagulopathy should be corrected before this procedure, unless there is severe respiratory failure.
3. Pleural adhesions increase the risk of perforation of the lung.
4. Hemodynamic or cardiac rhythm instability.
5. Chest wall infection at the insertion site.

EQUIPMENT

- Sterile drapes
- Antiseptic solution (povidone-iodine solution is usually used)
- Several sizes of needles (may use 18-gauge or 20-gauge spinal needles, or 16-gauge, 3-inch needle) or through-the-needle

catheters, for aspiration. (Through-the-needle catheters are preferable in patients who must remain in the supine position.)
- Syringes, 60-ml and 10-ml
- Needles, 25-gauge, $\frac{5}{8}$-inch; and 22-gauge, 1 $\frac{1}{2}$-inch
- Local anesthetic (1% lidocaine is usually used)
- Mask and goggles
- Sterile gloves
- Three-way stopcock
- Sponges, 4 × 4 gauze
- Three sterile specimen tubes
- Drainage tube and 500-ml vacuum bottle or collection bag (If these are unavailable, you may substitute IV tubing and a 500-ml bag of normal saline. Spike and drain the bag of fluid. Then invert the bag, maintaining sterility, and connect the sterile tubing to the three-way stopcock for drainage collection.)
- Puncture site bandage
  NOTE: Preassembled kits containing much of this equipment are available in many settings.

NURSING ACTIONS

1. Diagnostic x-ray examination is generally performed before the procedure to determine the highest level of the effusion.
2. Explain the procedure to the patient. Emphasize the need to remain still during the procedure.
3. Ideally, the patient should be placed in a seated position, leaning slightly forward, with his or her back to the person performing the procedure. One can achieve this by having the patient lean forward over a padded bedside table or the back of a chair. If the patient must be supine, the lateral approach may be used. For this approach, the affected side should face the person performing the procedure, and the patient's arm should be extended above the head to improve access to the site.
4. Prepare the site using antiseptic solution. For the removal of pleural fluid, the insertion site is the midscapular or posterior axillary line at a level overlying the fluid.[1] Use the second intercostal space, midclavicular line, for a tension pneumothorax.
5. Instruct the patient to refrain from coughing throughout the procedure.
  NOTE: At this point, the physician drapes the patient with sterile towels, exposing the site of the insertion. When the physician inserts

the needle and there is a return of fluid, the nurse connects the tubing (maintaining sterility) to the stopcock and fastens the tubing securely. A maximum of 1000 to 1500 ml of pleural fluid is withdrawn at one time.[1]

6. Provide verbal support and comfort measures during the procedure.

7. Sterility should be maintained throughout the procedure, and the sterile connection should not be broken to avoid contaminating the specimen. Record the amount, appearance, and consistency of all fluid obtained during the procedure.

8. After the procedure, apply pressure to the site to prevent bleeding. Apply a small dressing to the puncture site. Obtain a chest x-ray examination.

9. All specimens should be appropriately labeled and sent to the laboratory for analysis as ordered by the physician. Among the tests often ordered are a Gram stain, culture and sensitivity, cell count, cytology, pH, specific gravity, acid-fast staining, lactic dehydrogenase, and total protein tests.[2]

PATIENT CARE MANAGEMENT

1. Monitor vital signs every 15 minutes for 1 hour, every 30 minutes for 2 hours, and then every hour until the patient is stable.

2. Monitor the patient for signs and symptoms of complications such as pneumothorax, hemothorax, hypoxia, respiratory distress, and, later, infection. Symptoms may include dizziness, increased respirations, uncontrollable cough, tightness in the chest, frothy blood-tinged sputum, tachycardia, and shortness of breath.

3. Although rare, postexpansion pulmonary edema can occur if more than 1500 ml of fluid is withdrawn at one time.[1,2]

4. Assess volume status if a large amount of fluid has been withdrawn, especially if the patient had a fluid deficit before the procedure.

5. Continue to assess for pain, tenderness, redness, or drainage from the site.

PARACENTESIS

Paracentesis is a procedure for removing fluid from the peritoneal space with a large-bore needle and closed drainage system. It may be performed to obtain specimens used in the diagnosis of certain conditions or as a preparation for other procedures.

INDICATIONS

1. Accumulation of fluid or pressure in the abdominal cavity resulting from trauma or a disease process
   - Aspiration of fluid in the peritoneal space for analysis and culture
   - Drainage of fluid to relieve intraabdominal pressure
2. Preparation for other procedures, such as peritoneal dialysis or surgery

CONTRAINDICATIONS/CAUTIONS

1. Coagulopathy or thrombocytopenia should be corrected before this procedure to prevent bleeding.
2. The patient has severe bowel distension.
   - Placement of a nasogastric tube or rectal tube may be required for decompression before the procedure.
3. The patient has had previous abdominal surgery.

EQUIPMENT

The equipment for paracentesis is the same as the equipment for thoracentesis listed earlier in this procedure.

NURSING ACTIONS

1. Explain the procedure to the patient.
2. The bladder must be emptied before the procedure, either by voiding or by placement of a catheter.
3. Raise the head of the bed to a 45-degree angle (if tolerated). Allow at least 10 minutes for fluid to pool in the abdominal cavity.
4. Prepare the insertion site by cleansing the abdomen between the umbilicus and the symphysis pubis, including both lower quadrants, with antiseptic solution.
   NOTE: At this point the physician drapes the patient with sterile drapes, exposing the site of the insertion. Attach a collection device to the tubing and three-way stopcock. After insertion of the catheter and aspiration with syringe, connect the stopcock and tubing to the catheter. Generally up to 1500 ml of peritoneal fluid can be withdrawn without causing hemodynamic instability.
5. Be sure to record the amount, color, and consistency of all drainage.
6. Continue to assess vital signs during the procedure.

7. Apply pressure to the site for approximately 5 minutes, and place a small sterile dressing on the puncture site after the procedure.
8. Label all specimens appropriately, and send them to the laboratory for testing per physician request. Common laboratory tests include culture, Gram stain, amylase, white and red blood cell counts, total protein and albumin, lactate dehydrogenase (LDH), glucose, and cytology evaluation.

PATIENT CARE MANAGEMENT

1. Monitor the patient for pain or discomfort. Provide comfort measures.
2. Monitor vital signs every 30 minutes for 2 hours, then every hour until vital signs are stable.
3. Check the dressing for signs of leakage, bleeding, tenderness, swelling, or redness.

REFERENCES

1. Barefoot W: Performing thoracentesis. In Lynn-McHale DJ and Carlson KK, eds: *AACN Procedure manual for critical care*, ed 4, Philadelphia, 2001, Saunders, pp 145-150.
2. Gomella LG and Haist SA: *Clinician's pocket reference*, ed 10, New York, 2004, McGraw-Hill.

35 procedure

Vascular Access Devices

Debbie Smothers

DESCRIPTION

Emergency nurses may encounter patients with various vascular access devices (VADs). These devices generally are placed for long-term intermittent or continuous infusion of antibiotics, chemotherapy agents, or total parenteral nutrition (TPN). Patients with VADs may present to the ED because of catheter infection or occlusion, to have medications infused, or to have blood drawn.

There are two types of vascular access devices, implantable and nonimplantable. Implantable VADS include Port-a-Cath, Mediport, and Bard Implanted Port. Nonimplantable ports include peripherally inserted central catheters (PICCs), midlines, and central venous tunneled catheters such as the Hickman and the Groshong.

DEVICE DESCRIPTIONS

Peripherally Inserted Central Catheters
- Inserted into the upper arm or antecubital region
- Ideally, the distal tip rests in the central circulation in the lower third of the superior vena cava above the right atrial junction of the superior vena cava.
- The distal tip of PICC lines may be open ended or have a valve.
- PICC lines can be used for therapies with extreme pH, osmolality, and vesicant characteristics.
- A midline catheter is similar to a PICC line catheter, the difference being the location of the distal tip. The tip of a midline catheter is located peripherally in the basilic vein at the level of the axilla and therefore cannot be used for therapies with extreme pH, osmolality or vesicant characteristics. Midline catheters may be used for a term of 2 to 4 weeks. If a catheter is intentionally placed as a midline device, a shorter catheter can be used to reduce the amount of excess external catheter. Occasionally a midline may result from a PICC line insertion

when the catheter cannot be advanced into the central circulation.

Central Venous Tunneled Catheters
- Long-term indwelling catheters include the Hickman catheter (Figure P35-1) and the Groshong catheter (Figure P35-2).
- The catheter tip of both the Hickman and Groshong catheter is placed in the superior vena cava proximal to the right atrium. The catheter is then tunneled under the skin and exits between the fourth and fifth intercostal spaces onto the chest.
- The Hickman catheter is a silicone catheter and is open ended. It has a Dacron cuff subcutaneously at the exit site, which eventually adheres to tissue to hold the catheter in place and provide a barrier to infections.
- The Groshong catheter is a silicone catheter with a closed three-way valve on the end to prevent reflux of blood. It has an antimicrobial cuff under the subcutaneous tissue, which serves as a barrier to infection and holds the catheter in place.

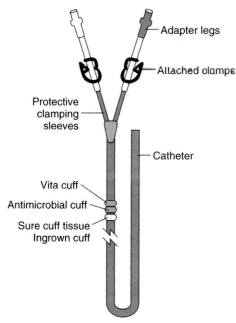

Figure P35-1 Hickman dual-lumen catheter.

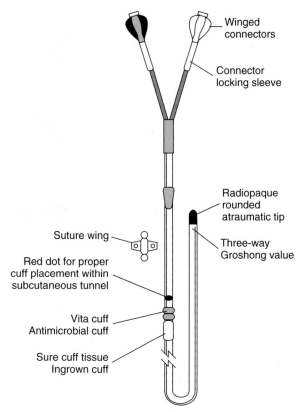

Figure P35-2   Groshong dual-lumen catheter.

Implantable Ports
- An implantable port consists of a catheter attached to a stainless steel, plastic, or titanium chamber that contains a self-sealing silicone diaphragm (Figure P35-3).
- The catheter tip is open ended and placed in the superior vena cava. The port usually lies subcutaneously near the second and fourth rib and is accessed through the skin.

INDICATIONS

In the emergency department:
- Intermittent infusion of:

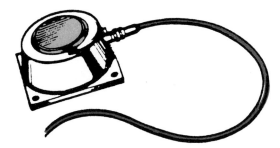

Figure P35-3   Implantable port.

NURSING ALERT

Manufacturers of metal ports recommend that the port not be exposed to the magnetic field in magnetic resonance imaging.

- ○ Antibiotics
- ○ Blood or blood products
- ○ Intravenous fluids
- Obtaining blood samples

CONTRAINDICATIONS/CAUTIONS

1. Peripherally inserted central catheter (PICC) lines can be ruptured if too much force is applied when flushing, infusing fluids, or performing an IV push of medications.
2. Midlines should not be used for hypertonic fluids or drugs that are extreme in pH or have vesicant properties.
3. Use of a syringe smaller than 10 ml can generate greater pressure and cause catheter rupture when flushing a PICC line.[1]

EQUIPMENT

- Alcohol and povidone-iodine swabs
- Noncoring 90-degree needle, such as a Huber or Lifeport needle for Port-a-Cath access
- Transparent dressing
- Needleless syringe device
- 2 × 2 gauze
- 10-ml syringe
- Extension tubing

- Blood tubes
- Normal saline flush
- Heparin flush solution

> ⧎ **N U R S I N G A L E R T** ⧏
>
> The concentration of heparin solution for adults is 100 units/ml and for children is 10 units/ml.

INITIAL NURSING ACTIONS (GENERAL)

1. See Table P35-1 for specific instruction in drawing blood and flushing each VAD.
2. Stop the infusion for 1 minute before obtaining blood.
3. Before injection of normal saline flush, IV solution, or medication, cleanse the injection cap with an antiseptic swab.
4. Strict aseptic technique and a transparent occlusive dressing should be applied to all VAD sites.

Accessing the Implantable Port

1. Open sterile gloves and use the glove package as a sterile field. Place the following on the sterile field:
   - Alcohol and povidone-iodine swabs
   - Noncoring 90-degree needle (Huber, Lifeport)
   - Transparent dressing
   - 20-gauge, 1-inch needle or needleless syringe device
   - 2 × 2 gauze
   - 10-ml syringes
   - Extension tubing

> ⧎ **N U R S I N G A L E R T** ⧏
>
> The noncoring needles vary in size from 19-gauge to 22-gauge and in length from $5/8$ to $1\,1/2$ inches. The larger gauge is preferred for administration of blood products.

---

2. Don sterile gloves.
3. Cleanse the skin over the injection port from the center of the device outward, with one to three alcohol swabs, using circular motions with each swab. Allow the alcohol to air dry.
4. Cleanse the same area with povidone-iodine swabs, allowing the area to dry for 1 to 2 minutes.

TABLE P35-1 Blood Draw and Flush Requirements for Vascular Access Devices

Type of VAD	Blood Draw	Flush
PICC	• Discard 2-3 ml of blood. • In a new syringe, pull plunger gently and slowly to avoid catheter collapse.	• Flush before and after a blood draw, before initiating an infusion or administering a medication, and after discontinuing an infusion or medication, with two 10-ml syringes of normal saline, using positive pressure flush method. • Open-ended catheters will require the normal saline flush plus 1 ml of heparin (100 units/ml)
Hickman catheter	• Use the proximal lumen (red) of the catheter. • Slowly withdraw and discard 5 ml of blood. • Obtain a new 10-ml syringe to draw the blood sample. • NOTE: A vacuum blood-collection system may be used to withdraw the waste (discard) sample and lab samples. Use at least a 5-ml tube to obtain the waste sample.	• Flush with 10-20 ml of normal saline between drug infusions and after drawing blood, using the positive pressure flush method. • Flush with 2-3 ml of heparin solution (per institutional protocol) in a 10-ml syringe before and after using the catheter. A heparin solution concentration of 100 units/ml is usually used for adults and a 10 units/ml concentration is used for pediatric patients. If more than one lumen is present, flush each lumen.
Groshong catheter	• A small slit near the tip stays closed under normal conditions, which prevents the backflow of blood.	• Flush with 10-20 ml of normal saline before and after drug infusions and blood draws.

Continued

TABLE P35-1   Blood Draw and Flush Requirements for Vascular Access Devices—cont'd

Type of VAD	Blood Draw	Flush
	• It is often helpful to pull back the plunger 1 to 2 ml, pause for a 2-second count, and then slowly withdraw blood. • A vacuum blood-collection system may be used as described with the Hickman catheter.	
Port-a-Cath	• Withdraw and discard 3-5 ml of blood. • Obtain the needed blood with another syringe and needle.	Flushing requirements for discontinuing infusion: • Flush with 10-20 ml of normal saline and continue IV infusion. If not infusing, additional flushing is necessary with 10-20 ml of normal saline. Flushing requirements for obtaining blood: • Flush with 10-20 ml of normal saline and continue IV infusion. If no infusion: • Flush with 10-20 ml of normal saline. • Administer 3-5 ml heparin (100 units/ml for adults and 10 units/ml for pediatric). Clamp the extension set while flushing the last 0.5 ml of solution. Discontinuation of an implantable port access needle: • Before discontinuation, flush with 10 ml heparin solution while stabilizing the port with a thumb and index finger. Begin pulling the needle out while pushing in the last 0.5 ml.

▶ **N U R S I N G   A L E R T** ◀

Omit the povidone-iodine swab if the patient has a known allergy or skin sensitivity to the agent.

5. Connect extension tubing to the 90-degree needle (some needles come with attached extension sets).
6. Withdraw 10 ml of normal saline and flush the extension tubing and needle.
7. Feel the injection site (port) with one hand by placing a thumb on one side of the port and an index finger on the other to stabilize the port.
8. With the other hand, hold the needle perpendicular to the skin. With firm, steady pressure, insert the needle through the skin and into the port until it touches the bottom of the chamber (Figure P35-4). When accessing an implantable port, do not rock or move the needle from side to side during insertion.
9. Gently pull back on the plunger of the syringe until blood return is noted. If there is no blood return with aspiration, try flushing the port with normal saline using a positive pressure flush method. It may be helpful to have the patient raise the arms above the head, turn head to the side, or cough. If there is still no blood return, remove the needle and repeat the process with a new needle.
10. Flush the port with normal saline using the positive pressure flush method.
11. Clamp the extension set. Place one sterile gauze pad under the needle and one above the needle. Cover with an occlusive dressing such as Tegaderm.

PATIENT CARE MANAGEMENT

1. Do not take blood pressures, draw blood, or insert a peripheral catheter in an extremity with a VAD.
2. Keep the insertion site covered with a sterile, occlusive dressing.
3. Assess for appropriate placement of the catheter.
   • If the length of the catheter is decreased, migration of the catheter into the right atrium may be suspected and can result in an unexplained increase in heart rate.
   • Complaints of a bubbling sound or an earache (on the same side as the catheter) as the flush solution is injected is indicative of catheter displacement into the jugular vein.

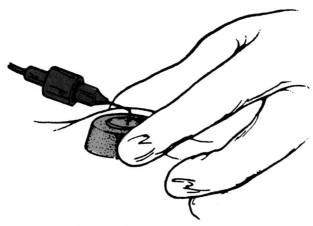

Figure P35-4 Accessing the port.

4. Infection is more common in catheters that are not tunneled under the skin, such as PICC lines. Signs and symptoms of catheter-related infection include:
   - Redness around the catheter or catheter insertion site
   - Drainage
   - Fever
   - Pain
5. If the patient presents with shortness of breath, tachycardia, anxiety, chest tightness, hypoxia, cyanosis, or hypotension, suspect an air embolism or, if the catheter has been newly placed, a pneumothorax.

Air Embolism
1. Clamp the catheter.
2. Turn the patient to the left side.
3. Place the patient in a head-down position (Trendelenburg position).
4. Administer oxygen.
   If air has entered the heart chambers, this position may keep the air in the right side of the heart, rather than allowing it to travel into the pulmonary system.

Pneumothorax
1. Note decreased or absent breath sounds on the affected side.
2. Perform chest x-ray.

3. Administer oxygen.
4. Allow the patient to remain in a position of comfort.
5. Prepare for chest tube insertion.
6. Catheter malfunction may be suspected if blood cannot be withdrawn and the catheter cannot be flushed. It may be helpful to have the patient raise the arms above the head, turn head to the side, or cough, and repeat the attempt to flush the catheter gently. If still unsuccessful, notify the physician.
7. If a Port-a-Cath is mobile, consider displacement and notify the physician.
8. Educate the patient and family in the appropriate care of the device as needed.

REFERENCES

1. Masooril S and Angeles T: Getting a line on central vascular access devices, *Nursing* (32) 4:36-43, 2002.

36 procedure

Visual Acuity

Tammy R. Higgins
Patty Ann Sturt

DESCRIPTION

Visual acuity (also called Snellen or eye testing) is a necessary component of a complete eye evaluation. Each eye is tested separately before consensual vision is tested.

INDICATIONS

- Documentation of baseline visual acuity
- Assessment of vision in patients with eye pain, facial/eye trauma, chemical exposure, or visual disturbances

CONTRAINDICATIONS/CAUTIONS

- In the event of chemical exposure, irrigation is the priority. Visual acuity should be postponed until the eye is thoroughly irrigated with copious amounts of normal saline. See Procedure 17, Eye Irrigation.
- Corneal abrasion or the presence of a foreign body may cause pain or tearing that can make obtaining an accurate visual acuity difficult. Instillation of a topical anesthetic may be necessary unless contraindicated because of the presence of penetrating trauma (see Chapter 12).

EQUIPMENT

- Snellen chart, Allencard (symbol card for children or illiterate patients), or Rosenbaum Pocket Vision Screener
- Marked distance of 20 feet (for use with Snellen chart or Allencard)
- Eye spoon or card (used to cover the eye not being tested)

NURSING ACTIONS

- Explain the procedure to the patient.
- Unless contraindicated by injury, have the patient keep corrective lenses in place during the exam and document whether they were used (i.e., write *corrected* or *uncorrected* on the chart).

- Place the patient 20 feet from a well-lit standard Snellen chart (or symbol chart for children or illiterate patients) at eye level.
- The eye that is not being tested should be occluded with an eye spoon, a card, or a hand with the fingers tightly held together. Instruct the patient not to place excessive pressure on the eye, as this may cause blurred vision.
- Test the unaffected eye first, then the affected eye, and then both eyes together.
- Have the patient read the smallest line possible.
- Document the lowest line read as a fraction along with the number of mistakes made on that line. For example, 20/40-2. This means that the patient read at 20 feet what a person with 20/20 vision can read at 40 feet. Document as OD (right eye), OS (left eye), or OU (both eyes).

ALTERNATIVE METHODS

- If the patient is unable to stand, a hand-held vision testing card called the Rosenbaum pocket screener can be used. The card is held 14 inches from the patient, and the test is performed in the same manner as the Snellen test.[1]
- If an eye chart is not available, have the patient read newspaper or similar print and document the furthest distance from which the patient can read it.
- If the patient is unable to read the top line of the eye chart, have the patient count the number of fingers held up from 3 feet away.
- If the patient is unable to detect the number of fingers held up at three feet, test and document whether the patient can perceive hand motion.
- If the patient is unable to detect hand motions, test and document whether the patient can perceive light.

REFERENCES

1. Bickley L: *Guide to physical examination and history taking,* Philadelphia, 2003, Lippincott Williams and Wilkins.

37 procedure

Wound Care

Ronald Stewart Gray

DESCRIPTION

Wound care in the emergency setting may range from treatment of minor injuries such as abrasions and skin tears, to more serious wounds such as evulsions and traumatic amputations. The goals of wound care are to stop the bleeding, minimize the risk of infection, minimize scarring, ensure adequate pain control, restore function, and ensure that the patient or the patient's caregiver understands the plan of treatment for all aspects of wound care.

INDICATIONS

Wound care is indicated when there has been a breach in skin integrity.

EQUIPMENT

- Proper lighting
- Protective gear: gloves, gown, goggles, mask, and shoe covers
- Sterile gloves
- Sterile towels
- Sterile bowls
- Sterile scissors and sterile pick ups
- Sterile scalpel and scalpel holder
- Skin disinfectant (See Table P37-1)
- Razor with recessed blade or clean scissors
- Cautery pin
- Analgesics (See Table P37-2)
- Needles (25-gauge and 27-gauge) for injecting anesthetic
- Intravenous catheter (18-gauge) for irrigation
- Syringe (20 to 60 ml)
- Splash guard
- Normal saline
- Suture material
- Wound tape
- Disposable skin stapler
- Triple antibiotic ointment

TABLE P37-1   Wound Cleansing Agents

Agents	Actions/Tissues Toxic	Indications and Contraindications
Alcohols	• Toxic to tissues	• No role in routine care
Chlorhexidine (Hibiclens)	• Fast-acting topical skin antiseptic. Toxic to wound defenses.	• Effective cleanser of intact skin. Keep away from face, eyes, ears, nose, and mouth.
Hexachlorophene (pHisoHex) (polychlorinated bisphenol)	• Little skin toxicity; scrub form is damaging to open wound	• Never use scrub solution in open wounds. Very good preoperative hand preparation
Hydrogen peroxide	• Toxic to open wounds	• Should not be used on wounds after the initial cleansing; may be used to clean intact skin
Nonionic detergents (Pluronic F-68, Shur-Clens)	• Wound cleanser. No toxicity to open wounds or eyes.	• Appears to be an effective, safe wound cleanser • Can be used on mucous membranes and in the eye
Phenols	• Extensive tissue necrosis and systemic toxicity	• Never use >2% aqueous phenol or >4% phenol plus glycerol.
Povidone-iodine solution (iodine complexes) (Betadine) supplied as a 10% solution.	• May cause systemic toxicity at higher concentrations; questionable toxicity at 1% concentration • Potent germicide in low concentrations • 10% solution is toxic to open wounds	• Probably a safe and effective wound cleanser at a 1% concentration • 10% solution is effective to prepare the skin about the wound

Adapted from Simon B and Hern HG Jr: Wound management principles. In Marx J, Hickenberger R, and Walls R, eds: *Rosen's emergency medicine, concepts and clinical practice*, ed 5, St. Louis, 2002, Mosby.

TABLE 37-2 Commonly Used Anesthetic Agents

Agent	Description	Onset	Duration	Comments
Lidocaine (Xylocaine)	Most common local and regional agent	• Onset for direct infiltration is seconds. • Onset for regional nerve block is 4-6 minutes.	• Direct infiltration: 20-60 minutes (up to 120 minutes) • Regional nerve block: 75 minutes	• Lidocaine is painful when injected because of its acidity. Inject slowly to lessen the pain. • Bicarbonate is sometimes added to lidocaine (1:10 volume ratio) to reduce pain during injection. • Lidocaine with epinephrine increases the duration of action. • Lidocaine with epinephrine should be avoided in wounds that are prone to infection.
Bupivacaine (Marcaine)	Local and regional agent	• Onset slightly slower than lidocaine	• 4-8 hours	• Bicarbonate can be added to bupivacaine (1:100 volume ratio) to reduce the pain of injection. • Also available with epinephrine.
LET (lidocaine, epinephrine, tetracaine)	Topical anesthetic	• 30 minutes	• Long duration • Specific time not established	• LET is placed directly in the wound, or a cotton ball or cotton-tipped applicator is soaked in the LET solution and placed into the wound.

EMLA	Local topical	• 1 hour	• 0.5-2 hours	• LET is never applied to mucous membranes (because of the rapid absorption from the membranes) or to wounds of the nose, ears, penis, digits, or eyelids (because of the vasoconstrictive properties of the epinephrine and lidocaine). • Primarily replacing the use of TAC • Used before a procedure such as starting an anesthetic IV. Applied to **intact** skin, and covered with an occlusive film dressing.
TAC (tetracaine, adrenaline, cocaine)	Topical anesthetic	• At least 8-10 minutes	• 30-120 minutes	• Soak a cotton ball and apply to the wound for 10-20 minutes.

Data from Simon B and Hern HG: Wound management principles. In Marx JA, Hockberger RS, and Walls RM, eds: *Rosen's emergency medicine and clinical practice*, ed 5, St Louis, 2002, Mosby, pp 737-751.

- Sterile gauze
- Nonadhering dressing
- Mesh gauze rolls for securing dressings
- Microporous tape

Much of this equipment can be found in prepackaged sterile instrument kits.

INITIAL NURSING ACTIONS

1. Bleeding may need to be controlled by direct pressure or a pressure bandage and elevation.
2. Review the patient's medical history for diseases that may affect healing (e.g., diabetes, peripheral vascular disease, and immunosuppression), allergies, and tetanus status (Reference Guide 23). Although a true allergy to local anesthetics is uncommon, obtaining a good history will help prevent an allergic reaction. There are two families of "caine" anesthetics, the ester and the amide families. Esters include procaine, tetracaine, and benzocaine. The amide family includes lidocaine and bupivacaine. There is no cross-reactivity between the two families.[1]
3. Radiographs may be ordered if the presence of a foreign body is suspected. However, if the suspected foreign body is organic (e.g., wood), xerograms, computed tomography scans, or ultrasonograms may be ordered because organic substances will not be seen on standard radiographs unless they displace tissues enough to produce a radiolucent shadow.[1]
4. Inform the patient of the procedure, and ensure patient comfort.
5. Ensure adequate pain control (see Table P37-2).
   - Anesthesia must be adequate for:
     - Exploration of the wound to determine wound depth and presence of foreign matter
     - Determination of damage to underlying tissue and structure
     - Preparation of the wound (debridement and cleansing)
     - Wound closure if needed
   - A topical anesthetic may be chosen for the repair of small lacerations (less than 5 cm), especially for children.

NURSING ALERT

Patients will require monitoring if sedation with analgesia is used (see Procedure 30).

- ○ *LET:* A solution of lidocaine, epinephrine (adrenaline), and tetracaine, used often
- ○ *TAC:* A solution of tetracaine, adrenaline (epinephrine), and cocaine, the first topical agent available for analgesia. Cocaine has been replaced by lidocaine in the newer formulation called LET, discussed above. LET gel is generally preferred over TAC because of its superior safety record and cost-effectiveness.
- ○ *EMLA:* (lidocaine 2.5%, prilocaine 2.5%) cream may be applied to the affected area but must be left in place for at least 60 minutes to achieve anesthesia.
- Local agents may be chosen to anesthetize the area surrounding the wound and the wound itself.
- Regional blocks may be used to produce greater anesthetic coverage by blocking the nerves supplying the area involved. For example, with puncture wounds, a regional block may be needed to anesthetize the area well enough to allow an excision of the wound for proper exploration and cleaning.

6. Clip hair around the wound. Using a razor can nick the skin or damage the hair follicle, creating an area for bacterial entrance and growth. If a razor must be used for hair removal, use one with a recessed blade. Areas of hair that provide an anatomic landmark useful in alignment of the wound edges, such as the eyebrows, should not be removed. Eyebrows do not always grow back or the regrowth may be inconsistent, which is another reason for avoiding shaving the eyebrows.

7. Disinfect the skin **surrounding the wound** with either povidone-iodine (Betadine) or chlorhexidine (Hibiclens) (Table P37-1). Both of these agents are fast acting and have a broad spectrum of antimicrobial activity.[1] Great care must be taken to prevent either of these substances from entering the wound because they impair the wound's defenses against infection.[1]

8. Wound debridement and removal of foreign matter and tissue that is nonviable is performed by the physician. Revision of the wound edges may be needed to allow better closure of the wound and to minimize the potential for scarring. Wound care may differ according to the severity of the wound.

9. After the wound has been debrided, it must be irrigated with copious amounts of normal saline under pressure. Cleansing of the wound before closure is one of the most important steps in minimizing wound infection. Normal saline (NS) is the

wound irrigant of choice because it is inexpensive, easy to prepare, and nontoxic to the wound's defense mechanisms.[1] Irrigating the wound with NS under high pressure (19-gauge IV catheter, with the needle removed, connected to a 20-ml to 35-ml syringe) within 1 inch of the wound is the most effective method of removing bacteria. Irrigation with bulb syringes, scrubbing of the wound, or soaking of the wound in an antiseptic solution will not clean the wound effectively.[1] Large-pore sponges can cause additional damage to cells. If a sponge is used, it should be a small-pore sponge with a surfactant (Polaximar 188). Abrasions may have dirt and gravel embedded in the dermis. After the area has been anesthetized, it requires meticulous cleaning to prevent an unsightly scar. Dirt and gravel remaining in the abrasion will cause permanent tattooing. Scrubbing in a circular pattern with a soft-bristled brush moistened with saline may be necessary to remove the debris.

10. Care must be taken when removing embedded glass, such as that from striking a windshield. Tweezers or the point of a #11 blade may help in removing glass from wounds.

11. Primary closure of wounds may be accomplished with tissue adhesive, wound tape, sutures, or staples (see Table 19-1, Surface Trauma). Certain types of wounds, such as some puncture wounds, some animal and human bites, and some avulsions, may be left to close by themselves because of a high risk of infection. If the delayed closure method is chosen, the wound is packed to prevent it from closing on its own. The pack is changed in 24 hours, and definitive closure is performed at 48 hours.

12. Apply a sterile dressing when indicated. Dressings should be impermeable to bacteria and prevent evaporation of water (drying of the wound causes a scab that delays healing). Dressings also can apply pressure to the wound site, minimizing edema and bleeding. Dressings may include petroleum-covered gauze placed over the wound and covered with a coarse mesh gauze; an occlusive transparent film dressing such as Tegaderm or Op-site; or a semiocclusive, semipermeable dressing such as Epi-lock or Biobrane. Dressings can be secured in place with mesh gauze rolls or microporous tape. Do not secure dressings with tape circumferentially because of the constriction that would result if the extremity swells.

13. Wounds in proximity to joints must be immobilized to prevent excessive stress on the wound.

PATIENT CARE MANAGEMENT

1. Administer antibiotics if ordered. Antibiotic treatment is usually reserved for exceptional circumstances, such as cat bites, human bites, some dog bites, through-and-through intraoral lacerations, some punctures to the foot, cases in which early signs of infection are present, grossly contaminated wounds, open fractures, and wounds exposing tendons or joints.[1]
2. Immunize the patient against tetanus if needed (Reference Guide 23).
3. Elevate the extremity above the level of the heart for the first 24 hours and apply ice packs to reduce edema. Use a barrier between the ice pack and the skin.
4. Immobilize the extremity, especially if the wound is near or over a joint, until the sutures are removed.
5. Injuries that carry high risk for infection must be evaluated in 48 hours.
6. Give the patient discharge instructions that include daily wound care, signs and symptoms of infection, suture removal dates (Procedure 33), and telephone numbers (e.g., private physician, clinics, emergency department) for follow-up appointments.

REFERENCES

1. Simon B and Hern HG Jr: Wound management principles. In Marx J, Hickenberger R, and Walls R, eds: *Rosen's emergency medicine, concepts and clinical practice*, ed 5, St Louis, 2002, Mosby.

index

Page numbers followed by "b" indicate boxes; page number followed by "f"
indicate figures; page number followed by "t" indicate tables.

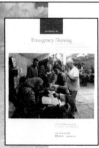